APPLIED BIOSTATISTICS
FOR THE HEALTH SCIENCES

APPLIED BIOSTATISTICS FOR THE HEALTH SCIENCES

RICHARD J. ROSSI
Montana Tech
Butte, Montana

WILEY

A JOHN WILEY & SONS, INC., PUBLICATION

Library of Congress Cataloging-in-Publication Data:

Rossi, Richard J., 1956-
    Applied biostatistics for the health sciences / Richard J. Rossi.
        p.   ;   cm.
    Includes bibliographical references and index.
    ISBN 978-0-470-14764-1 (cloth)
  1. Medical statistics. 2. Statistics. 3. Biometry. I. Title.
    [DNLM: 1. Biometry–methods. WA 950 R833 2010]
    R853.S7R67   2010
    610.72–dc22   2009019350

Printed in the United States of America

10 9 8 7 6 5 4 3 2 1

This book is dedicated to my parents, my wife, and my good friend Ray.

In loving memory of Maggie, Little Boy, Bayes, Ruth, Liz, Bonnie, and Duke.

CONTENTS

PREFACE

Applied Biostatistics for the Health Sciences is intended for use in an introductory biostatistics class for undergraduates in the health sciences including students studying premedicine, nursing, pharmacy, bioinformatics, healthcare informatics, biochemistry, and applied health sciences. This textbook is also appropriate for a first course in statistics for medical students or graduate students in public health. In fact, this book was written for introducing students to biostatistics as well as for preparing students for the material covered in upper division applied statistics courses. The only prerequisite for a course taught from this textbook is a typical course in high school algebra II or college algebra.

TOPIC COVERAGE

The topics chosen for this book were chosen for pedagogical reasons and have been tried, tested, and adjusted over the past 30 years of teaching introductory courses in statistics. Throughout *Applied Biostatistics for the Health Sciences*, the primary emphasis is placed on the correct usage, interpretation, and the conceptual ideas associated with each biostatistical method that is discussed.

The textbook is organized in two parts with Chapters 1–7 covering the basic inferential biostatistical methods used to describe sample data arising in a biomedical or health-related study. Chapters 8–13 cover several modeling approaches that are commonly used with biomedical and healthcare data. In particular, the following topics are presented in this textbook.

> *Chapter 1: Introduction to Biostatistics.* Chapter 1 provides an introduction to the ideas and basic terminology of biostatistics as well as the commonly used research protocols. Experiments are contrasted with observational studies and clinical trials are also discussed in Chapter 1. A description of the data sets used in several of the examples and exercises is given at the end of Chapter 1.
>
> *Chapter 2: Describing Populations.* Chapter 2 introduces variables, populations, population parameters, probability, and the binomial and normal probability models. Several biomedical parameters are introduced in Chapter 2 including the prevalence of a disease, the specificity and sensitivity of a diagnostic test, and the relative risk associated with a disease and risk factor.
>
> *Chapter 3: Random Sampling.* The basic ideas associated with random sampling are discussed in Chapter 3. In particular, the simple random sampling, stratified random sampling, random cluster sampling, and systematic random sampling plans are discussed including the determination of the appropriate sample size for estimating a mean or proportion with a prespecified bound on the error of estimation. The formulas for determining the overall sample size and its allocation for a stratified random sample may be considered as an optional topic and covered as time permits.
>
> *Chapter 4: Summarizing Random Samples.* Several important graphical and numerical summary statistics for qualitative and quantitative variables are presented. In

particular, along with the standard point estimators of the measures of location and dispersion, point estimators for estimating the prevalence of a disease, the sensitivity and specificity of a diagnostic test, the relative risk, and the coefficient of variation are presented in Chapter 4. The plug-in rule for estimating parameters is also included in this chapter.

Chapter 5: Measuring the Reliability of Statistics. The sampling distribution of an estimator is discussed in Chapter 5 with emphasis on evaluating the reliability of a point estimator. The topics discussed in Chapter 5 include properties of point estimators including the bias, standard error, bound on the error of estimation, and mean squared error associated with a point estimator. The Central Limit Theorem for the sample proportion and sample mean, the t distribution, and bootstrapping the sampling distribution of a point estimator are discussed in this chapter. The section on bootstrapping can be considered optional material to be covered if time permits.

Chapter 6: Confidence Intervals. Confidence intervals for a single proportion, a single mean, the difference of two proportions, the difference of two means, and the relative risk are presented in Chapter 6. Formulas for determining the sample size required for a prespecified margin of error are included for estimating a proportion, mean, and the difference between two proportions. Bootstrap confidence intervals are also discussed in this chapter and can be considered optional material.

Chapter 7: Testing Statistical Hypotheses. Chapter 7 includes a general discussion of hypothesis testing and significance testing that is followed by the hypothesis tests for testing hypotheses about a single proportion, t tests for a single mean, paired t-tests, and the two-sample t-test. Formulas for determining the approximate sample size required for a test having a prespecified size and power are also presented for each testing procedure.

Chapter 8: Simple Linear Regression. Chapter 8 is the first chapter in a series of chapters on modeling a response variable. The topics covered in Chapter 8 include analyzing scatterplots, correlation, the simple linear regression model, fitting and assessing the fit of a simple linear regression model, and statistical inferences drawn from a fitted model.

Chapter 9: Multiple Regression. Chapter 9 extends and broadens the methods discussed in Chapter 8 to multiple regression models. The multiple regression topics that are discussed in Chapter 9 include linear and nonlinear models, fitting and assessing the fit of a multiple regression model, drawing inferences from a fitted model, comparing nested regression models, dummy variable models, and variable selection procedures.

Chapter 10: Logistic Regression. Because building a logistic regression model is similar to building a linear regression model, the discussion of logistic regression follows immediately after the two chapters on linear regression. Topics discussed in Chapter 10 include the odds of an event, the odds ratio, logistic regression models, fitting and assessing the fit of a logistic regression model, drawing inferences from a logistic regression model, and variable selection.

Chapter 11: Design of Experiments. Chapter 11 provides an introduction to designing an experiment and precedes the typical chapter on analysis of variance. Topics covered in Chapter 11 include a discussion of experiments and observational studies, the completely randomized and randomized block designs, factorial experiments, and linear models for designed experiments.

Chapter 12: Analysis of Variance. Chapter 12 is the traditional chapter on analysis of variance. In Chapter 12, analysis of variance is discussed for single factor, randomized block, and factorial studies including discussions of the F-tests, the Bonferroni method of separating means, and methods for determining the number of replications needed for a study.

Chapter 13: Survival Analysis. Chapter 13 introduces methods for analyzing survival data. In particular, survival data, survivor functions, censoring, the Kaplan–Meier nonparametric estimator, the log-rank test, Cox's proportional hazards semiparametric estimator, and logistic regression for survival data are discussed.

This book was intended neither to cover all of the methods used in the statistical analysis of biomedical and healthcare data nor to be used as cookbook with recipes for several different statistical analyses. The primary emphasis of this book is to introduce students to the basic ideas of biostatistics and modeling approaches used in biostatistics.

It is also my experience that the order of presentation is appropriate for the nurture and development of the student's confidence and statistical maturity. I also believe that the statistical methods and ideas presented in *Applied Biostatistics for the Health Sciences* will provide a student with the necessary statistical tools required to succeed in advanced statistics courses such as linear or logistic regression, design and analysis of experimental data, multivariate statistics, analysis of microarray data, and survival analysis.

SPECIAL FEATURES

The special features of this book include the following:

- The importance of using/designing well-designed sampling plans is heavily emphasized throughout this text.

- Concepts are emphasized over computational formulas throughout this text.

- Several topics that are not usually covered in a first course in biostatistics are included in *Applied Biostatistics for the Health Sciences*, such as bootstrapping, sampling, sample size computations for two-sample confidence intervals and hypothesis tests, design of experiments, and survival analysis.

- A large number of the examples are based on real-life studies published in biomedical and healthcare journals.

- Bivariate data and bivariate analyses are presented early in the text. In particular, correlation, simple linear regression, and contingency tables are all introduced in Chapter 4.

- Logistic regression follows immediately after a discussion of linear regression, which seems natural.

- References are given to difficult problems that often occur when building and assessing a statistical model.

I have written this textbook with the expectation that access to a statistical computing package will be available to the students, and thus, the emphasis of this text is placed on the correct use, interpretation, and drawing statistical inferences from the output provided by a statistical computing package rather than the computational aspects required of the statistical methodology. While MINITAB® was used to produce the plots and computer output throughout the text, an introductory biostatistics course can be taught from *Applied*

Biostatistics for the Health Sciences using any of the commonly used statistical computing packages, such as SAS®, STATA®, and SPSS®. The vast majority of the exercises do not depend on the particular statistical computing package being used, and in fact, many of the exercises do not require a statistical computing package at all. I have also created several Microsoft® Office Excel® worksheets for *Applied Biostatistics for the Health Sciences* that can be used for determining sample sizes, computing confidence intervals, and computing test statistics and *p*-values that are available on the book's website.

PEDAGOGICAL FEATURES

The key pedagogical features of *Applied Biostatistics for the Health Sciences* include the following:

- The important formulas, procedures, and definitions are enclosed in site.
- There is a glossary at the end of each chapter containing the key terminology and ideas introduced in the chapter.
- Wherever possible the subscripts were dropped from the variables to simplify the notation used with many of the statistics.
- There are numerous worked out examples illustrating important concepts and proper use of a statistical method.
- Real-life data are used wherever possible in the examples and exercises, and the real-life data sets used throughout the book are available on the book's website.
- Computer output is provided in many of the examples and exercises to minimize the computational aspects of the statistical methods that have been used.

A large number of exercises have been included in each chapter, and the solutions to most of the exercises have also been included at the end of this text. I believe that the exercises accompanying this text do indeed cover a wide range of topics and levels of difficulty; there are many questions that deal with the conceptual aspects of the material discussed in each chapter that often lead to excellent classroom discussions. I believe that the successful completion of these exercises will help the student understand the statistical methods introduced in each chapter and gain the confidence necessary to be successful in upper division applied statistics courses, which, of course, are the goals of this textbook.

TEACHING FROM THIS BOOK

In teaching a one-semester introductory biostatistics course from this textbook it is possible to cover most of the Chapters 1–7; for a two-semester sequence most of the Chapters 1–7 can be covered in the first semester, and Chapters 8–13 can be covered in the second semester. While I have not taught a course from this book on the quarter system, I believe that by carefully selecting the topics to be covered in a single quarter most of Chapters 1–7 can be covered; for a two-quarter sequence, most of the material in Chapters 1–7 could be covered in the first quarter, with the remainder of the book covered in the second quarter. However, there are many different ways to teach from this book, and I leave that to the discretion and goals of the instructor.

WEBSITE

A website associated with *Applied Biostatistics for the Health Sciences* can be found at

http://www.mtech.edu//clsps/math/Faculty%20Links/rossi_book.htm

This website contains several of the data sets used in the examples and exercises included in *Applied Biostatistics for the Health Sciences*. The data sets are given in three formats, namely, as MINITAB worksheets, Microsoft Office Excel files, and text files. The website also contains several Microsoft Office Excel files that the students can use to simplify some of the computational aspects associated with sample sizes, confidence intervals, and *p*-values for Z and t-tests; these Microsoft Office Excel files are read only files that can be downloaded as needed for use by the instructor and the students.

ACKNOWLEDGMENTS

I would like to thank the following statisticians who motivated me to write this book: Ray Carroll, David Ruppert, Jay Devore, Roxy Peck, Fred Ramsey, Dan Schafer, and Chip Todd. I would also like to thank Lloyd Gavin and H. Dan Brunk, two very inspirational advisors from whom I learned so much, my editor Susanne Steitz-Filler for her help and guidance, and my family and friends for their support in this endeavor.

R. J. Rossi

Butte, Montana

CHAPTER 1

INTRODUCTION TO BIOSTATISTICS

PRIOR TO the twentieth century, medical research was primarily based on trial and error and empirical evidence. Diseases and the risk factors associated with a disease were not well understood. Drugs and treatments for treating diseases were generally untested. The rapid scientific breakthroughs and technological advances that took place in the latter half of the twentieth century have provided the modern tools and methods that are now being used in the study of the causes of diseases, the development and testing of new drugs and treatments, and the study of human genetics and have been instrumental in eradicating some infectious diseases.

Modern biomedical research is evidence-based research that relies on the scientific method, and in many biomedical studies it is the scientific method that guides the formulation of well-defined research hypotheses, the collection of data through experiments and observation, and the honest analysis whether the observed data support the research hypotheses. When the data in a biomedical study support a research hypothesis, the research hypothesis becomes a theory; however, when data do not support a research hypothesis, new hypotheses are generally developed and tested. Furthermore, because statistics is the science of collecting, analyzing, and interpreting data, statistics plays a very important role in medical research today. In fact, one of the fastest growing areas of statistical research is the development of specialized data collection and analysis methods for biomedical and healthcare data. The science of collecting, analyzing, and interpreting biomedical and healthcare data is called *biostatistics*.

1.1 WHAT IS BIOSTATISTICS?

Biostatistics is the area of statistics that covers and provides the specialized methodology for collecting and analyzing biomedical and healthcare data. In general, the purpose of using biostatistics is to gather data that can be used to provide honest information about unanswered biomedical questions. In particular, biostatistics is used to differentiate between chance occurrences and possible causal associations, for identifying and estimating the effects of risk factors, for identifying the causes or predispositions related to diseases, for estimating the incidence and prevalence of diseases, for testing and evaluating the efficacy of new drugs or treatments, and for exploring and describing the well being of the general public.

A biostatistician is a scientist trained in statistics who also works in disciplines related to medical research and public health, who designs data collection procedures, analyzes data, interprets data analyses, and helps summarize the results of the studies. Biostatisticians may also develop and apply new statistical methodology required for analyzing biomedical data. Generally, a biostatistician works with a team of medical researchers and is responsible for designing the statistical protocol to be used in a study.

Biostatisticians commonly participate in research in the biomedical fields such as epidemiology, toxicology, nutrition, and genetics, and also often work for pharmaceutical companies. In fact, biostatisticians are widely employed in government agencies such as the National Institutes of Health (NIH), the Centers for Disease Control and Prevention (CDC), the Food and Drug Administration (FDA), and the Environmental Protection Agency (EPA). Biostatisticians are also employed by pharmaceutical companies, medical research units such as the MAYO Clinic and Fred Hutchison Cancer Research Center, Sloan-Kettering Institute, and many research universities. Furthermore, some biostatisticians serve on the editorial boards of medical journals and many serve as referees for biomedical journal articles in an effort to ensure the quality and integrity of data-based biomedical results that are published.

1.2 POPULATIONS, SAMPLES, AND STATISTICS

In every biomedical study there will be research questions to define the particular population that is being studied. The population that is being studied is called the *target population*. The target population must be a well-defined population so that it is possible to collect representative data that can be used to provide information about the answers to the research questions. Finding the actual answer to a research question requires that the entire target population be observed, which is usually impractical or impossible. Thus, because it is generally impractical to observe the entire target population, biomedical researchers will use only a subset of the population units in their research study. A subset of the population is called a *sample*, and a sample may provide information about the answer to a research question but cannot definitively answer the question itself. That is, complete information on the target population is required to answer the research question, and because a sample is only a subset of the target population, it can only provide information about the answer. For this reason, statistics is often referred to as "the science of describing populations in the presence of uncertainty."

The first thing a biostatistician generally must do is to take the research question and determine a particular set of characteristics of the target population that are related to the research question being studied. A biostatistician then must determine the relevant statistical questions about these population characteristics that will provide answers or the best information about the research questions. A characteristic of the target population that can be summarized numerically is called a *parameter*. For example, in a study of the body mass index (BMI) of teenagers, the average BMI value for the target population is a parameter, as is the percentage of teenagers having a BMI value less than 25. The parameters of the target population are based on the information about the entire population, and hence, their values will be unknown to the researcher.

To have a meaningful statistical analysis, a researcher must have well-defined research questions, a well-defined target population, a well-designed sampling plan, and an observed sample that is representative of the target population. When the sample is representative of the target population, the resulting statistical analysis will provide useful information about the research questions; however, when the observed sample is not representative of the target population the resulting statistical analysis will often lead to misleading or incorrect inferences being drawn about the target population, and hence, about the research questions, also. Thus, one of the goals of a biostatistician is to obtain a sample that is representative of the target population for estimating or testing the unknown parameters.

Once a representative sample is obtained, any quantity computed from the information in the sample and known values is called *statistic*. Thus, because any estimate of the unknown parameters will be based only on the information in the sample, the estimates are also statistics. Statements made by extrapolating from the sample information (i.e., statistics) about the parameters of the population are called *statistical inferences*, and good statistical inferences will be based on sound statistical and scientific reasoning. Thus, the statistical methods used by a biostatistician for making inferences need to be based on sound statistical and scientific reasoning. Furthermore, statistical inferences are meaningful only when they are based on data that are truly representative of the target population. Statistics that are computed from a sample are often used for estimating the unknown values of the parameters of interest, for testing claims about the unknown parameters, and for modeling the unknown parameters.

1.2.1 The Basic Biostatistical Terminology

In developing the statistical protocol to be used in a research study, biostatisticians use the following basic terminology:

- The *target population* is the population that is being studied in the research project.
- The *units* of a target population are the objects on which the measurements will be taken. When the units of the population are human beings, they are referred to as *subjects* or *individuals*.
- A *subpopulation* of the target population is a well-defined subset of the population units.
- A *parameter* is a numerical measure of a characteristic of the target population.
- A *sample* is a subset of the target population units. A *census* is sample consisting of the entire set of population units.
- The *sample size* is the number of units observed in the sample.
- A *random sample* is a sample that is chosen according to a sampling plan where the probability of each possible sample that can be drawn from the target population is known.
- A *statistic* is any value that is computed using only the sample observations and known values.
- A *cohort* is a group of subjects having similar characteristics.
- A *variable* is a characteristic that will be recorded or measured on a unit in the target population.
- A *response variable* or *outcome variable* is the variable in a research study that is of primary interest or the variable that is being modeled. The response variable is also sometimes called the *dependent variable*.
- An *explanatory variable* is a variable that is used to explain or is believed to cause changes in the response variable. The explanatory variables are also called *independent variables* or *predictor variables*.

- A *treatment* is any experimental condition that is applied to the units.

- A *placebo* is an inert or inactive treatment that is applied to the units.

- A *statistical inference* is an estimate, conclusion, or generalization made about the target population from the information contained in an observed sample.

- A *statistical model* is a mathematical formula that relates the response variable to the explanatory variables.

One of the most misunderstood and abused concepts in statistics is the difference between a parameter and a statistic, and researchers who do not have a basic understanding of statistics often use these terms interchangeably, which is incorrect. Whether a number is a parameter or a statistic is determined by asking whether or not the number was computed from the entire set of units in the target population (parameter) or from a sample of the units in the target population (statistic). It is important to distinguish whether a number is a parameter or a statistic because a parameter will provide the answer to a statistical research question, while a statistic can provide information only regarding the answer, and there is a degree of uncertainty associated with the information contained in a statistic.

Example 1.1
In a study designed to determine the percentage of obese adults in the United States, the BMI of 500 adults was measured at several hospitals across the country. The resulting percentage of the 500 adults classified as obese was 24%.
   In this study, the target population was adults in the United States, 500 adults constitute a sample of the adults in the United States, the parameter of interest is the percentage of obese adults in the United States, and 24% is a statistic since it was computed from the sample, not the target population.

In designing a biomedical research study, the statistical protocol used in the study is usually determined by the research team in conjunction with the biostatistician. The statistical protocol should include the identification of the target population, the units in the population, the response variable and explanatory variables, the parameters of interest, the treatments or subpopulations being studied, the sample size, and models that will be fit to the observed data.

Example 1.2
In a study investigating the average survival time for stage IV melanoma patients receiving two different doses of interferon, $n = 150$ patients will be monitored. The age, sex, race, and tumor thickness of each patient will be recorded along with the time they survived after being diagnosed with stage IV melanoma. For this study, determine the following components of the statistical protocol:

a. The target population.
b. The units of target population.
c. The response variable.
d. The explanatory variables.
e. The parameter of interest.
f. The treatments.
g. The sample size.

Solutions

a. The target population in this study is individuals diagnosed with stage IV melanoma.
b. Units of the target population are the individuals diagnosed with stage IV melanoma.

c. The response variable in this study is the survival time after diagnosis with stage IV melanoma.

d. Explanatory variables in this study are age, sex, race, and tumor thickness.

e. The parameter of interest in this study is the average survival time after diagnosis with stage IV melanoma.

f. Treatments are the two different doses of interferon.

g. The sample size is $n = 150$.

1.2.2 Biomedical Studies

There are many different research protocols that are used in biomedical studies. Some protocols are forward looking studying what will happen in the future, some look at what has already occurred, and some are based on a cohort of subjects having similar characteristics. For example, the Framingham Heart Study is a large study conducted by the National Heart, Lung, and Blood Institute (NHLBI) that began in 1948 and continues today. The original goal of the Framingham Heart Study was to study the general causes of heart disease and stroke, and the three cohorts that have or are currently being studied in the Framingham Heart Study are

1. the original cohort that consists of a group of 5209 men and women between the ages of 30 and 62 recruited from Framingham, Massachusetts.
2. The second cohort, called the Offspring Cohort, consists of 5124 of the original participants' adult children and their spouses.
3. the third cohort that consists of children of the Offspring Cohort. The third cohort is recruited with a planned target study size of 3500 grandchildren from members of the original cohort.

Two other large ongoing biomedical studies are the Women's Health Initiative (WHI), which is a research study focusing on the health of women, and the National Health and Nutrition Examination Survey (NHANES), which is designed to assess the health and nutritional status of adults and children in the United States.

Several of the commonly used biomedical research protocols are described below.

- A *cohort study* is a research study carried out on a cohort of subjects. Cohort studies often involve studying the patients over a specified time period.
- A *prospective study* is a research study where the subjects are enrolled in the study and then followed forward over a period of time. In a prospective study, the outcome of interest has not yet occurred when the subjects are enrolled in the study.
- A *retrospective study* is a research study that looks backward in time. In a retrospective study, the outcome of interest has already occurred when the subjects are enrolled in the study.
- A *case–control study* is a research study in which subjects having a certain disease (cases) are compared with subjects who do not have the disease (controls).
- A *longitudinal study* is a research study where the same subjects are observed over an extended period of time.
- A *cross-sectional study* is a study to investigate the relationship between a response variable and the explanatory variables in a target population at a particular point in time.

- A *blinded study* is a research study where the subjects in the study are not told which treatment they are receiving. A research study is a *double-blind study* when neither the subject nor the staff administering the treatment know which treatment a subject is receiving.

- A *clinical trial* is a research study performed on humans and designed to evaluate a new treatment or drug or to investigate a specific health condition.

- A *randomized controlled study* is a research study in which the subjects are randomly assigned to the treatments with one of the treatments being a control treatment; a control treatment may be a standard treatment, a placebo, or no treatment at all.

It is important to note that a research study may actually involve more than one of these protocols. For example, a longitudinal study is often a cohort study, a case–control study is a retrospective study, a longitudinal study is a prospective study, and a clinical trial may be run as a double-blind randomized controlled study. Also, the nature of a particular research study will dictate the research protocol that is used. Finally, of all of the study protocols, the randomized controlled study is the gold standard in biomedical research because it provides more control over the external factors that can bias the results of a study.

Most of the medical journals that publish biomedical research require the authors of an article to describe the research protocol that was used in their study. In fact, during the peer-review process a journal article undergoes prior to publication, the research protocol will be carefully scrutinized and research based on poor research protocols will not be published. Several examples of the different research protocols used in published biomedical research articles are given in Examples 1.3–1.7.

Example 1.3

In the article "A prospective study of coffee consumption and the risk of symptomatic gallstone disease in men" published in the *Journal of the American Medical Association* (Leitzmann et al., 1999), the authors reported the results of a prospective cohort study designed to investigate whether coffee consumption helps prevent symptomatic gallstone disease. This study consisted of $n = 46,008$ men, aged 40–75 years in 1986, without any history of gallstone disease, and the subjects were monitored for a 10-year period from 1986 to 1996.

Example 1.4

In the article "Hospitalization before and after gastric bypass surgery" published in the *Journal of the American Medical Association* (Zingmond et al., 2005), the authors reported the results of a retrospective research study designed to investigate the amount of time spent in a hospital 1–3 years after an individual receives a Roux-en-Y gastric bypass (RYGB). This study consisted of $n = 60,077$ patients who underwent RYGB from 1995 to 2004 in California.

Example 1.5

In the article "Pesticides and risk of Parkinson disease: a population-based case–control study" published in the *Archives of Neurology* (Firestone et al., 2005), the authors reported the results of a case–control research study designed to investigate association between occupational and home-based pesticide exposure and idiopathic Parkinson disease. This study consisted of 250 subjects with Parkinson's disease and 388 healthy control subjects.

Example 1.6

In the article "Randomized, double-blind, placebo-controlled trial of 2 dosages of sustained-release bupropion for adolescent smoking cessation" published in the *Archives of Pediatric and Adolescent Medicine* (Muramoto et al., 2007), the authors reported the results of a randomized controlled double-blind research study designed to investigate the efficacy of sustained release of bupropion hydrochloride for adolescent smoking cessation. This study consisted of $n = 312$ subjects recruited through media and community venues from March 1, 1999 to December 31, 2002, who were aged 14–17 years, smoked at least six cigarettes per day, had an exhaled carbon monoxide level of 10 ppm or greater, had at least two previous quit attempts, and had no other current major psychiatric diagnosis.

Example 1.7
In the article "Antidepressant efficacy of the antimuscarinic drug scopolamine: a randomized, placebo-controlled clinical trial" published in *Archives of General Psychiatry* (Furey et al., 2006), the authors reported the results of a double-blind, placebo-controlled, dose finding clinical trial designed to investigate the antidepressant efficacy of scopolamine. This study consisted of $n = 19$ currently depressed outpatients aged 18–50 years with recurrent major depressive disorder or bipolar disorder.

1.2.3 Observational Studies Versus Experiments

When two or more subpopulations or treatments are to be compared in a biomedical research study, one of the most important aspects of the research protocol is whether the researchers can assign the units to the subpopulations or treatment groups that are being compared. When the researchers control the assignment of the units to the different treatments that are being compared, the study is called an *experiment*, and when units come to the researchers already assigned to the subpopulations or treatment groups, the study is called an *observational study*. Thus, in an experiment the researcher has the ability to assign the units to the groups that are being compared, while in an observational study the units come to the researcher already assigned to the groups.

One of the main reasons an observational study is used instead of an experiment in a biomedical research study is that it would be unethical to assign some subjects to a treatment that is known to be harmful and the remaining subjects to a treatment that is not harmful. For example, in a prospective 30-year study of the effects of smoking cigarettes, it would be unethical to assign some subjects to be smokers and others to be nonsmokers.

For ethical reasons, observational studies are often used in epidemiological studies designed to investigate the risk factors associated with a disease. Also, a retrospective study is always an observational study because it looks backward in time and the units have already been assigned to the groups being compared. On the other hand, a prospective study and a clinical trial can be run as either experiments or observational studies depending on whether it is possible for the researcher to assign the units to the groups.

Example 1.8
Determine whether it would be possible to perform an experiment in each of the scenarios given below.

   a. A nutritionist is interested in comparing several different diets in a prospective study. The treatments that will be compared are 10% fat in the diet, 15% fat in the diet, and 25% fat in the diet.

   b. A pediatrician is interested in studying the effects of a mother's use of tobacco on the birth weight of her baby. The two treatments that are to be compared are smoking during pregnancy and not smoking during pregnancy.

   c. A medical researcher is studying the efficacy of vitamin C as a preventive measure against the common cold. The two treatments that are being compared are 1000 mg vitamin C and 1000 mg placebo.

Solutions

a. Because the researcher can assign the subjects to each of the three diets in this study, it could be performed as an experiment.

b. Because smoking is known to have harmful effects on a fetus, it would be unethical for a pediatrician to assign some mothers smoke during pregnancy and others to not smoke during pregnancy. This study would have to be performed as an observational study by comparing the weights of babies born to mothers who chose to smoke during pregnancy with babies born to mothers who did not smoke during pregnancy.

c. Because the medical researcher could assign the subjects to these two treatments, it could be performed as an experiment.

An important advantage experiments have over observational studies is that it is possible in an experiment to control for external factors that might cause differences between the units of the target population. By controlling for the external factors in an experiment, it is possible to make the groups of units assigned to different treatments (i.e., treatment groups) as alike as possible before the treatments are applied. Moreover, in a well-designed experiment when the value of an explanatory variable is changed while no other changes take place in the experimental conditions, any differences in the responses are most likely due to the change in the value of this explanatory variable.

On the other hand, it is much harder to control external factors in an observational study because the units come to the researcher already assigned to the treatments, and thus, in an observational study there is no guarantee that the treatment groups were alike before the treatments were assigned to the units. Because experiments can be designed to control external factors, they can be used to establish evidence of causal relationships; an observational study generally cannot provide strong evidence of a causal relationship because uncontrolled external factors cannot be ruled out as the potential cause of the results.

Example 1.9

To study whether echinacea is effective in shortening the duration of the common cold, a random sample of 200 volunteers is taken. The 200 subjects are divided into two groups of size 100. Each group gets a supply of 300 mg pills and is instructed to take a 300 mg pill as soon as they recognize cold symptoms and to continue taking a pill each day until their cold symptoms go away. One group will receive 300 mg echinacea pills and the other group 300 mg placebo pills. The subjects are asked to record the duration of each cold they have in the following year.

a. Is this study an experiment or an observational study?

b. What is the target population in this study?

c. What is the response variable in this study?

d. What are the treatments in this study?

e. Is this a prospective or retrospective study?

Solutions

a. This study is an experiment because the researcher assigned the subjects to the treatments.

b. The target population in this study is people having the common cold.

c. The response variable in this study is the duration of the common cold.

d. The treatments in this study are 300 mg echinacea and 300 mg placebo.

e. This is a prospective study because the subjects are being followed forward in time.

Example 1.10

To study whether or not there is a relationship between childhood obesity and parental obesity in the United States, a random sample of 500 families was selected. The parents and children in each family were then classified as normal weight, overweight, or obese. The goal was to compare the percentage in each of the weight classifications of the children with normal weight parents against the percentages of the children with overweight and obese parents.

    a. Is this study an experiment or an observational study?

    b. What is the target population in this study?

    c. What is the response variable in this study?

    d. What are the treatments in this study?

Solutions

    a. This study is an observational study because the subjects came to the researcher assigned to their respective weight classifications.

    b. The target population in this study is parents with children living in the United States.

    c. The response variable in this study is weight classification of a child. The weight classification of the parent is an explanatory variable.

    d. The treatments in this study consist of weight classifications of the parents (normal, overweight, or obese).

1.3 CLINICAL TRIALS

Clinical trials are generally associated with biomedical research studies that are carried out on people for testing how well a new medical approach works, for testing the efficacy and safety of new drugs, for evaluating new biomedical procedures or technological advances, and for diagnosing, treating, managing, or preventing a disease. In the United States, a clinical trial is often highly regulated to ensure that it follows a well-designed research protocol that is ethical and preserves the safety of the participants.

For example, in the development of a new drug, a pharmaceutical company often begins by testing the drug on human cells and animals in a laboratory setting. If the initial laboratory research indicates that the drug may be beneficial to humans, the next step is to submit a new drug application (NDA) to the FDA. The NDA will contain information on the drug, the results of all prior test data on the drug, and descriptions of the manufacturing process used to make the drug. The FDA will then determine whether the drug is safe and effective for its proposed use(s), whether the benefits of the drug outweigh its risks, whether the drug's proposed labeling is appropriate, and, if not, what the drug's appropriate labeling is, and whether the methods used in manufacturing the drug and the controls used to maintain the drug's quality are adequate to preserve the drug's identity, strength, quality, and purity. Supervised clinical trials represent the final testing ground for a new drug, and the results of the clinical trials will be used in the final approval or disapproval of a new drug.

1.3.1 Safety and Ethical Considerations in a Clinical Trial

Every well-designed clinical trial will have a predetermined research protocol that outlines exactly how the clinical trial will be conducted. The clinical trial protocol will describe what will be done in the trial, the rules for determining who can participate, the specific research questions being investigated, the schedule of tests, procedures, medications, and dosages used in the trial, and the length of the trial. During the clinical trial, the participants are closely monitored by the research staff to determine the safety and effectiveness of their treatment. In fact, the ethical treatment and safety of the participants are carefully controlled in clinical trials performed in the United States.

In general, a clinical trial run in the United States must be preapproved by an independent committee of physicians, biostatisticians, and members of the community, which makes sure that the risks to the participants in the study are small and are worth the potential benefits of the new drug or treatment. Many, if not most, externally funded or university-based clinical trials must be reviewed and approved by an Institutional Review Board (IRB) associated with the funding agency. The IRB has the power to decide how often to review the clinical trial, and once started whether the clinical trial should continue as initially planned or modifications need to be made to the research protocol. Furthermore, the IRB may end a clinical trial when a researcher is not following the prescribed protocol, the trial is unsafe, or there is clear and strong evidence that the new drug or treatment is effective.

1.3.2 Types of Clinical Trials

Clinical trials can generally be classified as one of the following types of trials:

- Treatment trials that are clinical trials designed to test experimental treatments, new drugs, or new medical approaches or technology.
- Prevention trials that are clinical trials designed to investigate ways to prevent diseases or prevent the recurrence of a disease.
- Screening trials that are clinical trials designed to determine the best way to detect certain diseases or health conditions early on.
- Diagnostic trials that are clinical trials designed to determine tests or procedures that can be used for diagnosing a particular disease or condition.
- Quality-of-life trials that are clinical trials designed to explore ways to improve the comfort and quality of life for individuals with a chronic or terminal disease or condition.
- Genetic trials that are clinical trials designed to investigate the role genetics plays in the detection, diagnosis, or response to a drug or treatment.

Pharmaceutical companies commonly use treatment trials in the development and evaluation of new drugs, epidemiologists generally use prevention, screening, and diagnostic trials in their studies of diseases, public health officials often use quality-of-life trials, and geneticists often use genetic trials for studying tissue or blood samples from families or large groups of people to understand the role of genes in the development of a disease.

The results of a clinical trial are generally published in peer-reviewed scientific or medical journals. The peer-review process is carried out by experts who critically review a research report before it is published. In particular, the peer reviewers are charged with examining the research protocol, analysis, and conclusions drawn in a research report to ensure the integrity and quality of the research that is published. Following the publication of the results of a clinical trial or biomedical research study, further information is generally obtained as new studies are carried out independently by other researchers. The follow-up research is generally designed to validate or expand the previously published results.

1.3.3 The Phases of a Clinical Trial

Clinical research is often conducted in a series of steps, called phases. Because a new drug, medicine, or treatment must be safe, effective, and manufactured at a consistent quality, a series of rigorous clinical trials are usually required before the drug, medicine, or treatment can be made available to the general public. In the United States the FDA regulates and oversees the testing and approval of new drugs as well as dietary supplements, cosmetics, medical devices, blood products, and the content of health claims on food labels. The approval of a new drug by the FDA requires extensive testing and evaluation of the drug through a series of four clinical trials, which are referred to as *phase I, II, III,* and *IV* trials.

Each of the four phases is designed with a different purpose and to provide the necessary information to help biomedical researchers answer several different questions about a new drug, treatment, or biomedical procedure. After a clinical trial is completed, the researchers use biostatistical methods to analyze the data collected during the trial and make decisions and draw conclusions about the meaning of their findings and whether further studies are needed. After each phase in the study of a new drug or treatment, the research team must decide whether to proceed to the next phase or stop the investigation of the drug/treatment. Formal approval of a new drug or biomedical procedure generally cannot be made until a phase III trial is completed and there is strong evidence that the drug/treatment is safe and effective.

The purpose of a *phase I* clinical trial is to investigate the safety, efficacy, and side effects of a new drug or treatment. Phase I trials usually involve a small number of subjects and take place at a single or only a few different locations. In a drug trial, the goal of a phase I trial is often to investigate the metabolic and pharmacologic actions of the drug, the efficacy of the drug, and the side effects associated with different dosages of the drug. Phase I drug trials are also referred to as *dose finding trials*.

When the results of a phase I trial suggest that a treatment or drug appears to have promise, the treatment or drug is generally next studied in a *phase II* trial. In phase II clinical trials, the drug or treatment being studied is evaluated on a larger group of subjects to further investigate its effectiveness and safety. In general, the goal of a phase II trial is to study the feasibility and level of activity of the drug or treatment. Thus, phase II trials are designed to provide more information about the effective dosage of a drug, the severity of the side effects, and how to manage the side effects. Phase II trials are also referred to as *safety and efficacy trials* and usually involve more subjects than phase I trials.

When the preliminary results of a new drug or treatment from a phase II trial suggest the drug or treatment will be effective and safe, a *phase III* trial is designed to gather additional information that can be used in evaluating the overall benefit–risk relationship of the drug. Phase III trials are usually designed to compare the new drug/treatment with standard or commonly used drugs/treatments, to confirm its effectiveness, to further monitor side effects, and to determine how the new drug or treatment can be safely used. Phase III trials generally are large trials and may enroll subjects at a wide variety of locations. Phase III trials are also referred to as *comparative treatment efficacy trials*.

Finally, when a new drug or treatment has been examined in phase I, II, and III trials and has been approved for the general public, a *phase IV* trial is usually initiated. A phase IV trial is a postmarketing study designed to obtain additional information on the risks associated with the drug/treatment, its benefits, and its optimal use. The primary aim of a phase IV trial is to evaluate the long-term safety and effectiveness of a drug/treatment. Phase IV trials sometimes result in a drug being taken completely off the market or new restrictions being placed on the use of the drug. Phase IV trials are also referred to as *expanded safety trials* and usually involve a very large number of subjects.

Note that the number of subjects in a trial usually increases as the phases of the study progress. That is, a phase I trial usually involves fewer subjects than a phase II trial, a phase II trial usually involves fewer subjects than a phase III trial, and a phase III trial usually involves fewer subjects than a phase IV trial. Also, some research studies involving human subjects will have less than four phases. For example, it is not unusual for screening, prevention, diagnostic, genetic, and quality-of-life studies to be conducted in only phase I or II trials. However, new drugs and biomedical procedures almost always require phase I, II, and III clinical trials for approval and a phase IV trial to track the safety of the drug after its approval. The development of a new drug may take many years to proceed through the first three phases of the approval process, and following approval, the phase IV trial usually extends over a period of many years.

1.4   DATA SET DESCRIPTIONS

Throughout this book several data sets will be used in the examples and exercises. These data sets are given in Appendix B and are also available at http://www.mtech.edu/clsps/math/Faculty/rossi_book.htm as Excel files, text files, and MINITAB worksheets. Permission to use the Birth Weight, Intensive Care Unit, Coronary Heart Disease, UMASS Aids Research Unit, and Prostate Cancer data sets has been granted by John Wiley & Sons, Inc. These data sets were first published in *Applied Logistic Regression* (Hosmer, 2000). Permission to use the Body Fat data set has been provided by Roger W. Johnson, Department of Mathematics & Computer Science, South Dakota School of Mines & Technology and *Journal of Statistics Education*.

1.4.1   Birth Weight Data Set

The Birth Weight data set consists of data collected on 189 women to identify the risk factors associated with the birth of a low birth weight baby. The data set was collected at the Baystate Medical Center in Springfield, Massachusetts. The variables included in this data set are summarized in Table 1.1.

1.4.2   Body Fat Data Set

The Body Fat data set consists of data collected on 252 adult males. The data were originally collected to build a model relating body density and percentage of body fat in adult males to several body measurement variables. These data were originally used in the article "Generalized body composition prediction equation for men using simple measurement techniques," published in *Medicine and Science in Sports and Exercise* (Penrose et al., 1985). The variables included in this data set are summarized in Table 1.2.

1.4.3   Coronary Heart Disease Data Set

The Coronary Heart Disease data set consists of 100 observations on patients who were selected in a study on the relationship between the age and the presence of coronary heart disease. The variables included in this data set are summarized in Table 1.3.

TABLE 1.1   A Description of the Variables in the Birth Weight Data Set

Variable	Description	Codes/Values	Name
1	Identification code	ID number	ID
2	Low birth weight	1 = BWT ≤ 2500 g 0 = BWT > 2500 g	LOW
3	Age of mother	Years	AGE
4	Weight of mother at last menstrual period	Pounds	LWT
5	Race	1 = White 2 = Black 3 = Other	RACE
6	Smoking status during pregnancy	0 = No 1 = Yes	SMOKE
7	History of premature labor	0 = None 1 = One 2 = Two, etc.	PTL
8	History of hypertension	0 = No 1 = Yes	HT
9	Presence of uterine irritability	0 = No 1 = Yes	UI
10	Number of physician visits during the first trimester	0 = None 1 = One 2 = Two, etc.	FTV
11	Birth weight	Grams	BWT

1.4.4 Prostate Cancer Study Data Set

The Prostate Cancer Study data set consists of 380 patients in a study to determine whether the variables measured at a baseline medical examination can be used to predict whether the prostatic tumor has penetrated a prostatic capsule. The data were collected by Dr. Donn

TABLE 1.2   A Description of the Variables in the Body Fat Data Set

Variable	Description	Codes/Values	Name
1	Density determined from underwater weighing		Density
2	Percent body fat from Siri's (1956) equation	Percent	PCTBF
3	Age	Years	Age
4	Weight	Pounds	Weight
5	Height	Inches	Height
6	Neck circumference	Centimeters	Neck
7	Chest circumference	Centimeters	Chest
8	Abdomen circumference	Centimeters	Abdomen
9	Hip circumference	Centimeters	Hip
10	Thigh circumference	Centimeters	Thigh
11	Knee circumference	Centimeters	Knee
12	Ankle circumference	Centimeters	Ankle
13	Biceps extended circumference	Centimeters	Biceps
14	Forearm circumference	Centimeters	Forearm
15	Wrist circumference	Centimeters	Wrist

TABLE 1.3 A Description of the Variables in the Coronary Heart Disease Data Set

Variable	Description	Codes/Values	Name
1	Identification code	ID number	ID
2	Age in years	Years	Age
3	Coronary heart disease	0 = Absent 1 = Present	CHD

Young at the Ohio State University Comprehensive Cancer Center and the data have been modified to protect subject confidentiality. Variables included in this data set are summarized in Table 1.4.

1.4.5 Intensive Care Unit Data Set

The Intensive Care Unit data set consists of 200 observations on subjects involved in a study on the survival of patients following admission to an adult intensive care unit (ICU). The data set was collected at the Baystate Medical Center in Springfield, Massachusetts, and the variables included in this data set are summarized in Table 1.5.

1.4.6 Mammography Experience Study Data Set

The Mammography Experience Study data set consists of 412 observations on subjects from a study designed to investigate the factors associated with a woman's knowledge, attitude, and behavior toward mammography exams. The data were collected by Dr. J. Zapka and Ms. D. Spotts of the University of Massachusetts, Division of Public Health. The variables included in this data set are summarized in Table 1.6.

TABLE 1.4 A Description of the Variables in the Prostate Cancer Study Data Set

Variable	Description	Codes/values	Name
1	Identification code	ID number	ID
2	Tumor penetration of prostatic capsule	0 = No penetration 1 = Penetration	CAPSULE
3	Age	Years	AGE
4	Race	1= White 2 = Black	RACE
5	Results of the digital rectal exam	1 = No nodule 2 = Unilobar nodule (left) 3 = Unilobar nodule (right) 4 = Bilobar nodule	DPROS
6	Detection of capsular involvement in rectal exam	1 = No 2 = Yes	DCAPS
7	Prostatic-specific antigen value	mg/ml	PSA
8	Tumor volume obtained from ultrasound	cm^3	VOL
9	Total Gleason score	0–10	GLEASON

TABLE 1.5   A Description of the Variables in the Intensive Care Unit Data Set

Variable	Description	Codes/values	Name
1	Identification code	ID number	ID
2	Vital status	0 = Lived	STA
		1 = Died	
3	Age	Years	AGE
4	Sex	0 = Male	SEX
		1 = Female	
5	Race	1 = White	RACE
		2 = Black	
		3 = Other	
6	Service at ICU admission	0 = Medical	SER
		1 = Surgical	
7	Cancer part of	0 = No	CAN
	present problem	1 = Yes	
8	History of chronic	0 = No	CRN
	renal failure	1 = Yes	
9	Infection probable at	0 = No	INF
	ICU admission	1 = Yes	
10	CPR prior to	0 = No	CPR
	ICU admission	1 = Yes	
11	Systolic blood pressure	mmHg	SYS
	at ICU admission		
12	Heart rate at	Beats/min	HRA
	ICU admission		
13	Previous admission to an	0 = No	PRE
	ICU within 6 months	1 = Yes	
14	Type of admission	0 = Elective	TYP
		1 = Emergency	
15	Long bone, multiple, neck	0 = No	FRA
	single area, or hip fracture	1 = Yes	
16	pO_2 from initial	0 = > 60	PO2
	blood gases	1 = < 60	
17	pH from initial	0 = > 7.25	PH
	blood gases	1 = < 7.25	
18	pCO_2 from initial	0 = < 45	PCO
	blood gases	1 = > 45	
19	Bicarbonate from	0 = > 18	BIC
	Initial blood gases	1 = < 18	
20	Creatinine from	0 = < 2.0	CRE
	initial blood gases	1 = > 2.0	
21	Level of consciousness	0 = No coma or stupor	LOC
	at ICU admission	1 = Deep stupor	
		2 = Coma	

1.4.7 Benign Breast Disease Study

The Benign Breast Disease Study data set consists of data collected from 200 women in a case–control study designed to investigate the risk factors associated with benign breast disease at two hospitals in New Haven, Connecticut. The variables included in this data set are summarized in Table 1.7.

TABLE 1.6   A Description of the Variables in the Mammography Experience Data Set

Variable	Description	Codes/Values	Name
1	Identification code	ID number	OBS
2	Mammograph experience	0 = Never 1 = Within 1 year 2 = Over 1 year ago	ME
3	"You do not need a mammogram unless you develop symptoms"	1 = Strongly agree 2 = Agree 3 = Disagree 4 = Strongly disagree	SYMPT
4	Perceived benefit of mammography	5–20	PB
5	Mother or sister with a history of breast cancer	0 = No 1 = Yes	HIST
6	"Has anyone taught you how to examine your own breasts: that is BSE"	0 = No 1 = Yes	BSE
7	"How likely is it that a mammogram could find a new case of breast cancer"	1 = Not likely 2 = Somewhat likely 3 = Very likely	DETC

TABLE 1.7   A Description of the Variables in the Benign Breast Disease Study Data Set

Variable	Description	Codes/Values	Name
1	Stratum	1–50	STR
2	Observation within a stratum	1 = Case 2–4 = Control	OBS
3	Age of the subject at the interview	Years	AGMT
4	Final diagnosis	1 = Case 0 = Control	FNDX
5	Highest grade in school		HIGD
6	Degree	0 = None 1 = High school 2 = Jr. college 3 = College 4 = Masters 5 = Doctoral	DEG
7	Regular medical checkups	1 = Yes 2 = No	CHK
8	Age at first pregnancy	Years	AGP1
9	Age at menarche	Years	AGMN
10	No. of stillbirths, miscarriages, etc.		NLV
11	Number of live births		LIV
12	Weight of the subject	Pounds	WT
13	Age at last menstrual period	Years	AGLP
14	Marital status	1 = Married 2 = Divorced 3 = Separated 4 = Widowed 5 = Never married	MST

GLOSSARY

Biostatistics   Biostatistics is the science of collecting, an alyzing, and interpreting biomedical and healthcare data.

Blinded Study   A blinded study is a research study where the subjects in the study are not told which treatment they are receiving. A research study is a double-blind study when neither the subject nor the staff administering the treatment know which treatment a subject receives.

Case–Control Study   A case–control study is a retrospective study in which subjects having a certain disease or condition are compared with subjects who do not have the disease.

Census   A census is a sample consisting of the entire set of population units.

Clinical Trial   A clinical trial is a research study performed on humans and designed to evaluate a new treatment or drug or to investigate a specific health condition that follows a predefined protocol.

Cohort   A cohort is a group of subjects having similar characteristics.

Cross–Sectional Study   A cross-sectional study is a study to investigate the relationship between a response variable and the explanatory variables in a target population at a particular point in time.

Experiment   An experiment is a study where the researcher controls the assignment of the units to the treatments.

Explanatory Variable   An explanatory variable is a variable that is used to explain or is believed to cause changes in the response variable. The explanatory variables are also called independent variables or predictor variables.

Longitudinal Study   A longitudinal study is a study where the same subjects are observed over a specific period of time. A longitudinal study could be either a prospective or a retrospective study.

Observational Study   An observational study is any study where the units of the study come to the researchers already assigned to the subpopulations or treatment groups.

Parameter   A parameter is a numerical measure of a characteristic of the population.

Phase I Clinical Trial   A phase I clinical trial is designed for investigating the safety, efficacy, and side effects of a new drug or treatment. Phase I drug trials are also referred to as dose finding trials.

Phase II Clinical Trial   A phase II clinical trial follows a phase I trial and is used to further investigate the effectiveness, feasibility, and safety of a drug or treatment. Phase II trials are also referred to as safety and efficacy trials and usually have a larger sample size than a phase I trial.

Phase III Clinical Trial   A phase III clinical trial follows a phase II trial and is designed to gather additional information that will be used in evaluating the overall benefit–risk relationship of the drug. Phase III trials are generally large trials and are referred to as comparative treatment efficacy trials.

Phase IV Clinical Trial   A phase IV clinical trial is a postmarketing study designed to obtain additional information on the risks associated with the drug/treatment, its benefits, and its optimal use. The primary use of a phase IV trials is to evaluate the long-term safety and effectiveness of a drug/treatment. Phase IV trials are referred to as expanded safety trials and usually involve a large number of subjects.

Population Units   The units of a population are the objects on which measurements will be taken. When the units of the population are human beings, they are referred to as subjects or individuals.

Prospective Study   A prospective study is a study that monitors the units over a period of time and analyzes what happens to the units in the study.

Randomized Controlled Study   A randomized controlled study is a research study where the subjects are randomly assigned to the treatments with one of the treatments being a control treatment; a control treatment may be a standard treatment, a placebo, or no treatment at all.

Response Variable   A response variable is an observed variable or outcome variable in an experiment or study that is believed to depend on other variables in the study. The response variable is also called a dependent variable.

Retrospective Study   A retrospective study is a study that looks backward in time and analyzes what has happened to the units in the study.

Sample   A sample is a subset of the population units. A random sample is a sample that is chosen according to a sampling plan where the probability of each possible sample that can be drawn from the target population is known, where the probability of sampling each unit in the population is known.

Statistic   A statistic is any value that is computed from only the sample observations and known values.

Statistical Inferences   Statistical inferences are estimates, conclusions, or generalizations made about the target population from the information contained in an observed sample.

Statistical Model   A statistical model is a mathematical formula that relates the response variable to the explanatory variables.

Target Population   The target population is the population of units that is being studied.

Treatment   A treatment is any experimental condition that is applied to the units. A placebo treatment is an inert or inactive treatment that is applied to the units.

Variable   A variable is a characteristic that will be recorded or measured on a unit in the target population.

EXERCISES

1.1   What is biostatistics?

1.2   What does a biostatistician do?

1.3   What are three federal agencies that employ biostatisticians?

1.4   What is a
(**a**) target population?   (**b**) sample?
(**c**) census?

1.5   How is the target population different from a sample?

1.6   What is a
(**a**) parameter?   (**b**) statistic?

1.7   How is a statistic different from a parameter?

1.8 How can the value of an unknown parameter be
    (a) found exactly?   **(b)** estimated?

1.9 What is a numerical value that is computed from only the information contained in a sample called?

1.10 What is a numerical value that is computed from a census called?

1.11 What is a statistical inference?

1.12 What is a
    (a) random sample?   **(b)** cohort?
    (c) variable?   **(d)** treatment?
    (e) placebo?   **(f)** statistical model?

1.13 What is the difference between a response variable and an explanatory variable.

1.14 In a study designed to determine the percentage of understaffed hospitals in the United States, 250 of roughly 7500 hundred hospitals in the United States were surveyed. The resulting percentage of the understaffed hospitals was 41%.
    (a) What is the target population in this study?
    (b) Is 41% a statistic or a parameter? Explain.

1.15 In a study designed to determine the percentage of doctors belonging to the American Medical Association (AMA) who perform pro bono work, the AMA found from a census of its membership that 63% performed pro bono work. The AMA also found from a sample of 1000 members that the average number of pro bono hours worked by a doctor in a year was 223.
    (a) What is the target population in this study?
    (b) Is 63% a statistic or a parameter? Explain.
    (c) Is 223 a statistic or a parameter? Explain.

1.16 In a Red Cross sponsored laboratory study designed to investigate the average length of time blood can be stored safely in a blood bank in the United States, 20 freshly sampled 500 ml blood bags were monitored over a 6-month period. The results of this laboratory study showed that blood may be stored safely on average for 17 days.
    (a) What is the target population in this study?
    (b) Is 17 a statistic or a parameter? Explain.

1.17 In a study designed to investigate the effects of omega-3 fatty acids for lowering the risk of Alzheimer's disease, 300 participants aged 50 and older with mild to moderate Alzheimer's disease were selected for the study. The 300 participants were randomly assigned to two groups with one group receiving placebo pills and the other group receiving omega-3 supplement pills. Doctors and nurses will monitor the participants throughout the study, and neither the researchers conducting the trial nor the participants will know who is getting the omega-3 pills or the placebo pills.
    (a) What is the target population in this study?.
    (b) What are units of target population?
    (c) What are the treatments being used in this study?
    (d) What is the sample size in this study?
    (e) Is this a blinded study? Explain.
    (f) Is this a randomized controlled study? Explain.

1.18 To study whether vitamin C is effective in shortening the duration of a common cold, a random sample of 400 volunteers is taken. The 400 subjects are divided into two groups of size 200. Each group gets a supply of 1000 mg pills and is instructed to take a pill as soon as they recognize cold symptoms and to continue taking a pill each day until their cold symptoms go away. One group will receive 1000 mg vitamin C pills and the other group 1000 mg placebo pills. The subjects are asked to record the duration of each cold they have in the following year.

(a) What is the target population in this study?

(b) What is the response variable in this study?

(c) What are the treatments in this study?

(d) Could this be run as a double-blind study? Explain.

1.19 In a study designed to investigate the efficacy of three treatments for prostate cancer, $n = 1088$ patients were selected from Los Angeles public hospitals for the study. The treatments studied were surgery, hormone therapy, and radiation therapy. The goal of the study is to estimate the percentage of prostate cancer patients surviving at least 5 years for each of the treatments. The variables age, sex, and race were also recorded for each patient since they are believed to influence the survival time of a prostate cancer patient. Determine

(a) the target population in this study?.

(b) the unit of the target population?

(c) the parameters of interest in this study?

(d) the explanatory variables used in this study?

(e) the treatments being studied?

1.20 What is a

(a) retrospective study? **(b)** prospective study?

(c) longitudinal study? **(d)** case–control study?

(e) cross-sectional study? **(f)** clinical trial?

(g) blinded study? **(h)** double-blind study?

1.21 How do prospective and retrospective studies differ?

1.22 What is a randomized controlled study?

1.23 Use the Internet to find an article published in a biomedical journal where a prospective study was used and identify the target population, the units of the population, the response variable, the treatments used in the study, and the explanatory variables measured in the study.

1.24 Use the Internet to find an article published in a biomedical journal where a retrospective study was used and identify the target population, the units of the population, the response variable, the treatments used in the case–control study, and the explanatory variables measured in the study.

1.25 Use the Internet to find an article published in a biomedical journal where a cohort study was used and identify the target population, the units of the population, the response variable, the treatments used in the study, and the explanatory variables measured in the study.

1.26 Use the Internet to find an article published in a biomedical journal where a double-blind study was used and identify the target population, the units of the population, the response variable, the treatments used in the study, and the explanatory variables measured in the study.

1.27 Use the Internet to find an article published in a biomedical journal where a cross-sectional study was used and identify the target population, the units of the population, the response variable, the treatments used in the study, and the explanatory variables measured in the study.

1.28 Use the Internet to find an article published in a biomedical journal where a prospective case-control study was used and identify the target population, the units of the population, the response variable, the treatments used in the study, and the explanatory variables measured in the study.

1.29 What is an
    (a) experiment?   **(b)** observational study?

1.30 How is an experiment different from an observational study?

1.31 Why is an experiment preferred over an observation study?

1.32 Why are retrospective studies and case–control studies observational studies?

1.33 Explain why it would or would not be ethical to perform an experiment in each of the scenarios below.
    (a) A researcher is interested in the effects of smoking cigarettes on human health. The researcher would like to assign subjects to the treatments smoke cigarettes for 25 years and do not smoke at all in a 25-year prospective study.
    (b) A researcher is interested in determining the efficacy of a new HIV/AIDS drug. The researcher would like to assign subjects to standard treatment and the new drug in a randomized controlled study.
    (c) A researcher is interested in identifying the risk factors associated with Alzheimer's disease. The researcher would like to assign subjects to several different risk factors in a 20-year prospective study.
    (d) A researcher is interested in identifying the relationship between hormone therapy and breast cancer. The researcher would like to assign subjects to the treatments hormone therapy, time-reduced hormone therapy, and no hormone therapy at all in a 20-year prospective study.

1.34 What are the six different types of clinical trials that were discussed earlier in this chapter?

1.35 What is a
    (a) prevention trial?   **(b)** quality-of-life trial?
    (c) screening trial?   **(d)** treatment trial?

1.36 What are the four phases of clinical trials?

1.37 What is a
    (a) dose finding trial?
    (b) safety and efficacy trial?
    (c) comparative treatment efficacy trial?
    (d) expanded safety trial?

1.38   What phases must a new drug, treatment, or biomedical procedure go through to receive approval for widespread use in the United States?

1.39   What is the purpose of running a phase IV trial after a new drug, treatment, or biomedical procedure has been approved?

1.40   What reasons might be used for prematurely stopping a clinical trial?

1.41   Are all research studies based on clinical trials required to be studied in all four phases? Explain.

1.42   Use the Internet to find
    (a)   the FDA regulations for the approval of a new drug.
    (b)   the regulations used in the United Kingdom for the approval of a new drug.
    (c)   the regulations used in Japan for the approval of a new drug.
    (d)   two drugs that have been taken off the market for safety reasons after their approval.
    (e)   out what the CDER agency does with regard to drugs developed and marketed in the United States.

CHAPTER 2

DESCRIBING POPULATIONS

I N THE planning stages of a research project, a set of research questions is developed and refined. Once a well-defined set of research questions has been developed, a target population will be identified so that the goals of the research project can be attained by sampling the target population. The target population is the reference population about which the research questions apply, from which the sample data will be collected, and is the population that statistical inferences will be made about. The research questions will also define the set of variables that must be measured on each unit that is sampled. A *variable* is a characteristic that will be measured on the units of the target population.

It is important to note that each variable will then have its own population of values. That is, because the units of the population will differ to some degree, a variable will often reflect the differences between the population units and take on several different values. The research questions will also need to be converted into questions about the particular characteristics of the population of values of a variable. In particular, the research questions must be expressed as questions concerning the parameters of the population of values of the variable so that statistical methods can be used to estimate, test, or predict the values of the parameters of interest.

In converting the research questions to questions about the parameters of a population, it is critical for a biomedical researcher and a biostatistician to work together to identify the parameters of the population that are relevant to the research questions being asked. The biomedical research team will also need to determine all of the variables that will be measured before collecting the sample data. In a well-designed research project, it is likely that a biomedical researcher and a biostatistician will work together to design the appropriate sampling plan and to determine the appropriate statistical methodology that will provide meaningful and accurate statistical inferences about the target population and the research questions.

2.1 POPULATIONS AND VARIABLES

In a properly designed biomedical research study, a well-defined target population and a particular set of research questions dictate the variables that should be measured on the units being studied in the research project. In most research problems, there are many variables that must be measured on each unit in the population. The outcome variables that are of primary interest are called the *response variables*, and the variables that are believed to explain the response variables are called the *explanatory variables* or *predictor variables*. For example, in a clinical trial designed to study the efficacy of a specialized treatment designed to reduce the size of a malignant tumor, the following explanatory variables might be recorded for each patient in the study: age, gender, race, weight, height, blood type, blood pressure, and oxygen uptake. The response variable in this study might be change in the size of the tumor.

Variables come in a variety of different types; however, each variable can be classified as being either quantitative or qualitative in nature. A variable that takes on only numeric values is a *quantitative variable*, and a variable that takes on nonnumeric values is called a *qualitative variable* or a *categorical variable*. Note that a variable is a quantitative or qualitative variable based on the possible values the variable can take on.

Example 2.1

In a study of obesity in the population of children aged 10 or less in the United States, some possible quantitative variables that might be measured include age, height, weight, heart rate, body mass index, and percent body fat; some qualitative variables that might be measured on this population include gender, eye color, race, and blood type. A likely choice for the response variable in this study would be the qualitative variable Obese defined by

$$\text{Obese} = \begin{cases} \text{Yes} & \text{for a body mass index of} > 30 \\ \text{No} & \text{for a body mass index of} \leq 30 \end{cases}$$

2.1.1 Qualitative Variables

Qualitative variables take on nonnumeric values and are usually used to represent a distinct quality of a population unit. When the possible values of a qualitative variable have no intrinsic ordering, the variable is called a *nominal variable*; when there is a natural ordering of the possible values of the variable, then the variable is called an *ordinal variable*. An example of a nominal variable is Blood Type where the standard values for blood type are A, B, AB, and O. Clearly, there is no intrinsic ordering of these blood types, and hence, Blood Type is a nominal variable. An example of an ordinal variable is the variable Pain where a subject is asked to describe their pain verbally as

- No pain
- Mild pain
- Discomforting pain
- Distressing pain
- Intense pain
- Excruciating pain

In this case, since the verbal descriptions describe increasing levels of pain, there is a clear ordering of the possible values of the variable Pain levels, and therefore, Pain is an ordinal qualitative variable.

Example 2.2

In the Framingham Heart Study of coronary heart disease, the following two nominal qualitative variables were recorded:

$$\text{Smokes} = \begin{cases} \text{Yes} \\ \text{No} \end{cases}$$

and

$$\text{Diabetes} = \begin{cases} \text{Yes} \\ \text{No} \end{cases}$$

Example 2.3

An example of an ordinal variable is the variable Baldness when measured on the Norwood–Hamilton scale for male-pattern baldness. The variable Baldness is measured according to the seven categories listed below:

    I Full head of hair without any hair loss.

    II Minor recession at the front of the hairline.

    III Further loss at the front of the hairline, which is considered "cosmetically significant."

    IV Progressively more loss along the front hairline and at the crown.

    V Hair loss extends toward the vertex.

    VI Frontal and vertex balding areas merge into one and increase in size.

    VII All hair is lost along the front hairline and crown.

Clearly, the values of the variable Baldness indicate an increasing degree of hair loss, and thus, Baldness as measured on the Norwood–Hamilton scale is an ordinal variable. This variable is also measured on the Offspring Cohort in the Framingham Heart Study.

2.1.2 Quantitative Variables

A quantitative variable is a variable that takes only numeric values. The values of a quantitative variable are said to be measured on an *interval scale* when the difference between two values is meaningful; the values of a quantitative variable are said to be measured on a *ratio scale* when the ratio of two values is meaningful. The key difference between a variable measured on an interval scale and a ratio scale is that on a ratio scale there is a "natural zero" representing absence of the attribute being measured, while there is no natural zero for variables measured on only an interval scale. Some scales of measurement will have natural zero and some will not. When a measurement scale has a natural zero, then the ratio of two measurements is a meaningful measure of how many times larger one value is than the other. For example, the variable Fat that represents the grams of fat in a food product is measured on a ratio scale because the value Fat = 0 indicates that the unit contained absolutely no fat. When a scale of measurement does not have a natural zero, then only the difference between two measurements is a meaningful comparison of the values of the two measurements. For example, the variable Body Temperature is measured on a scale that has no natural zero since Body Temperature = 0 does not indicate that the body has no temperature.

    Since interval scales are ordered, the difference between two values measures how much larger one value is than another. A ratio scale is also an interval scale but has the additional property that the ratio of two values is meaningful. Thus, for a variable measured on an interval scale the difference of two values is the meaningful way to compare the values, and for a variable measured on a ratio scale both the difference and the ratio of two values are meaningful ways to compare difference values of the variable. For example, body temperature in degrees Fahrenheit is a variable that is measured on an interval scale so that it is meaningful to say that a body temperature of 98.6 and a body temperature of 102.3 differ by 3.7 degrees; however, it would not be meaningful to say that a temperature of 102.3 is 1.04 times as much as a temperature of 98.6. On the other hand, the variable weight in pounds is measured on a ratio scale, and therefore, it would be proper to say that a weight of 210 lb is 1.4 times a weight of 150 lb; it would also be meaningful to say that a weight of 210 lb is 60 lb more than a weight of 150 lb.

Example 2.4

The following questions were asked in the Framingham Heart Study on the Offspring Cohort and the corresponding variables recorded. The variables are listed in parentheses after each question. Determine which of these variables are qualitative and which quantitative. For the qualitative variables determine whether they are nominal or ordinal variables.

a. What is your gender? (Gender)
b. Systolic blood pressure (Systolic Blood Pressure)
c. Do you smoke? (Smoke)
d. How many cigarettes do you smoke per day? (No. Cigarettes)
e. What is your age? (Age)
f. How many times per week do you engage in intense physical activity? (No. Physical Activity)
g. How is your health now? (Health)

Solutions

a. Gender is a nominal qualitative variable.
b. Systolic Blood Pressure is a quantitative variable.
c. Smoke is a nominal qualitative variable.
d. No. Cigarettes is a quantitative variable.
e. Age is a quantitative variable.
f. No. Physical Activity is a quantitative variable.
g. Health is an ordinal qualitative variable.

A quantitative variable can also be classified as either a *discrete variable* or a *continuous variable*. A quantitative variable is a discrete variable when it can take on a finite or a countable number of values; a quantitative variable is a continuous variable when it can take on any value in one or more intervals. Note that the values that a discrete variable can take on are distinct, isolated, and can be counted. In the previous example, the variables Age, No. Cigarettes, and No. Physical Activity are discrete variables. A *counting variable* is a specialized discrete variable that simply counts how many times a particular event has occurred. The values a counting variables can take on are the values $0, 1, 2, 3, \ldots, \infty$. For example, in the Framingham Heart Study the variables No. Cigarettes and No. Physical Activity are counting variables.

Example 2.5

The following variables are all counting variables:

a. The number of cancer patients in remission following treatment at a hospital.
b. The number of laboratory mice that survive in an experiment.
c. The number of white blood cells in a 10 ml blood sample.

Continuous variables are variables that can take on any value in one or more intervals. Examples of continuous variables are the exact weight of a subject, the exact dose of a drug, and the exact height of a subject. In most problems, there will be variables of interest that are continuous variables, but because the variable can only be measured to a specific accuracy, a discrete version of the variable is used. For example, the weight of a subject is a continuous variable, but when it is measured only in pounds or tenths of pounds, it is a discrete variable.

Example 2.6
The following variables are continuous variables that might be measured on a discrete measurement scale:

a. Body temperature since it is usually measured in tenths of degrees.

b. Lung capacity since it is a volume and is usually measured in cubic centimeters.

c. Tumor size since it is measured as a depth in tenths of centimeters.

It is important that a variable truly reflects the characteristic being studied. A variable is said to be a *valid variable* when the measurements on the variable truly represent the characteristic the variable is supposed to be measuring. The validity of a variable depends on the characteristic being measured and the measuring device being used to measure the characteristic. When a characteristic of a unit is subjective in nature, it will be difficult to measure the characteristic accurately, and in this case, the validity of any variables used to measure this subjective characteristic is usually questionable.

Example 2.7
The intelligence of an individual is a subjectively measured characteristic. There are many tests that have been developed to measure intelligence. For example, the Fagan test measures the amount of time an infant spends inspecting a new object and compares this time with the time spent inspecting a familiar object (Fagan and Detterman, 1992). The validity of the Fagan test as a measure of intelligence, however, has been questioned by several scientists who have studied the relationship between intelligence and the Fagan test scores.

The diagram in Figure 2.1 summarizes the different types of variables/data that can be observed.

2.1.3 Multivariate Data

In most research problems, there will be many variables that need to be measured. When the collection of variables measured on each unit consists of two or more variables, a data set is called a *multivariate* data set, and a multivariate data set consisting of only two variables is called a *bivariate* data set. In a multivariate data set, there is usually one variable that is of primary interest to a research question that is believed to be explained

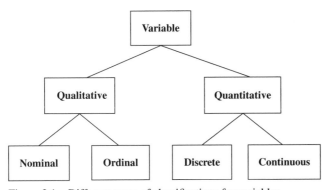

Figure 2.1   Different types of classifications for variables.

by some of the other variables measured in the study. The variable of primary interest is called a *response variable* and the variables believed to cause changes in the response are called *explanatory variables* or *predictor variables*. The explanatory variables are often referred to as the input variables and the response variable is often referred to as the output variable. Furthermore, in a statistical model, the response variable is the variable that is being modeled; the explanatory variables are the input variables in the model that are believed to cause or explain differences in the response variable. For example, in studying the survival of melanoma patients, the response variable might be Survival Time that is expected to be influenced by the explanatory variables Age, Gender, Clark's Stage, and Tumor Size. In this case, a model relating Survival Time to the explanatory variables Age, Gender, Clark's Stage, and Tumor Size might be investigated in the research study.

A multivariate data set often consists of a mixture of qualitative and quantitative variables. For example, in a biomedical study, several variables that are commonly measured are a subject's age, race, gender, height, and weight. When data have been collected, the multivariate data set is generally stored in a spreadsheet with the columns containing the data on each variable and the rows of the spreadsheet containing the observations on each subject in the study.

In studying the response variable, it is often the case that there are subpopulations that are determined by a particular set of values of the explanatory variables that will be important in answering the research questions. In this case, it is critical that a variable be included in the data set that identifies which subpopulation each unit belongs to. For example, in the National Health and Nutrition Examination Survey (NHANES) study, the distribution of the weight of female children was studied. The response variable in this study was weight and some of the explanatory variables measured in this study were height, age, and gender. The result of this part of the NHANES study was a distribution of the weights of females over a certain range of age. The resulting distributions were summarized in the chart given in Figure 2.2 that shows the weight ranges for females for several different ages.

Example 2.8
In the article "The validity of self-reported weight in US adults: a population based cross-sectional study" published in *BMC Public Health* (Villanueva, 2001), the author reported the results of a study on the validity of self-reported weight. The data set used in the study was a multivariate data set with response variable being the difference between the self-reported weight and the actual weight of an individual. The explanatory variables in this study were gender, age, race–ethnicity, highest educational attainment, level of activity, and perception of the individuals' current weight.

2.2 POPULATION DISTRIBUTIONS AND PARAMETERS

For a well-defined population of units and a variable, say X, the collection of all possible values of the variable X formed by measuring all of the units in the target population forms the population associated with the variable X. When multiple variables are recorded, each of the variables will generate its own population. Furthermore, since a variable may take on many different values, an important question concerning the population of values of the variable is "How can the population of values of a variable be described or summarized?" The two different approaches that can be used to describe the population of values of the variable are (1) to describe explicitly how the variable is distributed over its values and (2) to describe a set of characteristics that summarize the distribution of the values in the population.

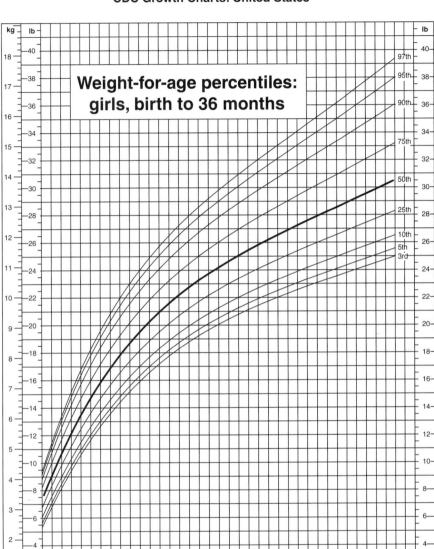

Figure 2.2   Weight-by-age chart for girls in the NHANES study.

2.2.1 Distributions

A statistical analysis of a population is centered on how the values of a variable are distributed, and the *distribution* of a variable or population is an explicit description of how the values of the variable are distributed often described in terms of percentages. The distribution of a variable is also called a *probability distribution* because it describes the probabilities that each of the possible values of the variable will occur. Moreover, the distribution of a variable is often presented in table or chart or modeled with a mathematical equation that

TABLE 2.1 **The Distribution of Blood Type According to the American Red Cross**

Blood Type	Percentage
O	45%
A	40%
B	11%
AB	4%

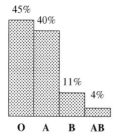

Figure 2.3   A bar chart of the distribution of blood types in the United States.

explicitly determines the percentage of the population taking on each possible value of the variable. The total percentage in a probability distribution is 100%. The distribution of a qualitative or a discrete variable is generally displayed in a bar chart or in a table, and the distribution of a continuous variable is generally displayed in a graph or is represented by a mathematical function.

Example 2.9

The four basic classifications of blood type are O, A, B, and AB. The distribution of blood type, according to the American Red Cross, is given in Table 2.1, and a bar chart representing this distribution is shown in Figure 2.3. Based on the information in Table 2.1, 45% of Americans have type O blood, 40% have type A, 11% have type B, and 4% have type AB blood.

Another method of classifying blood types is to represent blood type by type and Rh factor. A bivariate distribution of blood type for the variables type and Rh factor is given in Table 2.2 and the bar chart in Figure 2.4.

Example 2.10

One of the goals of the 1989 Wisconsin Behavioral Risk Factor Surveillance System (BRFS) was to estimate the distribution of adults who count calories. The distribution of male and female adults in Wisconsin who count calories is given in Table 2.3. Based on the information in Table 2.3, the

TABLE 2.2 **The Distribution of Blood Types with Rh Factor**

Type	Rh Factor	
	+	−
O	38%	7%
A	34%	6%
B	9%	2%
AB	3%	1%

TABLE 2.3   The Distribution of Adults who Count Calories Based on the 1989 Wisconsin BRFS by Age and Gender

Sex	Calories Eaten Per Day		
	% 1200 or Less	% > 1200	% Do Not Count
Male	4.6	10.6	84.8
Female	19.0	11.5	69.6

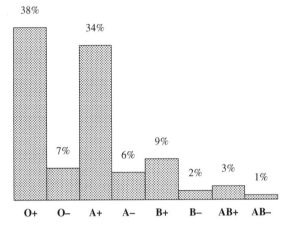

Figure 2.4   A bar chart of the distribution of blood types and Rh factor in the United States.

percentage of females who do not count calories is 69.6% and the percentage of males who do not count calories is 84.8%. Note that there are actually two distributions given in Table 2.3.

The distribution of a continuous quantitative variable is often modeled with a mathematical function called the *probability density function*. The probability density function explicitly describes the distribution of the values of the variable. A plot of the probability density function provides a graphical representation of the distribution of a variable, and the area under the curve defined by the probability density function corresponds to the percentage of the population falling between these two values. The height of the curve at a particular value of the variable measures the percentage per unit in the distribution at this point and is called the *density* of the population at this point. Regions where the values of the variable are more densely grouped are areas in the graph of a probability density function where it is tallest. Examples of the most common shapes of the distribution of a continuous variable are given in Figures 2.5–2.8.

The value of the population under the peak of a probability density graph is called a *mode*. A distribution can have more than one mode, and a distribution with more than one

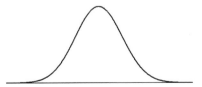

Figure 2.5   An example of a mound-shaped distribution.

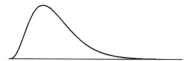

Figure 2.6   An example of a distribution with a long tail to the right.

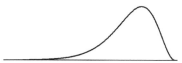

Figure 2.7   An example of a distribution with a long tail to the left.

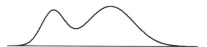

Figure 2.8   An example of a bimodal distribution.

mode is called a *multimodal* distribution. When a distribution has two or more modes, this usually indicates that there are distinct subpopulations clustering around each mode. In this case, it is often more informative to have separate graphs of the probability distributions for analyzing each of the subpopulations.

Example 2.11

In studying obsessive compulsive disorder (OCD), the age at onset is an important variable that is believed to be related to the neurobiological features of OCD; OCD is classified as being either Child Onset OCD or Adult Onset OCD. In the article "Is age at symptom onset associated with severity of memory impairment in adults with obsessive-compulsive disorder?" published in the *American Journal of Psychiatry* (Henin et al., 2001), the authors reported the distribution of the age for onset of OCD given in Figure 2.9. Because there are two modes (peaks) in Figure 2.9, the distribution is suggesting that there might be two different distributions for the age of onset of OCD, one for children and one for adults. Because the clinical diagnoses are Child Onset OCD and Adult Onset OCD, it is more informative to study each of these subpopulations separately. Thus, the distribution of age of onset of OCD has been separated into distributions for the distinct classifications as Child Onset OCD and Adult Onset OCD that are given in Figure 2.10.

The shape of the distribution of a discrete variable can also be described as long-tail right, mound shaped, long-tail left, or multimodal. For example, the 2005 National Health Interview Survey (NHIS) reports the distribution of the size of a family, a discrete variable, and the distribution according to the 2005 National Health Interview Survey is given in Figure 2.11. Note that the distribution of family size according to the 2005 NHIS data is a long-tail right discrete distribution.

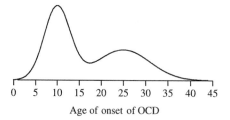

Age of onset of OCD

Figure 2.9   Distribution of age at which OCD is diagnosed.

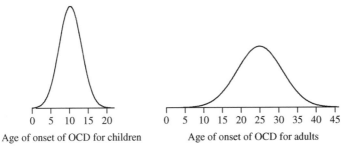

Age of onset of OCD for children   Age of onset of OCD for adults

Figure 2.10   Distribution of the age at which OCD is diagnosed for Child Onset OCD and Adult Onset OCD.

2.2.2 Describing a Population with Parameters

Because the distribution of a variable contains all of the information on how the units in the population are distributed, every question concerning the target population can be answered by studying the distribution of the target population. An alternative method of describing a population is to summarize specific characteristics of the population. That is, the target population can be summarized by determining the values of specific parameters such as the parameters that measure the typical value in the population, population percentages, the spread of the population, and the extremes of a population.

2.2.3 Proportions and Percentiles

Populations are often summarized by listing the important percentages or proportions associated with the population. The proportion of units in a population having a particular characteristic is a parameter of the population, and a population proportion will be denoted by p. The population proportion having a particular characteristic, say characteristic A, is defined to be

$$p = \frac{\text{number of units in population having characteristic A}}{N}$$

Note that the percentage of the population having characteristic A is $p \times 100\%$. Population proportions and percentages are often associated with the categories of a qualitative variable or with the values in the population falling in a specific ranges of values. For example, the distribution of a qualitative variable is usually displayed in a bar chart with the height of a bar representing either the proportion or percentage of the population having that particular value.

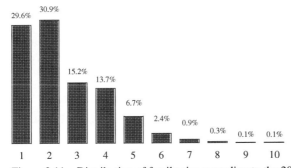

Figure 2.11   Distribution of family size according to the 2005 NHIS.

TABLE 2.4 The Proportions of Blood Type and Rh Factor

Blood Type	Rh Factor	
	+	−
O	0.38	0.07
A	0.34	0.06
B	0.09	0.02
AB	0.03	0.01

Example 2.12
The distribution of blood type according to the American Red Cross is given in Table 2.4 in terms of proportions.

An important proportion in many biomedical studies is the proportion of individuals having a particular disease, which is called the *prevalence of the disease*. The prevalence of a disease is defined to be

Prevalence = The proportion of individuals in a well-defined population having the disease of interest

For example, according to the Centers for Disease Control and Prevention (CDC) the prevalence of smoking among adults in the United States in January through June 2005 was 20.9%. Proportions also play important roles in the study of survival and cure rates, the occurrence of side effects of new drugs, the absolute and relative risks associated with a disease, and the efficacy of new treatments and drugs.

A parameter that is related to a population proportion for a quantitative variable is the *pth percentile* of the population. The *p*th percentile is the value in the population where *p* percent of the population falls below this value. The *p*th percentile will be denoted by x_p for values of *p* between 0 and 100. Note that the percentage of the population values falling below x_p is *p*. For example, if the 10th percentile is 2.2, then 10% of the population values fall below the value 2.2.

Percentiles can be used to describe many different characteristics of a population including the extreme values in the population, the typical values in the population, and the spread of the population. Commonly used percentiles include the

- deciles that are the 10th, 20th, 30th, 40th, 50th, 60th, 70th, 80th, and 90th percentiles;
- quartiles that are the 25th, 50th, and 75th percentiles;
- quintiles that are the 20th, 40th, 60th, and 80th percentiles.

The 50th percentile is called the *median*, and the median will be denoted by $\tilde{\mu}$. The median is a measure of the typical value in the population and is a very important parameter for distributions that have long tails. The median also plays an important role in the following studies:

- ID50 study that is designed to determine the median dose to infect a subject.
- LD50 study that is designed to determine the median lethal dose of a toxic material.
- LC50 study that is designed to determine the median lethal concentration of a toxic material.

TABLE 2.5   The Weight Classifications for Children Based Upon BMI

Classification	BMI Range
Underweight	BMI < 5th percentile
Normal weight	5th percentile $\leq$ BMI < 85th percentiles
At risk for overweight	85th $\leq$ BMI $\leq$ 95th percentiles
Overweight	BMI > 95th percentile

- IC50 study that is designed to determine the median inhibition value of a drug.
- EC50 study that is designed to determine the median concentration of a compound required to obtain the maximum effect *in vivo*.

Example 2.13

In studies investigating the prevalence of overweight and obesity among adults and children, the body mass index (BMI) is a commonly used measure of obesity. The formula for BMI is

$$\text{BMI} = \frac{\text{weight in kilograms}}{(\text{height in meters})^2}$$

Adults with BMI values exceeding the 85th percentile are classified as overweight. Children are classified according to the BMI breakdown given in Table 2.5.

Also, according to the article "Varying body mass index cutoff points to describe overweight prevalence among U.S. adults: NHANES III (1988 to 1994)" published in the *Journal of Obesity* (Kuczmarski et al., 1997)

The percentage of the population with BMI < 19.0 is 1.6% for men, 5.7% for women; BMI $\geq$ 19.0 to < 25.0 is 39.0% for men, 43.6% for women; BMI $\geq$ 25.0 is 59.4% for men, 50.7% for women. An estimated 97.1 million adults have a BMI $\geq$ >25.0. Additional prevalence estimates based on other BMI cutoff points and ages are presented.

A BMI calculator that computes BMI for any height and weight values and determines the percentile of the resulting BMI value can be found at the website http://www.halls.md/body-mass-index/bmi.htm.

2.2.4 Parameters Measuring Centrality

The two parameters in the population of values of a quantitative variable that summarize how the variable is distributed are the parameters that measure the typical or central values in the population and the parameters that measure the spread of the values within the population. Parameters describing the central values in a population and the spread of a population are often used for summarizing the distribution of the values in a population; however, it is important to note that most populations cannot be described very well with only the parameters that measure centrality and the spread of the population.

Measures of centrality, location, or the typical value are parameters that lie in the "center" or "middle" region of a distribution. Because the center or middle of a distribution is not easily determined due to the wide range of different shapes that are possible with a distribution, there are several different parameters that can be used to describe the center of a population. The three most commonly used parameters for describing the center of a population are the *mean*, *median*, and *mode*. For a quantitative variable X,

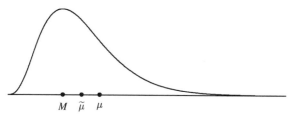

Figure 2.12   The relationships between μ, $\widetilde{\mu}$, and M for a long-tail right distribution.

- The *mean* of a population is the average of all of the units in the population, and will be denoted by μ. The mean of a variable X measured on a population consisting of N units is

$$\mu = \frac{\text{sum of the values of } X}{N} = \frac{\sum X}{N}$$

- The *median* of a population is the 50th percentile of the population, and will be denoted by $\widetilde{\mu}$. The median of a population is found by first listing all of the values of the variable X, including repeated X values, in ascending order. When the number of units in the population (i.e., N) is an odd number, the median is the middle observation in the list of ordered values of X; when N is an even number, the median will be the average of the two observations in the middle of the ordered list of X values.

- The *mode* of a population is the most frequent value in the population, and will be denoted by M. In a graph of the probability density function, the mode is the value of X under the peak of the graph, and a population can have more than one mode as shown in Figure 2.8.

The mean, median, and mode are three different parameters that can be used to measure the center of a population or to describe the typical values in a population. These three parameters will have nearly the same value when the distribution is symmetric or mound shaped. For long-tailed distributions, the mean, median, and mode will be different, and the difference in their values will depend on the length of the distribution's longer tail. Figures 2.12 and 2.13 illustrate the relationships between the values of the mean, median, and mode for long-tail right and long-tail left distributions.

In general, the mean is the most commonly used measure of centrality and is a good measure of the typical value in the population as long as the distribution does not have an extremely long tail or multiple modes. For long-tailed distributions, the mean is pulled out toward the extreme tail, and in this case it is better to use the median or mode to describe the typical value in the population. Furthermore, since the median of a population is based on the middle values in the population, it is not influenced at all by the length of the tails.

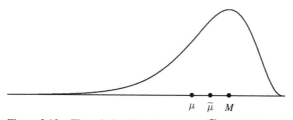

Figure 2.13   The relationships between μ, $\widetilde{\mu}$, and M for a long-tail left distribution.

Example 2.14

Consider the two populations that are listed below.

Population 1:   22, 24, 25, 27, 28, 28, 31, 32, 33, 35, 39, 41, 67

Population 2:   22, 24, 25, 27, 28, 28, 31, 32, 33, 35, 39, 41, 670

These two populations are identical except for their largest values, 67 and 670. For population 1, the mean is

$$\mu_1 = \frac{22 + 24 + 25 + 27 + 28 + 28 + 31 + 32 + 33 + 35 + 39 + 41 + 67}{13}$$

$$= \frac{432}{13} = 33.23$$

Now, because there are 11 units in population 1, the median is the sixth observation in the ordered list of population values. Thus, the median is 28. For population 2, the mean is

$$\mu_2 = \frac{22 + 24 + 25 + 27 + 28 + 28 + 31 + 32 + 33 + 35 + 39 + 41 + 670}{13}$$

$$= \frac{1035}{13} = 79.63$$

Since there are also 11 units in population 2, the median is also the sixth observation in the ordered list of population values. Thus, the median of population 2 is also 28.

Note that the mean of population 2 is more than twice the mean of population 1 even though the populations are identical except for their single largest values. The medians of these two populations are identical because the median is not influenced by extreme values in a population. In population 1, both the mean and median are representative of the central values of the population. In population 2, none of the population units is near the mean value, which is 79.63. Thus, the mean does not represent the value of a typical unit in population 2. The median does represent a fairly typical value in population 2 since all but one of the values in population 2 are relatively close to the value of the median.

The previous example illustrates the sensitivity of the mean to the extremes in a long-tailed distribution. Thus, in a distribution with an extremely long tail to the right or left, the mean will often be less representative than the median for describing the typical values in the population.

Recall that a multimodal distribution generally indicates there are distinct subpopulations and the subpopulations should be described separately. When the population consists of well-defined subpopulations, the mean, median, and mode of each subpopulation should be the parameters of interest rather than the mean, median, and mode of the overall population. Furthermore, in a study with a response variable and an explanatory variable, the mean of the subpopulation of response values for a particular value of the explanatory variable is called a *conditional mean* and will be denoted by $\mu_{Y|X}$. Conditional means are often modeled as functions of an explanatory variable. For example, if the response variable is the weight of a 10-year-old child and the explanatory variable is the height of the child, then the distribution of weights conditioned on height is a conditional distribution. In this case, the mean weight of the conditional distributions would be a conditional mean and could be modeled as a function of the explanatory variable height.

Example 2.15

The distribution of the age of onset of obsessive compulsive disorder given in Figure 2.14 is bimodal indicating there are possibly two subpopulations.

The mean value of the age of onset for OCD is $\mu = 16.2$, which is not representative of a typical value in either subpopulation. OCD has two clinical diagnoses, Child Onset OCD and Adult Onset OCD, and the mean values of these subpopulations are $\mu_C = 10.3$ and $\mu_A = 25$, respectively, and clearly, the subpopulation mean values provide more information about their typical values than

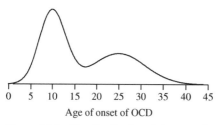

Figure 2.14   The distribution of the age of onset of obsessive compulsive disorder.

does the overall mean. The distributions of the Child Onset OCD and Adult Onset OCD are given in Figure 2.15.

Finally, for distributions with extremely long tails, another parameter that can be used to measure the center of the population is the *geometric mean*. The geometric mean is always less than or equal to the mean (μ) and is not as sensitive to the extreme values in the population as the mean is. The geometric mean will be denoted by GM and is defined as

$$GM = (\text{product of all of the } X \text{ values})^{1/N}$$

where N is the number of units in the population. That is,

$$GM = (X_1 \times X_2 \times X_3 \times \cdots \times X_N)^{1/N}$$

where the X values for the N units in the population are $X_1, X_2, X_3, \ldots, X_N$.

Example 2.16
The distribution given below has a long tail to the right.

$$22, 24, 25, 27, 28, 28, 31, 32, 33, 35, 39, 41, 670$$

In a previous example, μ was computed to be 79.63. The geometric mean for this population is

$$(22 \times 24 \times 25 \times 27 \times 28 \times 28 \times 31 \times 32 \times 33 \times 35 \times 39 \times 41 \times 670)^{\frac{1}{13}} = 29.4$$

Thus, even though there is an extremely large and atypical value in this population, the geometric mean is not sensitive to this value and is a more reasonable parameter for representing the typical value in this population. In fact, the geometric mean and median are very close for this population with GM = 29.4 and $\widetilde{\mu} = 28$.

2.2.5 Measures of Dispersion

While the mean, median, and mode of a population describe the typical values in the population, these parameters do not describe how the population is spread over its range of values. For example, Figure 2.16 shows two populations that have the same mean, median, and mode but different spreads.

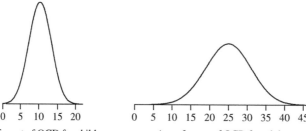

Age of onset of OCD for children   Age of onset of OCD for adults

Figure 2.15   The distributions of the age of onset of Child Onset and Adult Onset OCD.

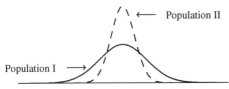

Figure 2.16   Two different populations having the same mean, median, and mode.

Even though the mean, median, and mode of these two populations are the same, clearly, population I is much more spread out than population II. The density of population II is greater at the mean, which means that population II is more concentrated at this point than population I.

When describing the typical values in the population, the more variation there is in a population the harder it is to measure the typical value, and just as there are several ways of measuring the center of a population there are also several ways to measure the variation in a population. The three most commonly used parameters for measuring the spread of a population are the *variance*, *standard deviation*, and *interquartile range*. For a quantitative variable X,

- the *variance* of a population is defined to be the average of the squared deviations from the mean and will be denoted by σ^2 or $\text{Var}(X)$. The variance of a variable X measured on a population consisting of N units is

$$\sigma^2 = \frac{\text{sum of all (deviations from } \mu)^2}{N} = \frac{\sum(X - \mu)^2}{N}$$

- the *standard deviation* of a population is defined to be the square root of the variance and will be denoted by σ or $\text{SD}(X)$.

$$\text{SD}(X) = \sigma = \sqrt{\sigma^2} = \sqrt{\text{Var}(X)}$$

- the *interquartile range* of a population is the distance between the 25th and 75th percentiles and will be denoted by IQR.

$$\text{IQR} = \text{75th percentile} - \text{25th percentile} = X_{75} - X_{25}$$

Note that each of these measures of spread is a positive number except in the rare case when there is absolutely no variation in the population, in which case they will all be equal to 0. Furthermore, the larger each of these values is the more variability there is in the population. For example, for the two populations in Figure 2.16 the standard deviation of population I is larger than the standard deviation of population II.

Because the standard deviation is the square root of the variance, both σ and σ^2 contain equivalent information about the variation in a population. That is, if the variance is known, then so is the standard deviation and vice versa. For example, if $\text{Var}(X) = \sigma^2 = 25$, then the standard deviation is $\sigma = \sqrt{25} = 5$, and if $\text{SD}(X) = \sigma = 20$, then $\text{Var}(X) = \sigma^2 = 20^2 = 400$. The standard deviation is generally used for describing the variation in a population because the units of the standard deviation are the same as the units of the variable; the units of the variance are the units of the variable squared. Also, the standard deviation is roughly the size of a typical deviation from the mean of the population. For example, if X is a variable measured in cubic centimeters (cc), then the standard deviation is also measured in cc's but the variance will be measured in cc^2 units.

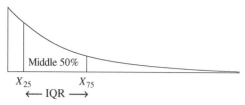

X_{25} X_{75}
← IQR →

Figure 2.17   IQR is the distance between X_{75} and X_{25}.

The interquartile range also measures the variability in a population by measuring the distance between the first and third quartiles (i.e., the 25th and 75th percentiles), and therefore, the interquartile range measures the distance over which the middle 50% of the population lies. The larger IQR is, the wider the range in which the middle 50% of the population lies. Figure 2.17 shows the relationship between the IQR and the quartiles of a population.

Like the median, the interquartile range is unaffected by the extremes in a population. On the other hand, the standard deviation and variance are heavily influenced by the extremes in a population. The shape of the distribution influences the parameters of a distribution and dictates which parameters provide meaningful descriptions of the characteristics of a population. However, for a mound-shaped distribution, the standard deviation and interquartile range are closely related with $\sigma \approx 0.75 \cdot IQR$.

Example 2.17
Consider the two populations listed below that were used in Example 2.14.

Population 1:   22, 24, 25, 27, 28, 28, 31, 32, 33, 35, 39, 41, 67

Population 2:   22, 24, 25, 27, 28, 28, 31, 32, 33, 35, 39, 41, 670

Again, these two populations are identical except for their largest values, 67 and 670. In Example 2.17, the mean values of populations 1 and 2 were found to be $\mu_1 = 33.23$ and $\mu_2 = 79.63$. The variances of these two populations are $\sigma_1^2 = 134.7$ and $\sigma_2^2 = 31498.4$, and the standard deviations are $\sigma_1 = \sqrt{134.7} = 11.6$ and $\sigma_2 = \sqrt{31498.4} = 177.5$. By changing the maximum value in the population from 67 to 670, the standard deviation increased by a factor of 15. In both populations, the 25th and 75th percentiles are 26 and 37, respectively, and thus, the interquartile range for both populations is $IQR = 37 - 26 = 11$.

For mound-shaped distributions, the standard deviation is a good measure of spread, and the mean and standard deviation can be used to summarize the distribution of a mound-shaped distribution reasonably well. The *Empirical Rules*, which are given below, illustrate how the mean and standard deviation can be used to summarize the percentage of the population units lying within one, two, or three standard deviations of the mean. The empirical rules are presented in Figures 2.18–2.20.

THE EMPIRICAL RULES

For populations having mound-shaped distributions,

1. roughly 68% of all of the population values fall within 1 standard deviation of the mean. That is, roughly 68% of the population values fall between the values $\mu - \sigma$ and $\mu + \sigma$.

2. roughly 95% of all the population values fall within 2 standard deviations of the mean. That is, roughly 95% of the population values fall between the values $\mu - 2\sigma$ and $\mu + 2\sigma$.

3. roughly 99% of all the population values fall within 3 standard deviations of the mean. That is, roughly 99% of the population values fall between the values $\mu - 3\sigma$ and $\mu + 3\sigma$.

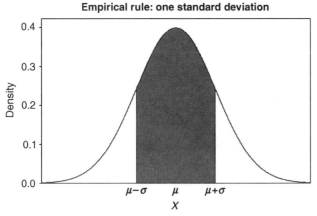

Figure 2.18   The one-standard deviation empirical rule; roughly 68% of a mound-shaped distribution lies between the values $\mu - \sigma$ and $\mu + \sigma$.

2.2.6 The Coefficient of Variation

The standard deviations of two populations resulting from measuring the same variable can be compared to determine which of the two populations is more variable. That is, when one standard deviation is substantially larger than the other (i.e., more than two times as large), then clearly the population with the larger standard deviation is much more variable than the other. It is also important to be able to determine whether a single population is highly variable or not. A parameter that measures the relative variability in a population is the *coefficient of variation*. The coefficient of variation will be denoted by CV and is defined to be

$$\mathrm{CV} = \frac{\sigma}{|\bar{x}|}$$

The coefficient of variation is also sometimes represented as a percentage in which case

$$\mathrm{CV} = \frac{\sigma}{|\bar{x}|} \times 100\%$$

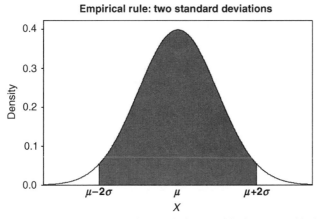

Figure 2.19   The two-standard deviation empirical rule; roughly 95% of a mound-shaped distribution lies between the values $\mu - 2\sigma$ and $\mu + 2\sigma$.

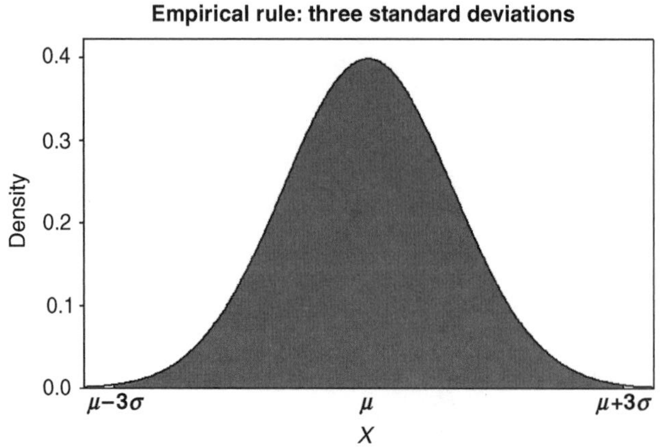

Empirical rule: three standard deviations

Figure 2.20   The three-standard deviation empirical rule; roughly 99% of a mound-shaped distribution lies between the values $\mu - 3\sigma$ and $\mu + 3\sigma$.

The coefficient of variation compares the size of the standard deviation with the size of the mean. When the coefficient of variation is small, this means that the variability in the population is relatively small compared to the size of the mean of the population. On the other hand, when the coefficient of variation is large, this indicates that the population varies greatly relative to the size of the mean. The standard for what is a large coefficient of variation differs from one discipline to another, and in some disciplines a coefficient of variation of less than 15% is considered reasonable, and in other disciplines larger or smaller cutoffs are used.

Because the standard deviation and the mean have the same units of measurement, the coefficient of variation is a unitless parameter. That is, the coefficient is unaffected by changes in the units of measurement. For example, if a variable X is measured in inches and the coefficient of variation is CV $= 2$, then coefficient of variation will also be 2 when the units of measurement are converted to centimeters. The coefficient of variation can also be used to compare the relative variability in two different and unrelated populations; the standard deviation can only be used to compare the variability in two different populations based on similar variables.

Example 2.18

Use the means and standard deviations given in Table 2.6 for the three variables that were measured on a population to answer the following questions:

a. Determine the value of the coefficient of variation for population I.
b. Determine the value of the coefficient of variation for population II.
c. Determine the value of the coefficient of variation for population III.
d. Compare the relative variability of each variable.

TABLE 2.6   The Means and Standard Deviations for Three Different Variables

Variable	μ	σ
I	100	25
II	10	5
III	0.10	0.05

Solutions

a. The value of the coefficient of variation for population I is $CV_I = \frac{25}{100} = 0.25$.

b. The value of the coefficient of variation for population II is $CV_{II} = \frac{5}{10} = 0.5$.

c. The value of the coefficient of variation for population III is $CV_{III} = \frac{0.05}{0.10} = 0.5$.

d. Populations II and III are relatively more variable than population I even though the standard deviations for populations II and III are smaller than the standard deviation of population I. Populations II and III have the same amount of relative variability even though the standard deviation of population III is one-hundredth that of population II.

The previous example illustrates how comparing the absolute size of the standard deviation is relevant only when comparing similar variables. Also, interpreting the size of a standard deviation should take into account the size of a typical value in a population. For example, a standard deviation of $\sigma = 0.01$ might appear to be a small standard deviation; however, if the mean was $\mu = 0.006$, then this would be a very large standard deviation ($CV = 167\%$); on the other hand, if the mean was $\mu = 5.2$, then $\sigma = 0.01$ would be a small standard deviation ($CV = 0.2\%$).

2.2.7 Parameters for Bivariate Populations

In most biomedical research studies, there are many variables that will be recorded on each individual in the study. A multivariate distribution can be formed by jointly tabulating, charting, or graphing the values of the variables over the N units in the population. For example, the *bivariate distribution* of two variables, say X and Y, is the collection of the ordered pairs

$$(X_1, Y_1), (X_2, Y_2), (X_3, Y_3), \ldots, (X_N, Y_N).$$

These N ordered pairs form the units of the bivariate distribution of X and Y and their joint distribution can be displayed in a two-way chart, table, or graph.

When the two variables are qualitative, the joint proportions in the bivariate distribution are often denoted by p_{ab}, where

$$p_{ab} = \text{proportion of pairs in population where } X = a \text{ and } Y = b$$

The joint proportions in the bivariate distribution are then displayed in a two-way table or two-way bar chart. For example, according to the American Red Cross, the joint distribution of blood type and Rh factor is given in Table 2.7 and presented as a bar chart in Figure 2.21.

In a bivariate distribution where one of the variables is quantitative and the other is qualitative, the best way to graphically present the distribution is to separate the distribution

TABLE 2.7 The Distribution of Blood Type by Rh Factor According to the American Red Cross

Blood Type	Rh Factor	
	+	−
O	38%	7%
A	34%	6%
B	9%	2%
AB	3%	1%

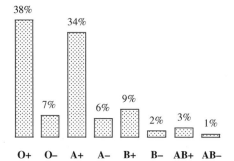

O+ O− A+ A− B+ B− AB+ AB−

Figure 2.21   The joint distribution of blood type and Rh factor according to the American Red Cross.

into subpopulations according to the values of the qualitative distribution. For example, if W = the weight of an individual and G = the sex of an individual, then the best way to present the bivariate distribution of weight and gender is to present the two subpopulations separately as shown in Figure 2.22.

In a multivariate population, the subpopulation remain important, and the subpopulation proportions, percentiles, mean, median, modes, standard deviation, variance, interquartile range are important parameters that can still be used to summarize each of the subpopulations.

In a bivariate distribution where both of the variables are quantitative, a three-dimensional graph can be used to represent the joint distribution of the variables. The joint distribution is displayed as a three-dimensional probability density graph with one axis for each of the variables and the third axis representing the joint density at each pair (X, Y); however, three-dimensional density plots are sometimes difficult to interpret. An example of a three-dimensional density plot is given in Figure 2.23.

To summarize the bivariate distribution of two quantitative variables, proportions, percentiles, mean, median, mode, standard deviation, variance, and interquartile range can be computed for each variable. In a bivariate distribution, the parameters associated with each separate variable are distinguished from each other by the use of subscripts. For example, if the two variables are labeled X and Y, then the mean, median, mode, standard deviation, variance, and interquartile range of the population associated with the variable X will be denoted by

$$\mu_x, \ \tilde{\mu}_x, \ M_x, \ \sigma_x, \ \sigma_x^2, \ \text{IQR}_x$$

and similarly for Y

$$\mu_y, \ \tilde{\mu}_y, \ M_y, \ \sigma_y, \ \sigma_y^2, \ \text{IQR}_y.$$

A parameter that measures the joint relationship between two quantitative variables, say X and Y, is the *correlation coefficient* that will be denoted by ρ. The correlation

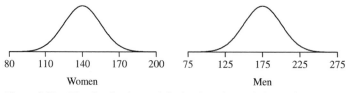

Figure 2.22   The distribution weight for the subpopulations of mean and women.

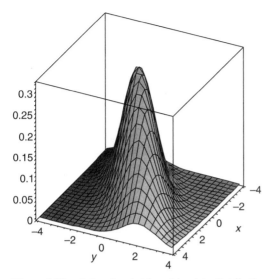

Figure 2.23   A density plot for a bivariate distribution.

coefficient measures the linear relationship between X and Y. That is, ρ measures the overall agreement between the pairs (X, Y) and the line $Y = aX + b$. The correlation coefficient is defined as

$$\text{Corr}(X, Y) = \rho = \frac{1/N \sum (X - \mu_x)(Y - \mu_y)}{\sigma_x \sigma_y}$$

where μ_x, μ_y and σ_x, σ_y are the means and standard deviations of X and Y, respectively.

The correlation coefficient is a unitless parameter that falls between -1 and 1. That is, the correlation between X and Y does not depend on the particular scales of units the variables are measured in. For example, if X is the height of an individual in pounds and Y is the height of an individual in inches, then the value of the correlation coefficient will be the same when X is measured in kilograms and Y is measured in centimeters. Also, the correlation between X and Y is the same as the correlation between Y and X (i.e., $\text{Corr}(X, Y) = \text{Corr}(Y, X)$).

It is important to note that the correlation coefficient can be used only with two quantitative variables and only measures the strength of the linear relationship between X and Y. A positive value of the correlation coefficient suggests that the larger values of X are more likely to occur with the larger values of Y and the smaller values of X with the smaller values of Y. A negative correlation indicates the larger values of X are more likely to occur with the smaller values of Y and the smaller values of X with the larger values of Y. Several properties of the correlation coefficient are listed below.

1. The value of the correlation coefficient is always between -1 and 1 (i.e., $-1 \leq \rho \leq 1$). When the correlation coefficient equals -1 or 1, the variables X and Y are said to be *perfectly correlated*. When two variables X and Y are perfectly correlated, the linear relationship is exact and $Y = aX + b$ for some values a and b. In this case, the value of Y is determined by the value of X. Furthermore, when $\rho = -1$ the value of b will be negative, and when $\rho = 1$ the value of b will be positive.

2. When $\rho \neq \pm 1$, the value of Y cannot be perfectly predicted from the value of X and the relationship is

$$Y = aX + b + \epsilon$$

where ϵ is an error term associated with the deviation from the linear relationship. The closer ρ is to ± 1, the stronger the linear relationship between the variables X and Y.

3. The strength of the linear relationship between X and Y is based on the value of the correlation coefficient and is often summarized according to the following guidelines:

   (a) $-0.30 \leq \rho < 0.30$ indicates at most a *very weak* linear relationship.

   (b) $-0.50 < \rho \leq -0.30$ or $0.30 \leq \rho < 0.50$ indicates a *weak* linear relationship.

   (c) $-0.80 < \rho \leq -0.50$ or $0.50 \leq \rho < 0.80$ indicates a *moderate* linear relationship.

   (d) $-0.90 < \rho \leq -0.80$ or $0.80 \leq \rho < 0.90$ indicates a *strong* linear relationship.

   (e) $\rho \leq -0.90$ or $\rho \geq 0.90$ indicates a *very strong* linear relationship.

   However, any discussion of the strength of the linear relationship between two variables must take into account the standards used in the discipline in which the research is being carried out.

4. When $\rho \approx 0$, there is no apparent linear relationship between the two variables. However, this does not exclude the possibility that there is a curvilinear relationship between the two variables.

In a multivariate distribution with more than two quantitative variables, the correlation coefficient can be computed for each pair of variables. For example, with three quantitative variables, say X, Y, and Z, the three correlation coefficients that can be computed are $\mathrm{Corr}(X, Y) = \rho_{xy}$, $\mathrm{Corr}(X, Z) = \rho_{xz}$, and $\mathrm{Corr}(Y, Z) = \rho_{yz}$. In most biomedical studies, there is a well-defined response variable and a set of explanatory variables. Since the changes in the explanatory variables are believed to cause changes in the response variable, the most important correlations to consider are those between the response variable and each of the explanatory variables.

Finally, correlation should not be confused with causation. A *causal relationship* exists when changing the value of X directly causes a change in the value of Y or vice versa. The correlation coefficient only measures the tendency for the value of Y to increase or decrease linearly with the values of X. Thus, a high correlation between X and Y does not necessarily indicate that changes in X will cause changes in Y. For example, there is a positive correlation between the number of times an individual on a diet weighs themselves in a week and their weight loss. Clearly, the number of times an individual weighs themselves does not cause a change in their weight. Causal relationships must be supported by honest logical and scientific reasoning. With the proper use of scientific principles and well-designed experiments, high correlations can often be used as evidence supporting a causal relationship.

2.3 PROBABILITY

In a data-based biomedical study, a random sample will be selected from the target population and a well-designed sampling plan requires knowing the chance of drawing a particular observation or set of observations. For example, it might be important to know the chance of drawing a female individual or an individual between the ages of 30 and 60. In other studies, it might be important to determine the likelihood that a particular genetic trait will be passed from the parents to their offspring.

A *probability* is a number between 0 and 1 that measures how likely it is for an event to occur. Probabilities are associated with tasks or experiment where the outcome cannot be determined without actually carrying out the task. A task where the outcome cannot be predetermined is called a *random experiment* or a *chance experiment*. For example, prior to treatment it cannot be determined whether chemotherapy will improve a cancer patient's health. Thus, the result of a chemotherapy treatment can be treated as a chance experiment before chemotherapy is started. Similarly, when drawing a random sample from the target population, the actual values of the sample will not be known until the sample is actually collected. Hence, drawing a random sample from the target population is a chance experiment.

Because statistical inferences are based on a sample from the population rather than a census of the population, the statistical inferences will have a degree of uncertainty associated with them. The measures of reliability for statistical inferences drawn from a sample are based on the underlying probabilities associated with the target population.

In a chance experiment, the actual outcome of the experiment cannot be predetermined, but it is important for the experimenter to identify all of the possible outcomes of the experiment before it is carried out. The set of all possible outcomes of a chance experiment is called the *sample space* and will be denoted by S. A subcollection of the outcomes in the sample space is called an *event*, and the probability of an event measures how likely the event is. An event is said to *occur* when a chance experiment is carried out and the chance experiment results in one of the outcomes in the event. For example, in a chance experiment consisting of randomly selecting an adult from a well-defined population, if A is the event that an individual between the ages of 30 and 60 is selected, then the event A will occur if and only if the age of the individual selected is between 30 and 60; if the age of the individual is not between 30 and 60, then the event A will not occur.

Probabilities are often used to determine the most likely outcome of a chance experiment and for assessing how likely it is for an observed data set to support a research hypothesis. The probability of an event A is denoted by $P(A)$, and the probability of an event is always a number between 0 and 1. Probabilities near 0 indicate an event rarely occurs and probabilities near 1 indicate an event is likely to occur. Probabilities are sometimes also expressed in terms of percentages in which case the percentage is simply the probability of the event times 100. When probabilities are expressed in terms of percentages, they will be between 0 and 100%.

Example 2.19

Suppose an individual is to be drawn at random and their blood type is identified. Prior to drawing a blood sample and typing it, an individual's blood type is unknown, and thus, this can be treated as a chance experiment. The four possible blood types are O, A, B, and AB, and hence, the sample space is $S = \{O, A, B, AB\}$. Furthermore, according to the American Red Cross, the probabilities of each blood type are

$$P(O) = 0.45, \ P(A) = 0.40, \ P(B) = 0.11, \ P(AB) = 0.04$$

Thus, if a person is drawn at random the probability that the person will have blood type AB is 0.04.

The probabilities associated with a chance experiment and a sample space S must satisfy the following three properties known as the *Axioms of Probability*.

THE AXIOMS OF PROBABILITY

- Probabilities are always greater than or equal to 0. That is, $P(A) \geq 0$ for any event A.
- The probability of the sample space is 1. That is, $P(S) = 1$, which means when the experiment is carried out it will result in one of the outcomes in S.
- The probability of every event is between 0 and 1. That is, $0 \leq P(A) \leq 1$ for every event A.

- When two events have no outcomes in common, then the probability that at least one of the two events occurs is the sum of their probabilities. That is,

$$P(A \text{ or } B) = P(A) + P(B)$$

when A and B have no outcomes in common.

Events that have no outcomes in common are called *disjoint events* or *mutually exclusive events*. If A and B are disjoint events, then the probability of the event "A and B" is 0. That is, it is impossible for the events to occur simultaneously.

2.3.1 Basic Probability Rules

Determining the probabilities associated with complex real-life events often requires a great deal of information and an extensive scientific understanding of the structure of the chance experiment being studied. In fact, even when the sample space and event are easily identified, the determination of the probability of an event can be an extremely difficult task. For example, in studying the side effects of a drug, the possible side effects can generally be anticipated and the sample space will be known. However, because humans react differently to drugs, the probabilities of the occurrence of the side effects are generally unknown. The probabilities of the side effects are often estimated in clinical trials.

The following basic probability rules are often useful in determining the probability of an event:

1. When the outcomes of a random experiment are equally likely to occur, the probability of an event A is the number of outcomes in A divided by the number of simple events in S. That is,

$$P(A) = \frac{\text{number of simple events in } A}{\text{number of simple events in } S} = \frac{N(A)}{N(S)}$$

2. For every event A, the probability of A is the sum of the probabilities of the outcomes comprising A. That is, when an event A is comprised of the outcomes $O_1, O_2, \ldots, O_k$, the probability of the event A is

$$P(A) = P(O_1) + P(O_2) + \cdots + P(O_k)$$

3. For any two events A and B, the probability that either event A or event B occurs is

$$P(A \text{ or } B) = P(A) + P(B) - P(A \text{ and } B)$$

4. The probability that the event A does not occur is 1 minus the probability that the event A does occur. That is,

$$P(A \text{ does not occur}) = 1 - P(A)$$

Example 2.20
Table 2.8 gives a breakdown of the pool of 242 volunteers for a university study on rapid eye movement (REM). Use Table 2.8 to determine the probability that

TABLE 2.8 **Summary table for the $n = 242$ volunteers in a university study of rapid eye movement (REM)**

Gender	Age			
	<18	18–20	21–25	>25
Female	3	58	42	25
Male	1	61	43	9

   a. a female volunteer is selected.

   b. a male volunteer younger than 21 is selected.

   c. a male volunteer or a volunteer older than 25 is selected.

Solutions Let F be the event a female volunteer is selected, M the event a male volunteer is selected, 21 the event a volunteer younger than 21 is selected, and 25 the event that a volunteer older than 25 is selected. Since a volunteer will be selected at random, each volunteer is equally likely to be selected, and thus,

   a. the probability that a female volunteer is selected is

$$P(F) = \frac{3 + 58 + 42 + 24}{242} = 0.53$$

   b. the probability that a male volunteer younger than 21 is selected is

$$P(M \text{ and } 21) = \frac{1 + 61}{242}$$

   c. the probability that a male volunteer or a volunteer older than 25 is selected is

$$P(M \text{ or } 25) = P(M) + P(25) - P(M \text{ and } 25)$$

$$= \frac{1 + 61 + 43 + 9}{242} + \frac{34}{242} - \frac{9}{242}$$

$$= 0.57$$

Example 2.21

Use table of percentages for blood type and Rh factor given in Table 2.9 to determine the probability that a randomly selected individual

   a. has Rh positive blood.

   b. has type A or type B blood.

   c. has type A blood or Rh positive blood.

Solutions Based on the percentages given in Table 2.9

   a. Rh positive blood is O+, A+, B+, and AB+, and thus, the probability that a randomly selected individual has Rh positive blood is

$$P(\text{Rh positive blood}) = P(O+) + P(A+) + P(B+) + P(AB+)$$

$$= 0.38 + 0.34 + 0.09 + 0.03 = 0.84$$

   b. type A or type B blood is A+, A−, B+, B−. Thus,

$$P(A \text{ or } B \text{ blood type}) = P(A+) + P(A-) + P(B+) + P(B-)$$

$$= 0.34 + 0.06 + 0.09 + 0.02 = 0.51$$

   c. the probability an individual has type A blood or Rh positive blood is

$$P(A \text{ or Rh positive}) = P(A) + P(\text{Rh positive}) - P(A \text{ and Rh positive})$$

$$= 0.40 + 0.84 - 0.34 = 0.90$$

TABLE 2.9 The Percentages of Each Blood Type and Rh Factor

Blood Type	Rh Factor	
	+	−
O	38%	7%
A	34%	6%
B	9%	2%
AB	3%	1%

2.3.2 Conditional Probability

In many biomedical studies, the probabilities associated with a qualitative variable will be modeled. A good probability model will take into account all of the factors believed to cause or explain the occurrence of the event. For example, the probability of survival for a melanoma patient depends on many factors including tumor thickness, tumor ulceration, gender, and age. Probabilities that are functions of a particular set of conditions are called *conditional probabilities.*

Conditional probabilities are simply probabilities based on well-defined subpopulations defined by a particular set of conditions (i.e., explanatory variables). The *conditional probability* of the event A given that the event B has occurred is denoted by $P(A|B)$ and is defined as

$$P(A|B) = \frac{P(A \cap B)}{P(B)}$$

provided that $P(B) \neq 0$. Specifying that the event B has occurred places restrictions on the outcomes of the chance experiment that are possible. Thus, the outcomes in the event B become the subpopulation upon which the probability of the event A is based.

Example 2.22
Suppose that in a population of 100 units 35 units are in event A, 48 of the units are in event B, and 22 units are in both events A and B. The unconditional probability of event A is $P(A) = \frac{35}{100} = 0.35$. The conditional probability of event A given that event B has occurred is

$$P(A|B) = \frac{0.22}{0.48} = 0.46$$

In this example, knowing that event B has occurred increases the probability that event A will occur from 0.35 to 0.46. That is, event A is more likely to occur if it is known that event B has occurred.

Since conditional probabilities are probabilities, the rules associated with conditional probabilities are similar to the rules of probability. In particular,

1. conditional probabilities are always between 0 and 1. That is, $0 \leq P(A|B) \leq 1$.
2. $P(A \text{ does not occur}|B) = 1 - P(A|B)$.
3. $P(A \text{ or } B|C) = P(A|C) + P(B|C) - P(A \text{ and } B|C)$.

Conditional probabilities play an important role in the detection of rare diseases and the development of screening tests for diseases. Two important conditional probabilities used in disease detection are the *sensitivity* and *specificity*. The sensitivity is defined to be the conditional probability of a positive test for the subpopulation of individuals having the disease (i.e., $P(+|D)$), and the specificity is defined to be the conditional probability of a negative test for the subpopulation of individuals who do not have the disease (i.e., $P(-|\text{not D})$). Thus, the sensitivity of a diagnostic test measures the accuracy of the test for an individual having the disease, and the specificity measures the accuracy of the test for individuals who do not have the disease. A good diagnostic test for the disease must have high sensitivity and specificity to ensure that it is unlikely that the test will report a false positive or a false negative result. Furthermore, when the prevalence of the disease, the sensitivity of the diagnostic test, and the specificity of the test are known, the probability that an individual has the disease given the test is positive is

$$P(D|+) = \frac{P(+|D) \times P(D)}{P(+|D) \times P(D) + P(+|\text{not D}) \times P(\text{not D})}$$

$$= \frac{\text{sensitivity} \times \text{prevalence}}{\text{sensitivity} \times \text{prevalence} + (1 - \text{specificity}) \times (1 - \text{prevalence})}$$

Also, the probability that an individual will test positive in a diagnostic test is

$$P(+) = P(+|D) \times P(D) + P(+|\text{not D}) \times P(\text{not D})$$

$$= \text{sensitivity} \times \text{prevalence} + (1 - \text{specificity}) \times (1 - \text{prevalence})$$

Example 2.23

Suppose the prevalence of HIV/AIDs is 5% among a particular population and an enzyme-linked immunosorbent assay (ELISA) test for diagnosing the presence of the HIV/AIDS virus has been developed. If the sensitivity of the ELISA test is 95% and the specificity is 99%, then the probability that an individual has the HIV/AIDS virus given the ELISA test is positive is

$$P(D|+) = \frac{P(+|D)P(D)}{P(+|D)P(D) + P(+|\text{not D})P(\text{not D})}$$

$$= \frac{0.95 \times 0.05}{0.95 \times 0.05 + 0.01 \times 0.95} = 0.83$$

Thus, an individual having a positive ELISA test has an 83% chance of having the HIV/AIDS virus.

Example 2.24

Suppose a new infectious disease has been identified, and the prevalence of this disease is $P(D) = 0.001$. Given that a person has the disease, the probability that the diagnostic test used to diagnose this disease is positive is $P(+|D) = 0.999$, and given that a person does not have the disease, the probability that the test is positive is $P(+|\text{not D}) = 0.01$. Then,

    a. the probability of a positive test result is

$$P(+) = P(+|D) \times P(D) + P(+|\text{not D})P(\text{not D})$$

$$= 0.999(0.001) + 0.01(.999) = 0.011$$

Thus, there is only a 1.1% chance that an individual will test positive for the disease. The reason why a positive test is so rare is that this disease is extremely rare since $P(D) = 0.001$.

    b. the probability that a person has the disease given the test is positive is

$$P(D|+) = \frac{P(+|D)P(D)}{P(+)}$$

$$= \frac{0.999(0.001)}{0.011} = 0.09$$

Thus, the probability of having the disease given the test is positive is roughly 100 times the unconditional probability of having the disease. Furthermore, in this example, it is still highly unlikely that an individual has the disease even when the test is positive ($P(D|+) = 0.09$, and hence, this is not a very informative diagnostic test.

2.3.3 Independence

In some cases, the unconditional probability and the conditional probability will be the same. In this case, knowing that the event B occurred does not change the likelihood that the event A will occur. When the unconditional probability of an event A is the same as the conditional probability of the event A given the event B, the events A and B are said to be *independent events*.

INDEPENDENT EVENTS

Two events A and B are independent if and only if one of the following conditions is met:

1. The probability of event A occurring is the same whether B occurred or not. That is,

$$P(A|B) = P(A)$$

2. The probability of event B occurring is the same whether A occurred or not. That is,

$$P(B|A) = P(B)$$

When two events are not independent, they are said to be *dependent events*. For example, the event that an individual has lung cancer and the event an individual has smoked a pack of cigarettes a day for several years are dependent events. On the other hand, the event an individual has lung cancer and the event an individual has blonde hair would be expected to be independent events.

If the events A and B are known to be independent, then the probability that A and B both occur is simply the product of their respective probabilities. That is, when A and B are independent

$$P(A \text{ and } B) = P(A)P(B)$$

Example 2.25

The genders of successive offspring of human parents are known to be independent events. If the probability of having a male offspring is 0.48, then probability of having

a. two male offspring is

$$P(\text{Male and Male}) = P(\text{Male})P(\text{Male}) = 0.48(0.48) = 0.23$$

b. a male followed by a female offspring is

$$P(\text{Male followed by a Female}) = P(\text{Male})P(\text{Female}) = 0.48(0.52)$$
$$= 0.25$$

c. a male and a female offspring is

$$P(\text{Male and Female}) = P(\text{Male then a Female}) + P(\text{Female then a Male})$$
$$= P(\text{Male})P(\text{Female}) + P(\text{Female})P(\text{Male})$$
$$= 0.48(0.52) + 0.52(0.48) = 0.23 + 0.25 = 0.48$$

d. five female offspring is

$$P(5 \text{ Female}) = P(\text{Female})P(\text{Female})P(\text{Female})P(\text{Female})P(\text{Female})$$
$$= (0.52)^5 = 0.04$$

e. the second offspring is a male given that the first was a female is 0.48 since successive births are independent. That is, since the successive offspring are independent

$$P(M|F) = P(M)$$

When the events A and B are independent so are the events A and not B, not A and B, and not A and not B. Thus,

$$P(A \text{ and not } B) = P(A)P(\text{not } B) = P(A)(1 - P(B))$$

$$P(\text{not } A \text{ and } B) = P(\text{not } A)P(B) = (1 - P(A))P(B)$$

$$P(\text{not } A \text{ and not } B) = P(\text{not } A)P(\text{not } B) = (1 - P(A))(1 - P(B))$$

Example 2.26
Achondroplasia is a genetic disorder related to dwarfism caused by an abnormal gene on one of the 23 chromosome pairs. Twenty percent of the individuals having achondroplasia inherit a mutated gene from their parents. An individual inherits one chromosome from each parent. It takes only one abnormal gene from a parent to cause dwarfism and two abnormal genes can cause death. If only one parent has a mutated gene then, there is a 50% chance that a child will receive this gene and inherit achondroplasia. On the other hand, if both parents have achondroplasia, there is a 50% chance that each parent will pass on the gene. Thus, because the parents' genes are passed on independently, there is a 25% chance that a child will inherit neither gene, a 50% chance that the child will inherit only one abnormal gene, and a 25% chance that the child will inherit two abnormal genes and be at risk of death. To see this, suppose each parent has achondroplasia and let

$$A = \text{the event the father passes on the abnormal gene}$$

and

$$B = \text{the event the mother passes on the abnormal gene}$$

Then, A and B are independent and $P(A) = P(B) = 0.5$, and the probability that the child inherits

a. no abnormal genes is

$$P(\text{not } A \text{ and not } B) = P(\text{not } A)P(\text{not } B) = (1 - 0.5)(1 - 0.5) = 0.25$$

b. only one abnormal gene is

$$= P(\text{not } A)P(B) + P(A)P(\text{not } B)$$

$$= (1 - 0.5)(0.5) + 0.5(1 - 0.5) = 0.25 + 0.25 = 0.5$$

c. inherits two abnormal genes is

$$P(A \text{ and } B) = P(A)P(B) = 0.5(0.5) = 0.25$$

Independence plays an important role in data collection and the analysis of the observed data. In most statistical applications, it is important that the observed data values are independent of each other. That is, knowing the value of one observation does not influence the value of any other observation.

2.4 PROBABILITY MODELS

The distribution of a quantitative variable is often modeled with a probability distribution. There is a wide range of mathematical probability models that are available for modeling the distribution of a quantitative variable; however, the particular probability model that is best used to model the distribution of a quantitative variable will depend on whether the variable of interest is discrete or continuous, the distribution of the variable, and any theoretical conditions or assumptions made about the population being modeled. Two of the most commonly used probability models in biomedical research are the *Binomial Probability*

Model, which is associated with a discrete counting variable, and the *Normal Probability Model*, which is often used to model the distribution of a continuous variable.

2.4.1 The Binomial Probability Model

The binomial probability model can be used for modeling the number of times a particular event occurs in a sequence of repeated trials. In particular, a binomial random variable is a discrete variable that is used to model chance experiments involving repeated dichotomous trials. That is, the binomial model is used to model repeated trials where the outcome of each trial is one of the two possible outcomes. The conditions under which the binomial probability model can be used are given below.

THE BINOMIAL CONDITIONS

The binomial distribution can be used to model the number of successes in n trials when

1. each trial of the experiment results in one of the two outcomes, denoted by S for success and F for failure.

2. the trials will be repeated n times under identical conditions and each trial is independent of the others.

3. the probability of a success is the same on each of the n trials.

4. the random variable of interest, say X, is the number of successes in the n trials.

A random variable satisfying the above conditions is called a *binomial random variable*. Note that a binomial random variable X simply counts the number of successes that occurred in n trials. The probability distribution for a binomial random variable X is given by the mathematical expression

$$p(x) = \frac{n!}{x!(n-x)!} p^x (1-p)^{n-x} \quad \text{for } x = 0, 1, \ldots, n$$

where $p(x)$ is the probability that X is equal to the value x. In this formula

- $\dfrac{n!}{x!(n-x)!}$ is the number of ways for there to be x successes in n trials,
- $n! = n(n-1)(n-2)\cdots 3\cdot 2\cdot 1$ and $0! = 1$ by definition,
- p is the probability of a success on any of the n trials,
- p^x is the probability of having x successes in n trials,
- $1 - p$ is the probability of a failure on any of the n trials,
- $(1-p)^{n-x}$ is the probability of getting $n - x$ failures in n trials.

Examples of the binomial distribution are given in Figure 2.24. Note that a binomial distribution will have a longer tail to the right when $p < 0.5$, a longer tail to the left when $p > 0.5$, and is symmetric when $p = 0.5$.

Because the computations for the probabilities associated with a binomial random variable are tedious, it is best to use a statistical computing package such as MINITAB for computing binomial probabilities.

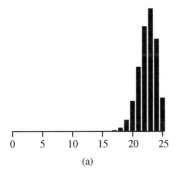

(a)

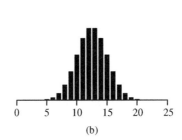

(b)

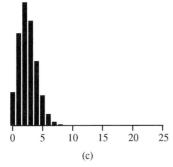

(c)

Figure 2.24   Three binomial distributions: (a) $n = 25$, $p = 0.1$; (b) $n = 25$, $p = 0.5$; (c) $n = 25$, $p = 0.9$.

Example 2.27

Hair loss is a common side effect of chemotherapy. Suppose that there is an 80% chance that an individual will lose their hair during or after receiving chemotherapy. Let X be the number of individuals who retain their hair during or after receiving chemotherapy. If 10 individuals are selected at random, use the MINITAB output given in Table 2.10 to determine

   a. the probability that exactly seven will retain their hair (i.e., $X = 7$).

   b. the probability that between four and eight (inclusive) will retain their hair (i.e., $4 \leq X \leq 8$).

   c. the probability that at most three will retain their hair (i.e., $X \leq 3$).

TABLE 2.10   The Binomial Distribution for $n = 10$ Trials and $p = 0.20$

```
Binomial with n = 10 and p = 0.2
  x     P( X = x )

  0       0.107374
  1       0.268435
  2       0.301990
  3       0.201327
  4       0.088080
  5       0.026424
  6       0.005505
  7       0.000786
  8       0.000074
  9       0.000004
 10       0.000000
```

d. the probability that at least six will retain their hair (i.e., $X \geq 6$).

e. the most likely number of patients to retain their hair (i.e., the mode).

Solutions Based on the MINITAB output in Table 2.10, the probability that

a. exactly seven will retain their hair (i.e., $X = 7$) is

$$P(X = 7) = p(7) = 0.000786$$

b. between four and eight (inclusive) will retain their hair (i.e., $4 \leq X \leq 8$) is

$$P(4 \leq X \leq 8) = p(4) + p(5) + p(6) + p(7) + p(8)$$
$$= 0.088080 + 0.026424 + 0.005505 + 0.000786 + 0.000074$$
$$= 0.12$$

c. at most three will retain their hair (i.e., $X \leq 3$) is

$$P(X \leq 3) = p(0) + p(1) + p(2) + p(3)$$
$$= 0.107374 + 0.268435 + 0.301990 + 0.201327$$
$$= 0.88$$

d. at least six will retain their hair (i.e., $X \geq 6$) is

$$P(X \geq 8) = p(6) + p(7) + p(8) + p(9) + p(10)$$
$$= 0.005505 + 0.000786 + 0.000074 + 0.000004 + 0.000000$$
$$= 0.0064$$

e. the most likely number of patients to retain their hair is $X = 2$.

The mean of a binomial random variable based on n trials and probability of success p is $\mu = np$ and the standard deviation is $\sigma = \sqrt{n \cdot p \cdot (1 - p)}$. The mean of a binomial is the expected number of successes in n trials, and the values of a binomial random variable are concentrated near its mean. The standard deviation measures the spread about the mean and is largest when $p = 0.5$; as p moves away from 0.5 toward 0 or 1, the variability of a binomial random variable decreases. Furthermore, when np and $n(1 - p)$ are both greater than 5, the Empirical Rules apply and

- roughly 68% of the binomial distribution lies between the values closest to the $np - \sqrt{n \cdot p \cdot (1 - p)}$ and $np + \sqrt{n \cdot p \cdot (1 - p)}$.
- roughly 95% of the binomial distribution lies between the values closest to $np - 2\sqrt{n \cdot p \cdot (1 - p)}$ and $np + 2\sqrt{n \cdot p \cdot (1 - p)}$.
- roughly 99% of the binomial distribution lies between the values closest to $np - 3\sqrt{n \cdot p \cdot (1 - p)}$ and $np + 3\sqrt{n \cdot p \cdot (1 - p)}$.

Example 2.28

Suppose the relapse rate within 3 months of treatment at a drug rehabilitation clinic is known to be 40%. If the clinic has 25 patients, then the mean number of patients to relapse within 3 months is $\mu = 25 \cdot 0.40 = 10$ and the standard deviation is $\sigma = \sqrt{25 \cdot 0.40 \cdot (1 - 0.40)} = 2.45$. Now, since $np = 25(0.4) = 10$ and $n(1 - p) = 25(0.6) = 15$, by applying the Empirical Rules roughly 95% of the time between 5 and 15 patients will relapse within 3 months of treatment. Using MINITAB, the actual percentage of a binomial distribution with $n = 25$ and $p = 0.40$ falling between 5 and 15 is 98%.

An important restriction in the setting for a binomial random variable is that the probability of success remains constant over the n trials. In many biomedical studies, the probability of success will be different for each individual in the experiment because the individuals are different. For example, in a study of the survival of patients having suffered heart attacks, the probability of survival will be influenced by many factors including severity of heart attack, delay in treatment, age, and ability to change diet and lifestyle following a heart attack. Because each individual is different, the probability of survival is not going to be constant over the n individuals in the study, and hence, the binomial probability model does not apply.

2.4.2 The Normal Probability Model

The choice of a probability model for continuous variables is generally based on historical data rather than a particular set of conditions. Just as there are many discrete probability models, there are also many different probability models that can be used to model the distribution of a continuous variable. The most commonly used continuous probability model in statistics is the *normal probability model*.

The normal probability model is often used to model distributions that are expected to be unimodal and symmetric, and the normal probability model forms the foundation for many of the classical statistical methods used in biostatistics. Moreover, the distribution of many natural phenomena can be modeled very well with the normal distribution. For example, the weights, heights, and IQs of adults are often modeled with normal distributions.

Several properties of a normal distribution are listed below.

PROPERTIES OF A NORMAL DISTRIBUTION

A normal distribution

- is a bell- or mound-shaped distribution.
- is completely characterized by its mean and standard deviation. The mean determines the center of the distribution and the standard deviation determines the spread about the mean.
- has probabilities and percentiles that are determined by the mean and standard deviation.

- is symmetric about the mean.
- has mean, median, and mode that are equal (i.e., $\mu = \tilde{\mu} = M$).
- has probability density function given by

$$f(x; \mu, \sigma) = \frac{1}{\sqrt{2\pi\sigma^2}} \cdot e^{-\frac{(x-\mu)^2}{2\sigma^2}} \quad \text{for}$$

$$-\infty < x < \infty$$

Example 2.29
The intelligence quotient (IQ) is based on a test of aptitude and is often used as a measure of an individual's intelligence. The distribution of IQ scores is approximately normally distributed with mean 100 and standard deviation 15. The normal probability model for IQ scores is given in Figure 2.25.

The standard normal, which will be denoted by Z, is a normal distribution having mean 0 and standard deviation 1. The standard normal is used as the reference distribution from which the probabilities and percentiles associated with any normal distribution will be determined. The cumulative probabilities for a standard normal are given in Tables A.1 and A.2; because 99.95% of the standard normal distribution lies between the values -3.49 and 3.49, the standard normal values are only tabulated for z values between -3.49 and 3.49. Thus, when the value of a standard normal, say z, is between -3.49 and 3.49, the

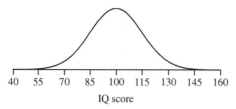

Figure 2.25 The approximate distribution of IQ scores with $\mu = 100$ and $\sigma = 15$.

tabled value for z represents the cumulative probability of z, which is $P(Z \leq z)$ and will be denoted by $\Phi(z)$. For values of z below -3.50, $\Phi(z)$ will be taken to be 0 and for values of z above 3.50, $\Phi(z)$ will be taken to be 1. Tables A.1 and A.2 can be used to compute all of the probabilities associated with a standard normal.

The values of z are referenced in Tables A.1 and A.2 by writing $z = a.bc$ as $z = a.b + 0.0c$. To locate a value of z in Table A.1 and A.2, first look up the value $a.b$ in the left-most column of the table and then locate $0.0c$ in the first row of the table. The value cross-referenced by $a.b$ and $0.c$ in Tables A.1 and A.2 is $\Phi(z) = P(Z \leq z)$. The rules for computing the probabilities for a standard normal are given below.

COMPUTING STANDARD NORMAL PROBABILITIES

1. For values of z between -3.49 and 3.49, the probability that $Z \leq z$ is read directly from the table. That is,

$$P(Z \leq z) = \Phi(z)$$

2. For $z \leq -3.50$ the probability that $Z \leq z$ is 0, and for $z \geq 3.50$ the probability that $Z \leq z$ is 1.

3. For values of z between -3.49 and 3.49, the probability that $Z \geq z$ is

$$P(Z \geq z) = 1 - P(Z \leq z) = 1 - \Phi(z)$$

4. For values of z between -3.49 and 3.49, the probability that $a \leq Z \leq b$ is

$$P(a \leq Z \leq b) = P(Z \leq b) - P(Z \leq a)$$
$$= \Phi(b) - \Phi(a)$$

Example 2.30
To determine the probability that a standard normal random variable is less than 1.65, which is the area shown in Figure 2.26, look up 1.6 in the left-most column of Table A.2 and 0.05 in the top row of this table, which yields $P(Z \leq 1.65) = 0.9505$.

Example 2.31
Determine the probability that a standard normal random variable lies between -1.35 and 1.51 (see Figure 2.27).

Solutions First, look up the cumulative probabilities for both -1.35 and 1.51 in Tables A.1 and A.2. The probability that $Z \leq -1.35$ and the probability that $Z \leq 1.51$ are shown in Figure 2.28. Subtracting these probabilities yields $P(-1.35 \leq Z \leq 1.51)$, and thus,

$$P(-1.35 \leq Z \leq 1.51) = \Phi(1.51) - \Phi(-1.35) = 0.9345 - 0.0885 = 0.8640$$

Example 2.32
Using the standard normal tables given in Tables A.1 and A.2, determine the following probabilities for a standard normal distribution:

   a. $P(Z \leq -2.28)$
   b. $P(Z \leq 3.08)$
   c. $P(-1.21 \leq Z \leq 2.28)$

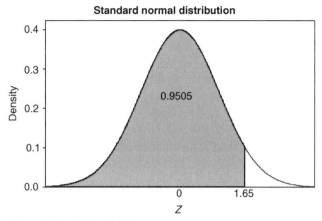

Figure 2.26 $P(Z \leq 1.65)$.

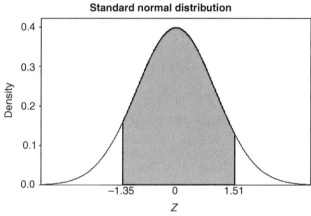

Figure 2.27 $P(-1.35 \leq Z \leq 1.51)$.

   d. $P(1.21 \leq Z \leq 6.28)$
   e. $P(-4.21 \leq Z \leq 0.84)$

Solutions Using the normal table in the appendix

   a. $P(Z \leq -2.28) = \Phi(-2.28) = 0.0113$
   b. $P(Z \geq 3.08) = 1 - \Phi(3.08) = 1 - 0.9990 = 0.0010$

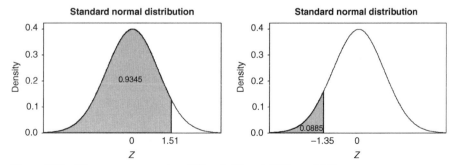

Figure 2.28   The areas representing $P(Z \leq 1.51)$ and $P(Z \leq -1.35)$.

TABLE 2.11 An Excerpted Section of the Cumulative Normal Table

					$\Phi(z) = P(Z \leq z)$					
z	0.00	0.01	0.02	0.03	0.04	0.05	0.06	0.07	0.08	0.09
					$\vdots$					
1.2	0.8849	0.8869	0.8888	0.8907	0.8925	0.8944	0.8962	0.8980	**0.8997**	0.9015
					$\vdots$					

c. $P(-1.21 \leq Z \leq 2.28) = \Phi(1.81) - \Phi(-1.21) = 0.9649 - 0.1131 = 0.8518$

d. $P(0.67 \leq Z \leq 6.28) = \Phi(6.28) - \Phi(0.67) = 1 - 0.7486 = 0.2514$

e. $P(-4.21 \leq Z \leq 0.84) = \Phi(0.84) - 0 = 0.7995$

The pth percentile of the standard normal can be found by looking up the cumulative probability $\frac{p}{100}$ inside of the standard normal tables given in Appendix A and then working backward to find the value of Z. Unfortunately, in some cases the value of $\frac{p}{100}$ will not be listed inside the table, and in this case, the value closest to $\frac{p}{100}$ inside of the table should be used for finding the approximate value of the pth percentile.

Example 2.33
Determine the 90th percentile of a standard normal distribution.

Solutions To find the 90th percentile, the first step is to find $\frac{90}{100} = 0.90$, or the value closest to 0.90, in the cumulative standard normal table. The row of the standard normal table containing the value 0.90 is given in Table 2.11. Since 0.8997 is the value closest to 0.90 that occurs in the row labeled 1.2 and the column labeled 0.08, the 90th percentile of a standard normal distribution is roughly $z = 1.2 + 0.08 = 1.28$.

The most commonly used percentiles of the standard normal are given in Table 2.12, and a more complete list of the percentiles of the standard normal distribution is given in Table A3. Note that for $p < 50$ the percentiles of a standard normal are negative, for $p = 50$ the 50th percentile is the median, and for $p > 50$ the percentiles of a standard normal are positive.

When X is a normal distribution with $\mu \neq 0$ or $\sigma \neq 1$, the distribution of X is called a *nonstandard normal distribution*. The standard normal distribution is the reference distribution for all normal distributions because all of the probabilities and percentiles for a nonstandard normal can be determined from the standard normal distribution. In particular, the following relationships between a nonstandard normal with mean μ and standard deviation σ and the standard normal can be used to convert a nonstandard normal value to a Z-value and vice versa.

TABLE 2.12 Selected Percentiles of a Standard Normal Distribution

p	1	5	10	20	25	50
pth percentile	−2.33	−1.645	−1.28	−0.84	−0.67	0.00

p	75	80	90	95	99	99.9
pth percentile	0.67	0.84	1.28	1.645	2.33	3.09

THE RELATIONSHIPS BETWEEN A STANDARD NORMAL AND A NONSTANDARD NORMAL

1. If X is a nonstandard normal with mean μ and standard deviation σ, then $Z = (X - \mu)/\sigma$.

2. If Z is a standard normal, then $X = \sigma \cdot Z + \mu$ is a nonstandard normal with mean μ and standard deviation σ.

Note that the value of a nonstandard normal X can be converted into a Z-value and vice versa. The first equation shows that centering and scaling the values of X converts them to Z-values, and the second equation shows how to convert a Z-value into an X-value. The relationship between a standard normal and a nonstandard normal is shown in Figure 2.29.

To determine the cumulative probability for the value of a nonstandard normal, say x, convert the value of x to its corresponding z value using $z = z - \mu/\sigma$; then determine the cumulative probability for this z value. That is,

$$P(X \le x) = P\left(Z \le \frac{x - \mu}{\sigma}\right)$$

To compute probabilities other than a cumulative probability for a nonstandard normal, note that the probability of being in any region can also be computed from the cumulative probabilities associated with the standard normal. The rules for computing the probabilities associated with a non-standard normal are given below.

NONSTANDARD NORMAL PROBABILITIES

If X is a nonstandard normal variable with mean μ and standard deviation σ, then

1. $P(X \ge x) = 1 - P(X \le x)$
$= 1 - P\left(Z \le \frac{x - \mu}{\sigma}\right)$

2. $P(a \le X \le b) = P(X \le b) - P(X \le b)$
$= P\left(Z \le \frac{b - \mu}{\sigma}\right) - P\left(Z \le \frac{a - \mu}{\sigma}\right)$

Note that each of the probabilities associated with a nonstandard normal distribution is based on the process of converting an x value to a z value using the formula $Z = (x - \mu)/\sigma$. The reason why the standard normal can be used for computing every probability concerning a nonstandard normal is that there is a one-to-one correspondence between the Z and X values (see Figure 2.29).

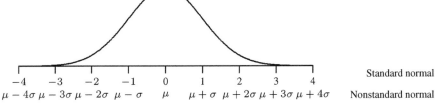

									Standard normal
-4	-3	-2	-1	0	1	2	3	4	
$\mu - 4\sigma$	$\mu - 3\sigma$	$\mu - 2\sigma$	$\mu - \sigma$	μ	$\mu + \sigma$	$\mu + 2\sigma$	$\mu + 3\sigma$	$\mu + 4\sigma$	Nonstandard normal

Figure 2.29   The correspondence between the values of a standard normal and a nonstandard normal.

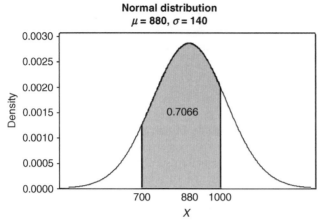

Figure 2.30 $P(700 \leq X \leq 1000)$.

Example 2.34

Suppose X has a nonstandard normal distribution with mean $\mu = 880$ and standard deviation $\sigma = 140$. The probability that X is between 700 and 1000 is represented by the area shown in Figure 2.30.

Converting the X values to Z-values leads to the corresponding probability, $P(-1.29 \leq Z \leq 0.86)$, for the standard normal shown in Figure 2.31.

Example 2.35

The distribution of IQ scores is approximately normal with $\mu = 100$ and $\sigma = 15$. Using this normal distribution to model the distribution of IQ scores,

a. an IQ score of 112 corresponds to a Z-value of

$$z = \frac{112 - 100}{15} = 0.8$$

b. the probability of having an IQ score of 112 or less is

$$P(X \leq 112) = P(Z \leq 0.80) = 0.7881$$

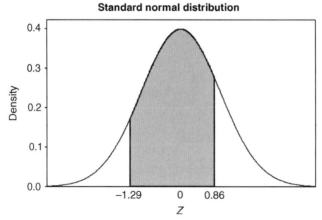

Figure 2.31   The Z region corresponding to $700 \leq X \leq 1000$.

c. the probability of having an IQ score between 90 and 120 is

$$P(90 \le X \le 120) = P\left(\frac{90-100}{15} \le Z \le \frac{120-100}{15}\right) = P(-0.67 \le Z \le 1.33)$$

$$= \Phi(1.33) - \Phi(-0.67) = 0.9082 - 0.2514$$

$$= 0.6568$$

e. the probability of having an IQ score of 150 or higher is

$$P(X \le 150) = P\left(Z \ge \frac{150-100}{15}\right) = P(Z \ge 3.33)$$

$$= 1 - \Phi(3.33) = 1 - 0.9996 = 0.0004$$

Example 2.36
In the article "Distribution of LDL particle size in a population-based sample of children and adolescents and relationship with other cardiovascular risk factors" published in *Clinical Chemistry* (Stan et al., 2005), the authors reported the results of a study on the peak particle size of low-density lipoprotein (LDL) in children and adolescents. It is known that smaller more dense particles (≤ 255 Å) of LDL are associated with cardiovascular disease.

The distribution of peak particle was reported to be approximately normal with mean particle size $\mu = 262$ Å and standard deviation $\sigma = 4$ Å. Based on this study, the probability that a child or adolescent will have a peak particle size of less than 255 Å is

$$P(X \le 255) = P\left(\frac{255-262}{4}\right) = P(Z \le -1.75) = 0.0401$$

Thus, there is only a 4% chance that a child or adolescent will have peak particle size less than 255 Å.

2.4.3 *Z* Scores

The result of converting a nonstandard normal value, a *raw value*, to a Z-value is a *Z score*. A Z score is a measure of the relative position a value has within its distribution. In particular, a Z score simply measures how many standard deviations a point is above or below the mean. When a Z score is negative the raw value lies below the mean of its distribution, and when a Z score is positive the raw value lies above the mean. Z scores are unitless measures of relative standing and provide a meaningful measure of relative standing only for mound-shaped distributions. Furthermore, Z scores can be used to compare the relative standing of individuals in two mound-shaped distributions.

Example 2.37
The weights of men and women both follow mound-shaped distributions with different means and standard deviations. In fact, the weight of a male adult in the United States is approximately normal with mean $\mu = 180$ and standard deviation $\sigma = 30$, and the weight of a female adult in the United States is approximately normal with mean $\mu = 145$ and standard deviation $\sigma = 15$. Given a male weighing 215 lb and a female weighing 170 lb, which individual weighs more relative to their respective population?

The answer to this question can be found by computing the Z scores associated with each of these weights to measure their relative standing. In this case,

$$z_{male} = \frac{215-180}{30} = 1.17$$

and

$$z_{\text{female}} = \frac{170 - 145}{15} = 1.67$$

Since the female's weight is 1.67 standard deviations from the mean weight of a female and the male's weight is 1.17 standard deviations from the mean weight of a male, relative to their respective populations a female weighing 170 lb is heavier than a male weighing 215 lb.

GLOSSARY

Binomial Probability Model   The binomial probability model is a probability model for a discrete random variable that counts the number of successes in n independent trials of a chance experiment having only two possible outcomes.

Chance Experiment   A task where the outcome cannot be predetermined is called a random experiment or a chance experiment.

Conditional Probability   The conditional probability of the event A given that the event B has occurred is denoted by $P(A|B)$ and is defined as

$$P(A|B) = \frac{P(A \cap B)}{P(B)}$$

Continuous Variable   A quantitative variable is a continuous variable when the variable can take on any value in one or more intervals.

Discrete Variable   A quantitative variable is a discrete variable when there are either a finite or a countable number of possible values for the variable.

Distribution   The distribution of a variable explicitly describes how the values of the variable are distributed in terms of percentages.

Event   An event is a subcollection of the outcomes in the sample space is associated with a chance experiment.

Explanatory Variable   An explanatory variable is a variable that is believed to cause changes in the response variable.

Independent Events   Two events A and B are independent when $P(A|B) = P(A)$ or $P(B|A) = P(B)$.

Interquartile Range   The Interquartile range of a population is the distance between the 25th and 75th percentiles and will be denoted by IQR.

Mean   The mean of a variable X measured on a population consisting of N units is

$$\mu = \frac{\text{sum of the values of } X}{N} = \frac{\sum X}{N}$$

Median   The median of a population is the 50th percentile of the possible values of the variable X and will be denoted by $\tilde{\mu}$.

Mode   The mode of a population is the most frequent value of the variable X in the population and will be denoted by M.

Multivariate Variable   A collection of variables that will be measured on each unit is called a multivariate variable.

Nominal Variable   A qualitative variable is called a nominal variable when the values of the variable have no intrinsic ordering.

Nonstandard Normal   A nonstandard normal is any normal distribution that does not have a standard normal distribution (i.e., either $\mu \neq 0$ or $\sigma \neq 1$).

Ordinal Variable A qualitative variable is called an ordinal variable when there is a natural ordering of the possible values of the variable.

Parameter A parameter is a numerical value that summarizes a particular characteristic of the population.

Percentile The pth percentile of a quantitative variable is the value in the population where p percent of the population falls below this value. The pth percentile is denoted by x_p for values of p between 0 and 100.

Probability A probability is a number between 0 and 1 that measures how likely it is for an event to occur.

Qualitative Variable A variable that takes on only numeric values is called a quantitative variable.

Quantitative Variable A variable that takes on nonnumeric values is called a qualitative variable or a categorical variable.

Response Variable The response variable is the outcome variable of primary interest to a researcher.

Sample Space The set of all possible outcomes of a chance experiment is called the sample space and is denoted by S.

Sensitivity The sensitivity is the conditional probability of a positive test for the subpopulation of individuals having the disease (i.e., $P(+|D)$).

Specificity The specificity is the conditional probability of a negative test for the subpopulation of individuals who do not have the disease (i.e., $P(-|\text{not D})$).

Standard Deviation The standard deviation of a population is defined to be the square root of the variance and will be denoted by σ.

Standard Normal The standard normal is a normal distribution with mean 0 and standard deviation 1.

Variance The variance of a variable X measured on a population consisting of N units is

$$\sigma^2 = \frac{\text{sum of all (deviations from } \mu)^2}{N} = \frac{\sum (X - \mu)^2}{N}$$

Z Score A Z score is a measure of relative position within a distribution and measures how many standard deviations a point is above or below the mean.

$$Z \text{ score} = \frac{X - \mu}{\sigma}$$

EXERCISES

2.1 What is the difference between a qualitative and a quantitative variable?

2.2 What is the difference between a discrete and a continuous variable?

2.3 What is the difference between a nominal and an ordinal variable?

2.4 Determine whether each of the following variables is a qualitative or quantitative variable.
  (**a**) Age
  (**b**) Systolic blood pressure
  (**c**) Race

(d) Gender

(e) Pain level

2.5   Determine whether each of the following variables is a qualitative or quantitative variable. If the variable is a quantitative variable, determine whether it is a discrete or continuous variable. If the variable is a qualitative variable determine whether it is a nominal or an ordinal variable.

(a) Smoking status

(b) Cancer stage

(c) Number of visits to the doctor

(d) Percentage body fat

(e) White blood cell count

(f) Body mass index

(g) Hair color

(h) Survival time after diagnosis with pancreatic cancer

(i) Number of months since last blood donation

(j) Number of sexual partners in last 6 months

2.6   Determine whether each of the following qualitative variables is a nominal or an ordinal variable. The values that the variable can take on are listed in parentheses following the name of the variable.

(a) Gender (M, F)

(b) Size of hospital (small, average, large)

(c) Blood type (A, B, AB, O)

(d) Radiation dosage (low, medium, high)

(e) Use of dietary supplements (yes, no)

(f) Fat in diet (low, medium, high)

(g) Eat lunch (always, sometimes, never)

2.7   The percentages given in Table 2.13 were extracted from a bar chart published in the article "Prevalence of overweight among persons aged 2–19 years, by sex—National Health and Nutrition Examination Survey (NHANES), United States, 1999–2000 through 2003–2004" in the November 17, 2006 issue of the *Morbidity and Mortality Weekly Report* (MMWR), a Centers for Disease Control and Prevention weekly publication.

(a) Create a side-by-side bar chart representing the percentages of overweight children for each gender by year.

(b) Create a side-by-side bar chart representing the percentages of overweight children for each year by gender.

TABLE 2.13   Prevalence of Overweight Children According to an Article in the November 17, 2006 Issue of MMWR

Gender	Year		
	1999–2000	2001–2002	2003–2004
Male	14	16.5	18.2
Female	13.8	14	16

TABLE 2.14 Percentages of Americans in the Blood Pressure Categories as Reported in the June 22, 2007 issue of MMWR

Ethnicity	Blood Pressure Category			
	Normal	Prehypertension Stage I	Hypertension Stage II	Hypertension
Mexican American	46	34	12	8
White	46	37	11	6
Black	36	38	16	10

2.8 The percentages in Table 2.14 were extracted from a bar chart published in the article "Percentage distribution of blood pressure categories among adults aged ≥ 18 years, by race/ethnicity—National Health and Nutrition Examination Survey, United States, 1999–2004" published in the June 22, 2007 issue of the *Morbidity and Mortality Weekly Report*, a Centers for Disease Control and Prevention weekly publication.

    (a) Create a side-by-side bar chart representing the percentages for each of the blood pressure categories by ethnicity category.

    (b) Create a side-by-side bar chart representing the percentages for each of the blood pressure categories within each ethnicity category.

    (c) Which ethnicity appears to have the largest percentage in the hypertension stage I and II categories?

2.9 The probability distribution of the continuous variable X is given in Figure 2.32. Which of the five points A, B, C, D, or E is the

    (a) mean of this distribution?

    (b) median of this distribution?

    (c) mode of this distribution?

    (d) value that only 25% of the X values in the population exceed?

    (e) value that 50% of the X values in the population exceed?

    (f) value that 75% of the X values in the population exceed?

2.10 If the 25th and 75th percentiles of the distribution given in Figure 2.32 are 67 and 125, determine the value of the interquartile range.

2.11 Use the distribution given in Figure 2.33 that represents a hypothetical distribution for the survival times for stage IV pancreatic cancer patients to answer the following questions:

    (a) Is this distribution symmetric, long-tailed right, or long-tailed left?

    (b) How many modes does this distribution have?

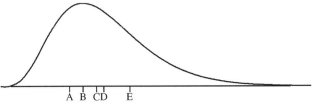

Figure 2.32   The probability distribution of the continuous variable X.

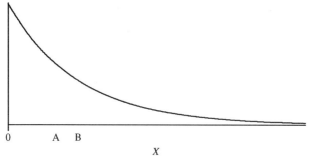

Figure 2.33   The distribution for Exercise 2.11.

   (c) Which of the two values A and B is the mean?
   (d) What is the value of the mode for this distribution?

2.12 In a bimodal distribution, which parameters best describe the typical values in the population?

2.13 What is the most common reason that a variable will have a bimodal distribution?

2.14 What is the prevalence of a disease?

2.15 How is a percentile different from a population percentage?

2.16 How do the mean and median differ?

2.17 When are the mean and median equal?

2.18 Is the
   (a) mean sensitive to the extreme values in the population?
   (b) median sensitive to the extreme values in the population?

2.19 Suppose the population of 250 doctors at a public hospital has been classified according to the variables Age and Gender and is summarized in the table below.

	25–40	41–55	56–70
Male	54	66	42
Female	24	41	23

   (a) Determine the percentage of doctors at this hospital that are female.
   (b) Determine the percentage of doctors at this hospital that are aged 56 or older.
   (c) Determine the percentage of doctors at this hospital that are female and aged 41 or older.
   (d) Determine the percentages of doctors at this hospital in each age group.
   (e) Determine the age group that the median age falls in.

2.20 Describe how the geometric mean (GM) is computed and why it might be used in place of the arithmetic mean.

2.21 What are three parameters that measure the

(a) typical values in a population.

(b) the spread of a population.

2.22 Which of the parameters

(a) measuring the typical value in a population are not sensitive to the extreme values in a population?

(b) measuring the spread of a population are not sensitive to the extreme values in a population?

2.23 Based on the National Health and Nutrition Examination Survey run from 1999 to 2002, the mean weight of an adult male in the United States is 190 lb. Suppose the distribution of weights of males is a mound-shaped distribution with standard deviation $\sigma = 25$. Determine

(a) the weight range that approximately 95% of the adult males in the United States fall in.

(b) the coefficient of variation for the weights of adult males in the United States.

2.24 For a mound-shaped distribution what is the approximate percentage of the population falling

(a) between the values $\mu - 2\sigma$ and $\mu + 2\sigma$.

(b) above the values $\mu + 3\sigma$.

(c) below the values $\mu - \sigma$.

2.25 Which parameter measures the relative spread in a population? How is this parameter computed?

2.26 What does it mean when there is a large distance between the

(a) 25th and 75th percentiles?

(b) 90th and 99th percentiles?

2.27 The approximate mean and standard deviations for the weights and heights for the U.S. population are given in Table 2.15 for men and women. Use the information in Table 2.15 to answer the following questions:

(a) Compute the coefficient of variation for the variable height for the population of adult males.

(b) Compute the coefficient of variation for the variable weight for the population of adult males.

(c) Compute the coefficient of variation for the variable height for the population of adult females.

TABLE 2.15 The Approximate Means and Standard Deviations for the Variables Weight and Height for the U.S. Population

Variable	Mean	Standard Deviation
Men		
Height (in.)	69.3	3.0
Weight (lb)	190	20
Women		
Height (in.)	63.8	2.2
Weight (lb)	163	18

     (d) Compute the coefficient of variation for the variable weight for the population of adult females.

     (e) For the variable height, determine which population, males or females, has a larger variability relative to the size of values in the population?

     (f) For the variable weight, determine which population, males or females, has a larger variability relative to the size of values in the population?

2.28   What does it mean when the value of the correlation coefficient for two quantitative variables is

     (a) $\rho = -1$.

     (b) $\rho = 0$.

     (c) $\rho = 1$.

2.29   What does the correlation coefficient measure?

2.30   What are the units of the correlation coefficient?

2.31   What does it mean when two events are said to be independent events?

2.32   Under what conditions is the probability of the event "A or B" equal to the sum of their respective probabilities?

2.33   Under what conditions is the probability of the event "A and B" equal to the product of their respective probabilities?

2.34   Suppose that $P(A) = 0.36$, $P(B) = 0.51$, and $P(A \text{ and } B) = 0.18$. Determine

     (a) the probability that event A does not occur.

     (b) the probability that event A or the event B occurs.

     (c) the probability that neither event A nor event B occurs.

     (d) the conditional probability that event A occurs given that event B has occurred.

     (e) the conditional probability that event B occurs given that event A has occurred.

2.35   Suppose that $P(A) = 0.4$, $P(B) = 0.5$, and A and B are disjoint events. Determine

     (a) the probability that event A does not occur.

     (b) the probability that event A or the event B occurs.

     (c) the probability that neither event A nor event B occurs.

     (d) the conditional probability that event A occurs given that event B has occurred.

     (e) the conditional probability that event B occurs given that event A has occurred.

2.36   Suppose that $P(A) = 0.4$, $P(B) = 0.5$, and A and B are independent events. Determine

     (a) the probability that event A does not occur.

     (b) the probability that both event A and event B occur.

     (c) the probability that either event A or event B occurs.

     (d) the conditional probability that event A occurs given that event B has occurred.

     (e) the conditional probability that event B occurs given that event A has occurred.

2.37   Suppose 40% of adults have had a tetanus shot in the last 10 years, 52% have had a flu shot in the last 5 years, and 33% have had both a tetanus shot in the last 10 years and a flu shot in the last 5 years. Determine the probability that

     (a) a randomly selected adult has had either a tetanus shot in the last 10 years or a flu shot in the last 5 years.

(**b**) a randomly selected adult has had a tetanus shot in the last 10 years given they have had a flu shot in the last 5 years.

(**c**) a randomly selected adult has had a flu shot in the last 5 years given they have had a tetanus shot in the last 10 years.

2.38   Suppose that a particular disease occurs with prevalence 0.05 (i.e., $P(D) = 0.05$), the probability that an individual has the disease and has a positive diagnostic test is 0.048 (i.e., $P(D$ and positive$) = 0.048$), and the probability that an individual has the disease and the test is negative is 0.94 (i.e., $P($not D and negative$) = 0.88$). Determine

(**a**) the sensitivity of this diagnostic test.

(**b**) the specificity of this diagnostic test.

(**c**) the probability that an individual has the disease given the test is positive.

2.39   According to the *Medscape Today* article "Standard of care for pap screening" (Lie, 2003), the sensitivity and specificity of the pap smear test for cervical cancer are at least 0.29 and 097, respectively. If the prevalence of cervical cancer is 0.01, determine the probability that a women

(**a**) has a positive test result.

(**b**) has cervical cancer given the result of the pap smear is positive for cervical cancer.

(**c**) does not have cervical cancer given the result of the pap smear is positive for cervical cancer.

2.40   In the article " Improved serodiagnostic testing for lyme disease: results of a multicenter serologic evaluation" published in the journal of *Emerging Infectious Diseases* (Craven et al., 1996), the authors report that in testing for Lyme disease the sensitivity of an ELISA test with a WCS antigen is 0.93 with specificity of 0.71. If the prevalence of Lyme disease in a particular region of the United States is 0.001, determine the probability that an individual being tested

(**a**) has a positive test result.

(**b**) has Lyme disease given the result of the ELISA test is positive for Lyme disease.

2.41   According to the American Red Cross, the percentage of Americans having type B blood is 11%. If four Americans are chosen at random and independently, determine the probability that

(**a**) all four have blood type B.

(**b**) none of the four has blood type B.

(**c**) exactly one of the four has blood type B.

2.42   The autosomal recessive genetic disorder sickle cell anemia is caused by a defect in the hemoglobin beta (HBB) gene. Two defective genes, denoted by SS, are needed for sickle cell anemia to occur in an individual. If each parent carries one sickle HBB gene (S) and one normal HBB gene (A), and a child receives exactly one gene independently from each parent, determine

(**a**) the probability that a child will have sickle cell anemia.

(**b**) the probability that a child will not have sickle cell anemia.

(**c**) the probability that a child will not have any sickle HBB genes.

2.43   What are the four conditions necessary to have a binomial distribution?

TABLE 2.16   The Binomial Probabilities for $n = 10$ Trials and $p = 0.25$

```
Binomial with n = 10 and p = 0.25
   x                    P( X = x)
   0                    0.056314
   1                    0.187712
   2                    0.281568
   3                    0.250282
   4                    0.145998
   5                    0.058399
   6                    0.016222
   7                    0.003090
   8                    0.000386
   9                    0.000029
  10                    0.000001
```

2.44   Suppose the variable X has a binomial distribution with $n = 10$ trials and probability of success $p = 0.25$. Using the probabilities given in Table 2.16, determine
(a) the most likely value of the random variable X.
(b) the probability that X is larger than 6.
(c) the probability that X is at least 6.
(d) the probability that X is between 3 and 6 (i.e., $3 \le X \le 6$).

2.45   Determine the mean and standard deviation for each of the following binomial distributions:
(a) $n = 25$ and $p = 0.80$
(b) $n = 40$ and $p = 0.60$
(c) $n = 50$ and $p = 0.10$

2.46   For what values of p will a binomial distribution
(a) have a long tail to the right?
(b) have a long tail to the left?
(c) be symmetric?
(d) have the largest value of σ?

2.47   Many studies investigating extrasensory perception (ESP) have been conducted. A typical ESP study is carried out by subjecting an individual claiming to have ESP to a series of trials and recording the number of correct identifications made by the subject. Furthermore, when a subject is strictly guessing on each trial, the number of correct identifications can be modeled by a binomial probability model with the probability of a correct identification being $p = 0.5$ on each trial. If a subject is guessing on each of 20 trials in a test of ESP, determine
(a) the probability of 20 correct identifications.
(b) the probability of 16 correct identifications.
(c) the probability of at least 16 correct identifications.
(d) the mean number of correct identifications.

2.48   Suppose an individual does actually have ESP and makes correct identifications with probability $p = 0.9$. If the individual is subjected to a series of 20 independent trials, determine the probability of making

(a) 20 correct identifications.

(b) at least 18 correct identifications.

2.49 Past studies have shown that 60% of the children of parents who both smoke cigarettes will also end up smoking cigarettes, and only 20% of children whose parents do not smoke cigarettes will end up smoking cigarettes. In a family with four children, use the binomial probability model to determine

(a) the probability that none of the children become smokers given that both parents are smokers.

(b) the probability that none of the children become smokers given that none of the parents are smokers.

2.50 In Exercise 2.49, is it reasonable to assume that each of the four children will or will not become a smoker independently of the other children? Explain.

2.51 Side effects are often encountered by patients receiving a placebo in a clinical trial. Suppose eight individuals were randomly and independently selected for the placebo group in a clinical trial. From past studies, it is known that the percentage of individuals experiencing significant side effects after receiving the placebo treatment is about 10%. Using the binomial probability model determine

(a) the probability that at least two of the eight patients in the placebo group experience significant side effects.

(b) the probability that no more than three of the eight patients in the placebo group experience significant side effects.

(c) the expected number of the eight patients in the placebo group experiencing significant side effects.

(d) the standard deviation of the number of the eight patients experiencing significant side effects.

2.52 If Z has a standard normal distribution, determine

(a) $P(Z \leq 0.82)$

(b) $P(Z < 1.99)$

(c) $P(Z < -2.04)$

(d) $P(Z > 0.04)$

(e) $P(Z \geq -2.45)$

(f) $P(Z > 3.21)$

(g) $P(-1.09 < Z \leq 2.33)$

(h) $P(-1.95 < Z < -1.33)$

(i) $P(2.04 < Z \leq 3.33)$

(j) $P(-2.35 < Z < 1.65)$

2.53 If Z has a standard normal distribution, determine

(a) the 5th percentile.

(b) the 25th percentile.

(c) the 75th percentile.

(d) the 98th percentile.

(e) the interquartile range.

2.54 Intelligence quotient scores are known to follow a normal distribution with mean 100 and standard deviation 15. Using the normal probability model, determine

(a) the probability that an individual has an IQ score of greater than 140.

(b) the probability that an individual has an IQ score of less than 80.

(c) the probability that an individual has an IQ score of between 105 and 125.

(d) the 95th percentile of IQ scores.

2.55 Suppose the birth weight of a full-term baby born in the United States follows a normal distribution with mean weight 3500 g and standard deviation 250 g. Determine

(a) the probability that a new-born baby weighs less than 3000 g.

(b) the probability that a new-born baby weighs more than 4100 g.

(c) the probability that a new-born baby weighs between 3100 and 3900 g.

(d) the 90th percentile of the distribution of birth weights for full-term babies.

2.56 Suppose the distribution of weights of women in the United States that are 63 in. tall follows a normal distribution with mean weight 128 lb and standard deviation 5 lb. Determine

(a) the probability that a 63 in. tall woman weighs more than 135 lb.

(b) the probability that a 63 in. tall woman weighs less than 120 lb.

(c) the probability that a 63 in. tall woman weighs between 112 and 140 lb.

(d) the 15th percentile of the distribution of weights for 63 in. tall women.

2.57 According to the National Health and Nutrition Examination Survey report "Healthy weight, overweight, and obesity among U.S. adults" (2003), the mean body mass index for an adult female in the United States is 26.5. Healthy weights for an adult female are indicated by BMI values between 18 and 25, women with a BMI values between 25 and 30 are considered overweight, and women with BMI values greater than 30 are considered obese. Assuming that the BMI for women in the United States is normally distributed with mean 26.5 and standard deviation 2.5, determine

(a) the probability that a woman has a BMI value of less than 25.

(b) the probability that a woman has a BMI value indicating she is overweight or obese.

(c) the probability that a woman has a BMI value indicating she is overweight but not obese.

(d) the 75th percentile of the distribution of BMI for women.

2.58 What are the units of a z score?

2.59 How many standard deviations below the mean does z score of -1.5 correspond to?

2.60 Under what conditions is it possible to determine the percentile associated with an observed z score?

2.61 Table 2.17 contains the standard weight classifications based on BMI values. Assuming that the BMI values are approximately normally distributed, determine the

TABLE 2.17 The Standard Weight Classifications Based on BMI Scores

Weight Classification	BMI Percentile Range
Underweight	Less than 5th percentile
Healthy weight	Between 5th and 85th percentiles
At risk of overweight	Between 85th and 95th percentiles
Overweight	Greater than the 95th percentile

TABLE 2.18   The Standard Weight Classifications Based on BMI Scores

	BMI	
Age	Mean	SD
10	16.6	2.3
15	19.8	3.1

(a) z score corresponding to the cutoff for the underweight classification.

(b) z scores corresponding to the cutoffs for the healthy weight classification.

(c) z scores corresponding to the cutoffs for the at-risk-of-overweight classification.

(d) z scores corresponding to the cutoff for the overweight classification.

2.62   Because a BMI value for a child depends on age and sex of the child, z scores are often used to compare children of different ages or sexes. Table 2.18 gives the mean and standard deviation for the distribution of BMI values for male children aged 10 and 15. Use the information in Table 2.18 to answer the following questions concerning two male children, a 10 and a 15 years old, each having a BMI value of 25:

(a) Compute the z score for the 10 years old.

(b) Compute the z score for the 15 years old.

(c) Which child has a larger BMI value relative to the population of males in their age group?

2.63   From the information given in Table 2.15, the approximate means and standard deviations for the variable weight for males and females in the United States are $\mu_m = 190$, $\sigma_m = 20$, $\mu_f = 163$, and $\sigma_f = 18$. For a male weighing 212 lb and a female weighing 181 lb, determine

(a) the z score for the male.

(b) the z score for the female.

(c) whether the male or the female is farther from the mean of their respective population.

CHAPTER 3

RANDOM SAMPLING

$\mathbf{O}$NE OF the most important requirements in any data-based research study is the data that are collected and analyzed are trustworthy and representative of the target population being studied. To have data that will provide reliable and accurate estimates of the unknown parameters, can be used to test the research hypotheses, and to ensure meaningful conclusions, a carefully designed sampling plan must be developed and used. A well-designed sampling plan can be used to produce highly accurate statistics while minimizing the cost of the study. The best way to obtain data that is representative of the target population is with a *random sample*. A random sample is also called a *probability sample* and utilizes a probability model in the selection of the population units that are sampled. In this chapter, the sampling process, probability samples, and several different types of random sampling plans will be discussed.

3.1 OBTAINING REPRESENTATIVE DATA

The purpose of sampling is to get a sufficient amount of data that is representative of target population so that statistical inferences can be made about the distribution and the parameters of the target population. Because a sample is only a subset of the units in the target population, it is generally impossible to guarantee that the sample data are representative of the target population; however, with a well-designed sampling plan, it will be unlikely to select a sample that is not representative of the target population. To ensure the likelihood that the sample data will be representative of the target population, the following components of the sampling process must be considered:

- *Target Population* The *target population* must be well defined, accessible, and the researcher should have a good understanding of the structure of the population. In particular, the researcher should be able to identify the units of the population, the approximate number of units in the population, subpopulations, the approximate shape of the distributions of the variables being studied, and the relevant parameters that need to be estimated.

- *Sampling Units* The *Sampling units* are the units of the population that will be sampled. A sampling unit may or may not be a unit of the population. In fact, in some sampling plans, the sampling unit is a collection of population units. The sampling unit is also the smallest unit in the target population that can be selected.

- *Sampling Element*   A *sampling element* is an object on which measurements will be made. A sampling element may or may not be a sampling unit. When the sampling unit consists of several population units, it is called a *cluster of units*. If each population unit in a cluster that will be measured, then the sampling elements are the population units within the sampled clusters. In this case, the sampling element is a subunit of the sampling unit.

- *Sampling Frame*   The *sampling frame* is the list of sampling units that are available for sampling. The sampling frame should be nearly equal to the target population. When the sampling frame is significantly different from the target population, it makes it less unlikely that a sample representative of the target population will be obtained, even with a well-designed sampling plan. Sampling frames that fail to include all of the units of the target population are said to *undercover* the target population and may lead to biased samples.

- *Sample Size*   The *sample size* is the number of sampling units that will be selected. The sample size will be denoted by n and must be sufficiently large enough to ensure the reliability of the statistical analysis. The variability in the target population plays a key role in determining the sample size necessary for the desired level of reliability associated with a statistical analysis.

Example 3.1
In studying the post-surgery infection rate, suppose the target population is the population of all individuals who had surgery in the past year. While it may be possible to obtain a sampling frame consisting of a list of all individuals who had surgery in the past year, it would be easier to obtain a list of the hospitals in the United States. In this case, an efficient way of samplign the population of individuals who had surgery in the past year is to use the list of hospitals in the United States as the sampling frame and let the sampling units be the collection of individuals who had surgery at each hospital. In this case, a sampling unit consists of many sampling elements, namely, the individuals who had surgery at a hospital.

In general, collecting data is easy, however, collecting data that is trustworthy and representative of the target population is a much harder task. Many researchers simply collect ad-hoc samples that are easy or convenient to collect; samples collected in an ad-hoc fashion are referred to as *samples of convenience*. Examples of samples of convenience include

- Observing data that are close at hand or data that are easy to obtain. This is known as *availability sampling*. A sample consisting of volunteers is an example of availability sampling.

- Observing data that are self-selected by the researcher. Self-selected sampling is also referred to as *expert sampling* or *judgment sampling*.

- Observing data from individuals who are previously referred to by previously sampled individuals. Sampling according to referrals from previously sampled units is known as *snowball sampling* or *chain referral sampling*.

Example 3.2
Suppose a physician at a clinic in Atlanta, Georgia wishes to study the relationship between the percentage fat in an individual's diet and the coronary heart disease. To obtain data for this study, the physician solicits volunteers by placing an advertisement in the local paper. In this case, the physician is using a sample of convenience consisting of volunteers. It is well documented that volunteers are generally very different from nonvolunteers, and hence, any result based on this sample could be biased.

While it is possible for a sample of convenience to produce data that are representative of the target population, there is no mechanism in this type of sampling process that ensures a high likelihood of obtaining representative data. In fact, it is unlikely that a sample of convenience will produce a sample that is representative of the target population. For this reason, inferences based on the statistical analysis of a sample of convenience cannot be considered trustworthy. Furthermore, in a sample of convenience, the mathematical theory that is used to develop and justify the statistical methods used in the analysis will not be valid.

3.1.1 The Sampling Plan

The goal of a well-designed sampling plan is to (1) ensure data that are representative of the target population will be observed and (2) the observed data will provide reliable information about the target population. A study is said to have *external validity* when the results of the study can be safely generalized about the target population. To have a study with external validity, it is critical that a representative sample be collected. Modern statistical theory makes it possible to design a sampling procedure that will almost surely produce a sample that is representative of the target population and will produce a statistical analysis that is highly accurate and reliable. A well-designed sampling plan should involve the following steps:

DESIGNING THE SAMPLING PLAN

A well-designed sampling plan should

1. have a set of well-defined research questions and hypotheses to be tested;

2. have a well-defined target population that is relevant to the questions of interest;

3. account for all of the variables that are believed to be important to the study;

4. have well-defined sampling units and sampling elements;

5. have a sampling frame that ensures a representative sample of the target population is possible;

6. have a sampling plan that will provide data that can be used to make reliable statistical inferences from the sample to the target population;

7. identify the statistical analysis that will be performed on the observed sample once it is collected;

8. have a predetermined sample size that is chosen to produce a prespecified level of accuracy for the statistics that will be computed from the information in the observed sample;

9. clearly outline all of the details involved in the sampling process including the timing of the sample, the data collection details, the measurement devices, and the training of the samplers.

Only after these steps have been carried out, should a researcher begin to collect the sample data.

3.1.2 Probability Samples

The statistical theory that provides the foundation for the estimation or testing of research hypotheses about the parameters of a population is based on the sampling structure known as *probability sampling*. A probability sample is a sample that is selected in a random fashion according to some probability model. In particular, a probability sample is a sample chosen so that each of the possible samples is known in advance and the probability of drawing each sampling unit is known. *Random samples* are samples that arise through a sampling plan based on probability sampling.

Probability sampling allows flexibility in the sampling plan and can be designed specifically for the target population being studied. That is, a probability sampling plan allows a sample to be designed so that it will be unlikely to produce a sample that is not representative of the target population. Furthermore, probability samples allow for confidence statements and hypothesis tests to be made from the observed sample with a high degree of reliability.

Samples of convenience are samples that are not based on probability samples and are also referred to as *nonprobability samples*. The statistical theory that justifies the use of confidence statements and tests of hypotheses does not apply to nonprobability samples; therefore, confidence statements and test of the research hypotheses based on nonprobability samples are erroneous applications of statistics and should not be trusted.

In a random sample, the chance that a particular unit of the population will be selected is known prior to sampling, and the units available for sampling are selected at random according to these probabilities. The procedure for drawing a random sample is outlined below.

THE PROCEDURE FOR DRAWING A RANDOM SAMPLE

---

1. Determine the sampling frame and sampling units.

2. Assign identification numbers to each of the sampling units in the sampling frame.

3. Program a computer to select a random sample of identification numbers according to the appropriate probabilities of the sampling plan.

4. Collect the data on the sampling units associated with the identification numbers selected in step 3.

To develop a good probability sampling plan, it is critical to have a sampling frame that covers the entire target population. When the sampling frame undercovers the target population, there is no probability sampling plan that can adjust for this undercoverage. Some of the important properties of a random sample that samples of convenience do not have are listed below.

PROPERTIES OF A RANDOM SAMPLE

---

1. Random samples generally produce samples that are representative of the target population.

2. Random samples are designed to be free from bias and do not favor any one portion of a population over another.

3. The results of a statistical analysis based on a random sample are repeatable from one sample to another. That is,

(a) statistics computed using a random sample have a predictable pattern of values in repeated sampling;

(b) many statistics computed from a random sample will not systematically over- or underestimate the parameters of interest;

(c) measures of the reliability of a statistic computed from a random sample can be computed.

Random sampling plans generally lead to meaningful statistical inferences because random samples produce data that are representative of the target population, and the statistical analyses based on two different random samples of size n selected from same target population should produce similar results.

3.2 COMMONLY USED SAMPLING PLANS

In practice, the appropriate sampling plan for a particular research problem will depend on the researcher's understanding of the target population, past research on the problem being studied, and any cost and logistical considerations involved in sampling the target population. Commonly used probability sampling plans include *simple random sampling*, *stratified random sampling*, *cluster sampling*, and *systematic random sampling*.

3.2.1 Simple Random Sampling

The first sampling plan that will be discussed is the *simple random sample*. A simple random sample of size n is a sample consisting of n sampling units selected in a fashion that every possible sample of n units has the same chance of being selected. In a simple random sample, every possible sample has the same chance of being selected, and moreover, each sampling unit has the same chance of being drawn in a sample. Simple random sampling is a reasonable sampling plan for sampling homogeneous or heterogeneous populations that do not have distinct subpopulations that are of interest to the researcher.

Example 3.3
Simple random sampling might be a reasonable sampling plan in the following scenarios:

a. A pharmaceutical company is checking the quality control issues of the tablet form of a new drug. Here, the company might take a random sample of tablets from a large pool of available drug tablets it has recently manufactured.

b. The Federal Food and Drug Administration (FDA) may take a simple random sample of a particular food product to check the validity of the information on the nutrition label.

c. A state might wish to take a simple random sample of medical doctors to review whether or not the state's continuing education requirements are being satisfied.

d. A federal or state environment agency may wish to take a simple random sample of homes in a mining town to investigate the general health of the town's inhabitants and contamination problems in the homes resulting from the mining operation.

The number of possible simple random samples of size n selected from a sampling frame listing of N sampling units is

$$\binom{N}{n} = \frac{N!}{n!(N-n)!}$$

The probability that any one of the possible simple random samples of n units selected from a sampling frame of N units is

$$\frac{1}{\frac{N!}{n!(N-n)!}} = \frac{n!(N-n)!}{N!}$$

In most research studies, the number of units in the target population is fairly large, and therefore, the number of possible simple random samples will also be extremely large. For example, suppose the sampling frame has $N = 100$ sampling units and a simple random sample of $n = 10$ units will be selected. The number of possible simple random samples of size $n = 10$ from this frame is

$$\binom{100}{10} = \frac{100!}{10!(100 - 10)!} = 17,310,309,456,440$$

That is, there are more than 17 trillion different possible simple random samples of size $n = 10$ that could be selected from a sampling frame consisting of $N = 100$ units. Furthermore, each of the possible samples would have a 1 in 17,310,309,456,440 chances of being selected in a simple random sample of size $n = 10$ drawn from this population.

Example 3.4
Determine the number of simple random samples possible when

   a. $N = 200$ and $n = 25$.
   b. $N = 500$ and $n = 15$.

Solutions The number of possible simple random samples when

   a. $N = 200$ and $n = 25$ is

$$\frac{50!(200 - 50)!}{200!} = 45,217,131,606,152,448,808,778,187,283,008$$

   That is, there are roughly 45 nontillion possible simple random samples of size $n = 25$ that can be drawn from a population consisting of 200 units.
   b. $N = 500$ and $n = 15$ is

$$\frac{15!(500 - 15)!}{500!} = 18,877,913,877,607,917,786,274,849,200$$

   That is, there are roughly 19 octillion possible simple random samples of size $n = 15$ that can be drawn from a population consisting of 500 units.

One of the reasons that statistics works so well is that random samples produce samples that are representative of the target population. That is, in most research studies there is an enormously large number of possible samples that could be drawn and most of these samples are representative of the target population being sampled. In fact, the number of possible samples that are representative of the target population is much larger than the number of samples that are not representative of the target population. Thus, in practice it is unlikely that a sample will be drawn that is not representative of the target population. The procedure for drawing a simple random sample of n units from a sampling frame consisting of N units is outlined below.

Many statistical packages such as MINITAB, SAS, SPSS, and Splus have sampling programs that can be used to select the identification numbers in a fashion that each number is equally likely to be selected.

> *THE SIMPLE RANDOM SAMPLING PROCEDURE*
>
> **1.** Determine the sampling frame and sampling units.
>
> **2.** Assign an identification number to each of the N units in the sampling frame.
>
> **3.** Determine the number of sampling units (n) that must be sampled to achieve the desired accuracy of the statistical analysis.
>
> **4.** Using a computer, select n identification numbers at random in a fashion that each unit has the same chance of being selected. These identification numbers identify the units to be selected in the sample.
>
> **5.** Collect and measure the units corresponding to the n units whose identification numbers were selected in step 4.

Simple random sampling is often used in the selection of individuals to be used in an experiment or a clinical trial. A researcher may be tempted to self-select the individuals for the experiment, but self-selection often introduces an unwanted source of bias into the sample. To draw honest conclusions from an experiment it is critical to have a sample that is free of bias and one that is representative of the target population being studied. When a researcher has a large pool of volunteers for an experiment, simple random sampling can be a reasonable way to obtain a representative sample from the pool of volunteers. Example 3.5 illustrates how to select a simple random sample.

Example 3.5

Suppose 10 individuals from a list of 25 carefully screened volunteers are to be selected for an experiment. The name of the volunteers, their age, and their gender are listed in Table 3.1.

This sampling frame contains 14 males (56%) and 11 females (44%) that have age ranging from 33 to 69. Identification number from 1 to 25 are assigned to each individual, and the list of volunteers with their identification numbers, age, and gender is given in Table 3.2.

Now there are

$$\binom{25}{10} = \frac{25!}{10!15!} = 3,268,760$$

TABLE 3.1 List of Volunteers from Which 10 Individuals Will be Selected

Name	Age	Gender	Name	Age	Gender
C. Smith	33	M	L. Griffin	49	F
T. Jones	53	F	S. Lufkin	39	F
R. Halmoth	63	M	K. Goren	59	M
A. Sadler	53	M	T. Green	69	M
P. Yawler	46	F	L. Samson	44	F
R. Tascher	52	M	M. Noone	55	F
W. Smythe	47	F	O. Reed	51	F
E. Morgan	61	M	J. Winston	59	F
C. Scott	66	M	F. Loomis	56	M
T. Johnson	58	F	H. Pengstrom	55	M
G. Abel	62	F	Y. Engolin	54	M
R. Rose	66	M	L. Howard	59	M
D. Donaldson	64	M			

TABLE 3.2   List of Volunteers with Identification Numbers

ID	Name	Age	Gender	ID	Name	Age	Gender
1	C. Smith	33	M	14	L. Griffin	49	F
2	T. Jones	53	F	15	S. Lufkin	39	F
3	R. Halmoth	63	M	16	K. Goren	59	M
4	A. Sadler	53	M	17	T. Green	69	M
5	P. Yawler	46	F	18	L. Samson	44	F
6	R. Tascher	52	M	19	M. Noone	55	F
7	W. Smythe	47	F	20	O. Reed	51	F
8	E. Morgan	61	M	21	J. Winston	59	F
9	C. Scott	66	M	22	F. Loomis	56	M
10	T. Johnson	58	23	23	H. Pengstrom	55	M
11	G. Abel	62	F	24	Y. Engolin	54	M
12	R. Rose	66	M	25	L. Howard	59	M
13	D. Donaldson	64	M				

TABLE 3.3   List of Individuals to be Sampled

ID	Name	Age	Gender	ID	Name	Age	Gender
8	E. Morgan	61	M	17	T. Green	69	M
3	R. Halmoth	63	M	4	A. Sadler	53	M
19	M. Noone	55	F	5	P. Yawler	46	F
15	S. Lufkin	39	F	22	F. Loomis	56	M
24	Y. Engolin	54	M	11	G. Abel	62	F

possible samples of size 10 that can be selected from this sampling frame. MINITAB was used to select 10 of the 25 identification numbers in a fashion so that each possible sample has the same chance of being selected. The 10 identification numbers selected by MINITAB for the simple random sample are 8, 17, 3, 4, 19, 5, 15, 22, 24, and 11, and a list of the individuals to be sampled is given in Table 3.3.

Note that the sample has 6 males (60%) and 4 females (40%) with ages ranging from 39 to 69. The mean and median of the original 25 individuals are $\mu = 54.9$ and $\tilde{\mu} = 55$, and the mean and median of the 10 individuals sampled are 55.8 and 55.5, respectively. Although the sample does not exactly mirror the population, it is fairly representative of the target population.

Several properties of a simple random sample are listed below.

PROPERTIES OF A SIMPLE RANDOM SAMPLE

1. Simple random samples are generally the easiest sampling plans to implement and generate data that are easily analyzed.

2. Simple random samples are likely to produce samples that are representative of a homogeneous or heterogeneous population.

3. Simple random samples are free from bias since no portion of the population is more likely to be sampled than any other portion of the population, provided the sampling frame covers the target population.

4. When the sample size is less than 5% of the number of units in the frame, the observations in a simple random sample are essentially independent of one another.

Although simple random samples are easy to implement and analyze, they are not always the most efficient sampling plans when there are distinct subpopulations that the researcher is interested in. In particular, when the target population has one or more small subpopulations, the simple random sampling plan is not designed to ensure these small subpopulations are adequately sampled. For example, suppose there is a clear genetic marker that predisposes an individual to a particular disease that only 1% of the general population has. If a simple random sample of $n = 100$ observations is to be selected from the general population, only one observation would be expected to have this genetic marker, and it is possible that none of the observations would be sampled from the subpopulation of individuals with this genetic marker. In fact, only 1% of any sample would be expected to be in this subpopulation. In this case, a simple random sample is not an efficient way of sampling the population with regard to the focus of this research, and a specialized sampling plan ensuring that the subpopulations are adequately represented in the sample is needed.

Example 3.6
Because only 1% of the US population has AB negative blood, it would take a simple random sample of approximately 10,000 individuals to obtain 100 individuals with the AB negative blood; if only 100 individuals were sampled, the sample may not even contain one individual having AB negative blood. Thus, to ensure that a sufficient number of individuals having AB negative blood are sampled, an alternative to the simple random sampling plan would be needed.

There are many specialized sampling plans that have been developed to take care of the situations where simple random sampling cannot be expected to produce a sample representative of the target population. It is important to keep in mind that the sampling plan that should be used in a particular research study will depend upon the structure of the population, the research questions, and any logistical considerations associated with sampling the population. Furthermore, prior information about the target population and sound professional judgment should be used in developing the sampling plan that will be used in place of a simple random sample.

3.2.2 Stratified Random Sampling

When a target population has well-defined subpopulations, the research questions are usually focused on the parameters of the subpopulations. In this case, it is important that the random sample contains sufficient data for estimating the parameters of interest in the subpopulations. Because a simple random sample cannot guarantee that each subpopulation is sufficiently represented in a sample, simple random sampling is generally not the most efficient method of sampling a target population with well-defined subpopulations.

A random sampling plan that is designed specifically for populations having distinct subpopulations is *stratified random sampling*. A stratified random sample should be used when the target population has well-defined and nonoverlapping subpopulations. The subpopulations of the target population are referred to as *strata* and a single subpopulation is called a *stratum*. A stratified random sample is a sample that is drawn by collecting a simple random sample from each stratum in the population. The process for drawing a stratified random sample is outlined below.

THE STRATIFIED RANDOM SAMPLING PROCEDURE

1. Identify the strata in the target population.
2. Develop a good sampling frame for each stratum.
3. Determine the overall sample size and the strata sample sizes.
4. Select a simple random sample from each of the strata.

Having good sampling frames for each strata and determining the appropriate sample sizes for each strata are critical components of a well-designed stratified random sampling plan. The cost of sampling within the strata and the variability within each stratum play important roles in the determination of the overall sample size and the strata sample sizes. Determination of the appropriate sample size for a stratified random sample and allocation of the sample to the strata will be discussed in detail Section 3.3.

In biomedical research studies, target populations having subpopulations are the norm rather than the exception. For example, studies involving humans often have subpopulations due to gender, race, blood type, and many other human characteristics. To investigate how these subpopulations of humans differ in a biomedical research problem, a stratified random sample can often be used to obtain the sample data that will be used in comparing the subpopulations of interest.

Example 3.7
Stratified random sampling might be the appropriate sampling plan in each of the following scenarios. Suppose the target population includes subpopulations defined by

a. male and female individuals;
b. hospitals in different regions of the country;
c. individuals with different blood types;
d. individuals of different races;
e. individuals in different age groups.

When a stratified random sample is properly used, the precision of the estimates based on stratified random sample will often be greater than the precision obtained through a simple random sample. Several properties of a stratified random sample are listed below.

PROPERTIES OF A STRATIFIED RANDOM SAMPLE

- A stratified random sample provides information on each subpopulations in the target population.
- A well-designed stratified random sample will produce sufficient evidence for estimating the parameters of the subpopulations.
- A stratified random sample is an efficient sampling plan and produces reliable estimates when there are well-defined subpopulations in the target population.
- A well-designed stratified random sample will reduce the costs associated with sampling the target population.
- The allocation of the overall sample size to the strata can be designed to satisfy several different constraints such as producing a sample that will minimize the cost of sampling or maximizes the reliability of an estimate.

Because the sampling plan for a stratified random sample is more complex than the sampling plan associated with a simple random sample, designing a stratified random sample requires information on each of the subpopulations. In particular, To have a stratified random sample, which is representative of the target population, it is critical that representative sampling frames are available for each of the strata.

When the research questions are based on studying or comparing the subpopulations in the target population, it is imperative that sufficient data are collected on individual subpopulations. Thus, because a well-designed stratified random sample can guarantee that a predetermined amount of data will be collected on the subpopulations, a stratified random sample should always be used as the sampling plan when the research questions center on the characteristics and parameters of the subpopulations in the target population.

3.2.3 Cluster Sampling

In many biomedical studies, a good sampling frame containing the units in the target population is extremely difficult to obtain. In some cases, the units of the population belong to clearly defined groups of units referred to as *clusters* of units. When a sampling frame that contains a list of clusters is available a random cluster sample can often be used to obtain a sample that is representative of the target population. For example, in surveying the general health of the people living in a particular town, a sampling frame consisting of the people living in the town would be difficult, if not impossible, to obtain. On the other hand, most towns will have a listing of the housing units within the town. In this case, the people living in the town are grouped in clusters according to housing units.

To use a random cluster sample, the clusters in a target population should be nonoverlapping and exhaustive so that a population unit belongs to only one cluster. Also, when the population units belong to well-defined clusters and a random cluster sample is selected, the cluster random sample will consist of *primary* and *secondary* units. The primary units in a cluster sampling plan are the clusters of population units and the secondary units are the units within the clusters. Thus, a primary unit is a sampling unit and a secondary unit is sampling element.

Example 3.8
A cluster random sample might be the appropriate sampling plan in each of the following scenarios:

a. Patient records from the hospitals in a state are being studied. Here, the hospitals are the clusters and patients are the secondary units in a cluster.

b. Infection rates on the floors of a hospital are being studied. The floors of a hospital are the clusters and the beds or rooms on a floor are the secondary units in a cluster.

c. The general health of the residents living in a city is being studied. Here, housing units might be used as the clusters and individuals living in a housing the secondary units in a cluster.

d. The care of patients living in nursing homes is being studied. Here, the nursing homes are the clusters and the patients in a nursing home are the secondary units in a cluster.

A cluster random sample is drawn by taking a simple random sample of clusters from the sampling frame and then measuring each of the secondary units within the clusters sampled. The process for drawing a cluster random sample is outlined below.

THE CLUSTER SAMPLING PROCEDURE

1. Determine the clusters of units in the target population.

2. Determine a sampling frame listing the clusters of population units. The sampling frame should cover the entire target population.

3. Assign identification numbers to the clusters in the sampling frame.

4. Determine the appropriate number of clusters to be sampled.

5. Using a computer, draw a simple random sample of the identification numbers.

6. Obtain the sample data from the clusters selected in step 5. In this step, the primary units (i.e., clusters) are sampled and the data are recorded by measuring each of the secondary units in a cluster that is sampled.

Note that the sampling frame used in a cluster sample is a list of the clusters available for sampling, and the sample size n is the number of clusters, and not the number of population units, that will be sampled. A cluster sample can also be designed as a two-stage sampling plan with first stage consisting of drawing a sample of n clusters and second stage consisting of drawing a random sample of the secondary units within a sampled cluster.

Example 3.9
In 2004, the World Health Organization (WHO) studied the mortality rate of internally displaced persons in Darfur, Sudan. Over one million residents of Darfur, Sudan sought refuge away from areas of conflict and 127 settlements of internally displaced persons were identified. Concern over the health status and mortality rate of internally displaced persons led to a WHO study in Darfur. The primary goal of this study was to estimate the crude mortality rate of internally displaced persons over the period June 15, 2004–August 15, 2004.

The sampling plan used to collect data for this study was a cluster random sample. The target population was all internally displaced persons in Darfur, Sudan and the clusters were settlements of internally displaced persons. The sampling frame consisted of internally displaced settlements listed by the World Food Programme (WFP) and the United Nations Office for the Coordination of Humanitarian Affairs (OCHA). Settlements that were not accessible due to poor roads or security reasons were deleted from the sampling frame. The sample size used in this study was $n = 50$ clusters, which were selected at random from the sampling frame.

Cluster random samples are typically used when a good sampling frame of population units is impossible or too expensive to obtain and there are well-defined clusters of units in the target population, which can be easily identified. Several properties of the cluster random sample are listed below.

PROPERTIES OF A RANDOM CLUSTER SAMPLE

1. Clusters of units can sometimes be defined by the geographic location of the units.

2. Cluster sampling is often less expensive than other methods of sampling.

3. Cluster sampling can be designed to handle subpopulations by using a stratified cluster random sample.

4. The collection and measuring of the sample data are often simpler in a cluster sample than in other sampling plans because the population units are sampled in clusters of units rather than as individual units.

The disadvantages of using random cluster sample are that cluster sampling may lead to biased results when the clusters of units sampled are not representative of whole population and the cost of a cluster sample will increase as the distance between the units in a cluster increases. Finally, when a sampling frame containing the population is available, a sampling plan other than a cluster sample should be used unless the cost benefits outweigh the loss of precision in the estimates obtained from the cluster sample.

3.2.4 Systematic Sampling

The final sampling plan that will be discussed is the *systematic random sampling* plan. A *1 in k systematic sample* is a probability sample obtained by randomly selecting one sampling unit from the first k units in the sampling frame and every kth unit thereafter. A systematic random sample is one of the most cost-effective and convenient sampling plans when the population units are randomly dispersed over the sampling frame. Systematic random sampling is also useful in quality control settings. For example, a pharmaceutical company may check the uniformity and quality of the drug tablets it manufactures. The ability to control the manufacturing process by sampling the output is an important aspect of quality control and may be monitored by selecting a systematic random sample of every 100th tablet produced.

The process for drawing a systematic random sample is outlined below.

THE SYSTEMATIC SAMPLE PROCEDURE

---

1. Determine the sampling interval k. Usually, the sampling interval k is the integer closest to $k = N/n$, where N is the number of units in the sampling frame and n is the desired sample size.

2. Select the starting point in the sampling frame by selecting a unit at random from the first k sampling units in the frame.

3. Select every kth unit in the sampling frame until n units have been selected.

4. Collect the data on the sampling units associated with the identification numbers selected in step 3. This is the data resulting from the systematic random sample.

The advantages of drawing a systematic random sample are that it is simple to collect, often less expensive than other sampling plans, spreads uniformly over the sampling frame, the statistical analysis of a systematic random sample is the same as the analysis used with a simple random sample, and when the size of the population is not fixed or is being monitored over time, a systematic random sample can be easily implemented without a sampling frame.

The only real disadvantage of using a systematic random sample occurs when a systematic sample isolates unwanted patterns in the population. That is, a systematic random sample may yield a biased sample when there is a periodic or cyclic pattern in the units listed in the sampling frame. Thus, it is critical to avoid the use of a systematic random sample when there could be cyclical patterns in the sampling frame or the sampling process. Cyclical patterns are often due to sampling the units over time.

Example 3.10

In the article "Insulin and gall stones: a population case–control study in southern Italy" published in *Gut* (Misciagna, 2000), the relationship between hyperinsulinaemia and gall stones was studied based on a systematic random sample was selected from a sampling frame consisting of the electoral register of Castellana, Italy. This systematic random sample yielded 2472 individuals who then had their gall bladder checked for gall stones and were contacted again between May 1992 and June 1993 for another gall stone screening.

3.3 DETERMINING THE SAMPLE SIZE

One of the most important aspects of any sampling plan is the determination of the number of units to sample. The sample size is denoted by n and is determined by several factors including

- the size of the population;
- the level of reliability required in the statistical analysis;
- the cost of sampling;
- whether or not subpopulations are present in the population;
- the variability in the population.

Of all the factors affecting the sample size, the most important factor to consider is the degree of reliability that will be required of the statistical analysis; The measures of reliability for a statistical analysis will depend on the statistical methods used in the analysis; however, one of the more commonly used measures of reliability for an estimate of a population proportion or mean is the *bound on the error of estimation*, which is denoted by B. The bound on the error of estimation is based on the two standard deviation empirical rule. Moreover, it is unlikely for an estimate of a proportion or a mean to be farther than B from the value of the population proportion or mean being estimated. Careful consideration must be given in prespecifying the value of B in designing a sampling plan with the appropriate sample size. That is, when n is too small, the estimates will not be reliable enough to provide useful information, and when the sample size is too large the benefits of having a large sample are not cost-effective.

In the following section, methods for determining the appropriate sample size for a given value of the bound on the error of estimation will be discussed only for simple random, stratified random, and systematic random samples. The determination of the sample size for a cluster sample is beyond the scope of this book but is covered in many specialized textbooks on sampling.

3.3.1 The Sample Size for a Simple Random Sample

In determining the sample size n that will produce a prespecified bound on the error of estimation, the number of units in the population (N) and the variance of the population (σ^2) must be known. When N and σ^2 are known, then the number of observations needed for estimating a mean (μ) with bound on the error of estimation of B is

$$n = \frac{N\sigma^2}{(N-1)D + \sigma^2}$$

where $D = B^2/4$. Note that this formula will not generally return a whole number for the sample size n; when the formula does not return a whole number for the sample size, the sample size should be taken to be the next largest whole number.

Example 3.11

Suppose a simple random sample is going to be taken from a population of $N = 5000$ units with a variance of $\sigma^2 = 50$. If the bound on the error of estimation of the mean is supposed to be $B = 1.5$, then the sample size required for the simple random sample selected from this population is

$$n = \frac{5000(50)}{4999 \left(\frac{1.5^2}{4} \right) + 50} = 87.35$$

Since 87.35 units cannot be sampled, the sample size that should be used is $n = 88$.

In many research projects, the values of N or σ^2 are often unknown. When either N or σ^2 is unknown, the formula for determining the sample size to produce a bound on the error of estimation for a simple random sample can still be used as long as the approximate values of N and σ^2 are available. In this case, the resulting sample size will produce a bound on the error of estimation that is close to B provided the approximate values of N and σ^2 are reasonably accurate.

The proportion of the units in the population that are sampled is n/N, which is called the *sampling proportion*. When a rough guess of the size of the population cannot be reasonably made, but it is clear that the sampling proportion will be less than 5%, then an alternative formula for determining the sample size is needed. In this case, the sample size required for a simple random sample having bound on the error of estimation of B for estimating the mean is approximately

$$n = \frac{4\sigma^2}{B^2}$$

Example 3.12

Suppose a simple random sample is going to be drawn from a large population with well over 1,000,000 units. Due to the cost of sampling this population, a sample of no more than 5000 units can be sampled. Thus, the sampling proportion is $n/N \leq 5000/1,000,000 \leq 0.005$. Suppose that the standard deviation is known to be roughly $\sigma = 100$, then the sample size needed to have a bound on the error of estimation of $B = 10$ for estimating the mean is roughly

$$n = \frac{4 \cdot 100^2}{10^2} = 400$$

To determine the sample size required in a study, the population variance must be known. Unfortunately, the variance of the target population is generally an unknown parameter. Thus, while a researcher might not know the exact value of the variance, it is likely that the researcher will have a rough idea of the variability in the target population. In particular, there are several methods that can be used to a obtain a rough estimate of population variance.

1. Previous research studies or prior knowledge about the target population can be used to develop a rough estimate of σ^2.

2. When the population is approximately normally distributed, a rough estimate of the standard deviation can be based on

$$\sigma \approx \frac{\text{maximum value in the population} - \text{minimum value in the population}}{4}$$

3. A small sample of the population units can be sampled in a pilot study for estimating the value of σ^2.

The population proportions are also often studied in biomedical research. The sample size required for estimating a population proportion, say p, with a bound on the error of estimation B will also depend on the values of N and σ^2. In this case, the variance is $\sigma^2 = p(1-p)$, and the number of observations needed for estimating a population proportion with bound on the error of estimation of B is

$$n = \frac{Np(1-p)}{(N-1)D + p(1-p)}$$

where $D = B^2/4$. However, since the value of p will be unknown to a researcher, a reasonable guess of the value of p is needed to use this formula because the variance will take on its largest value, $\sigma^2 = 0.25$, when $p = 0.5$, using $p = 0.5$ in the above formula will produce a conservative sample size that will guarantee the bound on the error of estimation does not exceed B. That is, the value of n found using $p = 0.5$ will be larger than the actual value needed to obtain a bound on the error of estimation. Furthermore, since the value of n is larger than necessary, the resulting value of B will be smaller than anticipated by the formula. Thus, the conservative sample size that will produce a bound on the error of estimation that does not exceed B is

$$n = \frac{(0.25)N}{(N-1)D + 0.25}$$

where $D = B^2/4$.

Example 3.13
Suppose a simple random sample is going to be taken from a population of $N = 80,000$ units to estimate an unknown proportion p. If the desired bound on the error of estimation for estimating the proportion is $B = 0.025$, then the conservative estimate of the sample size is

$$n = \frac{80,000(0.25)}{79,999 \left(\frac{0.025^2}{4}\right) + 0.25} = 1568.65$$

Thus, the sample size that should be used for this simple random sample is $n = 1569$.

When N is unknown and a rough guess of the size of the population cannot be made, an alternative formula for determining the sample size required to produce a bound on the error of estimation for estimating a proportion that does not exceed the value B is

$$n = \frac{1}{B^2}$$

Example 3.14
Suppose a simple random sample is going to be taken from a population with a large number of units to estimate a proportion p. If N is unknown and the desired bound on the error of estimation for estimating the proportion is $B = 0.025$, then the conservative estimate of the sample size is

$$n = \frac{1}{0.025^2} = 1600$$

Finally, the cost of sampling when using a simple random sample is

$$C = C_0 + nC_1$$

where C_0 is the initial cost of designing the sampling plan, obtaining a sampling frame, training samplers, and any other initial costs normally associated with the overhead cost of sampling, and C_1 is the cost incurred in the act of sampling a unit from the target population.

Example 3.15
Suppose the initial cost involved in sampling the target population is $12,000 and the cost of sampling a unit from the population is $25. A simple random sample of 581 units drawn from this population would have a total cost of

$$C = \$12,000 + 581(\$25) = \$26{,}525$$

In many biomedical research studies, a compromise must be made between the total cost of sampling and the number of units that need to be sampled. Clearly, a researcher cannot sample more units than can be afforded; however, when a specific bound on the error of estimation is required to have useful estimates, then sufficient funding must be ensured since the number of units cannot be reduced. When sufficient funding is not available for sampling, the best approach is to sample as many observations as can be afforded that will produce a larger value of B than was desired. Thus, when a researcher's budget does not allow an adequate number of units to be sampled, the researcher must decide whether the information gained from the smaller sample is even worth the expense and efforts of carrying out the research project.

Example 3.16
Suppose the initial cost involved in sampling the target population is $37,000, the cost of sampling a unit is $130, and the total budget available for sampling is $100,000. A simple random sample is to be selected from the target population with $N = 200,000$ and $\sigma^2 \approx 1200$. If the required bound on the error of estimation for estimating the mean is $B = 1.5$, based on the cost values the number of units that the researcher can afford to draw is

$$n_{\text{afford}} = \frac{100{,}000 - 37{,}000}{130} = 484.5$$

Thus, the researcher can afford to sample 484 units. However, the number of units required for a bound on the error of estimation equal to 1.5 is

$$\frac{200{,}000(1200)}{199{,}999 \left(\frac{1.5^2}{4} \right) + 1200} = 2110.8$$

Thus, the required sample size for $B = 1.5$ is $n = 2,111$, but the researcher can only afford to sample 484 units. The trade-off in this case is that with only 484 units the value of B would be roughly 3.1 rather than 1.5. At this point, the researcher would have to re-evaluate the need to have a value of $B = 1.5$; if a value of $B = 3.1$ would still provide meaningful information about the mean of the target population, then a sample of size $n = 484$ units would be acceptable. On the other hand, if it is critical for the estimate of the mean to be within $B = 1.5$ of the true value of μ, then the researcher must find more funds to facilitate a simple random sample of $n = 2111$ units.

3.3.2 The Sample Size for a Stratified Random Sample

Recall that a stratified random sample is simply a collection of simple random samples selected from the subpopulations in the target population. In a stratified random sample, there are two sample size considerations, namely, the overall sample size n and the allocation of n units over the strata. When there are k strata, the strata sample sizes will be denoted by $n_1, n_2, n_3, \ldots, n_k$, where the number to be sampled in strata 1 is n_1, the number to be sampled in strata 2 is n_2, and so on.

There are several different ways of determining the overall sample size and its allocation in a stratified random sample. In particular, *proportional allocation* and *optimal allocation* are two commonly used allocation plans. Throughout the discussion of these two allocation plans, it will be assumed that the target population has k strata, N units, and N_j is the number of units in the jth stratum.

The sample size used in a stratified random sample and the most efficient allocation of the sample will depend on several factors including the variability within each of the strata, the proportion of the target population in each of the strata, and the costs associated with sampling the units from the strata. Let σ_i be the standard deviation of the ith stratum, $W_i = N_i/N$ the proportion of the target population in the ith stratum, C_0 the initial cost of sampling, C_i the cost of obtaining an observation from the ith stratum, and C is the total cost of sampling. Then, the cost of sampling with a stratified random sample is

$$C = C_0 + C_1 n_1 + C_2 n_2 + \cdots + C_k n_k$$

The process of determining the sample size for a stratified random sample requires that the allocation of the sample be determined first. The allocation of the sample size n over the k strata is based on the *sampling proportions* that are denoted by $w_1, w_2, \ldots w_k$. Once the sampling proportions and the overall sample size n have been determined, the ith stratum sample size is $n_i = n \times w_i$.

The simplest allocation plan for a stratified random sample is *proportional allocation* that takes the sampling proportions to be proportional to the strata sizes. Thus, in proportional allocation, the sampling proportion for the ith stratum is equal to the proportion of the population in the ith stratum. That is, the sampling proportion for the ith stratum is

$$w_i = \frac{N_i}{N}$$

The overall sample size for a stratified random sample based on proportional allocation that will have bound on error of estimation for estimating the mean equal to B is

$$n = \frac{N_1 \sigma_1^2 + N_2 \sigma_2^2 + \cdots + N_k \sigma_k^2}{N \left[\frac{B^2}{4} \right] + \frac{1}{N} \left(N_1 \sigma_1^2 + N_2 \sigma_2^2 + \cdots + N_k \sigma_k^2 \right)}$$

The sample size for the simple random sample that will be selected from the ith stratum according to proportional allocation is

$$n \times w_i = n \times \frac{N_i}{N}$$

TABLE 3.4 Strata Size, Standard Deviation, and the Cost of Sampling for the Three Strata in the Target Population

Stratum	N	SD	Cost
1	1000	10	9
2	1500	12	4
3	2500	8	25

Example 3.17

Suppose the target population consists of three strata. Use Table 3.4 to determine the overall sample size and the proportional allocation for a stratified random sample that will have bound on the error of estimation for estimating the mean of $B = 1.5$. Also, determine the total cost of sampling when the initial cost associated with sampling is $C_0 = \$1000$. There are $N = 1000 + 1500 + 2500 = 5000$ units in the target population, and the proportional allocation sampling proportions are

$$w_1 = \frac{1000}{5000} = 0.2, \quad w_2 = \frac{1500}{5000} = 0.3, \quad \text{and } w_3 = \frac{2500}{5000} = 0.5$$

The overall sample size is

$$n = \frac{1000(10^2) + 1500(12^2) + 2500(8^2)}{5000 \left[\frac{1.5^2}{4} \right] + \frac{1}{5000} 1000(10^2) + 1500(12^2) + 2500(8^2)} = 163.7$$

and thus, the overall sample size is $n = 164$. The strata sample sizes according to proportional allocation are

$$n_1 = 0.2(164) = 32.8$$
$$n_2 = 0.3(164) = 49.2$$
$$n_3 = 0.5(164) = 82$$

When the overall cost of sampling is not fixed, the stratified random sampling the sizes can safely be rounded off to the nearest whole number, and thus, the sampling allocation for this stratified random sample is $n_1 = 33, n_2 = 49$, and $n_3 = 82$. The total cost of this sampling plan is

$$C = \$1000 + 33 \times \$9 + 49 \times \$4 + 82 \times \$25 = \$3543$$

When a stratified random sample will be used to estimate a population proportion with bound on the error of estimation equal to B, the overall sample size using proportional allocation is

$$n = \frac{N_1 p_1(1 - p_1) + N_2 p_2(1 - p_2) + \cdots + N_k p_k(1 - p_k)}{N \left[\frac{B^2}{4} \right] + \frac{1}{N} (N_1 p_1(1 - p_1) + N_2 p_2(1 - p_2) + \cdots + N_k p_k(1 - p_k))}$$

where p_i is the proportion of the ith stratum having the characteristic of interest. The ith stratum sample size is

$$n \times w_i = n \times \frac{N_i}{N}$$

Because the values of $p_1, p_2, \ldots, p_k$ are unknown, a conservative estimate of the overall sample size can be found by using $p_i = 0.5$. In this case,

$$n = \frac{N}{NB^2 + 1}$$

TABLE 3.5   Strata Size and the Cost of Sampling the Three Strata in the Target Population

Stratum	N	Cost
1	1000	5
2	1500	4
3	2500	11

Example 3.18

Suppose the target population consists of three strata. Use Table 3.5 to determine the overall sample size and the proportional allocation for a stratified random sample that will have a bound on the error of estimation for estimating a proportion of $B = 0.05$. Also, determine the total cost of sampling when the initial cost is $C_0 = \$2400$.

Because there is no information available on the values of p_1, p_2, and p_3, the conservative value for the overall sample size for n is

$$n = \frac{5000}{5000(0.05^2) + 1} = 370.4$$

Thus, the overall sample size is $n = 371$ and the strata sample sizes are

$$n_1 = 374 \times \frac{1000}{5000} = 74.8$$

$$n_2 = 374 \times \frac{1500}{5000} = 112.2$$

$$n_3 = 374 \times \frac{2500}{5000} = 187$$

Thus, take the strata sample sizes to be $n_1 = 75$, $n_2 = 112$, and $n_3 = 187$, and the total cost associated with this stratified random sample is

$$C = \$2400 + 75 \times \$5 + 112 \times \$4 + 187 \times \$11 = \$5280$$

Note that proportional allocation takes into consideration only the variability within the strata and the proportion of population units in each of the strata in determining the overall sample size. Thus, the cost of sampling each strata is not a factor in determining the overall sample size when proportional allocation is used. For example, in Example 3.18 the cost of sampling a unit in strata 3 was \$11 and the largest portion of the sample was allocated to strata 3 making the total cost of sampling high.

Optimal allocation is an allocation plan that takes into account the cost of sampling as well as the variability and proportion of the target population in each strata in determining the overall sample size. Furthermore, optimal allocation can be used to allocate the overall sample size n for either minimizing the bound on the error of estimation when the total cost of sampling is fixed or to minimize the total cost of sampling when the bound on the error of estimation is fixed. That is, when the total cost of sampling is fixed optimal allocation produces the sample size that minimizes the bound on the error of estimation, and when the value of the bound on the error of estimation is fixed prior to sampling optimal allocation will produce a sample that has a minimum total cost of sampling.

The overall sample size for estimating either a mean or proportion in a stratified random sample using optimal allocation when the total cost of sampling is a fixed value C is

$$n = \frac{(C - C_0)\left[\frac{N_1\sigma_1}{\sqrt{C_1}} + \frac{N_2\sigma_2}{\sqrt{C_2}} + \cdots + \frac{N_k\sigma_k}{\sqrt{C_k}}\right]}{N_1\sigma_1\sqrt{C_1} + N_2\sigma_2\sqrt{C_1} + \cdots + N_k\sigma_k\sqrt{C_k}}$$

where C_0 is the initial setup cost and C_i is the cost of sampling a unit from the ith stratum. Note that for estimating a proportion $\sigma_i = \sqrt{p_i(1 - p_i)}$ and $\sigma_i = 0.5$ should be used when no information on the values of the p_i's are available.

The optimal allocation sampling proportions are

$$w_i = \frac{\frac{N_i \sigma_i}{\sqrt{C_i}}}{\frac{N_1 \sigma_1}{\sqrt{C_1}} + \frac{N_2 \sigma_2}{\sqrt{C_2}} + \cdots + \frac{N_k \sigma_k}{\sqrt{C_k}}}$$

The strata sample sizes are again computed using the formula

$$n_i = n \times w_i$$

and the strata sample sizes are again $n_i = n \times w_i$.

Note that when optimal allocation is used to determine the sample size for a stratified random sample strata, sizes (N_i), the strata standard deviations (σ_i), the initial cost associated with sampling (C_0), and the cost of sampling each strata (C_i) must be available to determine the overall and strata sample sizes. When estimating a proportion with a stratified random sample, the strata standard deviations are $\sigma_i = \sqrt{p_i(1 - p_i)}$, and since p_i is unknown, the value of $p_i = 0.5$ is used to determine a conservative sample size.

Example 3.19

Suppose the target population consists of two strata. Use Table 3.6 to determine the overall sample size and the strata sample sizes using optimal allocation when the total cost is fixed at $20,000 and the initial cost is $C_0 = \$4800$.

The overall sample size is

$$n = \frac{15,200 \left(\frac{2500(25)}{5} + \frac{7500(12)}{4} \right)}{2500(25)5 + 7500(12)4} = 791.1$$

and because the budget for sampling is fixed at $20,000, the researcher will only be able to afford to sample 791 units. The optimal allocation sampling proportions are

$$w_1 = \frac{\frac{2500(25)}{5}}{\frac{2500(25)}{5} + \frac{7500(12)}{4}} = 0.36$$

$$w_2 = \frac{\frac{7500(12)}{4}}{\frac{2500(25)}{5} + \frac{7500(12)}{4}} = 0.64$$

Thus, the strata sample sizes are $n_1 = 791 \times 0.36 = 284$ and $n_2 = 791 \times 0.64 = 506$. Note that because the total cost of sampling is fixed, the strata sample sizes must be rounded off to the next lowest whole number. Thus, the total cost of sampling the 791 units when optimal allocation used is

$$C = \$4800 + 284 \times \$25 + 506 \times \$16 = \$19,996$$

TABLE 3.6   Strata Size, Standard Deviation, and the Cost of Sampling for the Two Strata in the Target Population

Stratum	N	SD	Cost
1	2500	25	25
2	7500	12	16

TABLE 3.7 Strata Size and Cost of Sampling the Two Strata in the Target Population

Stratum	N	Cost
1	5000	16
2	15000	25

Example 3.20

Suppose the target population consists of two strata. Use Table 3.7 to determine the conservative estimate of the overall sample size and the optimal allocation for a stratified random sample designed to estimate a proportion when the total cost of sampling is fixed at $10,000 with an initial cost of $C_0 = \$3600$.

The overall sample size is

$$n = \frac{6400 \left(\dfrac{5000(0.5)}{4} + \dfrac{15,000(0.5)}{5} \right)}{5000(0.5)4 + 15,000(0.5)5} = 286.3$$

and because the total cost of sampling is fixed at $10,000, the researcher will only be able to afford to sample 286 units. The optimal allocation sampling proportions are

$$w_1 = \frac{\dfrac{5000(0.5)}{4}}{\dfrac{5000(0.5)}{4} + \dfrac{15,000(0.5)}{5}} = 0.29$$

$$w_2 = \frac{\dfrac{15,000(0.5)}{5}}{\dfrac{5000(0.5)}{4} + \dfrac{15,000(0.5)}{5}} = 0.71$$

Thus, the optimal allocation for a stratified random sample having a minimum bound on the error of estimation for estimating a proportion with a fixed cost of $10,000 will be an overall sample size of $n = 286$. The strata sample sizes are $n_1 = 286 \times 0.29 = 82$ and $n_2 = 286 \times 0.71 = 203$. Again, because the total cost of sampling is fixed, the strata sample sizes must be rounded off to the next lowest whole number. Thus, the total cost of sampling 286 units with optimal allocation is

$$C = \$3600 + 82 \times \$16 + 203 \times \$25 = \$9987$$

When it is more important to control the bound on the error of estimation than it is to control the cost of sampling, the sample size computations are different; however, the computation of the strata sampling proportions is the same. Suppose the bound on the error of estimation for estimating the mean or a proportion is fixed at value B. The sample size required to attain a bound on the error of estimation equal to B that will minimize the total cost of sampling is

$$n = \frac{\left(\frac{N_1 \sigma_1}{\sqrt{C_1}} + \frac{N_2 \sigma_2}{\sqrt{C_2}} + \cdots + \frac{N_k \sigma_k}{\sqrt{C_k}} \right) \left(N_1 \sigma_1 \sqrt{C_1} + N_2 \sigma_2 \sqrt{C_2} + \cdots + N_k \sigma_k \sqrt{C_k} \right)}{N^2 D + (N_1 \sigma_1^2 + N_2 \sigma_2^2 + \cdots + N_k \sigma_k^2)}$$

where $D = B^2/4$. Again, when a proportion is being estimated, the value p_i can be replaced by $p_i = 0.5$ to produce a conservative estimate of n.

TABLE 3.8 Strata Size, Standard Deviation, and Cost of Sampling the Three Strata in the Target Population

Stratum	N	SD	Cost
1	5,000	10	9
2	7,500	12	4
3	12,500	8	16

When the value of B is fixed and the total cost of sampling is minimized, optimal allocation sampling proportions are

$$w_i = \frac{\frac{N_i \sigma_i}{\sqrt{C_i}}}{\frac{N_1 \sigma_1}{\sqrt{C_1}} + \frac{N_2 \sigma_2}{\sqrt{C_2}} + \cdots + \frac{N_k \sigma_k}{\sqrt{C_k}}}$$

Example 3.21

Suppose a stratified random sample is to be drawn from a population having three strata for the purpose of estimating the mean of the target population. Using Table 3.8, determine the overall sample size and the strata sample sizes that minimize the total cost of sampling when the bound on the error of estimation is fixed at $B = 2$ and the initial cost of sampling is $C_0 = \$5300$.

The sample size required to produce a bound of $B = 2$ is

$$n = \frac{\left(\frac{5000(10)}{\sqrt{9}} + \frac{7500(12)}{\sqrt{4}} + \frac{12,500(8)}{\sqrt{16}} \right) \left(5000(10)\sqrt{9} + 7500(12)\sqrt{4} + 12,500(8)\sqrt{16} \right)}{25,000^2 \left[\frac{2^2}{4} \right] + 5000(10^2) + 7500(12^2) + 12,500(8^2)}$$

$$= 100.8$$

Thus, the sample size required to have a bound on the error of estimation equal to 2 is $n = 101$. The optimal allocation sampling proportions are

$$w_1 = \frac{\dfrac{5000(10)}{\sqrt{9}}}{\dfrac{5000(10)}{\sqrt{9}} + \dfrac{7500(12)}{\sqrt{4}} + \dfrac{12,500(8)}{\sqrt{16}}} = 0.19$$

$$w_2 = \frac{\dfrac{7500(12)}{\sqrt{4}}}{\dfrac{5000(10)}{\sqrt{9}} + \dfrac{7500(12)}{\sqrt{4}} + \dfrac{12,500(8)}{\sqrt{16}}} = 0.52$$

$$w_3 = \frac{\dfrac{12,500(8)}{\sqrt{16}}}{\dfrac{5000(10)}{\sqrt{9}} + \dfrac{7500(12)}{\sqrt{4}} + \dfrac{12,500(8)}{\sqrt{16}}} = 0.29$$

and thus, the strata sample sizes are $n_1 = 101 \times 0.19 = 19$, $n_2 = 101 \times 0.52 = 53$, and $n_3 = 101 \times 0.29 = 29$. The total total cost of sampling is

$$C = \$5300 + 19 \times \$9 + 52 \times \$4 + 29 \times \$16 = \$6143$$

Example 3.22

Suppose a researcher is going to draw a stratified random sample from a population having three well-defined subpopulations for the purpose of estimating a proportion. Use Table 3.9 to determine a conservative value of the overall sample size and strata sample sizes that will minimize the total cost of sampling when the bound on the error of estimation is fixed at $B = 0.03$ and the initial cost of sampling is $C_0 = \$2800$.

TABLE 3.9   Strata Size and Cost of Sampling the Three Strata in the Target Population

Stratum	N	Cost
1	12000	10
2	8000	8
3	10000	12

The overall sample size required to produce a bound on the error of estimation equal to 0.03 is

$$n = \frac{\left(\dfrac{12,000(0.5)}{\sqrt{10}} + \dfrac{8000(0.5)}{\sqrt{8}} + \dfrac{10,000(0.5)}{\sqrt{12}}\right)\left(12,000(0.5)\sqrt{10} + 8000(0.5)\sqrt{8} + 10,000(0.5)\sqrt{12}\right)}{30,000^2\left[\dfrac{0.03^2}{4}\right] + 12,000(0.25) + 8000(.25) + 10,000(.25)}$$

$$= 1078.0$$

Thus, the overall sample size is $n = 1078$, and the optimal allocation sampling proportions are

$$w_1 = \frac{\dfrac{12,000(0.5)}{\sqrt{10}}}{\dfrac{12,000(.5)}{\sqrt{10}} + \dfrac{8000(0.5)}{\sqrt{8}} + \dfrac{10,000(0.5)}{\sqrt{12}}} = 0.40$$

$$w_2 = \frac{\dfrac{8000(0.5)}{\sqrt{8}}}{\dfrac{12,000(.5)}{\sqrt{10}} + \dfrac{8000(0.5)}{\sqrt{8}} + \dfrac{10,000(0.5)}{\sqrt{12}}} = 0.30$$

$$w_3 = \frac{\dfrac{10,000(0.5)}{\sqrt{12}}}{\dfrac{12,000(.5)}{\sqrt{10}} + \dfrac{8000(0.5)}{\sqrt{8}} + \dfrac{10,000(0.5)}{\sqrt{12}}} = 0.30$$

Thus, the strata sample sizes are $n_1 = 1078 \times 0.40 = 432$, $n_2 = 1078 \times 0.30 = 324$, and $n_3 = 1078 \times 0.30 = 324$, and the total cost of sampling is

$$C = \$2800 + 432 \times \$10 + 324 \times \$8 + 324 \times \$12 = \$13,600$$

Note that when the total cost of sampling is fixed, the strata sample sizes should always be rounded off to preserve to ensure that the total cost of sampling does not exceed; however, when the bound on the error of estimation is fixed the sample sizes should be rounded off to ensure that the value of B does not exceed.

3.3.3 Determining the Sample Size in a Systematic Random Sample

The sample size for a systematic random sample that produces a bound on the error of estimation of B for estimating a mean or a proportion is

$$n = \frac{N\sigma^2}{(N-1)D + \sigma^2}$$

where σ is a reasonable estimate of the population standard deviation and $D = B^2/4$. Note that the value of n that produces a bound on the error of estimation equal to B is the same value that would be used in a simple random sample. Once the sample size for a systematic random sample has been determined, the *sampling interval k* can be determined. The sampling interval is the integer k that is closest to the value of $\frac{N}{n}$.

The cost of drawing systematic random sample of size n is

$$C = C_0 + nC_1$$

where C_0 is the initial setup cost of sampling and C_1 is the actual cost of sampling a unit. Although the formula for total cost of sampling is the same for systematic and simple random sampling, the actual cost of a systematic random sample is usually lower than the cost of simple random sample due to lower initial costs (C_0) and a lower cost of sampling a unit (C_1) incurred in systematic random sampling.

Example 3.23

Suppose a 1 in k systematic random sample will be selected from a population of $N = 5000$ units. If $\sigma \approx 50$, the sample size necessary to have a bound on the error of estimation of the mean of $B = 5$ is

$$n = \frac{5000(50^2)}{(5000 - 1)\left[\frac{5^2}{4}\right] + 50^2} = 370.4$$

Thus, the sample size required to have a bound on the error of estimation equal to 5 is $n = 371$, and the sampling interval is the value of k closest to $\frac{5000}{371}$ that is 13. Thus, the sampling plan is a 1 in 13 systematic random sample. The first unit to be sampled should be randomly selected from the first 13 units, and then every 13th unit thereafter is to be sampled. If the initial cost of sampling is $C_0 = \$500$ and the cost of sampling a unit is $C_1 = \$2$, then the total cost of sampling for this sampling plan is

$$C = \$500 + 371 \times \$2 = \$1242$$

The sample size necessary to estimate a proportion p within a bound on the error of estimation of B is

$$n = \frac{Np(1 - p)}{(N - 1)D + p(1 - p)}$$

where p is a reasonable estimate of the population proportion and $D = B^2/4$; a conservative estimate of the sample size can be found by substituting $p = 0.5$ into this formula.

Example 3.24

Suppose the goal of a research project is to estimate a population proportion within a bound $B = 0.025$ for a population consisting of $N = 100,000$ units. The sample size necessary for a systematic random sample that will produce an estimate of p that having a bound on the error of estimation equal to 0.025 is

$$n = \frac{100,000(0.25)}{(100,000 - 1)\left[\frac{0.025^2}{4}\right] + 0.25} = 1574.8$$

Thus, a sample of $n = 1575$ units will produce an estimate of p with bound on the error of estimation $B = 0.025$. In this case, the sampling interval k is the integer closest to $\frac{100,000}{1575}$ that is 63. Thus, the sampling plan is a 1 in 63 systematic random sample. The first unit to be sampled should be randomly selected from the first 63 units, and then every 63rd unit thereafter is to be sampled.

GLOSSARY

1 in k Systematic Sample A 1 in k systematic sample is a probability sample obtained by randomly selecting one sampling unit from the first k units in the sampling frame and then every kth unit thereafter.

Availability Sampling A sample selected by observing data that are close at hand or data that are easy to obtain is called availability sampling.

Bound on the Error of Estimation The bound on the error of estimation is based on the two standard deviation empirical rule, and it is unlikely for an estimate to be farther from the true value of the parameter being estimated than the value of B.

Cluster A cluster of units is a clearly defined group of units in the target population.

Expert Sampling A sample by observing data that are self-selected by a researcher is referred to as expert sampling or judgment sampling.

External Validity A study is said to have external validity when the results of the study can safely be generalized to the target population.

Optimal Allocation Optimal allocation is an allocation plan that takes into account the cost of sampling as well as the variability and proportion of the population units in each of the strata.

Primary Units The primary units in a cluster sampling plan are the clusters of population units.

Probability Sample A probability sample is a sample that is selected in a random fashion where each of the possible samples and the probability of drawing each sampling unit are known prior to sampling.

Proportional Allocation In proportional allocation the sampling proportion for the ith stratum is

$$w_i = \frac{N_i}{N}$$

where N is the number of units in the population and N_i is the number of units in the ith stratum.

Random Sample A random sample is a sample that is chosen using a probability sample.

Sample Size The sample size is the number of sampling units that will be selected and is usually denoted by n.

Samples of Convenience Samples that are collected in an ad-hoc fashion are referred to as samples of convenience.

Sampling Element A sampling element is an object on which measurements will be made.

Sampling Frame A sampling frame is the list of sampling units that are available for sampling.

Sampling Proportion The sampling proportion for the ith stratum is the proportion of the overall sample allocated to the ith stratum and is denoted by w_i.

Sampling Units Sampling units are the units of the population that will be sampled.

Secondary Units The secondary units in a cluster sample are the units of the population contained in a cluster.

Simple Random Cluster Sample A simple random cluster sample is a sample selected by taking a simple random sample of n of the population clusters in the target population.

Simple Random Sample A simple random sample of size n consists of n sampling units selected in a fashion that every possible sample of n units has the same chance of being selected.

Snowball Sampling A sample that is selected by sampling according to referrals from previously sampled units is called snowball sampling or chain referral sampling.

Strata The different subpopulations making up the target population are referred to as strata and a single subpopulation is called a stratum.

Stratified Random Sample   A stratified random sample is a sample that is selected by collecting a simple random sample from each stratum in the population.

EXERCISES

3.1   What does it mean when a sample is said to be representative of the target population?

3.2   Why is it important to a have a sample that is representative of the target population?

3.3   How is a sample different from a population?

3.4   How is a statistic different from a parameter?

3.5   What is the difference between a sampling unit and a sampling element?

3.6   What is the sampling frame?

3.7   How does the sampling frame differ from the target population?

3.8   Why is it important to have a sampling frame that covers the target population?

3.9   What does it mean when a sampling frame is said to undercover the target population?

3.10   How is a random sample different from a sample of convenience?

3.11   What are the advantages of using a well-designed probability sample in place of a sample of convenience?

3.12   Does a large sample always provide more accurate information about a population than a small sample? Why?

3.13   Suppose a large sample of convenience is selected and then a simple random sample is selected from the sample of convenience.
   (a) Is this a probability sample? Why?
   (b) Does this sampling plan remove any of the concerns about making inferences about the target population from the sample of convenience? Why?

3.14   How many simple random samples are possible when the population consists of
   (a) $N = 100$ units and $n = 25$ units will be sampled?
   (b) $N = 500$ units and $n = 25$ units will be sampled?
   (c) $N = 1000$ units and $n = 50$ units will be sampled?
   (d) $N = 5000$ units and $n = 100$ units will be sampled?

3.15   What is a stratum in a target population?

3.16   When should a
   (a) simple random sample be used?
   (b) stratified random sample be used?
   (c) cluster random sample be used?
   (d) systematic random sample be used?
   (e) stratified cluster random sample be used?

3.17   Which sampling plan should be used when
   (a) there are well-defined subpopulations in the target population that need to be represented in the sample?

(b) information is needed on a small but important subset of the target population?

(c) the units in the population are homogeneously distributed?

(d) the units in the population are heterogeneously distributed?

3.18 Determine which sampling plan should be used in each of the following scenarios:

(a) A Food and Drug Administration (FDA) inspector needs to check the quality of a generic drug made by a pharmaceutical company by sampling the production line.

(b) A blood center in New York City plans on taking an annual sample of the center's inventory for a quality control study on each of the four blood types.

(c) A researcher must select, without bias, a sample of 25 individuals from a large pool of volunteers for a particular experiment.

(d) A researcher must select, without bias, a sample of 250 individuals from a large pool of volunteers for a particular experiment where one of the explanatory factors is gender.

(e) The Department of Health in a particular state is studying the distribution of Body Mass Index (BMI) for 10-year-old children. The sampling available for this study consists of a list of elementary schools in the state and home school associations.

3.19 Determine the sampling plan used in each of the following studies:

(a) In a study on head injuries reported in the article "Helmet Use and risk of head injuries in Alpine skiers and snowboarders" published in the *Journal of the American Medical Association* (Sulheim et al., 2005), the author sampled every 10th skier in line at the ski lifts at a ski resort every Wednesday and Sunday during the winter months.

(b) In a study on the hepatitis B and C viruses reported in the article "Frequency of vaccine-related and therapeutic injections—Romania, 1998" published in the *Morbidity and Mortality Weekly Report* (1998) the authors sampled 300 households and surveyed each of the residents in a household.

(c) In a study on secondhand smoking reported in the article "Exposure to secondhand smoke among students aged 13–15 years—worldwide, 2000–2007" published in the *Morbidity and Mortality Weekly Report* (2007), the authors collected sample data from participating schools by randomly selecting classes within a school and then surveying each of the students in the class.

(d) In a study of tuberculosis reported in the article "Tuberculin skin test screening practices among US colleges and universities" published in the *Journal of the American Medical association* (Hennessey et al., 1998), the authors randomly selected and surveyed 263 2-year colleges and 361 4-year universities.

3.20 How does a simple random cluster sample differ from a simple random sample?

3.21 How does a systematic sample differ from a simple random sample?

3.22 What is the special condition that must be investigated before using a systematic sample?

3.23 Under what conditions would it make sense to use a stratified

(a) cluster sample?   (b) systematic sample?

3.24 Which sampling plan should be used to sample a population that is known to have a bimodal distribution? Why?

3.25   For a population consisting of $N = 10,000$ units, determine the sample size that will result from using a
   (a) 1 in 25 systematic random sample.
   (b) 1 in 50 systematic random sample.
   (c) 1 in 200 systematic random sample.

3.26   A systematic random sample is going to be used to sample a population consisting of $N = 5000$ units. Determine the sampling interval for 1 in k systematic sample if the desired sample size is

   (a) 20   **(b)** 50
   (c) 100   **(d)** 200

3.27   Determine the starting unit that would be sampled for each of the systematic random samples in Exercise 3.26.

3.28   Draw a simple random sample of $n = 25$ units from the
   (a) Birth weight data set.   **(b)** Body fat data set.

3.29   Draw a simple random sample of $n = 50$ units from the
   (a) Birth Weight data set.   **(b)** Body Fat data set.

3.30   Using the Birth Weight data set, draw a stratified random sample of
   (a) 25 mothers who smoked during pregnancy and 25 mothers who did not smoke during pregnancy.
   (b) 10 units from each of the three races represented in the data set.

3.31   Using the Body Fat data set as the sampling frame, draw a systematic random sample consisting of

   (a) $n = 15$ units.   **(b)** $n = 25$ units.

3.32   How can an approximate value of the standard deviation be determined prior to sampling a target population?

3.33   Determine a reasonable estimate of the standard deviation when
   (a) the expected range of a mound-shaped distribution is 1000.
   (b) the expected range of a mound-shaped distribution is 5.
   (c) in two previous studies on populations that are fairly similar to the population to be sampled produced estimated standard deviations of 10.

3.34   What is the bound on the error of estimation?

3.35   Why is it important to have a prespecified bound on the error of estimation in developing a well-designed sampling frame?

3.36   Determine the sample size required for a simple random sample to attain the prespecified bound on the error of estimation for estimating a mean when

   (a) $N = 5000$, $\sigma = 100$, and $B = 5$.
   (b) $N = 1000$, $\sigma = 20$, and $B = 2$.
   (c) $N = 25,000$, $\sigma = 250$, and $B = 5$.
   (d) $N = 10,000$, $\sigma = 10$, and $B = 0.25$.

3.37 Determine the cost of sampling in each part of Exercise 3.36 if the initial cost involved with sampling the target population is $500 and the cost of sampling a unit is $5 per unit.

3.38 Determine the sample size required for a simple random sample to attain the pre-specified bound on the error of estimation for estimating a mean in each of the following scenarios where the number of units in the target population is unknown.
  (a) $\sigma = 100$ and $B = 5$.
  (b) $\sigma = 50$ and $B = 2$.
  (c) $\sigma = 250$ and $B = 10$.
  (d) $\sigma = 150$, and $B = 5$.

3.39 Determine the cost of sampling in each part of Exercise 3.38 if the initial cost involved in sampling the target population is $2500 and the cost of sampling a unit is $15 per unit.

3.40 Determine the conservative sample size required for a simple random sample to attain the prespecified bound on the error of estimation for estimating a proportion when
  (a) $N = 5000$ and $B = 0.05$.
  (b) $N = 1000$ and $B = 0.04$.
  (c) $N = 25,000$ and $B = 0.03$.
  (d) $N = 10,000$ and $B = 0.04$.

3.41 Determine the conservative sample size required for a simple random sample to attain the prespecified bound on the error of estimation for estimating a proportion when
  (a) $B = 0.05$.
  (b) $B = 0.04$.
  (c) $B = 0.03$.
  (d) $B = 0.025$.

3.42 Determine the cost of sampling for each part of Exercise 3.41 if the initial cost involved with sampling the target population is $10,500 and the cost of sampling a unit is $25 per unit.

3.43 A pharmaceutical company has developed a new pill that will mitigate the pain suffered during a migraine headache and needs to estimate the mean time it takes for the pill to begin mitigating a migraine headache. A simple random sample migraine sufferers will be drawn from a large pool of volunteers for this study. If it is known that the minimum time it will take for the pill to begin having an effect is 5 min and the maximum time is 85 min, determine
  (a) an estimate of the standard deviation σ.
  (b) the sample size required for estimating the mean time with a bound on the error of estimation of 2 min.
  (c) cost of sampling when the initial cost is $500 and the cost per sampled unit is $25.

3.44 A hospital auditor has been asked to estimate the proportion of patient accounts in which the hospital overcharged a patient during the last 25 years. If the auditor will use a simple random sample to estimate this proportion, determine

TABLE 3.10   Information on the Three Strata in the Target Population

Stratum	N	SD	Cost
1	5,000	25	5
2	7,500	36	3
3	2,500	16	7
	15,000		

(a) the sample size required for estimating the proportion with a bound on the error of estimation of 0.035.

(b) the cost of sampling if the initial cost is $40,000 and the cost of sampling a record is $5.

3.45 What are two different allocation plans that can be used in a stratified random sample?

3.46 How do the proportional and optimal allocation plans differ for a stratified random sample?

3.47 Suppose the target population consists of $N = 10,000$ units distributed over four strata. If the number of units in the four strata are $N_1 = 4000$, $N_2 = 1500$, $N_3 = 2500$, and $N_4 = 2000$, determine the

(a) sampling proportions for a stratified random sample using proportional allocation.

(b) strata sample sizes if the overall sample size is $n = 250$.

(c) the cost of sampling when the initial cost is $C_0 = \$2500$ and the cost associated with sampling a unit from each stratum are $C_1 = 3$, $C_2 = 5$, $C_3 = 8$, and $C_4 = 12$.

3.48 Use Table 3.10 to answer the following questions concerning a stratified random sample based on proportional allocation:

(a) Determine the sampling proportions.

(b) Determine the sample size that will produce a bound on the error of estimation for estimating the mean of $B = 2.5$.

(c) Determine the allocation of the sample (i.e., strata sample sizes).

(d) Determine the cost of sampling if the initial cost is $C_0 = \$10,900$ and the cost of sampling in each stratum is $C_1 = \$5$, $C_2 = \$3$, and $C_3 = \$7$, respectively.

3.49 Use Table 3.11 to answer the following questions concerning a stratified random sample using optimal allocation. If the goal of this study is to estimate the mean of the target population, determine

TABLE 3.11   Sampling Information on the Three Strata in the Target Population

Stratum	N	SD	Cost
1	25,000	50	10
2	50,000	75	15
3	25,000	40	13
	100,000		

TABLE 3.12 Sampling Information for Registered Nurses having 2-year and 4-year Degrees

Degree	N	SD	Cost
2-Year	6,000	25	10
4-Year	14,000	50	10
	20,000		

(a) the sampling proportions.

(b) the sample size that will have a total cost of $25,000 when the initial cost is $C_0 = \$21,000$.

(c) the allocation of the sample (i.e., strata sample sizes).

3.50 A state nursing association is studying the yearly overtime hours put in by registered nurses employed at hospitals. Since a registered nurse can have either a 2-year or a 4-year degree in nursing, a stratified random sample will be used. The goal of this study is to estimate the mean of yearly overtime hours put in by a registered nurse employed at a hospital. Using Table 3.12, determine

(a) the sampling proportions for a stratified random sample using optimal allocation.

(b) the sample size required to have a bound on the error of estimation for estimating the mean of $B = 5$.

(c) the strata sample sizes.

(d) the cost associated with this sampling plan if the initial cost of sampling is $C_0 = \$5000$.

3.51 An insurance company is interested in estimating the mean length of hospital stay following heart bypass surgery. A stratified random sample of public and private hospitals will be used for estimating the mean length of hospital stay following a heart bypass surgery. Suppose there is $15,000 available for the total cost of sampling, and the initial setup cost of sampling is $C_0 = \$10,000$. Use Table 3.13 to determine

(a) the optimal allocation sampling proportions.

(b) the sample size for a stratified sample using optimal allocation that produces the smallest bound on the error of estimation.

(c) the strata sample sizes.

3.52 The American Medical Association (AMA) wishes to estimate the mean number of hours per week surgeons and nonsurgical doctors work, and a stratified random sample using optimal allocation will be used for estimating the mean. Suppose that

TABLE 3.13 Sampling Information on Public and Private Hospitals

Hospital	N	SD	Cost
Private	10,000	1.2	25
Public	15,000	1.5	15
	25,000		

TABLE 3.14   Sampling Information on AMA Surgeons and Nonsurgical Doctors

Type of Doctor	N	SD	Cost
Surgeon	20,000	2	20
Nonsurgical	80,000	5	10
	100,000		

a bound on the error of estimation of $B = 0.5$ is desired, and the initial setup cost of sampling is $C_0 = \$6000$. Use Table 3.14 to determine

(a) the optimal allocation sampling proportions.

(b) the sample size for a stratified sample using optimal allocation that produces the smallest total cost for the desired bound on the error of estimation.

(c) the strata sample sizes.

(d) the total cost of sampling.

3.53   Using Exercise 3.52, determine the optimal allocation

(a) sampling proportions for estimating the proportion of doctors who work at least 30 h per week.

(b) sample size for a stratified sample using optimal allocation that produces the smallest total cost for a bound on the error of estimation of $B = 0.04$.

(c) strata sample sizes.

(d) total cost of sampling.

3.54   For estimating the mean of a particular population, a systematic random sample will be drawn. If the number of units in the population is $N = 2500$ and the standard deviation is $\sigma = 20$, determine

(a) the sample size required to have a bound on the error of estimation of $B = 2.5$

(b) the sampling interval k.

(c) the cost of sampling if $C_0 = \$250$ and the cost of sampling each unit is $\$1.50$.

3.55   For estimating a proportion in a particular population, a systematic random sample will be drawn. If the number of units in the population is $N = 6000$, determine

(a) the sample size required to have a bound on the error of estimation of $B = 0.05$

(b) the sampling interval k.

(c) the cost of sampling when $C_0 = \$490$ and the cost of sampling of each unit is $\$5.50$.

3.56   One of the several large federal facilities that are used to store the current version of the flu vaccine is to be sampled in a quality control investigation. A systematic sample will be used to estimate the proportion of damaged or improperly sealed vials of the flu vaccine. If the facility contains $N = 100,000$ vials of the flu vaccine, determine

(a) the number of vials to be sampled if the desired bound on the error of estimation is $B = 0.025$

(b) the sampling interval k.

(c) the cost of sampling when $C_0 = \$9000$ and the cost of sampling each unit is $\$25$.

CHAPTER 4

SUMMARIZING RANDOM SAMPLES

THE DISCIPLINE of statistics is concerned with making inferences about populations in the presence of uncertainty. The reason there is uncertainty in a statistical inference is that a statistical inference is based on a sample rather than a census of the entire population. That is, a census is required to find the true values of the population parameters, and since a statistic is simply a quantity that is computed from a sample drawn from the target population, the value of a parameter cannot be determined from the information contained in a sample. Furthermore, since a sample contains only a portion of the target population, a statistic will only be a reliable estimate of the value of an unknown parameter when the sampled portion of the population is truly representative of the entire population. Thus, it is critical that statistics are only computed from a sample collected from a well-designed sampling plan.

Statistical methods for estimating the unknown values of the population parameters for a univariate or a multivariate population will be discussed in this chapter. In particular, the two types of statistics discussed in this chapter are *graphical statistics* that result in plots, charts, or graphs to display the summarized sample information and *numerical statistics* that result in numbers that can be used to summarize a sample, estimate parameters, or test hypotheses concerning an unknown parameter.

Finally, the main emphasis of this chapter is the correct use and interpretation of a statistic. The formulas for computing the values of each of the statistics discussed in this chapter are presented and their use illustrated, but in most cases it is recommended that a statistical computing package be used when computing the values of the statistics.

4.1 SAMPLES AND INFERENTIAL STATISTICS

Recall, that a statistic is rule that depends only on the sample and known values. Thus, statistics are based on samples and can be used only to estimate the unknown parameters from the sample data. Parameters, on the other hand, are based upon a complete census of a population. The goal of a statistical analysis is to use the information contained in the observed sample to find out as much information about the target population as possible by estimating the unknown parameters of the target population. Also, since a parameter is only a numerical summary of a characteristic of the target population, to determine the

Applied Biostatistics for the Health Sciences. By Richard J. Rossi
Copyright © 2010 by John Wiley & Sons, Inc.

parameters that are meaningful in a biomedical research study, the distribution of the target population must also be estimated.

A well-planned statistical analysis will address each of the components described below.

THE COMPONENTS OF A STATISTICAL ANALYSIS

A proper statistical analysis consists of the following basic research components:

1. A set of well-posed research questions proposed by the research team.

2. A well-defined target population that is relevant to the research questions that will be sampled.

3. A set of variables that will be measured on the units that are sampled including a response variable, demographic variables, and explanatory variables. The demographic variables should be chosen to control for the effects of variables external to the study.

4. A set of parameters in the target population that will be estimated. The parameters must provide relevant information about the answers to the research questions.

5. A well-designed sampling plan that utilizes a probability sample that will produce a sample that is representative of the target population. In the sampling plan, the sample size n must be determined so that the statistics computed from the observed sample will be accurate and reliable.

6. A well-designed statistical analysis that explicitly outlines the statistical methods that will be used in analyzing the sample data.

7. A summary of the statistical analysis along with the appropriate measures of the reliability for the statistical analysis. The measures of reliability are important because they provide a measure of how accurate the statistical inferences are expected to be.

Note that each of the eight components of a statistical analysis is to be carried out before the observed sample is collected. Furthermore, the details of the first six components are often developed in an iterative process. For example, in many biomedical studies the original questions of interest are often too broad and in order to have a plausible study must be revised to narrow the research goals. In any case, extensive planning is key to a valid scientific study and an appropriate statistical analysis.

4.2 INFERENTIAL GRAPHICAL STATISTICS

Once the sample data have been collected, the first step in a statistical analysis is often to examine some descriptive graphical statistics. Graphical statistics are typically used for estimating the shape of a distribution, for describing the tails of a distribution, for estimating the number of modes in the distribution, for estimating the typical values and the spread of the distribution, and for suggesting a plausible probability model for the population distribution. Note that the appropriate graphical statistic for summarizing a sample will depend on the type of data that is collected. That is, there are graphical statistics that can be used for summarizing qualitative and quantitative data. The graphical statistic chosen to summarize a sample also depends on the particular goals and objectives of a research project.

4.2.1 Bar and Pie Charts

In the case of qualitative or discrete data, the graphical statistics that are most often used to summarize the data in the observed sample are the *bar chart* and the *pie chart* since the important parameters of the distribution of a qualitative variable are population proportions. Thus, for a qualitative variable the sample proportions are the values that will be displayed in a bar chart or a pie chart.

In Chapter 2, the distribution of a qualitative variable was often presented in a bar chart in which the height of a bar represented the proportion or the percentage of the population having each quality the variable takes on. With an observed sample, bar charts can be used to represent the sample proportions or percentages for each of the qualities the variable takes on and can be used to make statistical inferences about the population distribution of the variable.

There are many types of bar charts including simple bar charts, stacked bar charts, and comparative side-by-side bar charts. An example of a simple bar chart for the weight classification for babies, which takes on the values normal and low, in the Birth Weight data set is shown in Figure 4.1.

Note that a bar chart represents the category percentages or proportions with bars of height equal to the percentage or proportion of sample observations falling in a particular category. The widths of the bars should be equal and chosen so that an appealing chart is produced. Bar charts may be drawn with either horizontal or vertical bars, and the bars in a bar chart may or may not be separated by a gap. An example of a bar chart with horizontal bars is given in Figure 4.2 for the weight classification of babies in the Birth Weight data set.

In creating a bar chart it is important that

1. the proportions or percentages in each bar can be easily determined to make the bar chart easier to read and interpret.

2. the total percentage represented in the bar chart should be 100 since a distribution contains 100% of the population units.

3. the qualities associated with an ordinal variable are listed in the proper relative order! With a nominal variable the order of the categories is not important.

4. the bar chart has the axes of the bar chart clearly labeled so that it is clear whether the bars represent a percentage or a proportion.

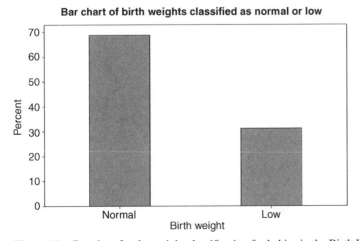

Figure 4.1   Bar chart for the weight classification for babies in the Birth Weight data set.

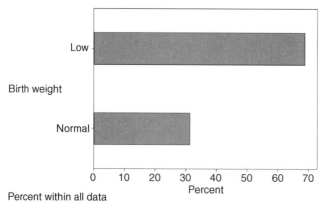

Figure 4.2   A horizontal bar chart for the birth weight data.

5. the bar chart has either a caption or a title that clearly describes the nature of the bar chart.

Because bar charts are often used for comparing two or more populations, it is not a good idea, use bars that reflect the frequency of a category. The proportion or percentage of the sample belonging to each of the categories should always be used in a comparative bar chart. That is, the percentage or proportion of the sample falling in a category does not depend on the sample size, whereas the frequency of a category strongly depends on the sample size. Also, since the heights of the bars in a bar chart are meant to provide estimates of the percentage or proportion of the population having a quality, the heights of the bars should not represent the frequency of a quality.

Comparative bar charts are often useful when the distribution of two or more populations is being compared. In particular, when a population contains well-defined subpopulations it is often useful to have a bar chart for each of the subpopulations. The two most commonly used comparative bar charts are the *side-by-side bar chart* and the *stacked bar chart*. Examples of the side-by-side and stacked bar charts are given in Figures 4.3 and 4.4.

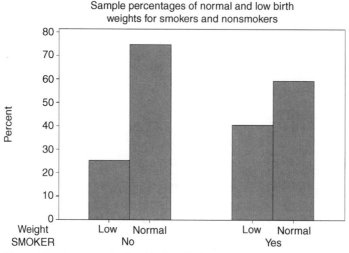

Figure 4.3   An example of a side-by-side bar chart.

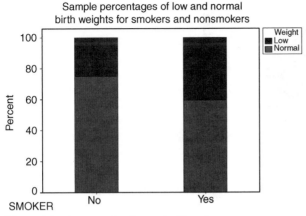

Figure 4.4   An example of a stacked bar chart.

When a qualitative variable has only two possible categories, a stacked bar chart can often be used to make quick comparisons between the percentages of each category for the two subpopulations; however, when a qualitative variable has several categories, a stacked bar chart is often harder to interpret than a side-by-side bar chart. Therefore, stacked bar charts should rarely be used. In fact, a stacked bar chart should be used only when the chart clearly shows that there are significant differences between the subpopulations being compared.

Example 4.1
The bar chart given in Figure 4.5 is based on the Birth Weight data set and a comparison of the relationship between a mother's smoking status during pregnancy and a baby's birth weight classification.
    Use this bar chart to estimate the

   a. percentage of low-weight babies for mothers who smoked during pregnancy.
   b. percentage low-weight babies for mothers who did not smoke during pregnancy.

Solutions   Based on the bar chart

   a. the estimate of the percentage of low-weight babies for mothers who smoked during pregnancy is about 40.

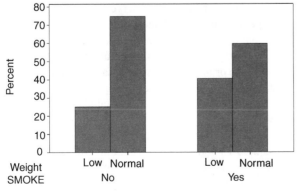

Percent within levels of SMOKE

Figure 4.5   A bar chart for mother's smoking status and baby's weight classification.

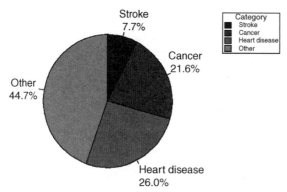

Figure 4.6 Pie chart showing the leading causes of death among women in 2003.

b. the estimate of the percentage of low-weight babies for mothers who did not smoke during pregnancy is about 25.

An alternative graphical statistic that can also be used to summarize the distribution of a qualitative variable is the *pie chart*. A pie chart conveys the same information as a bar chart. A pie chart is constructed by determining the percentage or proportion of the sample in each of the categories of a qualitative variable, and then slicing the pie into areas that are proportional to percentages observed in the categories. An example of a pie chart is provided in Figure 4.6 that shows the leading causes of death among women in the year 2003 according to the U.S. Department of Health Services.

Note that when subpopulations are being studied, pie charts for each of the subpopulations can be placed along side each other for comparison. One problem inherent to pie charts is that when the variable has a large number of categories some of the slices in the pie chart will become very small making the pie chart hard to read. Furthermore, small pie slices can be hard to label clearly. In any case, the percentages being represented by the slices of the pie should be included in the pie chart or provided in a companion table make it easier to interpret the information contained in the sample.

4.2.2 Boxplots

One of the most commonly used graphical statistics for estimating the distribution of a quantitative variable is the *boxplot*. A boxplot, also called a *box and whisker plot*, is a graphical statistic that can be used to summarize the observed sample data and can provide useful information on the shape and the tails of the population distribution. A boxplot is a simple graphical statistic that can be used to make inferences about the tails of the distribution, the typical values in the population, and the spread of the population. Boxplots are also useful in identifying extreme or unusual points in a sample, and a boxplot can also be used in comparing the distributions of two or more subpopulations.

A boxplot is based on the *five-number summary* associated with a sample. The five-number summary associated with a sample consists of the following statistics: the minimum of the sample, the maximum of the sample, the sample 25th percentile ($Q1$), the sample 50th percentile ($\tilde{x}$), and the sample 75 percentile ($Q3$). The five-number summary can be used to create two types of boxplots, namely, the *simple boxplot* and the *outlier boxplot*.

A simple boxplot is a graphical statistic based on the five-number summary and an outline for constructing a simple boxplot is given below.

TABLE 4.1   The Five-Number Summary for the Sample in Example 4.2

n	Minimum	$Q1$	Median	$Q3$	Maximum
112	3	12	18	31	49

CONSTRUCTING A SIMPLE BOXPLOT

1. Determine the five-number summary statistic associated with the observed sample.

2. Draw a box from $Q1$ to $Q3$. The width of the box is arbitrary but should be chosen so that a visually appealing plot is produced.

3. A vertical line is drawn inside the box at the value of the sample median.

4. Attach the lower and upper whiskers to the box. The lower whisker is a line drawn from the $Q1$ down to the minimum value in the sample, and the upper whisker is a line drawn from $Q3$ up to the maximum value in the sample.

Example 4.2
Suppose a simple random sample of $n = 112$ observations results in the five-number summary given in Table 4.1. The resulting boxplot based on this sample is shown in Figure 4.7.

In a simple boxplot, the box contains 50% of the sample observations, the length of the box is an estimate of the interquartile range, and the whiskers extend from the sample 25th and 75th percentiles to the extreme values in the sample. A boxplot may be drawn either horizontally or vertically, and the width of a boxplot should always be chosen so that the boxplot is visually appealing.

The statistical inferences that can be made from a simple boxplot include inferences about the

1. shape of the underlying distribution and the direction of the longer of the tails of the distribution.

2. population median.

3. minimum and maximum values in the distribution.

4. spread of the distribution.

A potential problem that can occur when making inferences about the tails of a distribution from a simple boxplot is that too much emphasis is placed on the maximum and the minimum values of the sample. That is, a simple boxplot utilizes none of the

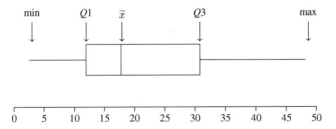

Figure 4.7   An example of a simple boxplot and its five-number summary.

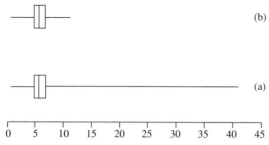

Figure 4.8 A simple boxplot with the observation in error (a) and with the observation in error corrected (b).

information between the ends of the box (i.e., $Q1$ and $Q3$) and the extreme values in the sample. Example 4.3 illustrates the nature of this potential problem.

Example 4.3
Suppose that in a simple random sample of $n = 213$ observations a mistake was made in entering the value of one of the observations. In particular, suppose that all of the observations fall between 0 and 12, but one observation had a measured value that was 4.12 that was recorded as 41.2. The boxplots given in Figure 4.8 illustrate how this single observation can influence the inferences made about the tails of a distribution.

Note that boxplot in Figure 4.8a indicates the distribution has a long tail to the right, while boxplot in Figure 4.8b indicates tails of the distribution have about the same length. Thus, boxplot in Figure 4.8a, which is based on the misrecorded observation, suggests the underlying distribution has a long tail to the right, while the boxplot in Figure 4.8b, which is based on the correct value of the observation, suggests the underlying distribution is approximately mound shaped.

Thus, it is always important to carefully inspect the recorded values in a sample so that incorrectly recorded values are corrected before they are used in a statistical analysis. However, in practice even the best scientist will make a mistake that will not be caught before plotting the data; an alternative version of a boxplot that places less emphasis on the maximum and minimum of the sample can be used. In particular, a *outlier boxplot* can be used to identify the extreme points in a sample. An outlier boxplot is also based on the five-number summary, and the procedure for constructing an outlier boxplot is outlined below.

CONSTRUCTING AN OUTLIER BOXPLOT

---

1. Determine the five-number summary associated with the observed sample.

2. Draw a box from $Q1$ to $Q3$. The width of the box should be chosen so that a visually appealing plot is produced.

3. A vertical line is drawn inside the box at the value of the sample median.

4. Attach the lower and upper whiskers to the box. The lower whisker in an outlier box a line is drawn from $Q1$ down to the larger of the minimum value in the sample and $Q1 - 1.5 \times (Q3 - Q1)$; the upper whisker in an outlier box is a line drawn from $Q3$ up the smaller of the maximum value in the sample and $Q3 + 1.5 \times (Q3 - Q1)$.

5. The observations in the sample falling below the lower whisker or above the upper whisker are represented with a special plotting symbol such as an asterisk.

The value of $Q3 - Q1$ can be used to estimate the value of the interquartile range and will be denoted by $\widehat{IQR}$. Many statisticians refer to the observed values falling more than a distance of $1.5 \times \widehat{IQR}$ from $Q1$ or $Q3$ as *outliers* and observations more than $3 \times \widehat{IQR}$ from $Q1$ or $Q3$ as *extreme outliers*. An outlier is a point that is judged to be unusually different from the rest of the data, and an outlier boxplot can be used to identify the outliers and extreme outliers in a sample.

An outlier boxplot can be used as the basis for making statistical inferences about

1. the shape of the underlying distribution and the direction of the longer of the tails of the distribution.
2. the extreme observations falling outside of the region $Q1 - 1.5 \times \widehat{IQR}$ and $Q3 + 1.5 \times \widehat{IQR}$.
3. the population median.
4. the minimum and maximum values of the distribution.
5. the first and third quartiles, X_{25} and X_{75}.

Note that there are several parameters in a distribution that cannot be estimated from the information contained in a boxplot. For example, reliable estimates of the mean, the modes, and the variance of a population cannot be obtained only from the information displayed in a boxplot. It is also impossible to estimate most of the percentiles of a distribution using only a boxplot.

Example 4.4
An outlier boxplot based on the five-number summary

$$min = 3.2, \ Q1 = 12.0, \ \tilde{x} = 17.6, \ Q3 = 30.7, \ \text{and max} = 49.1$$

is shown in Figure 4.9. Note that there are two extreme observations denoted by ($*$) that fall more than $1.5 \times \widehat{IQR}$ from the upper end of box ($Q3$). These extreme observations have values 44.9 and 49.1.

Note that an outlier boxplot is similar to a simple boxplot; however, an outlier boxplot contains more information on the extreme observations in a sample. Outliers can have a strong influence on the results of a statistical analysis, and an outlier should not be removed from a data set unless it is clearly an impossible value of the variable or it can be identified as a mistaken data point. Points declared to be outliers need to be carefully investigated since outliers may have strong influence on the statistical inferences drawn from a sample. Furthermore, when one or more outliers detected in the sample observations, it is often a good idea to investigate the observation points further. Observations deemed to be impossible values should be eliminated from the data set, and outliers that arise from

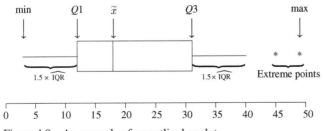

Figure 4.9   An example of an outlier boxplot.

mistakes in recording the value of an observation should be corrected. When an outlier cannot be legitimately removed from a data set or its value corrected, the influence of the outlier can be investigated by following the strategy outlined below.

A PROCEDURE FOR DEALING WITH OUTLIERS

1. First, try to determine whether the outlier is the result of a mistake in recording the data or an impossible value of the variable.

   (a) Outliers that are found to be recording errors should be replaced with their correct values.

   (b) Outliers that are found to be impossible values of the variable should be deleted from the data set.

2. When an outlier cannot be corrected or removed from the data set, the influence of the outlier can be investigated as follows:

   (a) Perform the statistical analysis on the entire data set (i.e., including the outlier).

   (b) Remove the outlier from the data set and rerun the statistical analysis on the reduced data set (i.e., without the outlier).

   (c) Examine the differences in the results of the two statistical analyses and summarize the results of both analyses.

Example 4.5
Determine whether the observation $x = 112.2$ is an outlier or an extreme outlier in each of the following scenarios:

a. $Q1 = 150$, $Q3 = 232$, and $\widehat{IQR} = 35$
b. $Q1 = 75$, $Q3 = 102$, and $\widehat{IQR} = 6$
c. $Q1 = 121$, $Q3 = 131$, and $\widehat{IQR} = 2.5$

Solutions The $x = 112.2$ is

a. not an outlier because $x = 112.2$ is within $1.5 \times 35 = 52.5$ of $Q1 = 150$.
b. an outlier because $x = 112.2$ is more than $1.5 \times 6 = 9$ from $Q3 = 102$ but not more than $3(6) = 27$ from $Q3 = 102$.
c. an extreme outlier because $x = 112.2$ is more than $3 \times 2.5 = 7.5$ from $Q1 = 121$.

Example 4.6
The outlier boxplot given in Figure 4.10 is based on the age of a mother (Age) in the Birth Weight data set. Use this boxplot to answer the questions below.

a. Estimate the median age of a mother.
b. Estimate the 75th percentile of the distribution of the variable Age.
c. Describe the shape of the underlying distribution of the variable Age.
d. Estimate the interquartile range in the distribution of the variable Age.
e. Are there any outliers or extreme outliers in this data set for the variable Age?

Solutions Based on the boxplot given in Figure 4.10

a. the estimate of the median age of a mother is about 23.5 years.
b. the estimate the 75th percentile for the distribution of the variable Age is 26.

Boxplot of Age

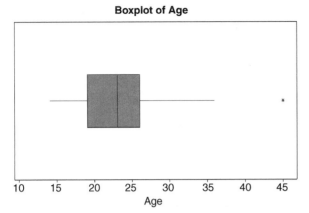

Figure 4.10   A boxplot for mother's age in the birth weight study.

    c. the shape of the underlying distribution of the variable Age appears to be long tailed to the right.

    d. the estimate of the interquartile range in the distribution of the variable Age is $\widehat{\text{IQR}} = 26 - 19 = 7$

    e. the observation Age $= 45$ is an outlier but not an extreme outlier since 45 more than $1.5\widehat{\text{IQR}} = 10.5$ from $Q3$ but not more than $3\widehat{\text{IQR}} = 21$ from $Q3$.

    When subpopulations are present in the target population and there is a categorical variable recorded in the sample that identifies the subpopulation each observation comes from, separate boxplots for each of the subpopulations can be drawn and compared. For example, the boxplots shown in Figure 4.19 are based on the Birth Weight data set for the weights of babies. The subpopulations accounted for in Figure 4.19 are mothers who smoked during pregnancy (Smoker) and mothers who did not smoke during pregnancy (Nonsmoker).

    Note that the boxplots in Figure 4.19 suggest that the distribution of birth weights of babies whose mothers smoked during pregnancy is shifted slightly to the left of the distribution for babies with nonsmoking mothers. In particular, the values of $Q1$, the sample

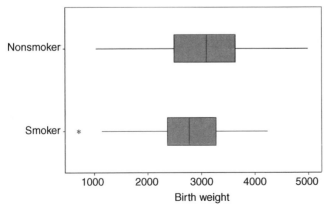

Figure 4.11   Boxplots for the birth weights of babies for mothers who smoked during pregnancy and mothers who did not smoke during pregnancy.

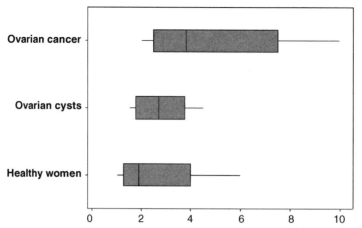

Figure 4.12 Boxplots of the serum Fas levels for women with ovarian cancer, women with ovarian cysts, and healthy women.

median, and $Q3$ are roughly 2700, 2400, and 3300 g, respectively, for the babies in the Smoker subpopulation and are 2500, 3000, and 3600 g, respectively, for the Nonsmoker subpopulation.

Example 4.7
Suppose the boxplots given in Figure 4.12 resulted from a study on the relationship between serum soluble Fas levels and ovarian cancer. The three boxplots in Figure 4.12 graphically summarize the sample data for women with ovarian cancer, women with benign ovarian cysts, and from healthy women.

   Thus, on the basis of these boxplots it appears that there might be a relationship between ovarian cancer and serum Fas levels. In particular, it appears that women with ovarian cancer and ovarian cysts have higher serum Fas levels than do healthy women.

4.2.3 Histograms

A second graphical statistic that provides statistical information about the distribution of a quantitative variable based on a sample is the *histogram*. A histogram is a vertical bar chart drawn over a set of class intervals that cover the range of the observed data. Furthermore, because the histogram is based on the entire sample and not just the five-number summary associated with the sample, a histogram generally will provide more information about a distribution than a boxplot will. An example of a histogram is given in Figure 4.13.

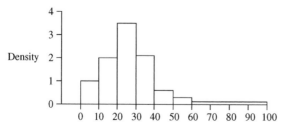

Figure 4.13   Example of a histogram.

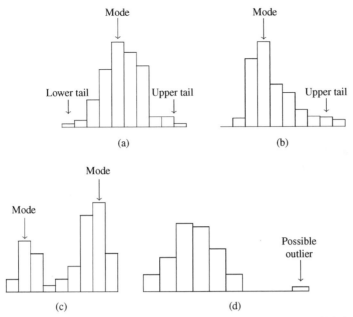

Figure 4.14   Examples of a mound-shaped histogram (a), a long tail right histogram (b), a bimodal histogram (c), and a histogram with an outlier (d).

Histograms are particularly useful for continuous variables and can be used to make statistical inferences about the shape of a distribution, the tails of the distribution, the modes of the distribution, the typical values in the distribution, the spread of the distribution, and the percentage of the distribution falling between a specified range of values. Histograms can also be used for determining a reasonable probability distribution for modeling the distribution of the target population. Several examples of histograms and their key features are given in Figure 4.14.

The most commonly used type of histogram is the *relative frequency histogram*. A relative frequency histogram is a histogram that displays the proportion or the percentage of the sample observations falling in a set of class intervals of equal width covering the range of the sample data; the relative frequency of each class is simply the proportion of the sample observations falling in that class. Thus, a relative frequency histogram is a histogram constructed with equal class intervals where the heights of the bars represent either the relative frequency or the percentage of the sample observations falling in the class interval. Note that in a relative frequency histogram the sum of the heights of the bars is either 1 or 100%, depending on whether relative frequency or percentage is used for the heights of the bars. The rules for constructing a relative frequency histogram are given below.

CONSTRUCTING A RELATIVE FREQUENCY HISTOGRAM

---

1. Determine the class intervals to be used in the histogram. The class intervals must have equal widths and completely cover the range of the sample data.

2. Compute the relative frequencies of each of the class intervals. The percentage of the sample observations in a class interval is found by multiplying the relative frequency by 100%.

3. Draw bars with heights equal to the relative frequency (or percentage) of each class over their respective class intervals.

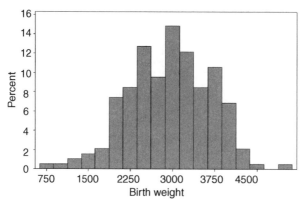

Figure 4.15   A relative frequency histogram for birth weight.

Example 4.8

A relative frequency histogram for the birth weights of babies in the Birth Weight data set is given in Figure 4.15.

Note that percentage associated with a class interval was used for the height of the bars in this histogram rather than relative frequency. Furthermore, this histogram suggests that the distribution is roughly mound-shaped distribution, and thus, a normal probability distribution might be a reasonable probability distribution for modeling for the underlying distribution of the variable birth weight (BWT).

In a relative frequency histogram, the class intervals must be of equal width; however, in many cases the research questions will suggest that class intervals with unequal class widths should be used. In particular, when the underlying distribution has a long tail to the right or left, it is often preferable to combine several equal width class intervals in the tail region into a single larger interval since larger class intervals will often eliminate empty class intervals in a histogram that unfairly suggest that outliers are present in the data set or the distribution is multimodal. For example, many types of cancer occur in individuals of all ages; however, most often cancers are detected in middle age and older adults. In this case, the age of detection may range from 0 to nearly 100; however, because of the scarcity of data in the lower ages, the single age class 0 to 30 might be used in the histogram. Also, when the incidence and detection of cancer are more prevalent for individuals aged 30–60 the researcher might choose to use the class intervals 0–30, 30–39, 40–49, 50–59, 60–69, and 70–100 in the histogram.

When unequal width class intervals are used in a histogram, the heights of the bars in the histogram must be adjusted to reflect that the relative frequencies of the classes occurred in classes of different widths. The correct scale to use for the heights of the bars in a histogram with unequal class intervals is the *density* scale where the density of a class is defined as

$$\text{Density of a class} = \frac{\text{relative frequency of the class}}{\text{class width}}$$

Note that the density of a class interval reflects the proportion of observations per one unit of width within a class interval. A *density histogram* is drawn with a bar equal to the density of each of the class intervals. The rules for constructing a density histogram are given below.

DENSITY HISTOGRAM

1. Determine the class intervals to be used in the histogram. The class intervals must cover the range of the sample data completely.

2. Compute the relative frequency of each of the class intervals.

3. Compute the density of each class interval

$$\text{Density} = \frac{\text{relative frequency}}{\text{class width}}$$

4. Draw a histogram with the bars having height equal to the class interval density over each of the class intervals.

Note that a density histogram can be constructed with equal or unequal class intervals and is constructed such that the total area under the histogram is 1; a density histogram can be based on the percentage in a class interval rather the relative frequency and in this case the total area under the histogram will be 100%.

Example 4.9
Examples of a density histogram and an adjusted relative frequency histogram with unequal class widths are given in Figures 4.16 and 4.17, respectively.

Clearly, the shape of relative frequency histogram suggests that the distribution has a different shape from that of the density histogram. Both histograms suggest that the distribution peaks in the 40–50 class interval and that 14% of the sample falls in the 60–100 class interval. On the other hand, the density histogram suggests that the distribution tapers off from 50 to 100, while the relative frequency histogram suggests a dip between 40 and 60 and a second peak somewhere between 60 and 100. In this case, the relative frequency histogram suggests a misleading shape for the underlying distribution by overemphasizing the percentage of the sample falling in the class interval 60–100.

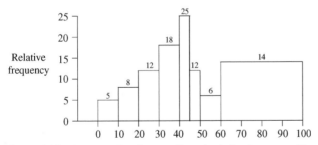

Figure 4.16   An example of an unadjusted relative frequency histogram with unequal class intervals.

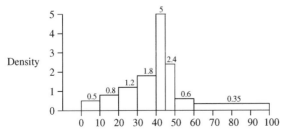

Figure 4.17   An example of an density histogram based on unequal width class intervals.

Thus, because a histogram should reflect the shape of the distribution that was sampled and the shape of the population distribution is based on the density of the units in the population, a density histogram should always be used when the class intervals have unequal class widths. Furthermore, when a density histogram is used, the area of the histogram covering any interval can be used as an estimate of the proportion of population units falling in the interval. Note that the area of a histogram over a class interval is found by multiplying the density of the interval times the width of the interval. That is,

$$\text{Area of interval in a histogram} = \text{density} \times \text{width of the interval}$$

For example, for the histogram in Figure 4.17 the density of the class interval 60–100 is 3.5, and therefore, the area of this interval is $40 \times 3.5 = 14$. Thus, 14% of the sample falls in the interval 60–100, and therefore, an estimate of the percentage of the population falling between 60 and 100 is 14%.

Example 4.10

Use the density histogram given in Figure 4.18 to estimate the percentage of the population falling

  a. below 25.
  b. between 25 and 40.

Solutions Based on the density histogram in Figure 4.18

  a. the estimate of the percentage of the population falling below 25 is found by computing the areas of the bars over the intervals 0–10, 10–20, and 20–25 and then summing these percentages. Thus, the estimated percentage of the population falling below the value 20 is

$$0.5 \times 10 + 0.8 \times 10 + 1.2 \times 5 = 19\%$$

  b. the estimate of the percentage of the population falling between 25 and 40 is found by computing the areas of the bars over the intervals 25–30 and 30–40 and then summing these percentages. Thus, the estimated percentage of the population falling between 25 and 40 is

$$1.2 \times 5 + 1.8 \times 10 = 24\%$$

When analyzing a histogram, sampling variation must be allowed since histograms tend to have small peaks and valleys that are simply because of sampling variation. The small peaks and valleys in a histogram should not be allowed to influence the shape of the distribution suggested by a histogram since small peaks and valleys due to sampling variability often disappear when larger samples are collected. Some final comments on

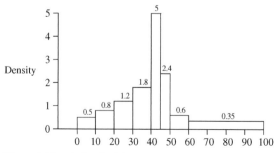

Figure 4.18   A density histogram.

using a histogram to make statistical inferences about the underlying population are listed below.

SOME COMMENTS ON USING HISTOGRAMS

---

1. When the class intervals have equal widths, both the density and the relative frequency histograms will suggest exactly the same shape for the underlying distribution.

2. When the histogram classes have unequal class widths, a density histogram must be used for making inferences about the shape of the underlying distribution.

3. In general, the larger the random sample is the more informative the histogram will be. With small samples, histograms and boxplots will often provide unreliable information about the population distribution and sampling variability may produce unwanted peaks and valleys.

4. Histograms provide more information about the underlying population than do boxplots. Thus, histograms and boxplots are best when used together in making inferences about the underlying distribution.

5. Histograms based on well-designed random samples can be used for

   (a) estimating the shape of underlying distribution.

   (b) identifying outliers.

   (c) estimating the modes of a population.

   (d) estimating the percentage of a population falling in a particular region.

   (e) suggesting probability models that might be used for modeling the underlying distribution.

   (f) comparing the distributions of two or more subpopulations.

Example 4.11

The histograms and boxplots given in Figures 4.19 and 4.20 were created from the birth weights (BWT) in the Birth Weight data set for each smoking status (Smoke). Use these graphical statistics to answer the following questions:

   a. Does the distribution of the variable birth weight appear to have the same general shape for mothers who smoked during pregnancy and mothers who did not smoke during pregnancy?

   b. Suggest a possible probability model that might be used to model each distribution.

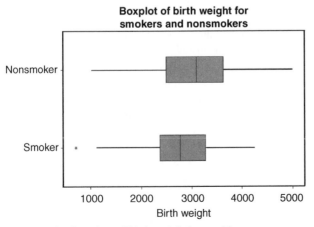

Figure 4.19   Boxplots of birth weight by smoking status.

Histogram of birth weight by mother's smoking status

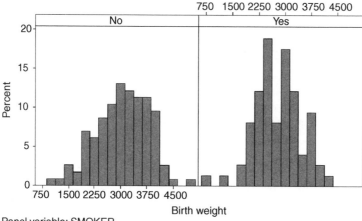

Panel variable: SMOKER

Figure 4.20   Histograms of birth weight by smoking status.

Solutions On the basis of the boxplots and histograms given in Figures 4.19 and 4.20

a. it appears that both distributions have the same general shape. In particular, both distributions appear to be mound shaped. Here, the peaks and valleys in the histogram for mothers who smoked during pregnancy are most likely due to sampling variation.

b. both histograms suggest a mound-shaped distribution, and thus, the normal probability model might be considered as a plausible probability model for both distributions. Thus, normal probability models with different means and standard deviations could be considered for modeling the distributions of the birth weights for these two subpopulations.

4.2.4 Normal Probability Plots

A boxplot and a histogram often suggest a plausible probability model that could be used for the underlying distribution. Moreover, in many cases the boxplot and histogram suggest that the distribution is mound shaped, and hence, the normal probability model should be considered a possible probability model for the distribution. A *normal probability plot* is a graphical statistic that can be used to assess the fit of a normal distribution to the observed data. A normal probability plot is also often referred to as a *normal plot*. An example of a normal probability plot is given in Figure 4.21 for the birth weights of babies in the Birth Weight data set for mothers who smoked during pregnancy.

There are many different forms of a normal probability plot, and since each statistical package handles a normal probability plot differently, the details of creating a normal plot will not be discussed here. Regardless of how a normal probability plot is created, each normal plot can be used visually to assess whether or not it is plausible that the sampled data for a continuous variable came from a normal distribution. Normal plots are basically plots of the sample percentiles versus the expected percentiles of the normal distribution that best fits the observed sample. When the points in a normal plot fall nearly on a straight line, it is reasonable to assume that the sample data came from a normal distribution; when the points in a normal plot deviate from a straight line, the normal probability plot is suggesting that data came from a distribution that is not normally distributed.

Normal plots are typically used as a visual assessment of how well the observed data fits a normal probability model, and thus, normal plots can be difficult to interpret and

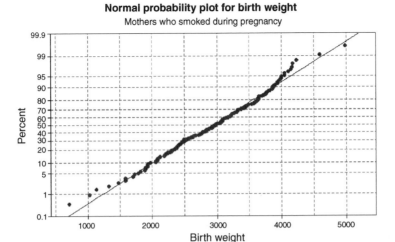

Figure 4.21 A normal probability plot of the birth weights for mothers who smoked during pregnancy.

should not be overanalyzed. In particular, due to sampling variation it is unlikely that the points will fall on a perfectly straight line even when the population sampled is normally distributed. One method determining whether the points in a normal plot are close enough to a straight line is to use the *fat pencil test*.

THE FAT PENCIL TEST

---

1. Imagine laying an imaginary fat pencil over the points in the normal plot.

2. When all of the points in the normal plot are covered by the imaginary pencil, the normal plot suggests that a normal probability model might be a reasonable model for the underlying distribution that was sampled; when some of the points in the normal plot are not covered by the imaginary pencil, the normal plot is suggesting that a normal probability model is not a reasonable model for the underlying distribution that was sampled.

Interpreting a normal plot is based on a subjective assessment of the plot, the fat pencil test can be used to remove some of the subjectivity encountered in evaluating the information contained in a normal plot. A histogram and a boxplot can also be used to back up inferences made from the normal plot. An example of a normal plot that would pass the fat pencil test is given in Figure 4.22a, and an example of a normal plot that does not pass the fat pencil test is given in Figure 4.22b,

Example 4.12
Use the fat pencil test to determine whether the data displayed in each of the normal plots given in Figure 4.23 suggests that a normal probability model is a reasonable model for the underlying distribution.

Solutions The normal plots in Figure 4.23a–d are fairly linear and do pass the fat pencil test; however, the normal plots in Figure 4.23b–c clearly deviate from a straight line and do not pass the

Normal probability plots

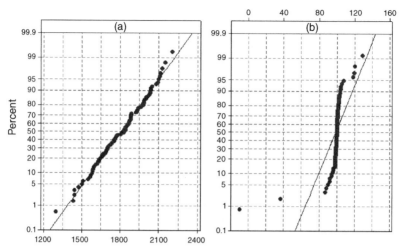

Figure 4.22   A normal plot that passes the fat pencil test (a) and a normal plot that does not pass the fat pencil test.

fat pencil test. Thus, a normal probability model is a reasonable model for only the distributions associated with the samples and normal probability plots displayed in Figure 4.23a–d.

Finally, several of the statistical methods that will be discussed in later chapters, such as confidence intervals, hypothesis tests, and statistical modeling will require that the underlying distribution of the data is approximately normally distributed. When a statistical procedure is appropriate only when the underlying distribution is approximately normally distributed, normal probability plots should be used to check whether or not the sample data support the hypothesis that the underlying distribution is normally distributed.

Normal probability plots

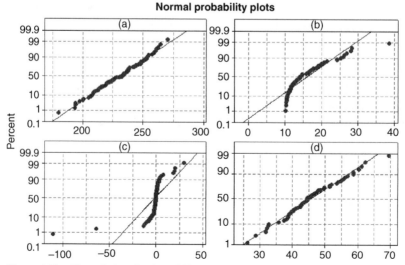

Figure 4.23   Normal plots for four different data sets.

4.3 NUMERICAL STATISTICS FOR UNIVARIATE DATA SETS

After performing a graphical statistical analysis of a sample data set, the next step in a typical statistical analysis is to compute the appropriate numerical statistics that will lead to estimates and statistical inferences for the unknown parameters of the population. Recall that a parameter is a numerical measure of a characteristic of the population and can be computed only by taking a census of the target population. On the other hand, a statistic is any quantity that is computed from the sample observations that are selected from the target population. Because statistics are based on samples, and samples contain only partial information on the population, the values of the computed statistics are not going to be equal to the values of the unknown parameters. However, the values of the estimates that are computed from a well-designed random sample should contain fairly reliable information about the values of unknown parameters.

A *point estimate* is a single-valued estimate of a parameter as a statistic computed from a sample. Simply put, a point estimate is a single number computed from the sample observations that is used to estimate the unknown value of a population parameter, and a *point estimator* is the rule or formula that is used to compute the value of the point estimate. Thus, a point estimator is a rule and a point estimate is the number that results from applying a point estimator to the sample data. Furthermore, point estimators are often based on rules similar to those used for computing the value of a parameter when the entire population is at hand. For example, the population mean is computed from a list of the N units in the population using the formula

$$\mu = \frac{\sum X}{N}$$

and the point estimator of μ is computed from the n sample observations according to the formula

$$\bar{x} = \frac{\sum x}{n}$$

4.3.1 Estimating Population Proportions

Population proportions, percentages, and probabilities such as the prevalence of a disease, the specificity and the sensitivity of a diagnostic test, the probability of being cured of a disease, and survival probabilities are often the focus of biomedical research studies. Thus, in many biostatistical analyses proportions, percentages, and probabilities will be estimated from an observed sample.

Recall that the proportion of the population having a particular characteristic, say characteristic A, is found by computing

$$p = \frac{\text{number of population units having characteristic } A}{N}$$

where N is the number of units in the population. The rule for estimating a population proportion from a random sample of n observations is given below.

ESTIMATING A PROPORTION

When p is the proportion of the population units with characteristic A, the point estimator of p is the proportion of the sample having characteristic A, and is denoted by $\widehat{p}$. The formula for computing $\widehat{p}$ is

$$\widehat{p} = \frac{\text{the number of sample observations with characteristic } A}{n}$$

where n is the sample size.

For estimation purposes, the formulas for estimating a proportion and a probability are essentially the same and both can be converted to estimates of a percentage by multiplying by 100%. That is, to estimate the percentage of the population units with characteristic A, use

$$\text{Estimated percentage} = \widehat{p} \times 100\%$$

Example 4.13

In the article "Cannabis smoking and peridontal disease among young adults" published in the *Journal of the American Medical Association* (Thomson et al., 2008), the authors reported the summary data given in Table 4.2 for $n = 903$ individuals monitored in a longitudinal study on the relationship between cannabis use and peridontal disease. The cohort in this study was identified in 1973 and last monitored in 2005.

Based on the summary data in Table 4.2 the estimate of the proportion of individuals who are the highest 20% users of cannabis is

$$\widehat{p} = \frac{182}{903} = 0.202$$

and the proportion of individuals who use cannabis (i.e., some use highest 20%) is

$$\widehat{p} = \frac{428 + 182}{903} = 0.676$$

Recall that the prevalence proportion P of a specific disease is the proportion of a particular population that has this disease at a given time. The following description of how the National Cancer Institute computes the complete prevalence proportion was taken from www.cancer.gov.

TABLE 4.2   Summarized Frequencies of Cannabis Use for a Longitudinal Study of Predontal Disease ($n = 903$)

Cannabis Use	Frequency
None	293
Some	428
Highest 20%	182
Total	903

Complete prevalence represents the proportion of people alive on a certain day who were diagnosed with the disease, regardless of how long ago the diagnosis was made. Complete prevalence can be estimated from self-reported population-based surveys (Byrne et al., 1992), although one must be concerned with underreporting and misclassification of disease. Direct computation (the counting method) of complete cancer prevalence requires registry data that has been collected over a sufficiently long period of time to capture all prevalent cases of the disease.

Thus, for a specific disease and target population, the prevalence proportion, say P, for a given time can be estimated using the formula

$$\widehat{P} = \frac{\text{the estimated number of individuals with the disease}}{\text{the number in the target population at the given time}}$$

or from a random sample using

$$\widehat{P} = \frac{\text{the number of individuals in the sample with the disease}}{\text{the number sampled}}$$

Example 4.14

In the article "Estimating the prevalence of chronic fatigue syndrome and associated symptoms in the community" published in *Public Health Reports* (Price et al., 1992), the authors report the results of a stratified random cluster sample of 13,185 individuals that are summarized in Table 4.3.

Based on the data given in Table 4.3, the estimates of the prevalence of chronic fatigue are

$$\widehat{P}_{\text{men}} = \frac{107}{5410} \times 100\% = 2.2\%$$

$$\widehat{P}_{\text{women}} = \frac{159}{7775} \times 100\% = 2.4\%$$

$$\widehat{P}_{\text{combined}} = \frac{266}{13185} \times 100\% = 2.3\%$$

Thus, based on the sample data it appears that the prevalence rates are roughly the same for men and women.

When a sample contains two qualitative variables, a *two-way cross-classification frequency table* or *two-way contingency table* is often used to display a summary of the sample data. A two-way contingency table is constructed by categorizing the sample data according to the two qualitative variables under consideration. In particular, suppose the qualitative variables are denoted by A and B. If A is the row variable and has r categories and B is the column variable with c categories, then the sample information is tabulated and the frequencies of the combined A and B categories are listed in a $r \times c$ contingency table. The process of categorizing the sample data according to two qualitative variables is called

TABLE 4.3   Results of the Chronic Fatigue Random Sample of Individuals

Criteria	Men	Women	Combined
Absence of fatigue	5,205	7,395	12,600
Fatigue	107	159	266

TABLE 4.4 An Example of a 2 × 3 Contingency Table

	Gender Smokers			
	Current smoker	Former smoker	Never smoked	Total
Male	27	13	45	85
Female	22	18	33	73
Total	49	35	78	158

cross classification. An example of a 2 × 3 contingency table is given in Table 4.4 for a hypothetical simple random sample cross-classified by the variables gender and smoking status.

A two-way contingency table can be used for estimating population proportions, percentages, and conditional probabilities. An estimate of the conditional probability that variable A takes on the value a (i.e., $A = a$) given that variable B takes on the value b (i.e., $B = b$) can be computed from a random sample summarized in an $r \times c$ table using

$$\widehat{P}(A = a | B = b) = \frac{\text{number of sample observations with } A = a \text{ and } B = b}{\text{number of sample observations with } B = b}$$

For example, using the contingency table given in Table 4.4, the estimate of the conditional probability that an individual is a former smoker given the individual is male is

$$\widehat{P}(\text{former smoker}|\text{male}) = \frac{\text{No. of former smokers and male in the sample}}{\text{no. of males in the sample}}$$

$$= \frac{13}{85} = 0.153$$

An estimate of the conditional probability that an individual is a former smoker given the individual is female is

$$\widehat{P}(\text{former smoker}|\text{female}) = \frac{\text{No. former smokers and female in the sample}}{\text{No. females in the sample}}$$

$$= \frac{18}{73} = 0.247$$

Example 4.15
The 2 × 2 contingency table given in Table 4.5 contains a summary of 189 individuals in the Birth Weight data set. In particular, the Table 4.5 contains the information on the qualitative variables low

TABLE 4.5 A 2 × 2 Contingency Table for the Birth Weight Data Cross-Classified According to Smoking Status and BWT

Low	Smoke		
	Yes	No	Total
1 (Below normal)	30	29	59
0 (Normal)	44	86	130
Total	74	115	189

and smoke where

$$Low = \begin{cases} 1 \text{ when birth weight} < 2500 \text{ grams} \\ 0 \text{ when birth weight} \geq 2500 \text{ grams} \end{cases}$$

and

$$Smoke = \begin{cases} Yes \text{ mother smoked during pregnancy} \\ No \text{ mother did not smoke during pregnancy} \end{cases}$$

Use the summary data given in Table 4.5 to estimate the proportion of low birth weight babies for

   a. all individuals (i.e., $P(low = 1)$)

   b. the subpopulation of mothers who were smokers (i.e., $P(low = 1|smoke = yes)$)

   c. the subpopulation of mothers who were nonsmokers (i.e., $P(low = 1|smoke = no)$)

Solutions Based on the data in Table 4.5

   a. the estimate of the proportion of low birth weight babies for all individuals is

$$\widehat{P}(low = 1) = \frac{59}{189} = 0.31$$

   b. the estimate of the proportion of low birth weight babies for the subpopulation of mothers who smoked during pregnancy (i.e., $P(low = 1|smoke = yes)$) is

$$\widehat{P}(low = 1|smoke = yes) = \frac{30}{74} = 0.41$$

   c. the estimate of the proportion of low birth weight babies for the subpopulation of mothers who did not smoke during pregnancy (i.e., $P(low = 1|smoke = no)$) is

$$\widehat{P}(low = 1|smoke = No) = \frac{29}{115} = 0.25$$

Sensitivity and specificity are conditional probabilities that play an important role in the development of diagnostic tests for diseases and investigating the efficacy of a new drug. Recall that the sensitivity and specificity of a test are defined to be the following conditional probabilities:

   Sensitivity = the probability of a positive test given the disease is present

       = $P(+|D)$

   Specificity = the probability of a negative test given the disease is absent

       = $P(-|D)$

The sensitivity and specificity of a diagnostic test can be estimated from the information contained in a 2×2 contingency table when a random sample of n observations is summarized in a table of the form given in Table 4.6. Then, based on the contingency table given

TABLE 4.6 A 2 × 2 Contingency Table for Estimating the Sensitivity and Specificity of a Diagnostic Test

Test Result	Diseased	
	Yes	No
Positive	a	b
Negative	c	d

in Table 4.6, the estimates of the sensitivity and specificity of the test are

$$\text{Estimated sensitivity} = \widehat{P}(+|\text{diseased}) \quad\quad = \tfrac{a}{a+c}$$

$$\text{Estimated specificity} = \widehat{P}(-|\text{not diseased}) = \tfrac{d}{b+d}$$

Example 4.16

Suppose a diagnostic test for detecting Alzheimer's disease is being developed. A preliminary evaluation of the test based on a sample of 120 individuals results in the 2 × 2 contingency table given in Table 4.7. Use the information in Table 4.7 to estimate the sensitivity and specificity of this diagnostic test.

Solutions Based on the data in Table 4.7, the estimates of the sensitivity and specificity for this diagnostic test are

$$\widehat{P}(+|D) = \frac{58}{60} = 0.967$$

$$\widehat{P}(-|D) = \frac{55}{60} = .917$$

The relative risk of a disease for exposure to a specific risk factor is another parameter that is often studied in biomedical research studies. The relative risk of a disease is defined to be the ratio of the probability of the disease for exposure to the risk factor and the probability of not having the disease for those not exposed to this risk factor. That is, the relative risk of a disease for exposure to a risk factor is

$$RR = \frac{P(\text{disease}|\text{exposure to the risk factor is present})}{P(\text{disease}|\text{exposure to the risk factor is absent})}$$

The relative risk of a disease for exposure to a risk factor can also be estimated from a 2 × 2 contingency table. Suppose the sample data are summarized in a 2 × 2 contin-

TABLE 4.7 Result of the 120 Individuals Sampled in a Study on the Diagnostic Test for Alzheimer's Disease

Test Result	Diseased	
	Yes	No
Positive	58	5
Negative	2	55

TABLE 4.8   A 2 × 2 Contingency Table for Estimating the Relative Risk of a Disease for a Particular Exposure Factor

Risk Factor	Disease	
	Present	Absent
Present	a	b
Absent	c	d

gency table of the form given in Table 4.8. Then, the estimate of the relative risk (RR) is given by

$$\widehat{\text{RR}} = \frac{a(c+d)}{c(a+b)}$$

Example 4.17
In the Birth Weight study, one of the research goals might be to estimate the relative risk of having a low birth weight baby for a mother who smoked during pregnancy. The Birth Weight data set has been cross-classified according to smoking status and the coded birth weights (i.e., the variables smoke and low) in Table 4.9.

   Use the information in Table 4.9 to estimate the relative risk of a below-normal birth weight baby for mothers who smoked during pregnancy.

Solutions   The estimated relative risk of having a below normal birth weight baby for mothers who smoked during pregnancy is

$$\widehat{RR} = \frac{0.405}{0.252} = 1.61$$

Thus, the relative risk of having a below normal birth weight baby for a mother who smoked during pregnancy is 1.6 times that of a mother who did not smoke during pregnancy.

   Finally, the proportion or percentage of the population falling below a particular value of a quantitative variable, say x^*, is another type of parameter that is often of interest in a biomedical research study. For example, in the Birth Weight study the researchers might be interested in knowing the proportion of babies born with birth weights less than 2000 g. In this case, an estimate of this proportion could be found by simply determining the number of babies in the sample with birth weights below 2000 g and dividing by the sample size. In the Birth Weight data set there are 19 observations below 2000 and hence, an estimate of the proportion of babies with birth weights less than 2000 g is $\frac{19}{189} = 0.10$.

TABLE 4.9   A 2 × 2 Contingency Table for Low and Smoke Status for the Birth Weight Data Set

Smoke	Low	
	1 (Below Normal)	0 (Normal)
Yes	30	44
No	29	76

4.3.2 Estimating Population Percentiles

A set of parameters often used to describe maximum exposure levels, thresholds, benchmarks, or for comparing the status of a patient against the norms of a reference population are the *percentiles* of a population. For example, percentiles are now used in evaluating whether or not a child is overweight or obese. In particular, a child is considered to have normal weight when its Body Mass Index (BMI) falls between the 5th and 85th percentiles, and a child is considered overweight when its BMI exceeds the 95th percentile. The *p*th *percentile* of a variable X is the value of the variable such that $p\%$ of the population falls below this value and is denoted by x_p. The 50th percentile is called the *median* and the 25th and 75th percentiles are called the first and third quartiles of the population.

The *p*th percentile can be estimated from the raw data or a plot such as a normal probability plot. In either case, the percentage of sample points falling below the estimate of the *p*th percentile will be $p\%$. The rule for computing the *p*th percentile is given below.

ESTIMATING A PERCENTILE

The point estimator of a population percentile is the *sample p*th *percentile* that is denoted by $\widehat{x}_p$. To compute the value of $\widehat{x}_p$, determine the observed value in the sample where $p\%$ of the sample lies below this value.

In general, it is best to use a statistical package or probability plot for computing the estimates of the percentiles, but a boxplot can be used for estimating the 25th, 50th, and 75th percentiles of a population.

Example 4.18
In the Birth Weight data set the 10th, 25th, 50th, and 75th, and 90th percentiles for mothers who smoked during pregnancy and mothers who did not smoke during pregnancy are summarized in Table 4.10.

Note that the sample percentiles given in Table 4.10 indicate that babies born to mothers who smoked during pregnancy tend to have lower birth weights than the babies born to mothers who did not smoke during pregnancy. That is, the sample percentiles for the birth weights of babies born to mothers who smoked during pregnancy are less than the corresponding percentiles for the birth weights of babies born to mothers who did not smoke during pregnancy.

Note that the values of the sample 25th, 50th, and 75th percentiles could be read directly from a boxplot; however, the values of the 10th and 90th sample percentiles can-

TABLE 4.10 Estimates of Selected Birth Weight Percentiles by Smoking Status in the Birth Weight Study

Smoking Status	Percentiles				
	10th	25th	50th	75th	90th
Mother who smoked	1927	2363.5	2775.5	3270.8	3619
Mother who did not smoke	2091	2495	3100	3629	4019

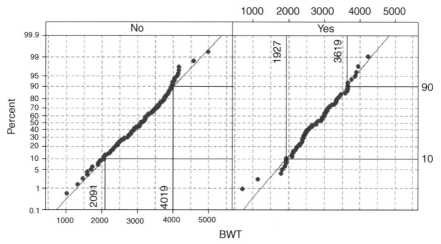

Panel variable: SMOKER

Figure 4.24   Normal plots for birth weight according to mother's smoking status.

not be found using the information conveyed by a boxplot. It is possible to obtain estimates of the population percentiles from some forms of a normal probability plot. In particular, the normal probability plots that the statistical computing package MINITAB produces are particularly good for this purpose. For example, using the normal probability plot for the birth weights (BWT) of the babies in the Birth Weight data set, given in Figure 4.24, the estimates of the 10th and 90th percentiles can be read off the normal plot.

In this example, MINITAB was instructed to put in reference lines for the values corresponding to the percentages equal to 10% and 90%. Thus, the sample 10th and 90th percentiles of birth weights for babies with mothers who did not smoke during pregnancy are 2091 and 4019, respectively; the sample 10th and 90th percentiles of birth weights for babies whose mothers did smoke during pregnancy are 1927 and 3619, respectively.

4.3.3 Estimating the Mean, Median, and Mode

Recall that the mean, median, and mode of a population are all measures of the typical value in a population. The mean, median, and mode are also referred to as measures of location because they provide information on the central values of the population. It is important to note that the shape of the underlying distribution dictates which of the mean, median, and mode will be the most meaningful measure of the central or typical value in a population. For example, since the mean is always pulled out in the direction of the longest tail, when a distribution has an extremely long tail the median and the mode are more meaningful parameters for describing the typical value in a population than is the mean. Thus, in deciding on which parameters to estimate it is very important to investigate the underlying shape of the distribution with a histogram and boxplot. In general, the following recommendations can be helpful in determining which location parameters best measure the typical value in a population, and thus, should be estimated.

PARAMETERS OF CENTRALITY AND DISTRIBUTIONAL SHAPES

---

1. When the boxplot and histogram suggest that the underlying distribution is mound shaped, then the mean, median, and mode should be nearly equal. In this case, it is appropriate to estimate the mean, median, and mode.

2. When the boxplot and histogram suggest the underlying distribution has an extremely long tail to the right or left the mean is pulled out toward the longer tail, and in this case, the median and mode are the appropriate parameters for representing the typical or central values in the population. In this case, it is best to estimate the median and the mode.

3. When the boxplot and histogram suggest a distribution with more than one mode this suggests that there may be well-defined subpopulations present in the underlying distribution. In this case, the modes are generally more appropriate descriptors of the typical values in each subpopulation. Furthermore, the mean and median of a bimodal population often do not provide any relevant information on the individual subpopulation means and medians. In this case, the modes are the appropriate parameters to estimate.

The recommendations on which of the mean, median, and mode should be estimated are based on the fact that a long tail pulls the mean away from the center (i.e., typical) value in the population and that a multimodal distribution is usually due to having well-defined subpopulations in the underlying population. Figure 4.25 illustrates the relationships between the mean (μ), the median ($\widetilde{\mu}$), and the mode (M) for distributions that are long tail left, long tail right, mound shaped, or multimodal.

Recall that the mode represents the value in the population that has the largest probability for a discrete variable or the largest density for a continuous variable. While the mode is generally not the primary parameter that a researcher will be interested in, the mode is often an important parameter in multimodal distributions. The best statistic for estimating the modes (M) of a population is the histogram. Because a histogram may indicate there is more than one mode in a population, it is important to identify

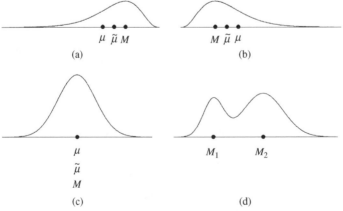

Figure 4.25   The four most common distributional shapes (a) long tail left; (b) long tail right; (c) mound shaped; (d) bimodal.

only the obvious modes in a histogram. The sample mode is the most frequent value in the sample and will be denoted by $\widehat{M}$, and when there are two modes in a histogram they are denoted by $\widehat{M}_1$ and $\widehat{M}_2$. A method for finding the value of $\widehat{M}$ is outlined below.

ESTIMATING A MODE

The sample mode $\widehat{M}$ can be found by

    1. Locating the class interval in a histogram that is the tallest.

2. The sample median, $\widehat{M}$, is the midpoint of this class interval.

Example 4.19
The histogram given in Figure 4.26 is based on Body Fat data set for the variable percentage of body fat (PCTBF) calculated by an underwater weighing technique for a sample of $n = 252$ men.

    Since the tallest class in this histogram covers the interval 20–25, the estimate of the mode is the midpoint of the interval 20–25 which is 22.5, Thus, the estimate of the mode of the distribution of percentage of body fat for men is $\widehat{M} = 22.5$.

    Provided that the distribution is not multimodal or extremely long tailed, the mean of the population can be used for describing the typical or central values in a population. Recall that the mean of a population X is found by averaging all of the values of X in the population. That is,

$$\mu = \frac{\sum X}{N}$$

The estimator of the mean is called the *sample mean* and is denoted by $\bar{x}$. The formula for computing the value of $\bar{x}$ from the information contained in a simple random sample is given below.

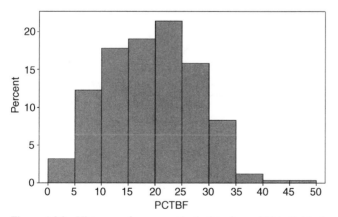

Figure 4.26   Histogram for percent body fat of $n = 252$ individuals.

ESTIMATING THE MEAN

The point estimator of the population mean μ is sample mean $\bar{x}$. The value of $\bar{x}$ is the average of the observed values in the sample.

$$\bar{x} = \frac{\text{sum of the observed data values}}{\text{the sample size}} = \frac{\sum x}{n}$$

Note that both $\bar{x}$ and μ are arithmetic averages; the sample mean is computed for a sample selected from the population, and the population mean is found from a census of the population. Since the value of a parameter can be found only from a census and a sample is not a census, $\bar{x}$ is only an estimate of μ and is not equal to the unknown value of μ. Simply put, $\bar{x}$ is a "mathematical guess" of the unknown value of μ based on an observed sample.

Example 4.20

Suppose a nutritionist is studying the caloric content of a 4-ounce serving of a new low-fat ice-cream that is under development. A random sample of 12 observations yields the following data on caloric content of a 4-ounce serving of this ice-cream. Use the data given in Table 4.11 to estimate the mean caloric content for a 4-ounce serving of this ice-cream.

The estimated mean caloric content for a 4-ounce serving of this ice-cream is

$$\bar{x} = \frac{124 + 125 + 127 + \cdots + 117 + 119}{12}$$

$$= \frac{1499}{12} = 124.92$$

The sample mean is also the balancing point or center of gravity of a histogram. Three examples of the balancing point of a histogram ($\bar{x}$) are given in Figure 4.27. Note that the balancing point of a histogram is $\bar{x}$ that is pulled out toward the longest tail of a histogram, and the longer the tail is, the farther the sample mean will be pulled from the center of the distribution.

When the variable of interest is a discrete variable and the sample information is presented in a table listing each observed x value and its frequency, the value of $\bar{x}$ can be computed by using the formula

$$\bar{x} = \frac{\sum (\text{frequency of an } x \text{ value}) \times (\text{the } x \text{ value})}{n}$$

TABLE 4.11   Values of a Sample of $n = 12$ Caloric Contents of a New Low-Fat Ice-Cream

Obs.	Caloric content	Obs.	Caloric content	Obs.	Caloric content
1	124	5	116	9	131
2	125	6	134	10	130
3	127	7	125	11	117
4	126	8	125	12	119

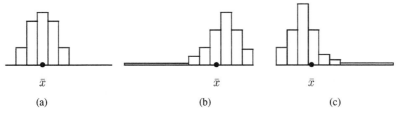

Figure 4.27 The balancing points of three histograms: (a) mound shaped; (b) long tail left; and (c) long tail right.

Example 4.21
Suppose that a random survey of $n = 75$ heads of household was conducted in a study on the use of a local clinic. Table 7.10 contains the number of visits to the clinic by a family and the frequency of each number of visits. Use the information in Table 7.10 to estimate the mean number of family visits to this clinic.
Based on the data summarized in Table 7.10, the estimate of the mean number of visits per year to this clinic for a family is

$$\bar{x} = \frac{5 \cdot 0 + 12 \cdot 1 + 22 \cdot 2 + 17 \cdot 3 + 18 \cdot 4 + 1 \cdot 5}{75}$$

$$= \frac{184}{75} = 2.45$$

The median of a population ($\widetilde{\mu}$) is the value in the population that divides the population into two halves with 50% of the population falling at or below the median and 50% of the population falling at or above the median. Thus, the $\widetilde{\mu}$ is the 50th percentile in a population. Unlike the mean, the median is not sensitive to the values in the tails of the distribution, and thus, the median as the parameter of that should be used for describing the center of a long-tailed distribution. The estimate of the population median is called the *sample median* and is denoted by $\widetilde{x}$. The rule for computing the value of the sample median is given below.

TABLE 4.12 The Number of Sampled Visits to the Clinic Summarized According to Frequency of Visit

No. of Visits	Frequency
0	5
1	12
2	22
3	17
4	18
5	1
	75

ESTIMATING THE MEDIAN

The point estimator of the population median $\widetilde{\mu}$ is the sample median $\widetilde{x}$ that is the middle value in the ordered sample. To find the value of the sample median $\widetilde{x}$:

1. List the sample observations in order from lowest value to highest value, including all of the values that are repeated in the sample.

2. Determine the middle observation in this ordered list.

(a) When the sample size n is an odd number, then there will be exactly one observation in the middle of the ranked sample. In this case, the value of $\widetilde{x}$ is equal to the value of this middle observation.

(b) On the other hand, when n is an even number there will be no middle observation. In this case, the value of $\widetilde{x}$ is the average of the two middle observations in the ranked sample.

Note that to find the value of the sample median, the values of the sample must be ranked in either ascending or descending order. The sample median can found from the information contained in a boxplot and a normal probability plot.

Example 4.22
Using the random sample of the 12 observations on caloric content of a 4-ounce serving of the low-fat ice-cream in Example 4.20, the estimate of the median caloric content for a 4-ounce serving of this ice-cream is found by (1) sorting the values listed below in ascending order and (2) by averaging the two middle values. The sorted sample values are listed below.

$$116,\ 117,\ 119,\ 124,\ 125,\ 125,\ 125,\ 126,\ 127,\ 130,\ 131,\ 134$$

Because the number of observations is even (i.e., $n = 12$), the estimate of the median caloric content for a 4-ounce serving of this low-fat ice-cream is the average of the two middle values, 125 and 125. Thus, the value of the sample median is $\widetilde{x} = \frac{125+125}{2} = 125$.

Example 4.23
The boxplot and histogram given in Figure 4.28 are based on the 252 observations on the variable body density (Density) found in the Body Fat data set.
Use the histogram and boxplot in Figure 4.28 along with $\sum x = 266$ to

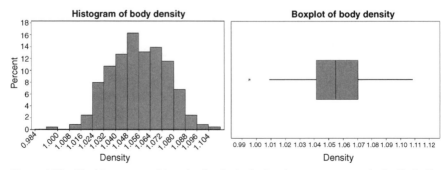

Figure 4.28   The histogram and boxplot for the body density measurements in the Body Fat data set.

a. estimate the general shape of the underlying distribution of the variable density.

b. estimate of the mode of the distribution of the variable density.

c. determine whether it is reasonable to use the mean as a measure of the central value in the distribution of the variable density.

d. estimate of the mean and the median of the variable density.

Solutions

a. Based on the histogram and boxplot in Figure 4.28, the general shape of the underlying distribution of body density appears to be mound shaped.

b. The estimate of the mode of the distribution of body density is the midpoint of the class interval 1.048–1.056 that is $\widehat{M} = 1.052$.

c. Because the histogram and boxplot in Figure 4.28 suggest that the underlying distribution is mound shaped, it is reasonable to use the mean as a measure of the central value.

d. The estimate of the mean is $\bar{x} = \dfrac{\sum x}{n} = \dfrac{266}{252} = 1.056$ and the estimate of the median is $\tilde{x} = 1.055$. Note that because the histogram and boxplot for this sample are indicating a mound-shaped distribution, it follows that $\bar{x}$ and $\tilde{x}$ will be nearly equal, which they are in this case.

Finally, in a well-designed statistical analysis before estimating the parameters that measure the central values in a population, graphical statistics such as boxplots, histograms, and normal probability plots should first be examined. Only after analyzing the graphical statistics should a centrality parameter be estimated. In general, it is reasonable to use the mean and median as measures of the central values in the population, unless there is evidence that one of the tails in the distribution is extremely long. In the presence of a long-tailed distribution the median is a more meaningful measure of the central or typical value in a population than the mean is since the mean is sensitive to the longer tail in a distribution.

A statistic is said to be *robust* or *resistant* to the extremes of a sample if it is not affected by the extreme values in a sample. The sample median is robust to the extremes of a sample; however, the sample mean is not robust to the extremes. In the presence of an outlier, special care must be given to avoid blindly reporting the value of any statistic that is not robust to the extremes. The histogram and boxplot can be used to identify observations that might be highly influential when estimating the mean or any other statistic that is not robust to the extremes of a sample.

4.3.4 Estimating the Variance and Standard Deviation

While it is important in most research studies to estimate the central values in the target population, it is possible to have two different populations with the same means and medians that have very different distributions. For example, consider the two distributions shown in Figure 4.29 that have the same mean and median.

Even though the distributions shown in Figure 4.29 have the same means and medians, clearly one population is much more spread out than the other population. In fact, the values in one population range from about 80 to 120, while the values in the other population range from 70 to 130, and clearly, the standard deviations of these two mound-shaped distributions are different. Thus, the spread of a population is also an important characteristic to consider when summarizing the distribution of a particular population.

The three population parameters that measure the spread of a population for a quantitative variable are the variance (σ^2), the standard deviation (σ), and the interquartile range.

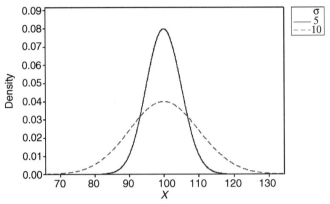

Figure 4.29   Two mound-shaped distributions with the same mean but different standard deviations.

Recall that the variance of a population of N units is

$$\sigma^2 = \frac{\sum (X - \mu)^2}{N}$$

the standard deviation is $\sigma = \sqrt{\sigma^2}$, and the IQR is the distance between the 75th and 25th percentiles. In practice, the standard deviation is usually reported as the measure of spread because the units of the standard deviation are also the units of measurement, while the units of the variance are the units of measurement squared. Furthermore, the standard deviation is interpreted as roughly the size of the typical deviation of a population unit from the mean.

The formulas for estimating the variance and standard deviation of the distribution of a variable X from a random sample are given below.

ESTIMATING THE VARIANCE AND STANDARD DEVIATION

The point estimator of the population variance (σ^2) is the *sample variance* that is denoted by s^2, and the point estimator of the population standard deviation (σ) is the *sample standard deviation* that is denoted by s. The values of estimators s^2 and s are computed using

$$s^2 = \frac{\sum (x_i - \bar{x})^2}{n - 1}$$

$$s = \sqrt{s^2}$$

Note that the formula for computing the sample variance is very similar to the formula used for computing the value of the population variance; however, there are two key differences in these formulas. First, because the value of μ is unknown, $\bar{x}$ is in place of μ. Second, in the formula for σ^2 the divisor is N and in the formula for s^2 the divisor is $n - 1$, not n. It turns out that a slightly better estimator of σ^2 results from dividing by $n - 1$ rather than by n. In particular, dividing by $n - 1$ rather than by n produces an estimator that does not systematically over- or underestimate the variance of a population. The sample variance and sample standard deviation are said to have $n - 1$ *degrees of freedom*; the degrees of freedom are important in several statistical procedures that will be discussed in Chapters 6, 7, 8, 9, and 12.

Note that like most of the statistics that have been previously discussed, the estimates of the standard deviation and variance are best computed using a statistical computing package. However, for small samples, the value of s^2 can be computed by following the steps outlined below.

COMPUTING THE VALUE OF s^2

1. Compute the sample mean $\bar{x}$.

2. For each observation in the sample, compute the deviation from the sample mean.

3. Square each of the n deviations from the mean.

4. Sum the squared deviations from the mean.

5. Divide the sum of the squared deviations by $n - 1$ to determine the value of

$$s^2 = \frac{\sum(x - \bar{x})^2}{n - 1}$$

Example 4.24 illustrates how the sample variance and sample standard deviation can be computed from the information in a small random sample.

Example 4.24

Use the sample data for the study on the caloric content of a new low-fat ice-cream that is given in Table 4.11 Example 4.20 to estimate the variance and standard deviation of the caloric content of a 4-ounce serving of this new ice-cream.

Solutions

1. From Example 4.20, the value of the sample mean is $\bar{x} = 124.92$.

2. The 12 deviations from the sample mean are

```
124-124.92  =  -0.92        125-124.92  =   0.08
127-124.92  =   2.08        116-124.92  =  -8.92
134-124.92  =   9.08        125-124.92  =   0.08
131-124.92  =   6.08        130-124.92  =   5.08
117-124.92  =  -7.92        126-124.92  =   1.08
125-124.92  =   0.08        119-124.92  =  -5.92
```

3. The squared deviations are

$$(-0.92)^2, \ (0.08)^2, \ (2.08)^2, \ (-8.92)^2, \ (9.08)^2, \ (0.08)^2$$

$$(6.08)^2, \ (5.08)^2, \ (-7.92)^2, \ (1.08)^2, \ (0.08)^2, \ (-5.92)^2$$

4. The sum of the squared deviations is

$$\sum(x - \bar{x})^2 = (-0.92)^2 + (0.08)^2 + (2.08)^2 + (-8.92)^2 + (9.08)^2 + (0.08)^2$$

$$+(6.08)^2 + (5.08)^2 + (-7.92)^2 + (1.08)^2 + (0.08)^2 + (-5.92)^2$$

$$= 328.9168$$

5. Thus, $s^2 = \dfrac{\sum(x - \bar{x})^2}{n - 1} = \dfrac{328.9168}{12 - 1} = 29.90$ and $s = \sqrt{29.90} = 5.47$

Thus, the estimate of the variance of the caloric content of a 4-ounce serving of this low-fat ice cream is $s^2 = 29.90$, and the estimate of the standard deviation is $s = 5.47$.

For larger samples, the following alternative forms of s^2 are more efficient formulas for computing the value of s^2.

COMPUTATIONAL FORMULAS FOR s^2

$$s^2 = \frac{\sum x_i^2 - \frac{\left(\sum x_i\right)^2}{n}}{n-1}$$

$$= \frac{\sum x_i^2 - n(\bar{x})^2}{n-1}$$

These alternative formulas for computing the value of s^2 given above are algebraically equivalent to $s^2 = \dfrac{\sum(x-\bar{x})^2}{n-1}$; however, they are more efficient in computing formulas. In general, the values of s^2 and s should be computed using a statistical computing package to ensure the accuracy of the computed values, regardless of the sample size.

Example 4.25
Compute the value of s^2 for the data on the caloric content of the low-fat ice-cream given in Example 4.20 using

a. $s^2 = \dfrac{1}{n-1}\left[\sum x_i^2 - \dfrac{(\sum x_i)^2}{n}\right]$

b. $s^2 = \dfrac{1}{n-1}\left[\sum x_i^2 - n(\bar{x})^2\right]$

Solutions First, it is necessary to compute the values of $\sum x$ and $\sum x^2$.

$$\sum x = 124 + 125 + \cdots + 126 + 125 + 119$$

$$= 1499$$

$$\sum x^2 = 124^2 + 125^2 + \cdots + 125^2 + 119^2$$

$$= 187579$$

a. $s^2 = \dfrac{1}{12-1}\left[187579 - \dfrac{1499^2}{12}\right] = 29.90$

b. $s^2 = \dfrac{1}{12-1}\left[187579 - 12(124.92)^2\right] = 28.99$

The estimates in parts (a) and (b) are slightly different because the value of $\bar{x}$ was rounded to 124.92 in part (b). The actual value of $\bar{x}$ is $\bar{x} = \dfrac{1499}{12} = 124.91\bar{6}$, and when $\bar{x} = 124.9167$ has been used in place of $\bar{x} = 124.92$, the resulting value of s^2 in part (b) would be $s^2 = 29.89$. While the differences in the values of s^2 are small, this is again strong evidence of why a statistical computing package should be used for computing the values of any statistics. Furthermore, statistical packages are designed to produce the most accurate values of the statistics possible.

Because the sample variance and the sample standard deviation utilize all of the observations in a sample, like the sample mean they are statistics that are sensitive to the extremes in a sample. That is, when there is at least one extreme point in the sample, these extreme values will have a large influence on the values of s^2 and s.

The interquartile range is a parameter that measures the spread of a population and is not sensitive to the extreme values in a population. Recall that the population IQR measures the distance between the first and third population quartiles. That is,

$$\text{IQR} = \text{75th percentile} - \text{25th percentile} = X_{0.75} - X_{0.25}$$

The formula for the sample interquartile range is given below.

ESTIMATING THE INTERQUARTILE RANGE

The point estimator of the population interquartile range is the *sample interquartile range* that is denoted by $\widehat{\text{IQR}}$. To compute the value of $\widehat{\text{IQR}}$

1. determine the 25th and 75th sample percentiles, $Q1$ and $Q3$.

2. the value of $\widehat{\text{IQR}}$ is found by subtracting $Q1$ from $Q3$. That is,

$$\widehat{\text{IQR}} = Q3 - Q1$$

Note that the value of $\widehat{\text{IQR}}$ is easily computed from the information in a boxplot since the lower boundary of the box in a boxplot is $Q1$ and the upper boundary is $Q3$, and therefore, $\widehat{\text{IQR}}$ is simply the width of the box in the boxplot. Furthermore, the values of $Q1$ and $Q3$ are often included in the standard summary statistics provided by a statistical computing package for summarizing a sample.

Example 4.26
Use the outlier boxplot given in Figure 4.30 based on $n = 252$ values of percentage of body fat (PCTBF) in the Body Fat data set to estimate of the interquartile range of the variable PCTBF.

From the boxplot it appears that $Q1 \approx 12.5$ and $Q3 \approx 25$, and therefore, an estimate of the interquartile range of PCTBF is $\widehat{\text{IQR}} = 25 - 12.5 = 12.5$.

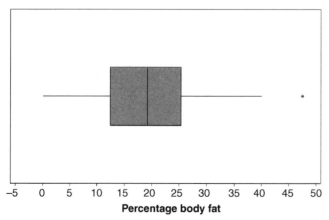

Percentage body fat

Figure 4.30   A boxplot of the percentage body fat (PCTBF) for a sample of $n = 252$ men.

Variable	N	Mean	SD	Minimum	Q1	Median	Q3	Maximum
Sample 1	13	7.46	4.45	3.00	3.50	4.00	12.00	13.00
Sample 2	13	7.46	2.11	3.00	7.00	7.00	8.00	13.00

When the target population follows a normal distribution with mean μ and standard deviation σ, the interquartile range is

$$\underbrace{\mu + 0.67 \times \sigma}_{Q3} - \underbrace{(\mu - .67 \times \sigma)}_{Q1} = 1.34 \times \sigma$$

Thus, for a normal distribution it follows that

$$\sigma = \frac{IQR}{1.34} \approx 0.75 \times IQR$$

Hence, when the boxplot and histogram suggest that the population that is approximately normally distributed, a robust estimator of σ is

$$\widehat{\sigma} = 0.75 \times \widehat{IQR}$$

Thus, in the presence of a single outlier and an otherwise mound-shaped histogram, $\widehat{\sigma}$ is an estimator of the standard deviation σ that will not be affected by the value of this single outlier.

Finally, the distance between the minimum and the maximum values in a sample is called the *sample range* and is often reported as an estimate of the spread of the population; however, because the range only uses the information on the minimum and maximum values in the sample it does not accurately reflect the spread of values in the sample. For example, consider the following two samples that have the same mean and range.

```
Sample 1:  3  3  3  4  4  4  4  10 12 12 12 13 13

Sample 2:  3  7  7  7  7  7  7   7  8  8  8  8 13
```

In both samples, the range is $13 - 3 = 10$; however sample 2 is clearly more concentrated around the sample mean ($\bar{x} = 7.46$) than is sample 1. The summary statistics provided by the statistical computing package MINITAB for each of these samples is given below in Table 4.26. Note that ranges and the sample means are equal for these two samples; however, the sample standard deviation for sample 1 is more than twice the sample standard deviation for sample 2. The sample interquartile ranges also differ greatly with sample 1 having $\widehat{IQR} = 8.5$ and sample 2 having $\widehat{IQR} = 1$. The differences in the values of the sample standard deviations and sample interquartile ranges clearly demonstrate that there is a difference in variability in these two samples; however, the sample range does not.

4.3.5 Linear Transformations

Because biomedical research is being performed all over the world, it is sometimes necessary for a researcher to convert from one scale of measurement to another. For example, Body Mass Index (BMI) is computed using the International System of Units as

$$BMI = \frac{weight \text{ (kg)}}{height^2 (m^2)}$$

which can be converted to the units used in the United States by

$$\text{BMI} = 703 \times \frac{\text{weight (lb)}}{\text{height}^2 \text{ (in}^2)}$$

or units used in the United Kingdom by

$$\text{BMI} = 6.35 \times \frac{\text{weight (stone)}}{\text{height}^2 (\text{m}^2)}.$$

Other variables frequently measured in biomedical research where the units are often region specific include temperature, weight, height, and volume among others.

When the conversion from one set of units to another is performed on a variable by simply adding a constant to the variable and/or multiplying the variable by a constant, the conversion process is said to be a *linear transformation*. That is, a linear transformation Y of a variable X is defined to be

$$Y = aX + b$$

where a and b are constants.

Example 4.27
In the article "Defining the relationship between plasma glucose and HbA1c: analysis of glucose profiles and HbA1c in the diabetes control and complications trial" published in *Diabetes Care* (Rohlfing et al., 2002), the authors reported that the relationship between mean plasma glucose level (MPG) and HbA_{1c} is approximately

$$\text{MPG (mg/dl)} = 35.6 \times \text{HbA}_{1c} - 77.3$$

Thus, there is an approximate linear transformation that can be used to convert an HbA_{1c} level to a corresponding mean plasma glucose level.

When two variables X and Y are related by the linear transformation $Y = aX + b$, the distribution of Y can be completely determined from the distribution of X. In particular, the mean, median, standard deviation, interquartile range, and percentiles of Y can be determined from the corresponding parameters in the distribution of X. For example, the mean value of Y is $\mu_Y = a\mu_x + b$ where μ_X is the mean of the X variable. The formulas for determining the parameters in the distribution of Y from the parameters of the distribution of X are given below for the linear transformation $Y = aX + b$.

LINEAR TRANSFORMATIONS OF PARAMETERS

For the linear transformation $Y = aX + b$	$\sigma_Y = |a| \times \sigma_X$
$\mu_Y = a\mu_x + b$	$\text{IQR}_Y = |a| \times \text{IQR}_X$
$\tilde{\mu} = a\tilde{\mu}_X + b$	$Y_p = aX_p + b \ (a > 0)$
$\sigma_Y^2 = a^2\sigma_X^2$	$Y_p = aX_{1-p} + b \ (a < 0)$

Note that formulas for the variance, standard deviation, and interquartile range are not affected by the size of the constant b. On the other hand, multiplying by a constant a will increase the variation in the new variable Y when $|a| > 1$ and will decrease the variation in the new variable Y when $-1 < a < 1$. For example, the transformation $Y = X + 3$ simply amounts to shifting the every value in the distribution to the right three units that does not change the variability among the values; however, the transformation $Y = 3X$ increases the spread of the values by a factor of 3 according to the standard deviation and interquartile range.

Given a random sample on a variable X, the following rules show how to compute the estimates of the corresponding parameters of the variable $Y = aX + b$ from the estimates $\bar{x}, \tilde{x}, s_X^2, s_X, \widehat{\text{IQR}}_X$, and $\widehat{x}_p$.

LINEAR TRANSFORMATIONS OF THE ESTIMATED PARAMETERS

For the linear transformation $Y = aX + b$ $\qquad$ $\widehat{\text{IQR}}_Y = |a| \times \widehat{\text{IQR}}_X$

$$\bar{y} = a\bar{x} + b$$

$$\tilde{y} = a\tilde{x}_X + b$$

$$s_Y^2 = a^2 s_x^2$$

$$s_Y = |a| \times s_x$$

$$\widehat{y}_p = a\widehat{x}_p + b \quad (a > 0)$$

$$\widehat{y}_p = a\widehat{x}_{1-p} + b \quad (a < 0)$$

Example 4.28

Body temperature is often measured in degrees Celsius or degrees Fahrenheit. Let C be the variable representing the body temperature of an adult in degrees Celsius and F the variable representing the body temperature of an adult in degrees Fahrenheit. The conversion formula $F = 1.8\,C + 32$ is used to convert temperatures from degrees Celsius to degrees Fahrenheit. Use the following estimates that were computed from a random sample on the variable C to estimate the

a. mean body temperature for an adult in degrees Fahrenheit.

b. standard deviation of body temperatures for an adult in degrees Fahrenheit.

c. Interquartile range of body temperatures for an adult in degrees Fahrenheit.

d. 95th percentile of body temperatures for an adult in degrees Fahrenheit.

$$\bar{C} = 37°\text{C}, s_C = 0.7°\text{C}, \widehat{\text{IQR}}_C = 0.5°\text{C}, \widehat{C}_{0.95} = 38.2°\text{C}$$

Solutions The estimate of the

a. mean body temperature for an adult in degrees Fahrenheit is

$$\bar{F} = 1.8 \times \bar{C} + 32 = 1.8 \times 37 + 32 = 98.6°\text{F}$$

b. standard deviation of body temperatures for an adult in degrees Fahrenheit is

$$s_F = |1.8| \times s_C = 1.8 \times 0.7 = 1.26°\text{F}$$

c. Interquartile range of body temperatures for an adult in degrees Fahrenheit is

$$\widehat{\text{IQR}}_F = |1.8| \times \widehat{\text{IQR}}_C = 1.8 \times 0.5 = 0.9°\text{F}$$

d. 95th percentile of body temperatures for an adult in degrees Fahrenheit is

$$\widehat{F}_{0.95} = 1.8 \times \widehat{C}_{0.95} + 32 = 1.8 \times 38.2 + 32 = 100.76°\text{F}$$

Example 4.29

In some studies, the measuring device used to measure a particular characteristic on a sampled unit will be biased leading to inaccurate observations. A common form of bias encountered with a measuring device occurs when each observed measurement deviates from the true value by the same amount that is known as a *calibration error*. In this case,

$$\text{Observed value} = \text{true value} + \text{constant bias}$$

For example, the weights reported by a scale may be the true weight of an individual plus 1 lb in which case

$$\text{Observed weight} = \text{true weight} + 1$$

In this case, the observed sample mean would 1 lb larger than the true sample mean; however, the sample standard deviation based on the observed weights would be the correct value. Thus, when the bias in a measuring device is constant, the value of the sample mean will be off by an amount equal to this constant; however the sample standard deviation, sample variance, and sample interquartile range will be unaffected by this type of bias. In any case, a measuring device should be checked for accuracy, and calibrated when needed, before collecting any sample data to avoid biased observations that could lead to unreliable statistical inferences.

4.3.6 The Plug-in Rule for Estimation

In some research problems, one of the parameters of interest will be based on a function of one or more parameters. When a specific quantity is a function of one or more parameters of the population, a reasonable approach to estimate the quantity is to replace the unknown parameters in the formula with their corresponding estimates. This approach is known as the *plug-in rule* of estimation. For example, the *coefficient of variation* is defined to be

$$\text{CV} = \frac{\sigma}{|\mu|}$$

Thus, using the plug-in rule of estimation, a reasonable estimate of the coefficient of variation is

$$\widehat{\text{CV}} = \frac{s}{|\bar{x}|}$$

Note that the plug-in-rule has been used previously in this section in the following ways:

1. $\bar{x}$ was substituted for μ in the formula for estimating σ^2 (i.e., s^2).

2. $Q1$ and $Q3$ were substituted for the 25th and 75th percentiles in the formula for estimating IQR (i.e., $\widehat{\text{IQR}}$).

3. estimates of the population proportions were used in the formula for estimating the relative risk (i.e., $\widehat{\text{RR}}$).

Example 4.30

The histogram and boxplot given in Figure 4.31, the normal plot given in Figure 4.32, and the descriptive statistics given in Table 4.13 were computed from the $n = 252$ observations in the Body Fat data set for the variable body density (Density).

On the basis of the histogram, boxplot, and normal probability plot of body density, it appears reasonable to assume that the underlying distribution of the variable body density is approximately

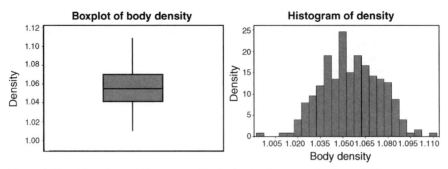

Figure 4.31   A boxplot and histogram of body density for a sample of $n = 252$ men.

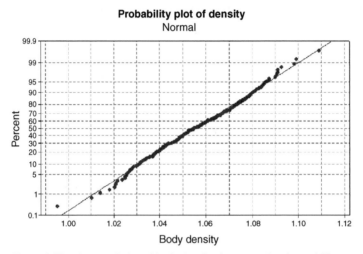

Figure 4.32   A normal plot of body density for a sample of $n = 252$ men.

normal. Since the percentiles of a normal are $X_p = \mu + \sigma Z_p$, a reasonable approach for estimating the percentiles based on the observed sample is to use $\bar{x}$ and s in place of μ and σ in the formula for X_p. That is, an estimate of X_p can be computed using the formula $\widehat{x}_p = \bar{x} + s Z_p$. In particular, based on the summary statistics in Table 4.13, an estimate of the 95th percentile of the variable density is

$$\widehat{x}_{0.95} = 1.0556 + 0.019 \times 1.645 = 1.086855$$

It is also possible to estimate the percentage of individuals with a body density of more than 1.10 using the normal probability model. To do this, first convert 1.10 to an approximate Z score

TABLE 4.13   Summary Statistics for the Variable Body Density

Variable	n	$\bar{x}$	s	$Q1$	$\widetilde{x}$	$Q3$
Density	252	1.0556	0.0190	1.0414	1.0549	1.0704

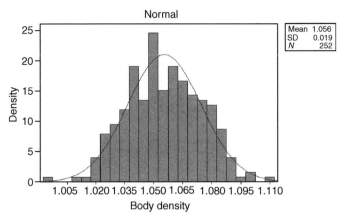

Figure 4.33   A histogram of body density with fitted normal probability model.

using the formula $Z = \frac{x - \bar{x}}{s}$. This yields

$$Z = \frac{1.10 - 1.0556}{0.019} = 2.34.$$

Then, $\widehat{P}$(body density > 1.10) is found by determining $P(Z > 2.34)$ using the normal table, which gives $P(Z > 2.34) = 1 - P(Z \leq 2.34) = 1 - 0.9904 = 0.0096$. Thus, an estimate of the percentage of individuals with a body density of more than 1.10 is $100 \times 0.0096 = 0.96\%$.

The plug-in-rule can also be used to investigate the fit of a particular probability model to a data set. In fact, it is common in a statistical analysis to present a histogram with a fitted probability distribution superimposed over it. In fact, most statistical computing packages can fit a wide variety of probability models to the observed data and superimpose the fitted model over the histogram of the observed data. Moreover, a histogram with a particular probability model fitted to the data can be used as a visual evidence to support or refute the probability model under consideration.

For instance, in Example 4.30 the sample data for the variable Density in the Body Fat data set suggest that the variable Density is approximately normally distributed. The histogram in Figure 4.33 has a normal curve with mean $\bar{x} = 1.0556$ and standard deviation $s = 0.019$ superimposed over the histogram of Density that seems to fit reasonably well to the observed data. That is, there is no strong disagreement between the observed data (i.e., the histogram) and the fitted normal distribution.

4.4 STATISTICS FOR MULTIVARIATE DATA SETS

When a sample consists of records for more than one variable on each unit sampled, the sample is called a *multivariate sample* and the resulting data set is referred to as a *multivariate data set*. A *bivariate sample* is a sample where two variables are recorded for each unit sampled. A multivariate data set often contains both qualitative and quantitative variables. The analysis of a multivariate data set can be based on the summary statistics discussed in the previous section as well as some specialized statistics that describe the joint distribution of two or more variables. For example, in most multivariate analyses the sample mean,

TABLE 4.14 Summary Statistics for the Quantitative Variables Measured in the Body Fat Data Set

Variable	N	Mean	SD	Q1	Median	Q3	IQR
Age	252	47.48	43.120	35.500	43.000	54.000	18.500
Neck	252	37.99	2.431	36.400	38.000	39.475	3.075
Chest	252	100.82	8.430	94.250	99.650	105.530	11.270
Abdomen	252	92.56	10.783	84.525	90.950	99.575	15.050
Hip	252	99.91	7.164	95.500	99.300	103.575	8.075
Thigh	252	59.41	5.250	56.000	59.000	62.450	6.450
Knee	252	38.59	2.412	36.925	38.500	39.975	3.050
Ankle	252	23.10	1.695	22.000	22.800	24.000	2.000
Biceps	252	32.27	3.021	30.200	32.050	34.375	4.175
Forearm	252	28.66	2.021	27.300	28.700	30.000	2.700
Wrist	252	18.23	0.934	17.600	18.300	18.800	1.200
Density	252	1.06	0.019	1.041	1.055	1.070	0.029

median, and standard deviation, among other statistics, are computed for every quantitative variable and sample proportions and frequencies are computed for the qualitative variables observed in the sample.

Example 4.31
The summary statistics given in Table 4.14 were computed for the quantitative variables measured in the Body Fat data set.

4.4.1 Graphical Statistics for Bivariate Data Sets

When a multivariate data set consists of a quantitative response variable and a set of quantitative explanatory variables, then pair-wise relationships between the response variable and each of the explanatory variables can be explored graphically with a *scatterplot*. A scatterplot of a variable Y versus a variable X is a two-dimensional plot of the observed ordered pairs (X, Y). For example, suppose the data given in Table 4.15 represents a random sample collected in a study designed to investigate the relationship between the height and weight of a male high school student, and a scatterplot of weight versus height based on the data in Table 4.15 is given in Figure 4.34.

TABLE 4.15 A Random Sample of Heights and Weights of $n = 18$ Male High School Students

Ht. (in.)	Wt. (lb)	Ht. (in.)	Wt. (lb)
67	145	69	173
71	175	63	123
76	245	61	113
67	158	70	191
68	166	70	188
78	205	65	143
62	125	69	163
73	202	64	153
63	133	69	184

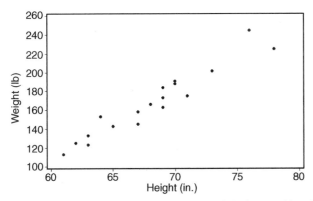

Figure 4.34   Scatterplot for weight versus height for $n = 18$ male high school students.

A scatterplot can be used to visually inspect the relationship between two variables, and the scatter of points in a scatterplot is referred to as a *data cloud*. The key to analyzing a scatterplot is to look for any obvious or strong patterns in the data cloud. In particular, the typical patterns to look for in a scatterplot include a linear data cloud sloping upward, a linear data cloud sloping downward, data cloud that is curved, or a data cloud revealing no obvious pattern. Examples of the typical data cloud patterns that are seen in a scatterplot are shown in Figure 4.35.

It is also important to consider the strength of the relationship indicated by the data cloud in a scatterplot. That is, strong linear or curvilinear relationships will be obvious in a scatterplot, and the more concentrated the data cloud is around a line or a curve the stronger the relationship between the two variables is. In particular, when the points in a scatterplot lie very close to a straight line or a curve, the data cloud is indicating that there is a strong relationship between the variables being studied; when the points are widely scattered about a line or a curve, the data cloud is suggesting that the relationship between the two variables is weak. And finally, when there is no apparent pattern in the data cloud in a scatterplot, there may be no direct relationship between the two variables.

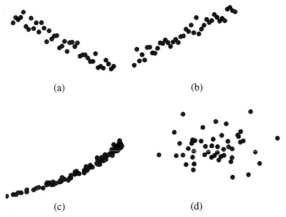

Figure 4.35   Examples of the four types of commonly encountered scatterplots: (a) linear sloping downward; (b) linear sloping upward; (c) curvilinear; (d) no obvious pattern.

4.4.2 Numerical Summaries for Bivariate Data Sets

The population *correlation coefficient* is a parameter that measures the strength of the linear relationship between two quantitative variables. The correlation coefficient for two quantitative variables X and Y is denoted by ρ and is defined by

---

THE POPULATION CORRELATION COEFFICIENT

$$\rho = \frac{1}{N} \sum \frac{(X - \mu_X)(Y - \mu_Y)}{\sigma_X \sigma_Y}$$

where μ_X, and μ_Y, σ_X, σ_Y are the means and standard deviations of the X and Y variables, respectively, and N is the number of pairs of units (X, Y) in the population.

The correlation coefficient ρ is a unitless parameter. That is, the value of ρ is independent of the units of the variables X and Y. For example, if X is height in inches and Y is weight in pounds, then the value of ρ will be exactly the same when X is measured in centimeters and Y is measured in kilograms. A positive value of ρ indicates that as the values of X increase the value of Y tends to increase, also; a negative value of ρ indicates that values of Y tend to decrease as the value of X increases. When the relationship between Y and X is a perfect linear relationship (i.e., $Y = aX + b$), ρ will be either $+1$ ($a > 0$) or -1 ($a < 0$) and X and Y are said to be *perfectly correlated*. When X and Y are not perfectly correlated (i.e., $\rho \neq \pm 1$), the closer ρ is to -1 or $+1$, the stronger the linear relationship between X and Y is.

FACTS ABOUT THE CORRELATION COEFFICIENT

1. ρ is a unitless parameter.
2. ρ is always between -1 and 1.
3. $\rho = \pm 1$ if and only if X and Y are perfectly related to one another by $Y = aX + b$.
4. ρ only measures the strength of the linear relationship between two variables. The closer ρ is to ± 1 the stronger the linear relationship between X and Y.
5. The value of ρ is 0 when X and Y are independent variables.
6. When X and Y are not independent, the value of ρ can be 0 even when there is a strong relationship between two variables.

Note that two variables can be strongly related even though they are uncorrelated (i.e., $\rho = 0$). For example, the variables plotted in Figure 4.36 are uncorrelated and clearly there is a strong relationship between these two variables; however, it is not a linear relationship. Because the variables plotted in Figure 4.36 are clearly not linearly related the value of the correlation coefficient cannot be used as a measure of the strength of the relationship between these variables. Even though $\rho = 0$ for the two variables plotted in Figure 4.36, there is clearly a strong curvilinear relationship between these two variables. In fact, the relationship between the variables in

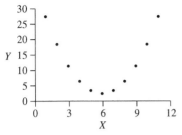

Figure 4.36   An example of a strong curvilinear relationship between X and Y where $\rho = 0$.

Figure 4.36 is given by the quadratic relationship $Y = 2 + (X - 6)^2$. Thus, since the correlation coefficient only measures the strength of the linear relationship between two variables, it cannot be used as a measure of the strength of a nonlinear relationship between two variables.

Given a sample of n bivariate observations (X, Y), *Pearson's sample correlation coefficient*, which is denoted by r, is a statistic that can be used for estimating the population correlation coefficient ρ. The formula for the sample correlation coefficient is derived from the definition of ρ and the plug-in rule. The formula for computing the sample correlation coefficient r is

$$r = \frac{1}{n-1} \sum \frac{(x - \bar{x})(y - \bar{y})}{s_x s_y}$$

where $\bar{x}$, $\bar{y}$, s_x and s_y are the sample means and sample standard deviations for the X and Y variables, respectively.

The sample correlation coefficient has many properties similar to those of the population correlation coefficient that are summarized below.

FACTS ABOUT THE SAMPLE CORRELATION COEFFICIENT

1. r is a unitless measure.

2. r is always between -1 and 1.

3. $r = \pm 1$ if and only if all of the sample observations line on a straight line.

4. r only measures the strength of the linear relationship suggested by the sample observations on two variables. Values of r close to ± 1 are associated with data clouds tightly grouped about a straight line.

5. Values of r close to 0 are associated with data clouds that are not tightly grouped

about any straight line.

6. A value of $r > 0$ indicates the variable Y tends to increase as the X variable increases, which means the data cloud is upward sloping (i.e., a positive slope).

7. A value of $r < 0$ indicates the variable Y tends to decrease as the X variable increases, which means the data cloud is downward sloping (i.e., a negative slope).

Since r only measures the strength of the linear relationship, it is entirely possible for two variables to have a strong nonlinear relationship even when $r \approx 0$. Thus, before computing the value of r, a scatterplot should be examined to determine whether the data cloud is linear. Moreover, when the data cloud is nonlinear, there is no need to compute the value of r since it would be meaningless to measure the strength of a linear relationship for a data cloud that is not linear.

The procedure outlining how to compute the value of r is described below.

COMPUTING THE SAMPLE CORRELATION COEFFICIENT

---

1. Compute the values of the scaled deviations using the sample means and sample standard deviations for the observed X and Y values. That is, compute $\dfrac{x - \bar{x}}{s_X}$ and $\dfrac{y - \bar{y}}{s_Y}$ for each of the observed pairs (x, y).

2. For each pair (x, y), multiply the scaled X deviation by the scaled Y deviation. That is, compute $\dfrac{x - \bar{x}}{s_X} \times \dfrac{y - \bar{y}}{s_Y}$ for each of the observed pairs (x, y).

3. The value of r is found by summing the product of the scaled deviations and then dividing by $n - 1$.

$$r = \frac{1}{n-1} \sum \frac{(x - \bar{x})(y - \bar{y})}{s_x s_y}$$

As is the case with most statistics, the value of r is best found using a statistical computing package. Also, the value of r should be only computed and used as a measure of the relationship between two variables only when the data cloud in a scatterplot suggests there is a linear relationship. The scatterplots shown in Figure 4.37 provide examples of scatterplots with sample correlations $r = -1, 1, 0, 0.8, 0.4$ when there is a linear relationship and $r = 0$ when there is a nonlinear relationship between the variables X and Y.

Many researchers confuse correlation, which measures the association between two variables, and causation that means the value of one variable depends on the value of

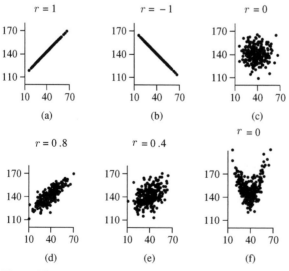

Figure 4.37 Examples of scatterplots. (a) $r = -1$; (b) $r = 1$; (c) $r = 0$; (d) $r = 0.8$; (e) $r = 0.4$; (f) $r = 0$ for a nonlinear relationship.

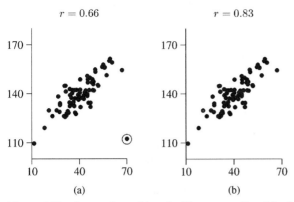

Figure 4.38   Scatterplots with and without an outlier: (a) with the outlier $r = 0.66$; (b) without the outlier $r = 0.83$

the other variable. The difficult question of whether a high correlation suggests a cause-and-effect relationship is often encountered in biomedical studies and can be answered only through a thorough scientific investigation. There is an important distinction between association and cause-and-effect relationships, namely, cause-and-effect relationships can be tested with sample data and associations cannot. That is, cause-and-effect relationships are often tested by using well-designed experiments, but they cannot be tested using the data from observational study.

A *bivariate outlier* is any point that is not consistent with the remaining points in the sample, and a bivariate outlier can usually be detected by examining a scatterplot. The value of r is sensitive to bivariate outliers; however, the influence of a bivariate outlier will decrease rapidly as the sample size increases. The scatterplots in Figure 4.38 illustrate the influence an outlier has on the value of the sample correlation coefficient for a random sample of $n = 78$ observations. Note that the circled point in Figure 4.38a does not appear to be consistent with the rest of the sample points in the data cloud, and therefore, the circled point is a bivariate outlier. The sample correlation coefficient for all 78 observations is $r = 0.66$; however, if the outlier was not present in the data set the value of r would have been $r = 0.83$.

The identification of bivariate outliers in a scatterplot is fairly easy; however, dealing with outliers is not an easy task. The first step in dealing with an outlier is to investigate whether the value of the outlier is because of a data entry mistake or is an impossible value; if the outlier is an impossible value, it should be deleted from the data set and the statistical analysis can continue as planned. On the other hand, when an outlier is not a data entry mistake or an impossible value and the deletion of an outlier from a data set cannot be justified on sound scientific reasons, the influence of the outlier should be examined. The influence of an outlier on the sample correlation coefficient can be assessed by computing the value of r with and without the outlier present in the data set. When the value of r does not change much for these two data sets, the outlier should be kept in the data set. However, when the value of r is dramatically different for these two data sets, more advanced measures will be required for minimizing the influence of the outlier.

In a multivariate data set, there are often many relationships that will be investigated. One approach for exploring the relationships among the variables in the data set is to consider all of the pairwise relationships between the quantitative variables.

The steps for investigating pairwise relationships in a multivariate data set are outlined below.

INVESTIGATING PAIRWISE RELATIONSHIPS IN A MULTIVARIATE DATA SET

---

1. Compute the summary statistics for each of the variables. Usually, this includes sample means, medians, standard deviations, and some percentiles along with a boxplot and histogram.

2. Summarize the sample data for each pair of variables in a scatterplot.

3. Identify and deal with any bivariate outliers clearly visible in the scatterplots.

4. For the scatterplots with linear data clouds, compute the sample correlation coefficient r.

5. Identify and summarize any curvilinear pattern in the scatterplots.

Note that three-way or higher level multivariate relationships will often be hidden in the pairwise scatterplots. Methods for investigating multivariate relationships will be discussed in Chapter 9.

Example 4.32

In the Body Fat, study, the following variables were recorded for studying the percentage of body fat (PCTBF) in an adult male and the variables that might be used to explain PCTBF.

```
Age (years)
Weight (lb)
Height (in.)
Neck circumference (cm)
Chest circumference (cm)
Abdomen circumference (cm)
Hip circumference (cm)
Thigh circumference (cm)
Knee circumference (cm)
Ankle circumference (cm)
Biceps (extended) circumference (cm)
Forearm circumference (cm)
Wrist circumference (cm)
Percent Body Fat
```

The response variable in this data set is percent body fat (PCTBF) and the other variables are explanatory variables that are believed to be useful in explaining the percentage of body fat in an adult male. Because, it is known that percent body fat tends to increase with weight, but it is not as clear how the other variables in the study affect percent body fat, scatterplots were created to investigate the relationship between percent body fat and each of the explanatory variables. The scatterplots for percent body fat versus age, height, abdomen circumference, and forearm circumference are given in Figure 4.39.

Notice that there is a single observation in the scatterplot of percent body fat versus height that is quite different from the remaining points in the data cloud; the bivariate outlier in this plot occurs at a height of roughly 30 in. This point seems to be an obvious mistake since the weight for this individual is 205 lb and it would be extremely unlikely for a 30 in. tall individual to weigh 205 lb. Thus, further investigation of this point is needed to determine whether it is a recording error that can be corrected. If it is not a fixable recording error, then this point should be removed from the data set since it appears to be an impossible value.

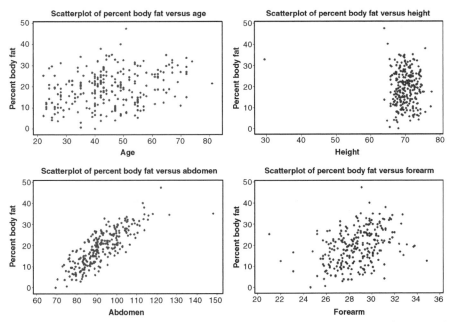

Figure 4.39   Scatterplots of percent body fat versus age, height, abdomen circumference, and forearm circumference.

Each of the four scatterplots in Figure 4.39 reveal data clouds that could be described as either linear upward sloping data clouds or data clouds with no obvious patterns. The correlations corresponding to the scatterplots in Figure 4.39 are

	PCTBF
Age	0.291
Height	-0.089
Abdomen	0.813
Forearm	0.361

Now, from the scatterplots in Figure 4.39 and the values of r, it is clear that the abdomen circumference has the strongest linear relationship with percent body fat and there is no obvious linear relationship between percent body fat and height.

4.4.3 Fitting Lines to Scatterplots

When the data cloud and its associated sample correlation indicate that there is a strong linear relationship between the response and the explanatory variable, they are suggesting that there might be a straight line $Y = a + bX$ that may explain the relationship between these two variables. Furthermore, once the equation of the line has been derived it may be used for predicting the value of the response variable for a particular value of the explanatory variable.

One method for determining the equation of the line that "best" fits a data cloud is the *least squares procedure*. Recall that the equation of a line is $y = a + bx$, where a is the y intercept and b is the slope of the line. The least squares procedure determines the equation of the line that minimizes the sum of the squared deviations from the line to the observed bivariate points. That is, for a random sample of n observed bivariate points $(x_1, y_1), (x_2, y_2), \ldots, (x_n, y_n)$ the *least squares regression line* is the line that minimizes the sum of squares given by

$$SS(a, b) = \left[y_1 - (a + bx_1) \right]^2 + \left[y_2 - (a + bx_2) \right]^2 + \cdots + \left[y_n - (a + bx_n) \right]^2$$

$$= \sum \left[y - (a + bx) \right]^2$$

The least squares regression line is found by determining the values of a and b that produce the smallest sum of squared deviation, $SS(a, b)$, and the resulting least squares line is denoted by $\widehat{y} = b_0 + b_1 x$, where b_0 is the least squares estimate of the y intercept and b_1 is the least squares estimate of the slope. The equation of the least squares regression line is computed from the five bivariate summary statistics $\bar{x}$, $\bar{y}$, s_X, s_Y, and r, and the formulas for the values of b_0 and b_1 are given below.

THE LEAST SQUARES REGRESSION LINE

The least squares regression line is $\widehat{y} = b_0 + b_1 x$, where

$$b_1 = r \times \frac{s_Y}{s_X}$$

$$b_0 = \bar{y} - b_1 \bar{x}$$

Note that the slope of the least squares regression line is b_1 and estimates the expected change in the Y variable for a one unit increase in the X variable. The y intercept of the least squares regression line is b_0, which estimates the mean value of Y when $X = 0$. The least squares regression line can also be used to predict the value of Y for a particular value of X, provided the value of X is in the range of the observed data.

Example 4.33

In Example 4.32, a strong linear relationship ($r = 0.813$) between percent body fat (PCTBF) and abdomen circumference (Abdomen) was found using the data in the Body Fat data set. Using the summary statistics given in Table 4.16, answer the following:

    a. Determine the equation of the least squares regression line.

    b. Determine the predicted value of the percentage of body fat for a 95 cm abdomen circumference (i.e., $A = 95$) based on the least squares regression line.

    c. Determine the estimated expected change in percent body fat for an increase of one cm in abdomen circumference.

TABLE 4.16 Summary Statistics for the Variables Abdomen and PCTBF

Statistic	Abdomen (X)	PCTBF (Y)
Sample mean	92.56	10.783
Sample SD	19.15	8.369

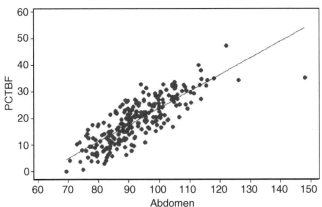

PCTBF = −39.28 + 0.6313 Abdomen

Figure 4.40   A scatterplot with the least squares regression line for relating percent body fat to abdomen circumference.

Solutions   First, the values of the least squares estimated b_1 and b_0 are

$$b_1 = r \times \frac{s_Y}{s_X} = 0.813 \times \frac{8.369}{10.783} = 0.63$$

$$b_0 = \bar{x} - b_1 \bar{y} = 19.15 - 0.63 \times 92.56 = -39.16$$

a. The equation of the least squares regression line is $\widehat{\mathrm{PCTBF}} = -39.16 + 0.63$ Abdomen.

b. The predicted percentage of body fat for an adult male having an abdomen circumference of 95 cm is

$$\widehat{\mathrm{PCTBF}}_{95} = -39.16 + 0.63 \times 95 = 20.69\%$$

c. The estimated expected change in percent body fat for an increase of 1 cm in abdomen circumference is $b_1 = 0.63$.

A scatterplot of percent body fat versus abdomen circumference with the least squares regression line is shown in Figure 4.40.

GLOSSARY

Bar Chart   A bar chart is a graphical statistic that represents the category percentages or proportions with bars of height equal to the percentage or proportion of sample observations falling in each category.

Bivariate Outlier   A bivariate outlier is any point that is not consistent with the remaining points in the sample.

Bivariate Sample   A bivariate sample is a sample where two variables are recorded on each unit in the sample.

Boxplot   A boxplot is a graphical statistic for a quantitative variable that is based on the five-number summary that can be used to make inferences about the tails of the distribution, the typical values in the population, and the spread of the population.

Coefficient of Variation   The coefficient of variation is defined to be

$$CV = \frac{\sigma}{|\mu|}$$

and using the plug-in rule a reasonable estimate of the coefficient of variation is

$$\widehat{CV} = \frac{s}{|\bar{x}|}$$

Cross-classification The process of categorizing the sample data according to two qualitative variables is called cross-classification.

Data Cloud The scatter of points in a scatterplot is called a data cloud.

Density The density of a class interval reflects the proportion or percentage of the sample observations per unit of width in a class interval.

$$\text{Density of a class} = \frac{\text{relative frequency of the class}}{\text{class width}}$$

Fat Pencil Test The fat pencil test is a method of analyzing a normal probability plot. When all of the points in the normal probability plot are covered by an imaginary pencil, the normal probability plot suggests that a normal probability model might be a reasonable model for the underlying distribution; when some of the points in the normal probability plot are not covered by the imaginary pencil, the normal probability plot is suggesting that the sample data do not support the hypothesis that the underlying distribution is normally distributed.

Five-number Summary The five-number summary associated with a sample consists of the minimum of the sample, the maximum of the sample, the sample 25th percentile (Q1), the sample 50th percentile ($\tilde{x}$), and the sample 75 percentile (Q3).

Graphical Statistics Graphical statistics are statistics that display the summarized sample information in plots, charts, or graphs.

Histogram A histogram is a graphical statistic for a quantitative variable that is a vertical bar chart drawn over a set of class intervals that cover the range of the observed data.

Least Squares Procedure The least squares procedure is a method for determining the equation of the line that "best" fits the data cloud in a scatterplot. The least squares regression line is the line that results from using the least squares procedure.

Linear Transformation A linear transformation of a variable X is $Y = aX + b$, where a and b are constants, for any numbers a and b.

Multivariate Sample A sample that consists of records on more than one variable on each unit sampled is called a multivariate sample and the resulting data set is referred to as a multivariate data set.

Normal Probability Plot A normal probability plot is a plot of the sample percentiles versus the expected percentiles of the best fitting normal distribution.

Numerical Statistics Numerical statistics are statistics that result in numbers that can be used to summarize a sample, estimate parameters, or test hypotheses concerning an unknown parameter.

Outlier An outlier is a point that is judged to be unusually different from the rest of the data. Data points falling more than a distance of $1.5 \times \widehat{IQR}$ from Q1 or Q3 are called outliers, and points falling more than a distance of $3 \times \widehat{IQR}$ from Q1 or Q3 are called extreme outliers.

Pearson's Sample Correlation Coefficient   Pearson's sample correlation coefficient r is the point estimator of the population correlation coefficient.

$$r = \frac{1}{n-1} \sum \frac{(x - \bar{x})(y - \bar{y})}{s_x s_y}$$

Pie Chart   A pie chart is constructed by determining the percentage or proportion of the sample in each possible category and then drawing a pie with the slices having area proportional to the category percentages.

Plug-in-rule   The approach to estimate an unknown quantity by replacing the unknown parameters in the formula with their corresponding estimates is known as the plug-in rule of estimation.

Population Correlation Coefficient   The population correlation coefficient is a parameter that measures the strength of the linear relationship between two quantitative variables. The correlation coefficient for two quantitative variables X and Y is denoted by ρ.

Robust Estimator   A statistic is said to be robust or resistant to the extremes of a sample when it is not sensitive to the extreme values in a sample.

Sample Interquartile Range   The sample interquartile range $\widehat{\text{IQR}}$ is the point estimator of the population interquartile range.

$$\widehat{\text{IQR}} = Q3 - Q1$$

Sample Mean   The sample mean $\bar{x}$ is the average of the observed values in the sample and is the point estimator of the population mean.

$$\bar{x} = \frac{\text{sum of the observed data values}}{\text{the sample size}} = \frac{\sum x}{n}$$

Sample Median   The sample median $\tilde{x}$ is the point estimator of the population median and is the middle value in the ordered sample.

Sample Mode   The sample mode is the most frequent value in the sample and is denoted by $\widehat{M}$.

Sample Percentile   The point estimator of a population percentile is the sample pth percentile that is denoted by $\widehat{x}_p$. The value of $\widehat{x}_p$ is the observed value in the sample where $p\%$ of the sample lies below this value.

Sample Proportion   The sample proportion is the point estimator of a population proportion.

$$\widehat{p} = \frac{\text{the number of sample observations having characteristic } A}{n}$$

Sample Range   The sample range is the distance between the minimum and the maximum values in a sample.

Sample Standard Deviation   The sample standard deviation s is the point estimator of the population standard deviation.

$$s = \sqrt{s^2}$$

Sample Variance   The sample variance s^2 is the point estimator of the population variance.

$$s^2 = \frac{1}{n-1}\left[\sum (x_i - \bar{x})^2\right]$$

Scatterplot   A scatterplot of a variable Y versus a variable X is a two-dimensional plot of the observed ordered pairs (X, Y).

Statistic   A statistic is any value that is computed from the sample and known values.

Two-way Contingency Table   A two-way contingency table summarizes the sample data that have been cross-classified according to two qualitative variables.

EXERCISES

4.1   Why is it important to use a well-designed sampling plan when making inferences from a sample to the target population?

4.2   Can reliable inferences be drawn from a sample of convenience? Why?

4.3   How does a statistic differ from a parameter?

4.4   Can the value of a parameter be determined from the information contained in a sample? Explain.

4.5   Which graphical statistics can be used with

    (a) qualitative data?   **(b)** quantitative data?

4.6   What are three different types of bar charts?

4.7   What does the height of a bar in a bar chart represent?

4.8   How should a bar chart be constructed when there is sample information on two or more subpopulations that needs to be displayed?

4.9   In the Mammography Experience Study, individuals were asked to respond to the statement "You do not need a mammogram unless you develop symptoms" (strongly agree, agree, disagree, strongly disagree). Use the bar chart in Figure 4.41, based on the $n = 412$ responses of the women included in the Mammography Experience data set, to answer the following:

    (a) Estimate the percentage of women who agree or strongly agree with the statement "You do not need a mammogram unless you develop symptoms."

    (b) Estimate the percentage of women who disagree or strongly disagree with the statement "You do not need a mammogram unless you develop symptoms."

4.10   In the Mammography Experience Study, individuals were asked about their prior experience with mammography (never, within 1 year, over 1 year). Use the summarized data in Table 4.17, based on the $n = 412$ responses of the women included in the Mammography Experience data set, to answer the following:

    (a) Convert the raw counts into estimates of the percentage in each of the three mammography experience categories.

    (b) Create a bar chart displaying the estimated percentages.

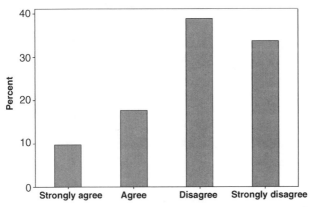

Figure 4.41   Bar chart of $n = 412$ responses to the statement "You do not need a mammogram unless you develop symptoms" in the Mammography Experience Study.

4.11 In the Mammography Experience Study individuals were surveyed on their mammography experience (never, within 1 year, over 1 year) and whether or not they have a mother or sister with a history of breast cancer (No, Yes). Use the bar chart in Figure 4.42, based on the $n = 412$ responses of the women included in the Mammography Experience data set, to answer the following.

   (a) Estimate the percentage of women who have a mother or sister with a history of breast cancer.

   (b) Estimate the percentage of women who have had a mammography experience and have a mother or sister with a history of breast cancer.

   (c) Estimate the percentage of women who have never had a mammography experience and whose mother and sister have no history of breast cancer.

4.12 In the Benign Breast Disease Study, the sample consists of $n = 50$ women diagnosed with fibrocystic breast disease and $n = 150$ women without fibrocystic breast disease. One of the variables recorded on each women in the study was whether or not they had regular checkups (Yes, No). Using the data in the Benign Breast Disease data set

   (a) create a bar chart showing the percentage of women in each group who did or did not get regular checkups.

   (b) determine whether women with fibrocystic breast disease one more or less likely to get a regular checkup than women without fibrocystic breast cancer.

4.13 What are the five statistics that make up the five-number summary?

TABLE 4.17   **A Frequency Table Based on Two Survey Items for the $n = 412$ Women in the Mammography Experience Study**

Mammography Experience	Count
Never	234
Within 1 year	104
Over 1 year	74
	412

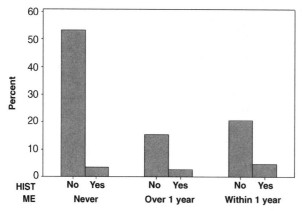

Figure 4.42   Bar chart for mammography experience and family history for the $n = 412$ women in the Mammography Experience Study.

4.14 Which quartiles can be estimated from the information displayed in a boxplot?

4.15 What is an outlier?

4.16 How can an outlier boxplot be used to identify an

(**a**) outlier?   (**b**) extreme outlier?

4.17 How should an outlier or extreme outlier in a sample be handled?

4.18 Using the five-number summary given in Table 4.18
(**a**) construct a boxplot.
(**b**) describe the shape of the distribution suggested by the boxplot in part (a).
(**c**) estimate the interquartile range.
(**d**) determine whether there are outliers or extreme outliers suggested by this boxplot?

4.19 Use the outlier boxplot given in Figure 4.43, based on the weights of the $n = 200$ women in the Benign Breast Disease data set, to answer the following:
(**a**) Describe the shape of the distribution of weights of women suggested by boxplot in Figure 4.43.
(**b**) Estimate the median weight of a woman.
(**c**) Estimate the interquartile range.
(**d**) Determine whether there are outliers or extreme outliers suggested by this boxplot?

TABLE 4.18   The Five-Number Summary for Exercise 4.18

	Statistic
Minimum	12
Maximum	208
Sample median	54
$Q1$	23
$Q3$	77

Boxplot of WT

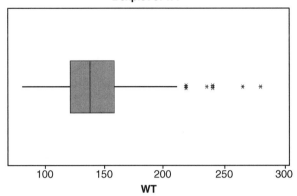

Figure 4.43   An outlier boxplot of the weights of women in the Benign Breast Disease data set.

4.20   Can a boxplot be used for estimating the modes in a bimodal distribution? Explain.

4.21   Can the mean of a population be estimated from the information contained in a boxplot? Explain.

4.22   How is a histogram different from a bar chart?

4.23   Which graphical statistic provides more information about the underlying distribution of a quantitative variable, a boxplot or a histogram? Explain.

4.24   What inference would you make about the relationship between the mean and the median when the sample histogram and boxplot suggest the population has an extremely long tail to the

    (a) right?   **(b)** left?

4.25   If a sample of $n = 250$ observations has 45 observations falling in the interval 0–25, compute the
    (a) percentage of the sample falling between 0 and 25.
    (b) density of the histogram class over the class interval 0–25.

4.26   Why should the density scale be used in histograms having classes of unequal widths?

4.27   Use the density histogram shown in Figure 4.44, based on the $n = 252$ observations on the variable Height contained in the Body Fat data set, to answer the following:
    (a) Does this histogram indicate any potential outliers?
    (b) Ignoring any potential outliers, does this histogram support the use of a normal probability model for modeling the distribution of height for adult males? Explain.

4.28   Use the density histogram shown in Figure 4.45, based on the $n = 200$ observations on the variable AGMT contained in the Benign Breast Disease data set, to answer the following:
    (a) Describe the shape of the underlying distribution of the variable Age suggested by the histogram in Figure 4.45.
    (b) Estimate the primary and secondary modes of the distribution of the variable Age.

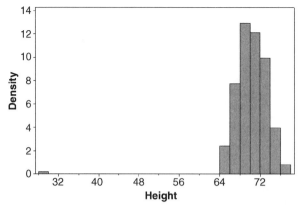

Figure 4.44   Density histogram of the $n = 252$ heights of adult males in the Body Fat data set.

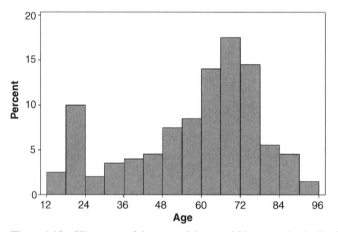

Figure 4.45   Histogram of the ages of the $n = 200$ women in the Benign Breast Disease data set.

(c) Does this histogram support the use of a normal probability model for modeling the distribution of the variable Age? Explain.

4.29   Use the percent relative frequency histograms in Figure 4.46, based on the variable weight (WT) for the case and control subpopulations for the $n = 200$ subjects in the Benign Breast Disease data set, to answer the following.

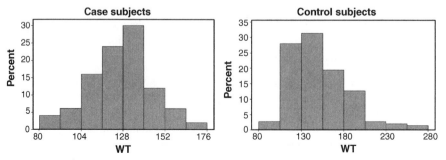

Figure 4.46   Percent histograms for the weight of the case and control subjects in the Benign Breast Disease Study.

(a) Describe the shape suggested by each of the histograms in Figure 4.46.

(b) Do the histograms in Figure 4.46 appear to indicate that the same probability model can be used for modeling the weights of women in these two subpopulations? Explain.

(c) Does either histogram in Figure 4.46 support the use of a normal probability model?

(d) Which subpopulation appears to have a higher percentage of women weighing more than 130 lb?

4.30   Using the Body Fat data set, create a boxplot and histogram for each of the following variables:

(a) PCTBF

(b) Density

(c) Weight

(d) Height

(e) Abdomen

4.31   Interpret the boxplots and histograms for each of the variables in Exercise 4.30. Be sure to comment on the general shape of the distribution, long tails in either direction, report estimates of the median and interquartile range, and identify any outliers in the data set.

4.32   Which of the two normal probability plots in Figure 4.47 supports the use of a normal probability model for modeling the underlying distribution of the variable being measured? Explain.

4.33   Use the normal probability plot in Figure 4.48, based on the $n = 252$ observations on the variable Density contained in the Body Fat data set, to answer the following:

(a) Does the normal probability plot in Figure 4.48 pass the "fat pencil test"? Explain.

(b) Does the normal probability plot in Figure 4.48 support the use of a normal probability model? Explain.

(c) Estimate the median of the distribution of the variable density.

(d) Estimate the 90th percentile of the distribution of the variable density.

4.34   Use the normal probability plot in Figure 4.49, based on the variable systolic blood pressure in the Intensive Care Unit data set, to answer the following:

(a) Does the normal probability plot in Figure 4.49 pass the "fat pencil test"? Explain.

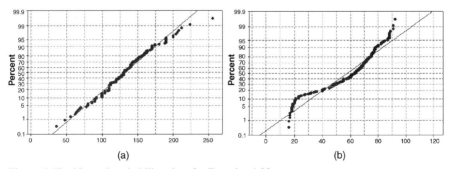

Figure 4.47   Normal probability plots for Exercise 4.32.

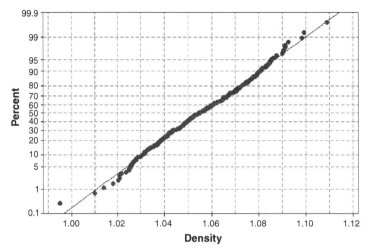

Figure 4.48   Normal probability plot for the $n = 252$ observations on the variable density in the Body Fat data set.

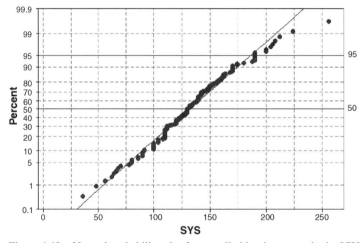

Figure 4.49   Normal probability plot for systolic blood pressure in the ICU data set.

(b) Does the normal probability plot in Figure 4.49 support the use of a normal probability model? Explain.

(c) Estimate the median of the distribution of the variable systolic blood pressure.

(d) Estimate the 95th percentile of the distribution of the variable systolic blood pressure.

4.35   Use the Coronary Heart Disease data set and the variable Age to answer the following:

(a) Create a normal probability plot of Age for the subpopulations where heart disease is present and absent.

(b) Interpret the normal probability plots created in part (a). Do these normal plots pass the "fat pencil test"?

(c) Estimate the median age in each of these subpopulations.

(d) Does there appear to be a difference in the distribution of the variable Age for these two subpopulations? Explain.

4.36   Using the Body Fat data set create normal probability plots for each of the following variables:

(a) Percent body fat (PCTBF)

(b) Density

(c) Ankle

(d) Thigh

(e) Biceps

4.37   Interpret the normal probability plots for each of the variables in Exercise 4.36. Be sure to comment on whether the normal probability plot supports the use of a normal probability model.

4.38   Use the data in Table 4.19 that summarizes the $n = 200$ observations on the variable age at menarche (AGMN) in the Benign Breast Disease data set to answer the following:

(a) Estimate the proportion of women experiencing menarche before age 10.

(b) Estimate the proportion of women experiencing menarche after their 13th birthday.

(c) Estimate the median age at which women experience menarche.

(d) Estimate the mean age at which women experience menarche.

(e) Estimate the 25th percentile of the distribution of the variable age at which a woman experiences menarche.

4.39   A diagnostic test is being developed for a particular disease and the final results of a study of this diagnostic test are presented in the 2×2 contingency table shown in Table 4.20. Use the information in Table 4.20 to answer the following:

(a) Estimate the sensitivity for this diagnostic test.

(b) Estimate the specificity for this diagnostic test.

TABLE 4.19   Frequency Table for the Age at Menarche of the $n = 200$ Observations in the Benign Breast Disease Data Set

Age Menarche	Count
8	1
9	1
10	7
11	31
12	50
13	42
14	31
15	17
16	13
17	7
	200

TABLE 4.20 The Results of a Diagnostic Test for 60 Diseased and 100 Nondiseased Subjects

Test Result	Diseased	
	Yes	No
Positive	54	7
Negative	6	93

4.40 A diagnostic test is being developed for a particular disease and the final results of a study of this diagnostic test are presented in the 2×2 contingency table shown in Table 4.21. Use the information in Table 4.21 to answer the following:
(a) estimate P(positive test result|diseased).
(b) estimate P(positive test result|not diseased).
(c) estimate P(negative test result|not diseased).
(d) What are the estimated values of the sensitivity and specificity of this diagnostic test?
(e) If the prevalence of this disease is $p = 0.05$, what is the estimated probability that an individual testing positive actually has the disease?

4.41 In the article "Comparable specificity of 2 commercial tuberculin reagents in persons at low risk for tuberculosis infection" published in the *Journal of the American Medical Association* (Villarino et al., 1999), the specificity of skin testing for tuberculosis with the reagents Aplisol and Tubersol was investigated. Use the information in Table 4.22, containing a summary of the $n = 1555$ participants not infected with tuberculosis in this study, to estimate the specificity of the skin test using the reagent
(a) Aplisol
(b) Tubersol

4.42 Suppose that in studying the factors related to a particular disease, say disease A, a new risk factor has been identified and studied. Use the summary data in Table 4.23 to estimate the relative risk of disease A for this new risk factor.

4.43 In the article "Aspirin and the treatment of heart failure in the elderly" published in *Archives of Internal Medicine* (Krumholz et al., 2001), the authors reported the results of their study on the use of aspirin as a discharge medication for patients 65 years or older who were hospitalized with heart failure or coronary artery disease. Using the summary data in Table 4.24 that was extracted from this article, compute the relative risk of death associated with not using aspirin.

TABLE 4.21 Results of a Diagnostic Test for 100 Diseased and 220 Nondiseased Subjects

Test Result	Diseased	
	Yes	No
Positive	87	17
Negative	13	213

TABLE 4.22   The Number of False Positives in a Skin Test for Tuberculosis

Test Result	Aplisol	Tubersol
Positive	17	28
Negative	1538	1527

TABLE 4.23   Results of a Study on a New Risk Factor That is Believed to be Associated with Disease A.

Factor	Disease	
	Present	Absent
Present	12	2
Absent	87	59

TABLE 4.24   A Summary of the Number of Deaths (i.e., 1-year Mortality) in a Study on Aspirin and Heart Failure

Aspririn Use	No. of Deaths	No. of Survivors
No	174	480
Yes	90	366

4.44   What inference can be drawn about the shape of the population when the sample mean is much larger than the sample median?

4.45   What does it mean when an estimator is said to be robust to the extreme values in a sample?

4.46   Give an example of a statistic that is

(**a**) robust to the extremes   (**b**) not robust to the extremes.

4.47   What is the difference between

(**a**) μ and $\bar{x}$?   (**b**) $\tilde{x}$ and $\tilde{\mu}$?

(**c**) IQR and $\widehat{\text{IQR}}$?   (**d**) $\hat{x}_p$ and X_p?

(**e**) σ and s?   (**f**) p and $\hat{p}$?

(**g**) s and $\hat{\sigma}$ (**h**) σ^2 and s^2?

4.48   What is the difference between $\bar{x}$ and $\tilde{x}$?

4.49   Is the estimate of the

(**a**) 1st percentile robust to the extremes in a sample? Explain.

(**b**) 45th percentile robust to the extremes in a sample? Explain.

(**c**) 99th percentile robust to the extremes in a sample? Explain.

(**d**) the mean robust to the extremes in a sample? Explain.

(**e**) interquartile range robust to the extremes in a sample? Explain.

4.50   Compute the values of $\bar{x}$, s^2, s, and the coefficient of variation (CV) when

(a) $n = 25$, $\sum x = 512$, and $\sum (x - \bar{x})^2 = 498$.
(b) $n = 50$, $\sum x = 6025$, and $\sum (x - \bar{x})^2 = 11025$.
(c) $n = 65$, $\sum x = 23.4$, and $\sum (x - \bar{x})^2 = 8.584$.
(d) $n = 250$, $\sum x = 5475$, and $\sum (x - \bar{x})^2 = 120462.75$.

4.51   Can the sample median be computed from the summary statistics n, $\sum x$, and $\sum x^2$? Explain.

4.52   In the article "Birth size and accelerated growth during infancy are associated with increased odds of childhood overweight in Mexican children" published in the *Journal of the American Dietetic Association* (Jones-Smith et al., 2007), two of the baseline variables measured on the $n = 163$ Mexican children sampled are birth weight (kg) and birth length (cm). Use the summary statistics in Table 4.25 to answer the following:
(a) Estimate the mean birth weight of a Mexican child.
(b) Estimate the standard deviation of the birth weight of a Mexican child.
(c) Estimate the coefficient of variation for the birth weight of a Mexican child.
(d) Estimate the mean birth length of a Mexican child.
(e) Estimate the standard deviation of the birth length of a Mexican child.
(f) Estimate the coefficient of variation for the birth length of a Mexican child.

4.53   Using the results of Exercise 4.52, convert the estimates of the mean, standard deviation, and coefficient of variation
(a) of the birth weight of a Mexican child from kilograms to pounds.
(b) of the birth length of a Mexican child from centimeters to inches.

4.54   Explain why the coefficients of variation are the same in Exercises 4.52 and 4.53.

4.55   Using the Body Fat data set,
(a) create a boxplot, histogram, and normal probability plot for variable percent body fat (PCTBF).
(b) Describe the shape of the distribution that is suggested by the graphical statistics in part (a).
(c) Are there any outliers or extreme outliers suggested by the graphical statistics in part (a)?
(d) Estimate the median of the variable percent body fat.
(e) Estimate the 25th percentile of percent body fat.
(f) Estimate mean of the variable percent body fat.
(g) Estimate variance and standard deviation of the variable percent body fat.
(h) Estimate coefficient of variation for the variable percent body fat.
(i) Estimate percentage of adult males having a percent body fat value less than 30%.

TABLE 4.25   Summary Statistics for the $n = 163$ Mexican Children in a Study on Accelerated Growth and Obesity

Variable	$\sum x$	$\sum x^2$
Birth weight (kg)	495.5	1533.6
Birth length (cm)	7905.5	384039.1

4.56 Use the Intensive Care Unit data set to identify potential differences in the subpopulations of systolic blood pressure (SYS) due to each survival status (STA) by

(a) creating histograms and boxplots of systolic blood pressure for each survival status.

(b) estimating the mean, median, and standard deviation of the variable systolic blood pressure for each survival status.

(c) using the information in part (b) to estimate the boundaries of the two standard deviation empirical rule (i.e., $\mu \pm 2\sigma$).

(d) using parts (a)–(d) to estimate potential differences in the systolic blood pressure of patients admitted to the intensive care unit who survived and who did not survive.

4.57 Using the estimates from Exercise 4.56 and assuming that the distribution of systolic blood pressure is approximately normally distributed for each survival status, estimate the

(a) probability that a patient who will survive will have a systolic blood pressure of more than 150.

(b) probability that a patient who will not survive will have a systolic blood pressure of more than 150.

4.58 Suppose an electronic scale used in an obesity study is inaccurate in that it under-reports an individual's weight by 2 lb. If the mean and standard deviation of the $n = 100$ adult males involved in the study are reported to be $\bar{x} = 218$ and $s = 30$, determine the correct values of $\bar{x}$ and s.

4.59 Suppose an electronic scale used in an obesity study is inaccurate in that it over-reports an individual's weight by 2%. If the mean and standard deviation of the $n = 100$ adult males involved in the study are reported to be $\bar{x} = 218$ and $s = 30$, determine the correct values of $\bar{x}$ and s.

4.60 What are three typical patterns seen in a scatterplot?

4.61 What is a bivariate outlier?

4.62 How are bivariate outliers be identified?

4.63 How are ρ and r different?

4.64 Describe each of the scatterplots in Figure 4.50. Be sure to identify any patterns, the strength of the pattern, and any bivariate outliers in each of these scatterplots.

4.65 Which of the scatterplots in Exercise 4.64 have

(a) positive sample correlation coefficients?

(b) negative sample correlation coefficients?

(c) sample correlation coefficients that are approximately 0?

4.66 What are the units of the sample correlation coefficient?

4.67 Why is it inappropriate to report the value of the sample correlation coefficient without discussing the scatterplot?

4.68 What can be said about the value of the sample correlation coefficient r when a scatterplot

(a) slopes downward in a linear fashion?

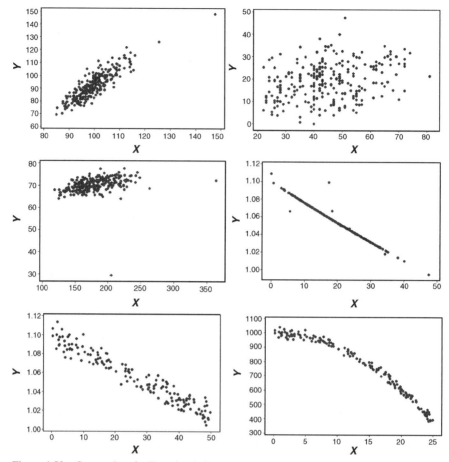

Figure 4.50   Scatterplots for Exercise 4.64.

(b) slopes upward in a linear fashion?
(c) reveals a curvilinear pattern?
(d) reveals no pattern at all?

4.69   What can be said about a scatterplot with a sample correlation coefficient of

(a) $r = 1$ **(b)** $r = 0$
(c) $r = 0.90$ **(d)** $r = -0.95$

4.70   Use the scatterplot in Figure 4.51 and the summary statistics for a bivariate random sample of $n = 150$ observations given in Table 4.26 to answer the following questions:

TABLE 4.26   **Summary Statistics for Exercise 4.70.**

Variable	Mean	SD
X	$\bar{x} = 6.6$	$s_X = 4.4$
Y	$\bar{y} = 35.8$	$s_Y = 7.9$

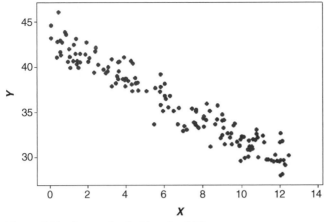

Figure 4.51   Scatterplot for Exercise 4.70.

    (a) Based on the scatterplot in Figure 4.51, is it reasonable to believe there is a linear relationship between Y and X? Explain.

    (b) If the sample correlation coefficient for Y and X is $r = -0.96$, determine the equation of the least squares regression line.

4.71   Use the Body Fat data set with the response variable weight and the explanatory variable height to answer the following:

    (a) Create a scatterplot for exploring the relationship between weight and height.

    (b) Does the data cloud in the scatterplot of weight versus height appear to be linear?

    (c) Compute the sample correlation coefficient between weight and height.

    (d) Fit the least squares regression line for weight as a linear function of height.

4.72   Use the Body Fat data set with the response variable percent body fat (PCTBF) to answer the following:

    (a) Create scatterplots of percent body fat versus each of the explanatory variables weight, abdomen circumference, hip circumference, and thigh circumference.

    (b) Compute the sample correlation coefficient associated with each of the scatterplots in part (a).

    (c) Identify any patterns or bivariate outliers in the scatterplots in part (a).

    (d) Determine which of the explanatory variables weight, abdomen circumference, hip circumference, and thigh circumference appears to have the strongest linear relationship with percent body fat.

    (e) Fit the least squares regression line for percent body fat with the explanatory variable identified in part (d).

4.73   Use the Body Fat data set with the response variable density to answer the following:

    (a) Create scatterplots of density versus each of the explanatory variables weight, abdomen circumference, hip circumference, and thigh circumference.

    (b) Compute the sample correlation coefficient associated with each of the scatterplots in part (a).

(c) Identify any pattern or bivariate outlier in the scatterplots in part (a).

(d) Determine which of the explanatory variables weight, abdomen circumference, hip circumference, and thigh circumference appears to have the strongest linear relationship with density.

(e) Fit the least squares regression line for density with the explanatory variable identified in part (d).

CHAPTER 5

MEASURING THE RELIABILITY OF STATISTICS

THE DISCIPLINE of Statistics deals with the science/art of describing populations from the information only on a portion of the population, namely, a random sample. Thus, statistical inferences are made about the population from a random sample, and statistics and estimators are not designed to determine the true values of the unknown population parameters. That is, a statistic is computed from an observed sample and provides a mathematical "guess" of the value of an unknown parameter. Furthermore, the observed value of a statistic that is used to estimate an unknown parameter is based on a particular observed sample, and a different random sample would be expected to produce a different value of the estimate of the unknown parameter. For example, the summary statistics in Table 5.1 were computed from three simple random samples of size $n = 25$ drawn from a normal population with mean 100 and standard deviation 20.

The different values of the estimates are due to the fact that the samples are slightly different, and the degree to which the possible samples differ depends on the underlying variability in the target population. The differences in the values of a statistic that result from the samples that could be drawn from a particular target population are called *sampling variability*. One of the most important considerations in any statistical analysis is the accuracy of any estimate and statistical inference that are made about the target population from a random sample. The answer to this question depends on the behavior of the estimator over all possible samples from the target population. In particular, the behavior of an estimator under random sampling will be affected by the sample size n, sampling variability, and the underlying variability in the target population. Moreover, understanding the behavior of an estimator under random sampling provides the necessary information for assessing the accuracy of the estimator.

5.1 SAMPLING DISTRIBUTIONS

Recall that a simple random sample is a sample of size n drawn from a population of N units and chosen in a fashion so that each possible sample of size n has the same chance of being selected. When a population is sampled, the observed sample that is obtained is just one of the many possible samples from this population. For example, even with a small

TABLE 5.1 **The Basic Summary Statistics Computed for Three Simple Random Samples of $n = 25$ Observations From a Normal Population with $\mu = 100$ and $\sigma = 20$**

Sample	$\bar{x}$	s	Minimum	$Q1$	$\tilde{x}$	$Q3$	Maximum
1	103.02	16.52	76.14	87.69	101.80	115.87	144.18
2	95.98	15.54	70.77	84.47	94.56	107.15	135.01
3	94.50	19.73	59.20	81.77	92.51	110.31	131.10

population of 100 units there are 17,310,309,456,440 (17 trillion!) possible different simple random samples of size $n = 10$ and 242,519,269,720,337,121,015,504 (242 sextillion!) possible different simple random samples of size $n = 25$. Also, because a simple random sample does not favor any one portion of the population over another, it is highly likely that the observed sample will be representative of the target population. Several properties of simple random samples are listed below.

PROPERTIES OF SIMPLE RANDOM SAMPLES

1. Well-designed simple random samples are meant to produce data that is representative of the target population.

2. When the sampling frame contains the entire population, the values of many statistics, such as $\bar{x}$, s^2, and p, computed from a simple random sample, will not systematically over or underestimate the parameter of interest.

3. Statistics computed from simple random samples have a predictable pattern of possible values.

4. Statistics computed from simple random samples can be made as accurate as is desired.

Note that because stratified random samples are collections of simple random samples they have the same properties as do simple random samples.

The values of the statistics and estimates computed from a sample will depend on the particular sample that is obtained; however, statistics that are computed from a simple random sample will also have a known and predictable pattern of behavior in repeated sampling. Furthermore, the predictable pattern of behavior of an estimator can be used to judge how reliable the estimator is in practice.

The predictable pattern of behavior of a statistic or an estimator is described by the *sampling distribution* associated with the statistic. The sampling distribution of a statistic, based on a sample of n measurements, is the probability distribution of the statistic. In particular, the sampling distribution of a statistic is formed by computing the values of the statistic for all possible samples of size n that could be selected from the target population. For example, suppose a simple random sample of size $n = 2$ is to be drawn from a population consisting of five units with values 1, 3, 5, 5, and 6. The sampling distribution of $\bar{x}$ would be found by determining all of the possible simple random samples of size $n = 2$ and computing the value of $\bar{x}$ for each possible sample. In this case, the sampling distribution of $\bar{x}$ would be found by tabulating the relative frequency of each possible value of $\bar{x}$.

Example 5.1

Suppose a simple random sample of size $n = 2$ is to be drawn from a population consisting of five units with values 1, 3, 5, 5, and 6. Determine the sampling distribution of $\bar{x}$.

TABLE 5.2   Basic Summary Statistics Computed for Three Samples of $n = 25$ Observations from a Normal Population with $\mu = 100$ and $\sigma = 20$

$\bar{x}$	2	3	3.5	4	4.5	5	5.5
$p(\bar{x})$	0.1	0.2	0.1	0.2	0.1	0.1	0.2

Solution First, the possible simple random samples of size $n = 2$ that can be selected from these five population units are

$$
\begin{array}{cccccccccc}
1.3 & 1.5 & 1.5 & 1.6 & 3.1 & 3.5 & 3.5 & 3.6 & 5.1 & 5.3 \\
5.5 & 5.6 & 5.1 & 5.3 & 5.5 & 5.6 & 6.1 & 6.3 & 6.5 & 6.5
\end{array}
$$

Thus, the possible values of $\bar{x}$ for these 20 possible samples are

$$
\begin{array}{cccccccccc}
2 & 3 & 3 & 3.5 & 2 & 4 & 4 & 4.5 & 3 & 4 \\
5 & 5.5 & 3 & 4 & 5 & 5.5 & 3.5 & 4.5 & 5.5 & 5.5
\end{array}
$$

Thus, based on the possible values of $\bar{x}$, the sampling distribution of $\bar{x}$ is given in Table 5.2

The sampling distribution of an estimator describes the long-run behavior of the estimator over repeated sampling from the target population. As is the case with most distributions, two of the most important characteristics of the sampling distribution are the mean and the standard deviation. In particular, the mean of the sampling distribution is the average value of the estimator computed over all possible samples, and the standard deviation of the sampling distribution measures the spread of the possible values of the statistic. An accurate estimator will have a sampling distribution with mean near the parameter it estimates and a small standard deviation.

5.1.1 Unbiased Estimators

When the mean of the sampling distribution is equal to the parameter being estimated, the estimator is said to be an *unbiased estimator*, and when the mean of the sampling distribution is not equal to the parameter of interest, the estimator is said to be a *biased estimator*. An unbiased estimator is an estimator that does not systematically over or underestimate the parameter of interest on the average, while a biased estimator is an estimator that does tend to over or underestimate the parameter of interest on the average. When T is an estimator of a parameter θ and μ_T is the mean of the sampling distribution of T, then the *bias* of T for estimating θ is defined to be the difference between μ_T and θ and is denoted by Bias(T, θ). Thus, the bias of an estimator T for estimating a parameter θ is

$$\text{Bias}(T, \theta) = \mu_T - \theta$$

Note that when Bias(T, θ) = 0, T is an unbiased estimator of θ. On the other hand, when Bias(T, θ) > 0, T tends to systematically overestimate θ, and when Bias(T, θ) < 0, T tends to systematically underestimate θ. A good estimator will be unbiased or have a small bias that decreases rapidly as the sample size increases.

Example 5.2

For the population given in Example 5.1 with values 1, 3, 5, 5, and 6, the mean of the population is

$$\mu = \frac{1 + 3 + 5 + 5 + 6}{5} = 4$$

Using the sampling distribution of $\bar{x}$ given in Table 5.2, the mean of the sampling distribution of $\bar{x}$ is

$$\mu_{\bar{x}} = 2(0.1) + 3(0.2) + 3.5(0.1) + 4(0.2) + 4.5(0.1) + 5(0.1) + 5.5(0.2) = 4$$

Thus, $\mu_{\bar{x}} = \mu = 4$, and hence, $\bar{x}$ is an unbiased estimator of μ for simple random samples of size $n = 2$.

In Example 5.2, the estimator $\bar{x}$ was found to be an unbiased estimator of μ for the population consisting of the values 1, 3,5, 5, and 6. In fact, it turns out that the mean of the sampling distribution of $\bar{x}$ will be μ for every population having mean μ. Thus, the estimator $\bar{x}$ is always an unbiased estimator of the population mean μ. Some of the estimators that were discussed in Chapter 4 that are also unbiased estimators are listed below.

UNBIASED ESTIMATORS

- $\bar{x}$ is an unbiased estimator of μ because $\mu_{\bar{x}} = \mu$.
- $\hat{p}$ is an unbiased estimator of a population proportion p because $\mu_{\hat{p}} = p$.
- s^2 is an unbiased estimator of a σ^2 because $\mu_{s^2} = \sigma^2$.

Recall that $s^2 = (1/(n-1))\left[\sum x^2 - n\bar{x}^2\right]$, and dividing by $n-1$ rather than n in the formula for s^2 produces an unbiased estimator of σ^2. In fact, another estimator of σ^2 that is sometimes used for estimating σ^2 is

$$\hat{\sigma}_n^2 = \frac{1}{n}\left[\sum x^2 - n\bar{x}^2\right] = \frac{n-1}{n}s^2$$

Now, $\hat{\sigma}_n^2$ is biased since the mean of the sampling distribution of $\hat{\sigma}_n^2$ is $\frac{n-1}{n}\sigma^2 \neq \sigma^2$. The bias of $\hat{\sigma}_n^2$ is

$$\text{Bias}(\hat{\sigma}_n^2, \sigma^2) = \frac{n-1}{n}\sigma^2 - \sigma^2 = \frac{-\sigma^2}{n} < 0$$

and thus $\hat{\sigma}_n^2$ tends to underestimate the value of σ^2 on the average.

Even though s^2 is an unbiased estimator of σ^2, it turns out that the sample standard deviation s is a biased estimator of σ, and s tends to underestimate the population standard deviation on the average. In general, creating an unbiased estimator of σ is difficult; however, since the bias of s is usually small and decreases rapidly as n increases, s is the most commonly used estimator of the population standard deviation σ.

5.1.2 Measuring the Accuracy of an Estimator

The sampling distribution of an estimator also contains information on the precision and accuracy of the estimator. In particular, the standard deviation of the sampling distribution measures the typical deviation of the estimator from the mean of the sampling distribution. The standard deviation of the sampling distribution of an estimator is called the *standard error* of the estimator, and the standard error of an estimator T will be denoted by $\text{SE}(T)$ or SE_T. The standard error measures the precision of an estimator and is a measure of the reliability of an unbiased estimator. The reliability of a biased estimator is measured by the *mean squared error* (MSE) of the estimator that is the average squared distance the estimator is from the parameter it estimates. The mean squared error of an estimator T of a parameter θ is a function of the estimator's bias and precision. In particular, the mean squared error of an estimator T for estimating a parameter θ is denoted by $\mathrm{MSE}(T < \theta)$ and is defined as

$$\mathrm{MSE}(T, \theta) = \mathrm{Bias}(T, \theta)^2 + \mathrm{SE}(T)^2$$

Note that for an unbiased estimator the mean squared error is equal to the square of the standard error of the estimator T since the bias is 0. Thus, only estimators that are unbiased or have a low bias that decreases as n increases and have a small standard error should be used for estimating an unknown parameter. Finally, when comparing two estimators of a parameter the estimator with the smallest mean squared error is the more accurate of the two estimators.

Example 5.3

Estimators s^2 and $\widehat{\sigma}_n^2$ are often used for estimating σ^2 when the population that is sampled is normally distributed. In this case,

1. s^2 is unbiased and $\mathrm{Bias}(\widehat{\sigma}_n^2, \sigma^2) = \dfrac{-\sigma^2}{n}$.

2. $\mathrm{SE}(s^2) = \sqrt{\dfrac{2\sigma^4}{n-1}}$.

3. $\mathrm{SE}(\widehat{\sigma}_n^2) = \sqrt{\dfrac{2(n-1)\sigma^4}{n^2)}}$.

Thus, the MSE of s^2 is

$$\mathrm{MSE}(s^2, \sigma^2) = \mathrm{Bias}(s^2, \sigma^2)^2 + \mathrm{SE}(s^2)^2$$

$$= 0^2 + \frac{2\sigma^4}{n-1} = \frac{2\sigma^4}{n-1}$$

and the MSE of $\widehat{\sigma}_n^2$ is

$$\mathrm{MSE}(\widehat{\sigma}_n^2, \sigma^2) = \mathrm{Bias}(\widehat{\sigma}_n^2, \sigma^2)^2 + \mathrm{SE}(\widehat{\sigma}_n^2)^2$$

$$= \left(\frac{-\sigma^2}{n}\right)^2 + \frac{2(n-1)\sigma^4}{n^2}$$

$$= \frac{(2n-1)\sigma^4}{n^2}$$

Table 5.3 shows the values of MSE for s^2 and $\widehat{\sigma}_n^2$ for several different values of n when $\sigma^2 = 25$.

Note that the mean squared error of $\widehat{\sigma}_n^2$ is always smaller than the MSE of s^2 even though $\widehat{\sigma}_n^2$ is a biased estimator of σ^2. Thus, $\widehat{\sigma}_n^2$ is a more accurate estimator than s^2 when the target population is normally distributed; however, the difference in accuracy rapidly decreases as n increases.

Also, the mean squared errors of both estimators decrease as n increases, and the bias of $\widehat{\sigma}_n^2$ decreases as n increases, also.

TABLE 5.3 The Standard Errors, Bias, and MSE's for s^2 and $\widehat{\sigma}_n^2$ for $n = 15, 25, 50, 100$

n	$\mathrm{SE}(s^2)$	$\mathrm{MSE}(s^2, \sigma^2)$	Bias of $\widehat{\sigma}_n^2$	$\mathrm{SE}(\widehat{\sigma}_n^2)$	$\mathrm{MSE}(\widehat{\sigma}_n^2, \sigma^2)$
15	9.45	89.29	-1.67	8.82	80.56
25	7.22	52.08	-1.00	6.92	49.00
50	5.05	25.51	-0.50	4.95	24.75
100	3.55	17.63	-0.25	3.52	12.44

In practice, the standard error of an estimator will usually depend on one or more unknown parameters, and thus the standard error will need to be estimated using the plug-in-rule. To distinguish between the true standard error and the estimated standard error, the estimated standard error will be denoted by se rather than SE. For example, the standard error of $\bar{x}$ is $SE(\bar{x}) = \sigma/\sqrt{n}$, but since the value of σ is almost always unknown, the estimated standard error is found by replacing the value of σ with the sample standard deviation s. In this case, the estimated standard error of $\bar{x}$ is

$$se(\bar{x}) = \frac{s}{\sqrt{n}}$$

5.1.3 The Bound on the Error of Estimation

The most commonly used measure of the reliability for an unbiased estimator is the *bound on the error of estimation* (*B*). The bound on the error of estimation is simply two times the standard error of the estimator. That is,

$$B = 2 \times SE(T)$$

Because the standard error is the standard deviation of the sampling distribution, at least 75% of the possible values of the estimator fall within B of the mean of the sampling distribution; if the sampling distribution is mound shaped, then roughly 95% of the possible values of the estimator fall within B of the mean. Thus, it is unlikely for an unbiased estimator to be more than a distance of B from the true value of the parameter being estimated. The empirical rules for an unbiased estimator are given below.

THE EMPIRICAL RULES FOR AN UNBIASED ESTIMATOR

When the sampling distribution of an unbiased estimator of θ is mound shaped

1. roughly 68% of the possible values of the estimator lie within one standard error of θ.

2. roughly 95% of the possible values of a statistics lie within two standard errors (i.e., B) of θ.

3. roughly 99% of the possible values of a statistics lie within three standard errors of θ.

Thus, for many unbiased estimators roughly 95% of all of the possible random samples will produce estimates that are within B of the true value of the parameter. In practice, there is no guarantee that an observed value of the estimator will actually be within B of the true value, however, there is only about a 5% chance that the sample will produce a value of the estimator that is farther than B from the true value under random sampling. On the other hand, when a sample of convenience is used, the bound on the error of estimation B has no meaning as a measure of the reliability of an estimator since the empirical rules only apply with random sampling.

Example 5.4

The sampling distribution of $\bar{x}$ is generally mound shaped, and thus, it is unlikely to observe a value of $\bar{x}$ more than

$$B = 2SE(\bar{x}) = 2 \times \frac{\sigma}{\sqrt{n}}$$

from the true value of μ. For example, when a random sample of $n = 50$ observations selected from a population with $\sigma = 10$, it will be unlikely for the observed value of $\bar{x}$ to be more than a distance of

$$B = 2 \times \frac{10}{\sqrt{50}} = 2.83$$

from the true value of the mean.

The formula for the bound on the error of estimation for an unbiased estimator can also be used for determining the sample size required for a prespecified level of reliability. For example, suppose a random sample is going to be drawn from a population with $\sigma \approx 5$ for estimating the mean of the population. If the observed value of $\bar{x}$ should be within $B = 0.5$ of μ, the sample size required to obtain this bound can be found by solving the equation

$$B = 2 \times \frac{\sigma}{\sqrt{n}}$$

for n. Thus, the value of n required for a random sample to have a bound on the error of estimation of $\bar{x}$ equal to B is

$$n = \left(\frac{2 \times \sigma}{B} \right)^2$$

Example 5.5
The sample size needed to have a bound on the error of estimation for $\bar{x}$ equal to 0.5 when $\sigma = 5$ is

$$n = \left(\frac{2 \times 5}{0.5} \right)^2 = 400$$

Thus, when a simple random sample of $n = 400$ observations is drawn from this population, the observed value of $\bar{x}$ will most likely be within $B = 0.5$ of the true value of μ.

5.2 THE SAMPLING DISTRIBUTION OF A SAMPLE PROPORTION

Recall that $\widehat{p}$ is the sample proportion that is the estimator used to estimate a population proportion. The sampling distribution of $\widehat{p}$, for a simple random sample of n observations, consists of all of the possible values of $\widehat{p}$ computed over all possible simple random samples of size n that could be selected from the target population. The sampling distribution of $\widehat{p}$ plays an important role in determining the reliability of any statistical inferences based on $\widehat{p}$.

5.2.1 The Mean and Standard Deviation of the Sampling Distribution of $\widehat{p}$

The mean of the sampling distribution of $\widehat{p}$ is always equal to p, so $\widehat{p}$ is an unbiased estimator of p, and therefore, $\widehat{p}$ is an unbiased estimator of the population proportion p. The formula for the standard error of $\widehat{p}$ depends on the proportion of the population sampled, and when the sampling proportion is more than 5%, (i.e, $\frac{n}{N} \geq 0.05$, the standard error of $\widehat{p}$ is

$$\text{SE}(\widehat{p}) = \sqrt{\frac{N - n}{N - 1}} \sqrt{\frac{p(1 - p)}{n}}$$

The term $\sqrt{\frac{N-n}{N-1}}$ is called the *finite population correction factor* and should always be used when the sampling proportion is at least 5%. If the number of units in the population, N, is unknown then finite population correction factor cannot be used. When the sampling proportion is less than 5%, the finite population correction factor is almost equal to 1 and does not have much effect on the value of the standard error. Thus, when the number of units in the population is unknown or the sampling proportion is less than 5%, the standard error of $\hat{p}$ will be approximately

$$SE(\hat{p}) = \sqrt{\frac{p(1-p)}{n}}$$

The standard error of $\hat{p}$ decreases as the sample size n increases in both forms of the standard error. In fact, as n approaches the number of units in the population N, the standard error approaches 0; when $n = N$ the standard error is exactly equal to 0 and the value of $\hat{p}$ will be p. Thus, $\hat{p}$ can be made as accurate as desired by choosing a sufficiently large sample size.

Example 5.6

Determine the standard error of $\hat{p}$ when

  a. $N = 1000$, $n = 100$, and $p = 0.25$.
  b. $N = 10,000$, $n = 100$, and $p = 0.56$.
  c. $N = 10,000$, $n = 2,000$, and $p = 0.43$.
  d. $n = 250$, $p = 0.68$, and N is unknown.

Solutions

  a. The sampling proportion is $\dfrac{100}{1000} = 0.1 \geq 0.05$, so the standard error of $\hat{p}$ should be computed using the finite population correction factor. Thus,

$$SE(\hat{p}) = \sqrt{\frac{1000 - 100}{1000 - 1}} \sqrt{\frac{0.25(1 - 0.25)}{100}} = 0.041$$

  b. The sampling proportion is $\dfrac{100}{10,000} = 0.01 < 0.05$ so the standard error of $\hat{p}$ can be computed without the finite population correction factor. Thus,

$$SE(\hat{p}) = \sqrt{\frac{0.56(1 - 0.56)}{100}} = 0.049$$

Note that is the finite population correction used, the true standard error is

$$SE(\hat{p}) = \sqrt{\frac{10,000 - 100}{10,000}} \sqrt{\frac{0.56(1 - 0.56)}{100}} = 0.0488$$

  c. The sampling proportion is $\dfrac{2000}{10,000} = 0.2 \geq 0.05$ so the standard error of $\hat{p}$ should be computed using the finite population correction factor. Thus,

$$SE(\hat{p}) = \sqrt{\frac{10,000 - 2000}{10,000 - 1}} \sqrt{\frac{0.43(1 - 0.43)}{100}} = 0.044$$

  d. Since N is unknown, the sampling proportion is also unknown, and thus, the standard error of $\hat{p}$ will be computed without the finite population correction factor. In this case,

$$SE(\hat{p}) = \sqrt{\frac{0.68(1 - 0.68)}{250}} = 0.030$$

In many research studies, the number of units in the target population will be unknown, and thus, in this case the standard error of $\widehat{p}$ must be computed without using the finite population correction factor. When the finite population correction factor is not used, the value of the approximate standard error of $\widehat{p}$ is a *conservative* value of the standard error. That is, the true standard error computed with the finite population correction factor will be smaller than the approximate standard error computed without the finite population correction factor.

When the value of p is unknown the standard error of $\widehat{p}$ must be estimated since it depends on the value of p. The estimated standard error of $\widehat{p}$ is denoted by $\text{se}(\widehat{p})$ and is computed using $\widehat{p}$ in place of p in the formulas for the standard error of $\widehat{p}$. Thus, the formulas for estimated standard errors of $\widehat{p}$ are

$$1.\ \ \text{se}(\widehat{p}) = \sqrt{\frac{N-n}{N}}\sqrt{\frac{\widehat{p}(1-\widehat{p})}{n}} \ \ \text{when} \ \ \frac{n}{N} \geq 0.05$$

$$2.\ \ \text{se}(\widehat{p}) = \sqrt{\frac{\widehat{p}(1-\widehat{p})}{n}} \ \ \text{when} \ \ \frac{n}{N} < 0.05 \ \text{or N is unknown.}$$

Example 5.7
In the article "Mortality associated with central nervous system tuberculosis" published in *Journal of Infection* (El Sahly et al., 2007), the authors reported the sample proportions in Table 5.4 for a study of central nervous system tuberculosis (CNSTB). The sample size for the CNSTB subpopulation is $n = 92$ and the sample size for the non-CNSTB subpopulation is $n = 3570$. Use the information in Table 5.4 to determine the standard error and bound on error of estimation for

  a. the estimated proportion of CNSTB individuals with daily alcohol use.

  b. the estimated proportion of non-CNSTB individuals that are current smokers.

Solutions Since the sampling proportion is unknown, the standard error of the sample proportions will be computed without the finite population correction factor. Thus,

  a. the standard error and bound on the error of estimation for the estimated proportion of CNSTB individuals with daily alcohol use are

$$\text{se}(\widehat{p}) = \sqrt{\frac{0.267(1-0.267)}{92}} = 0.046$$

and

$$B = 2 \times 0.046 = 0.092$$

  b. the standard error and bound on the error of estimation for the estimated proportion of non-CNSTB individuals that are current smokers are

$$\text{se}(\widehat{p}) = \sqrt{\frac{0.417(1-0.417)}{3570}} = 0.008$$

TABLE 5.4 Sample percentages for CNSTB and Non-CNSTB Individuals Reported in the *Journal of Infection* (El Sahly, 2007)

Factor	CNSTB	Non-CNSTB
Daily alcohol use	26.7%	33.7%
Current smoker	29.3%	41.7%

and

$$B = 2 \times 0.008 = 0.016$$

Note that the bound on the error of estimation for the estimated proportion of non-CNSTB individuals that are current smokers is much smaller than the bound on the error of estimation for the estimated proportion of CNSTB who use alcohol daily. The difference in these bounds on the error of estimation is primarily due to the difference in the sample sizes. In particular, since nearly 40 times as many non-CNSTB individuals were sampled, the standard errors and bounds on the error of estimation for the non-CNSTB proportions are much smaller than they are for the CNSTB proportions.

5.2.2 Determining the Sample Size for a Prespecified Value of the Bound on the Error Estimation

One of the most important aspects of planning a study or an experiment is the number of units that will be sampled. When a prespecified bound on the error of estimation is available, the sample size needed to attain this bound can usually be determined by solving the equation

$$B = 2 \times \mathrm{SE}$$

for n. In particular, the sample size for a prespecified bound on the error of estimation for estimating a proportion can be found by solving $B = 2\mathrm{SE}(\widehat{p})$ for n; however, because the standard error depends on the unknown value of p, a conservative (i.e., larger than necessary) value of n can be found by replacing p by 0.5 in the formula for the standard error of $\widehat{p}$. The sample size n that produces a bound on the error of estimation of no larger than B for a simple random sample is

---

THE SAMPLE SIZE REQUIRED FOR ESTIMATING A PROPORTION

When the bound on the error of the sample proportion should be no larger than B, the sample size is

1. $n = \dfrac{N}{(N-1)B^2 + 1}$ when N is known.

2. $n = \dfrac{1}{B^2}$ when N is unknown.

Note that the formulas for the sample size will not generally produce an integer value of n, and thus, the resulting value of n must be rounded off to the next largest integer to ensure that the value of B is attained. For example, if a simple random sample of n observations is to be taken from a population of $N = 50,000$ units and the desired bound on the error of estimation is $B = 0.01$, then the value of n is

$$n = \frac{50{,}000}{49{,}999(0.01)^2 + 1} = 8333.5$$

Hence, the estimator $\widehat{p}$ based on a simple random sample of $n = 8334$ units will have a bound on the error of estimation no larger than $B = 0.01$.

Example 5.8

Determine the sample size required to attain the value of B for estimating a proportion when

    a. $N = 5000$ and $B = 0.05$.

    b. $N = 5000$ and $B = 0.025$.

    c. N is unknown and $B = 0.05$.

    d. N is unknown and $B = 0.035$.

Solutions The value of n is

    a. $n = \dfrac{5000}{4999(0.05)^2 + 1} = 371$ because N is known.

    b. $n = \dfrac{5000}{4999(0.025)^2 + 1} = 1213$ because N is known.

    c. $n = \dfrac{1}{(0.05)^2} = 400$ because N is unknown.

    d. $n = \dfrac{1}{(0.035)^2} = 817$ because N is unknown.

    Note that the bound on the error of estimation B of $\widehat{p}$ is governed by the *square root law*, which says that the accuracy of the estimator $\widehat{p}$ is inversely proportional to the square root of the sample size n. Thus, decreasing the value of B by a factor of two requires a sample consisting of four times as many observations. For example, if the value of B is $B = 0.05$ for a sample of $n = 300$ observations, then it would require a sample of $n = 1200$ observations to produce a value of $B = 0.025$.

Example 5.9

Suppose a random sample of $n = 56$ observations yields an estimate $\widehat{p} = 0.42$. Determine the estimated standard error of $\widehat{p}$ and the bound on the error of estimation of $\widehat{p}$.

Solution With a sample of $n = 56$ observations and $\widehat{p} = 0.42$ and no information on N given, the standard error of $\widehat{p}$ is

$$\mathrm{se}(\widehat{p}) = \sqrt{\frac{0.42(1 - 0.42)}{56}} = 0.066$$

and the bound on the error of estimation of $\widehat{p}$ is

$$B = 2 \times \mathrm{se}(\widehat{p}) = 2(0.066) = 0.132$$

5.2.3 The Central Limit Theorem for $\widehat{p}$

Finally, the sampling distribution of $\widehat{p}$ will be approximately normally distributed for a sufficiently large random sample. In particular, when np and $n(1 - p)$ are both greater than 5, the sampling distribution of $\widehat{p}$ is approximately a normal distribution with mean p and standard deviation $\sqrt{p(1 - p)/n}$.

CENTRAL LIMIT THEOREM (CLT) FOR $\widehat{p}$

When both np and $n(1 - p)5$ are greater than   is approximately a standard normal distribution.
5, the distribution of

$$Z = \frac{\widehat{p} - p}{\mathrm{SE}(\widehat{p})}$$

    Thus, when n is sufficiently large, the Central Limit Theorem can be used for determining probabilities concerning $\widehat{p}$. The Central Limit Theorem will also form the basis for the confidence statements and hypothesis tests based on $\widehat{p}$ that will be discussed in Chapters 6 and 7.

Example 5.10

Suppose a simple random sample of n observations is to be taken from a population with unknown proportion p. If n is assumed to be sufficiently large so that the Central Limit Theorem applies, determine the approximate probability that $\widehat{p}$ is within B of p.

Solution   The probability that the observed value of $\widehat{p}$ is within B of p is

$$P(p - B \leq \widehat{p} \leq p + B) = P(-B \leq \widehat{p} - p \leq B)$$

$$= P(-2\mathrm{SE}(\widehat{p}) \leq \widehat{p} - p \leq 2\mathrm{SE}(\widehat{p}))$$

$$= P\left(-2 \leq \frac{\widehat{p} - p}{\mathrm{SE}(\widehat{p})} \leq 2\right)$$

$$\approx \underbrace{P(-2 \leq Z \leq 2)}_{\text{by the CLT}}$$

$$= 0.9544$$

Therefore, when the Central Limit Theorem applies, the probability that the observed value of $\widehat{p}$ is within B of p is about 0.95. That is, about 95% of all of the possible simple random samples would produce a value of $\widehat{p}$ within B of the unknown value of p.

5.2.4 Some Final Notes on the Sampling Distribution of $\widehat{p}$

In summary, several key properties of sample proportion $\widehat{p}$ are listed below.

PROPERTIES OF $\widehat{p}$

---

1. The mean of the sampling distribution of $\widehat{p}$ is p and thus, $\widehat{p}$ is an unbiased estimator of a population proportion p.

2. When the number of units in the target population is known, the standard error of $\widehat{p}$ is

$$\mathrm{SE}(\widehat{p}) = \sqrt{\frac{N - n}{N - 1}} \sqrt{\frac{p(1 - p)}{n}}$$

3. When the number of units in the target population is unknown or the sampling proportion is less than 0.05, the approximate value of the standard error of $\widehat{p}$ is

$$\mathrm{SE}(\widehat{p}) = \sqrt{\frac{p(1 - p)}{n}}$$

4. Because $\widehat{p}$ is an unbiased estimator of p and the standard error of $\widehat{p}$ decreases as the sample size n increases, $\widehat{p}$ can be made as accurate an estimator of p as is desired by choosing a sufficiently large sample size.

5. When the number of units in the target population is known the estimated standard error of $\widehat{p}$ is

$$\mathrm{se}(\widehat{p}) = \sqrt{\frac{N - n}{N}} \sqrt{\frac{\widehat{p}(1 - \widehat{p})}{n}}$$

6. When the number of units in the target population is unknown or the sampling proportion is less than 0.05 the estimated standard error of $\widehat{p}$ is

$$\mathrm{se}(\widehat{p}) = \sqrt{\frac{\widehat{p}(1 - \widehat{p})}{n}}$$

7. When both np and $n(1 - p)$ are greater than 5 the sampling distribution of $\widehat{p}$ is approximately normal with mean p and standard deviation $\mathrm{SE}(\widehat{p})$.

5.3 THE SAMPLING DISTRIBUTION OF $\bar{X}$

Recall that $\bar{x}$ is the sample mean and the sampling distribution of $\bar{x}$ consists of all of the possible values of $\bar{x}$ computed over all possible simple random samples of size n that could be selected from the target population. The sampling distribution of $\bar{x}$ plays an important role in judging the accuracy of the sample mean, making confidence statements about a population mean, and in testing hypotheses about the population mean.

5.3.1 The Mean and Standard Deviation of the Sampling Distribution of $\bar{x}$

The mean of the sampling distribution of $\bar{x}$ is μ, and thus, $\bar{x}$ is an unbiased estimator of μ. Since $\bar{x}$ is an unbiased estimator of μ the standard error of $\bar{x}$, denoted by $SE(\bar{x})$, will measure the accuracy of $\bar{x}$. The value of the standard error of $\bar{x}$ depends on the value of the standard deviation in the target population, the number of units in the population, and the sample size. When the number of units in the population is known, the standard error of $\bar{x}$ for a sample of n units is

$$SE(\bar{x}) = \sqrt{\frac{N-n}{N-1}} \times \frac{\sigma}{\sqrt{n}}$$

where σ is the standard deviation of the target population and $\sqrt{\frac{N-n}{N-1}}$ is the finite population correction factor.

Example 5.11
Suppose a simple random sample of $n = 100$ observations will be drawn from a population with $N = 800$ units and standard deviation $\sigma = 12$. The standard error of $\bar{x}$ is

$$SE(\bar{x}) = \sqrt{\frac{800-100}{800-1}} \times \frac{12}{\sqrt{10}} = 1.12$$

In many studies, the number of units in the population is unknown or the sampling proportion is less than 5%. In these cases, the finite population correction factor is generally not used, and the standard error of $\bar{x}$ for a sample of n units is approximated by

$$SE(\bar{x}) = \frac{\sigma}{\sqrt{n}}$$

Computing the standard error of $\bar{x}$ without the finite population correction factor produces a conservative standard error since the finite population correction factor is always less than 1. For example, if $N = 5000$, $n = 400$, and $\sigma = 10$, the value of the standard error with finite population correction factor is

$$SE(\bar{x}) = \sqrt{\frac{5000-400}{5000-1}} \times \frac{10}{\sqrt{400}} = 0.48$$

and without the finite population correction factor the conservative value of the standard error is

$$SE(\bar{x}) = \frac{10}{\sqrt{400}} = 0.50$$

In practice, whether or not the finite population correction factor is used in computing, the standard error of $\bar{x}$ does not significantly affect the value of the standard error unless the sampling proportion is quite large. In fact, the finite population correction factor is rarely used when the sampling proportion is less that 0.05. In either case, the bound on the error of estimation of $\bar{x}$ is

$$B = 2 \times \text{SE}(\bar{x})$$

Furthermore, since $\bar{x}$ is an unbiased estimator of μ, the bound on the error of estimation measures the accuracy of $\bar{x}$, and for most populations it is unlikely for the observed value of $\bar{x}$ to be more than B from the true value of μ. Also, the bound on the error of estimation of $\bar{x}$ follows the Square Root Law, and therefore, halving the value of B will require quadrupling the number of observations to be sampled.

Example 5.12

Compute the standard error of $\bar{x}$ and the bound on the error of estimation for $\bar{x}$ when

   a. $N = 1000$, $n = 100$, and $\sigma = 25$.
   b. $N = 5000$, $n = 800$, and $\sigma = 15$.
   c. $N = 100,000$, $n = 1200$, and $\sigma = 75$.
   d. N is unknown, $n = 20$, and $\sigma = 20$.
   e. N is unknown, $n = 120$, and $\sigma = 60$.

Solutions Since

   a. the sampling proportion is $\dfrac{100}{1000} = 0.10 > 0.05$, the finite population correction factor will be used and

$$\text{SE}(\bar{x}) = \sqrt{\frac{1000 - 100}{1000 - 1}} \times \frac{25}{\sqrt{100}} = 2.37$$

and $B = 2 \times 2.37 = 4.74$.

   b. the sampling proportion is $\dfrac{800}{5000} = 0.16 > 0.05$, the finite population correction factor will be used and

$$\text{SE}(\bar{x}) = \sqrt{\frac{5000 - 800}{5000 - 1}} \times \frac{15}{\sqrt{800}} = 0.49$$

and $B = 2 \times 0.49 = 0.98$.

   c. the sampling proportion is $\dfrac{1200}{100,000} = 0.012 < 0.05$, the finite population correction factor will not be used and

$$\text{SE}(\bar{x}) = \frac{75}{\sqrt{1200}} = 2.17$$

and $B = 2 \times 2.17 = 4.34$.

   d. the value of N is unknown, the standard error is approximately

$$\text{SE}(\bar{x}) = \frac{20}{\sqrt{20}} = 4.47$$

and $B = 2 \times 4.47 = 8.94$.

   e. the value of N is unknown, the standard error is approximately

$$\text{SE}(\bar{x}) = \frac{60}{\sqrt{120}} = 5.48$$

and $B = 2 \times 5.48 = 10.96$.

In practice, the value of σ will be unknown, and thus, the standard error of $\bar{x}$ must be estimated. Using the plug-in rule, the estimated standard error of $\bar{x}$ is found by substituting the value of the sample standard deviation, s, in the unknown value of σ. Thus, using the plug-in rule the estimated standard error of $\bar{x}$ is

$$\text{se}(\bar{x}) = \sqrt{\frac{N-n}{N-1}} \times \frac{s}{\sqrt{n}}$$

when the sampling proportion is greater than 0.05. The finite population correction factor should always be used when the sampling proportion is at least 5%. If the number of units in the population, N, is unknown, then finite population correction factor cannot be used, and when the sampling proportion is less than 5%, the finite population correction factor is almost 1 and does not affect the value of the standard error significantly. Furthermore, when the number of units in the population is unknown or the sampling proportion is less than 5%, the estimated standard error of $\bar{x}$ can be approximated using

$$\text{se}(\bar{x}) = \frac{s}{\sqrt{n}}$$

Note that the standard error of $\bar{x}$ decreases as the sample size n increases according to the Square Root Law for both forms of the standard error. In fact, as n approaches the number of units in the population N, the standard error approaches 0, and when $n = N$ the standard error of $\bar{x}$ is 0 and $\bar{x} = \mu$. Thus, as was the case with the sample proportion $\hat{p}$, the sample mean $\bar{x}$ can be made as accurate as desired by choosing a sufficiently large sample size.

Most statistical packages include the estimated standard error of the $\bar{x}$, computed as se $= s/\sqrt{n}$, as part of their basic summary statistics for a sample. For example, the summary statistics listed in Table 5.5 were generated by MINITAB for the quantitative variables AGE and BWT (birth weight) for the $n = 189$ observations in the Birth Weight data set. The column labeled "SE Mean" contains the estimated standard errors of the sample means computed without using the finite population correction factors. For example, for the variable BWT the estimated standard error is 53.0 that was computed by MINITAB as $\text{se}(\bar{x}) = 729.0/\sqrt{189} = 53.03$.

Also, it is possible to create an interval of reasonable estimates of μ from the values of $\bar{x}$ and se$(\bar{x})$ by taking $\bar{x} \pm B$. For example, using the summary statistics for the variable BWT listed in Table 5.5, the interval of reasonable estimates of the mean birthweight is $2944.7 \pm 2 \times 53$. That is, based on this sample the reasonable estimates of the mean birthweight range from a low of 2838.7 to a high of 3050.7.

Example 5.13
Suppose a random sample of $n = 105$ observations yields a sample mean of $\bar{x} = 12.2$ and a sample standard deviation of $s = 1.72$. Determine

a. the estimated standard error of $\bar{x}$.

b. the bound on the error of estimation of $\bar{x}$.

c. the interval of reasonable estimates of μ suggested by this sample.

TABLE 5.5   The Standard Summary Statistics Generated by MINITAB for the Variables Age and BWT in the Birth Weight Data Set

Variable	Total Count	Mean	SE Mean	StDev	Q1	Median	Q3
AGE	189	23.238	0.385	5.299	19.000	23.000	26.000
BWT	189	2944.7	53.0	729.0	2412.0	2977.0	3481.0

Solutions   Because N is unknown the finite population correction factor cannot be used in computing the value of se($\bar{x}$). Now, with a sample of $n = 105$ observations, $\bar{x} = 12.2$, and $s = 1.72$

    a. the estimated standard error of $\bar{x}$ is se($\bar{x}$) $= \dfrac{1.72}{\sqrt{105}} = 0.168$.

    b. the bound on the error of estimation of $\bar{x}$ is $B = 2 \times$ se($\bar{x}$) $= 2 \times 0.168 = 0.336$.

    c. based on this sample, interval of reasonable estimates of μ is 12.2 ± 0.336. That is, based on the observed sample the reasonable estimates of the mean fall between 11.864 and 12.536.

5.3.2 Determining the Sample Size for a Prespecified Value of the Bound on the Error Estimation

Before collecting the sample data, it is always important to determine the sample size n that will be necessary to produce the prespecified level of accuracy associated with the statistical analysis. Using B as the measure of accuracy of $\bar{x}$, the sample size required for a prespecified value of B can easily be determined by solving

$$B = 2 \times \text{SE}(\bar{x})$$

for n. Thus, the components that are required for determining the value of n for a given value of B are the standard deviation of the population σ and the number of units in the population N. The sample size n for a simple random sample that will produce a bound on the error of estimation of $\bar{x}$ having the prespecified value B is

---

THE SAMPLE SIZE REQUIRED FOR ESTIMATING A MEAN

1. $n = \dfrac{N\sigma^2}{(N-1)\frac{B^2}{4} + \sigma^2}$ when N is known.   **2.** $n = \left[\dfrac{2\sigma}{B}\right]^2$ when N is unknown.

      Note that both of the computational formulas for n depend on the unknown value of σ. Thus, a reasonable guess or estimate of σ must be available in the planning stage of the study to determine the sample size that will produce the prespecified accuracy. Experienced researchers often have prior studies or knowledge that is used in developing a reasonable guess of the value of σ that will be used in determining the sample size. Also, the formulas will not generally produce an integer value of n so the resulting value of n must be rounded off to the next largest integer to ensure the value of B is attained.

Example 5.14
Determine the sample size required to attain the prespecified value of B when

    a. $N = 20,000$, $\sigma \approx 500$, and $B = 25$.
    b. $N = 5,000$, $\sigma \approx 250$, and $B = 15$.
    c. N is unknown, $\sigma \approx 50$, and $B = 5$.
    d. N is unknown, $\sigma \approx 120$, and $B = 5$.

Solutions   The sample size required to attain a value of $B = 5$ is

    a. $n = 1482$ since N is known and the formula for n yields

$$n = \frac{20,000(500)^2}{(20,000-1)\frac{25^2}{4} + 500^2} = 1481.55$$

b. $n = 910$ since N is known and the formula for n yields

$$n = \frac{5000(250)^2}{(5000-1)\frac{15^2}{4} + 250^2} = 909.2$$

c. $n = 400$ since N is unknown and the formula for n yields

$$n = \left[\frac{2(500)}{5}\right]^2 = 400$$

d. $n = 2304$ since N is unknown and the formula for n yields

$$n = \left[\frac{2(120)}{5}\right]^2 = 2304$$

5.3.3 The Central Limit Theorem for $\bar{x}$

Although the probability distribution of the sampling distribution of $\bar{x}$ is usually unknown, when the sample size is sufficiently large the *Central Limit Theorem* will apply and the sampling distribution of $\bar{x}$ will be approximately normally distributed with mean μ and standard deviation $SE(\bar{x})$. The Central Limit Theorem for the sample mean is stated below.

THE CENTRAL LIMIT THEOREM FOR $\bar{x}$

When a random sample of n observations is selected from a population with standard deviation σ, then when the sample size n is sufficiently large, the sampling distribution of $\bar{x}$ will be approximately a normal distribution with mean equal to μ and standard deviation equal to $SE(\bar{x}) = \sigma/\sqrt{n}$. Thus, for a sufficiently large sample size n,

$$Z = \frac{\bar{x} - \mu}{\sigma/\sqrt{n}}$$

is approximately distributed as a standard normal distribution.

Note that the Central Limit Theorem states that for a sufficiently large sample the distribution of the sample mean will be approximately normal regardless of the shape of the underlying distribution being sampled. The following example illustrates the Central Limit Theorem when the target population follows an exponential distribution.

Example 5.15

The sampling distribution of $\bar{x}$ is simulated by drawing 500 simple random samples from an exponential distribution with mean $\mu = 20$ for each of the sample sizes $n = 20, 30, 50$, and 250. The exponential distribution being sampled is shown in Figure 5.1.

Figure 5.1 shows the histograms of the sample means computed from 500 random samples of sample sizes $n = 20, 30, 50$, and 250 drawn from this exponential distribution. The normal distribution suggested by the Central Limit Theorem with mean $\mu = 20$ and standard deviation $\sigma = SE(\bar{x})$ is superimposed over each histogram.

Note that as n increases the histograms behave more and more like a normal distribution. Also, note that the spread of the values of $\bar{x}$ decreases as n increases. The accuracy of $\bar{x}$ increases as n increases because the standard error of $\bar{x}$ is $SE(\bar{x}) = \sigma/\sqrt{n}$ that decreases according to the Square Root Law as n increases. Thus, the spread of the values of $\bar{x}$ for $n = 250$ is $\sqrt{5} = 2.24$ times less than the spread of values for $\bar{x}$ when $n = 50$.

The larger the sample size is the more close the sampling distribution of $\bar{x}$ will be to the limiting normal distribution given in the Central Limit Theorem. For a fixed sample

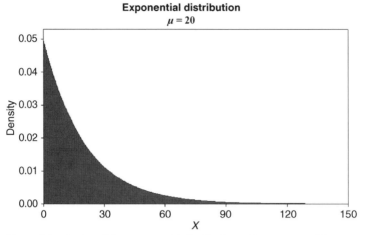

Figure 5.1 A plot of the exponential distribution with mean $\mu = 20$.

size n, the degree to which a normal distribution will approximate the sampling distribution of $\bar{x}$ will depend on the shape and the variability in the underlying distribution sampled. Underlying distributions that have extremely long tails in one direction or are extremely variable will require a larger sample size for the normal distribution to approximate the sampling distribution of $\bar{x}$. For many populations it is reasonable to use the normal distribution for approximating the sampling distribution of $\bar{x}$ when $n \geq 30$, and for almost all populations it is reasonable to use the normal distribution for approximating the sampling distribution of $\bar{x}$ when $n \geq 100$.

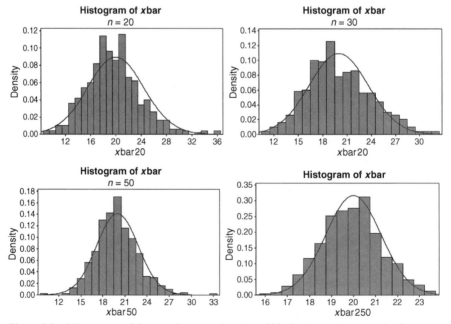

Figure 5.2 Histograms of the sample means based on 500 simple random samples from an exponential distribution with $\mu = 20$ for $n = 20, 30, 50,$ and 250.

The sampling distribution of $\bar{x}$ has mean of μ, standard deviation $\sigma/\sqrt{n}$, and the sampling distribution is roughly mound shaped for a sufficiently large sample size, and thus, the Empirical Rules apply to $\bar{x}$.

EMPIRICAL RULES FOR THE SAMPLING DISTRIBUTION OF $\bar{x}$

For sampling most populations

1. roughly 68% of the possible values of $\bar{x}$ lie within one standard error of μ. That is, roughly 68% of all possible random samples will produce a value of $\bar{x}$ between
$$\mu - \frac{\sigma}{\sqrt{n}} \text{ and } \mu + \frac{\sigma}{\sqrt{n}}.$$

2. roughly 95% of the possible values of $\bar{x}$ lie within two standard errors (i.e., B) of μ.

That is, roughly 95% of all possible random samples will produce a value of $\bar{x}$ between $\mu - 2 \times \frac{\sigma}{\sqrt{n}}$ and $\mu + 2 \times \frac{\sigma}{\sqrt{n}}$.

3. roughly 99% of the possible values of $\bar{x}$ lie within three standard errors of μ. That is, roughly 99% of all possible random samples will produce a value of $\bar{x}$ between
$$\mu - 3 \times \frac{\sigma}{\sqrt{n}} \text{ and } \mu + 3 \times \frac{\sigma}{\sqrt{n}}.$$

The Empirical Rules show that it is unlikely for an observed value of $\bar{x}$ to be more than two standard errors (i.e., B) from the true value of μ when a random sampling plan is used. On the other hand, when nonrandom sampling plans are used there is no predictable pattern for the possible values of $\bar{x}$, the Central Limit Theorem does not apply, and the bound on the error of estimation computed as $B = 2 \times \text{SE}(\bar{x})$ is meaningless.

5.3.4 The *t* Distribution

The *Central Limit Theorem* provides the approximate distribution of the sampling distribution of $\bar{x}$ when the SD is known; however, in practice the standard deviation is usually unknown. Thus, the Central Limit Theorem is a useful tool for planning statistical analyses, but it is not very useful once the data have been observed. If the sample size is greater than 100, a reasonable approach for estimating the sampling distribution of $\bar{x}$ is to use the sample standard deviation s in place of the unknown parameter σ. In this case, it is reasonable to approximate to the sampling distribution of $\bar{x}$ with a normal probability distribution having standard deviation $s/\sqrt{n}$.

For smaller values of n and an underlying distribution that is normally distributed, the distribution of

$$\frac{\bar{x} - \mu}{s/\sqrt{n}}$$

will follow a *t distribution* with $v = n - 1$ *degrees of freedom*. The *t* distribution was developed by W.S. Gosset, a mathematician at the Guinness Brewery in Dublin, Ireland. The *t* distribution is a mound-shaped symmetric distribution. The *t* distribution is similar in shape to a standard normal distribution (Z) but has heavier and longer tails than the standard normal distribution does; however, as the degrees of freedom of the *t* distribution increase, the *t* distribution becomes more like a standard normal distribution. The main difference between the Z distribution and the *t* distribution formed from $\bar{x}$ is that Z formula uses the true standard deviation σ and *t* uses the estimated standard deviation s. That is,

$$Z = \frac{\bar{x} - \mu}{\sigma/\sqrt{n}}$$

and

$$t = \frac{\bar{x} - \mu}{s/\sqrt{n}}$$

Moreover, the longer and heavier tails in the t distribution are because of the extra source of variation due to estimating σ in the t formula.

THE t DISTRIBUTION

When a random sample of n observations is drawn from a normal distribution, the sampling distribution of

$$\frac{\bar{x} - \mu}{s/\sqrt{n}}$$

is distributed as a t distribution with $\nu = n - 1$ degrees of freedom.

A t distribution with $\nu = 5$ degrees of freedom is shown along with a standard normal distribution in Figure 5.3, and Figure 5.4 illustrates the difference between t distributions with $\nu = 5$ and $\nu = 15$ degrees of freedom.

In practice, the t distribution is more frequently used in statistical applications than is the Z distribution because the standard deviation σ in most problems is unknown. However, because the t distribution approaches a standard normal distribution when the degrees of freedom become large, in practice the Z distribution can be used in place of the t distribution when $n > 100$. A table of some commonly used values of the t distribution is given in Table A.7.

Example 5.16
Suppose a sample of n observations is to be selected from a population that is normally distributed with unknown standard deviation. Consider the probability that a t distribution with $n - 1$ degrees of freedom falls between the values $-a$ and a, where $P(-a \leq t) = P(t \geq a) = 0.025$. Then, $P(-a \leq$

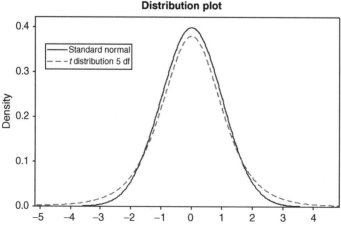

Figure 5.3 A plot showing the difference between a t distribution with $\nu = 5$ degrees of freedom and a standard normal distribution.

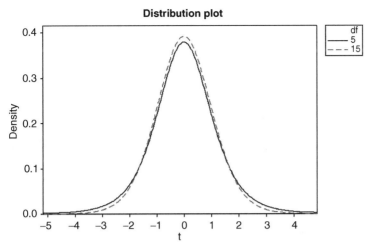

Distribution plot

Figure 5.4 t distributions with $\nu = 5$ and $\nu = 15$ degrees of freedom.

$t \leq a) = 0.95$ and substituting $\dfrac{\bar{x} - \mu}{s/\sqrt{n}}$ for t yields

$$0.95 = P\left(-a \leq \frac{\bar{x} - \mu}{s/\sqrt{n}} \leq a\right)$$

$$= P\left(-a \times \frac{s}{\sqrt{n}} \leq \bar{x} - \mu \leq a \times \frac{s}{\sqrt{n}}\right)$$

$$= P\left(-a \times \frac{s}{\sqrt{n}} - \bar{x} \leq -\mu \leq a \times \frac{s}{\sqrt{n}} - \bar{x}\right)$$

$$= P\left(\bar{x} - a \times \frac{s}{\sqrt{n}} \leq \mu \leq \bar{x} + a \times \frac{s}{\sqrt{n}}\right)$$

Thus, there is a 95% chance of drawing a sample that will produce a value of $\bar{x}$ such that the interval $\bar{x} + a \times s/\sqrt{n}$ to $\bar{x} + a \times s/\sqrt{n}$ captures the unknown value of μ. The interval $\bar{x} + a \times s/\sqrt{n}$ to $\bar{x} + a \times s/\sqrt{n}$ is called a *95% confidence interval for* μ and will be discussed in detail in Chapter 6.

It is important to note that the value of a in the confidence interval in Example 6.8 depends on the degrees of freedom of the t distribution that in turn is based on the sample size n. For example, if $n = 25$ the value of a used in a 95% confidence interval for μ is $a = 2.064$, and if $n = 11$ then $a = 2.228$. The values of a can be found in Table A.7 by locating the column for a 95% confidence level and the appropriate row listing the degrees of freedom associated with s.

The t distribution is an important sampling distribution that will be used in several of the statistical procedures that are presented in Chapters 6, 7, 8, 9, and 12. In particular, the t distribution will be used in computing confidence intervals and testing hypotheses about specific population parameters.

5.3.5 Some Final Notes on the Sampling Distribution of $\bar{x}$

In summary, $\bar{x}$ is an estimator of the population mean, and several key properties of the sample mean $\bar{x}$ are listed below.

THE KEY PROPERTIES OF $\bar{x}$

---

1. The mean of the sampling distribution of $\bar{x}$ is μ and thus, $\bar{x}$ is an unbiased estimator of the population mean μ.

2. When the number of units in the target population is known, the standard error of $\bar{x}$ is

$$\mathrm{SE}(\bar{x}) = \sqrt{\frac{N-n}{N-1}} \frac{\sigma}{\sqrt{n}}$$

3. When the number of units in the target population is unknown or the sampling proportion is less than 0.05 the standard error of $\bar{x}$ is

$$\mathrm{SE}(\bar{x}) = \frac{\sigma}{\sqrt{n}}$$

4. Because $\bar{x}$ is an unbiased estimator of μ and the standard error of $\bar{x}$ decreases as the sample size n increases, $\bar{x}$ can be made as accurate an estimator of μ as is desired by choosing a sufficiently large sample size.

5. When the number of units in the target population is known, the estimated stan-

dard error of $\bar{x}$ is

$$\mathrm{se}(\bar{x}) = \sqrt{\frac{N-n}{N}} \frac{s}{\sqrt{n}}$$

6. When the number of units in the target population is unknown or the sampling proportion is less than 0.05, the estimated standard error of $\bar{x}$ is

$$\mathrm{se}(\bar{x}) = \frac{s}{\sqrt{n}}$$

7. In many cases, when $n \geq 30$ the sampling distribution of $\bar{x}$ is approximately normal with mean μ and standard deviation $\mathrm{SE}(\bar{x})$. In most cases, when $n \geq 100$ the sampling distribution of $\bar{x}$ can be approximated by a normal with mean μ and standard deviation $\mathrm{se}(\bar{x})$.

8. When the underlying population being sampled is normally distributed, then

$$t = \frac{\bar{x} - \mu}{s/\sqrt{n}}$$

follows a t distribution with $\nu = n - 1$ degrees of freedom.

5.4 COMPARISONS BASED ON TWO SAMPLES

In many research studies, the goal is to estimate and compare the parameters of two different populations or to estimate and compare the parameters for two distinct subpopulations. For example, in a study investigating the relationship between diet and breast cancer, the proportion of women diagnosed with breast cancer whose everyday diet is classified as a high-fat diet (p_{high}) might be compared with the proportion of women diagnosed with breast cancer classified as having a low-fat diet (p_{low}). In this case, the parameters p_{high} and p_{low} could be estimated and the comparison of the proportions would be based on the difference between the two estimates, $\widehat{p}_{high} - \widehat{p}_{low}$. In many biomedical research studies, the population proportions or the population means are the parameters that will be compared in order to answer the research questions.

In studying two separate well-defined populations, a stratified random sample is typically used for collecting the sample data for which the parameters of the two populations will be estimated and compared. Since a stratified random sample consists of independently selected simple random samples from each population, a stratified random sample that provides good data and accurate estimates for both populations should be designed in the planning stages of the study.

It is also possible that when two distinct well-defined subpopulations within the target population are being studied, a simple random sample will be used and the data will be stratified according to subpopulation after they have been collected; this approach is called *poststratifying a sample.* Poststratification can be a useful technique when estimating the subpopulation parameters from a simple random sample; however, poststratification does not always provide the most accurate estimates of the subpopulation parameters. Thus, poststratification should only be used when each of the subpopulations consists of roughly the same number of units so that roughly equal amounts of data are collected on each of the subpopulations when a simple random sample is used.

5.4.1 Comparing Two Population Proportions

When two distinct populations, represented by X and Y, are being studied and the parameter of interest is the proportion of each population having a particular attribute, say p_X and p_Y, it is likely that a researcher will want to know whether there is evidence suggesting $p_X > p_Y$, $p_X < p_Y$, or $p_X = p_Y$. Once the samples have been collected from X and Y population, the sample proportions $\widehat{p}_X$ and $\widehat{p}_Y$ can be computed and used to estimate the difference between the population proportions p_X and p_Y.

Suppose that independent random samples are collected from X and Y populations, and n_X is the number of observations sampled from population X and n_Y is the number sampled from population Y. Then, the sample proportions are

$$\widehat{p}_X = \frac{\text{number of } X \text{ observations having the attribute}}{n_x}$$

$$\widehat{p}_Y = \frac{\text{number of } Y \text{ observations having the attribute}}{n_y}$$

The estimators $\widehat{p}_X$ and $\widehat{p}_Y$ are unbiased estimators of p_X and p_Y, respectively, and the standard errors of these estimators can be computed using the formulas presented in Section 5.2.

The comparison of p_X and p_Y will be based on the difference $p_X - p_Y$, and the point estimator of $p_X - p_y$ is $\widehat{p}_X - \widehat{p}_Y$ that is an unbiased estimator of $p_X - p_Y$. Because the samples are independently collected, the standard error of $\widehat{p}_X - \widehat{p}_Y$ is

$$\text{SE}(\widehat{p}_X - \widehat{p}_Y) = \sqrt{\text{SE}(\widehat{p}_X)^2 + \text{SE}(\widehat{p}_Y)^2}$$

The finite population correction factor is usually ignored in the computation of the standard error of $\widehat{p}_X - \widehat{p}_Y$, and in this case,

$$\text{SE}(\widehat{p}_X - \widehat{p}_Y) = \sqrt{\frac{p_X(1 - p_X)}{n_X} + \frac{p_Y(1 - p_Y)}{n_Y}}$$

The bound on the error of estimation of $\widehat{p}_X - \widehat{p}_Y$ is

$$B = 2 \times \text{SE}(\widehat{p}_X - \widehat{p}_Y)$$

and it is unlikely for $\widehat{p}_X - \widehat{p}_Y$ to be more than B from the unknown value of $p_X - p_Y$ when random samples from the X and Y populations are used.

The sampling distribution of $\widehat{p}_X - \widehat{p}_Y$ will be approximately normal when the four quantities

$$n_X p_X, \ n_X(1 - p_X) n_Y p_Y, \ \text{and } n_Y(1 - p_Y)$$

are all greater than equal to 5. In this case, there is roughly a 95% chance of observing a value of $\widehat{p}_X - \widehat{p}_Y$ that is within B of the unknown value of $p_X - p_Y$. Because p_X and p_Y are unknown and must be estimated, the standard error of $\widehat{p}_X - \widehat{p}_Y$ must also be estimated and is estimated according the plug-in rule. The estimated standard error of $\hat{p}_X - \hat{p}_Y$ is

$$se(\hat{p}_X - \hat{p}_Y) = \sqrt{\frac{\hat{p}_X(1 - \hat{p}_X)}{n_X} + \frac{\hat{p}_Y(1 - \hat{p}_Y)}{n_Y}}$$

and the bound on the error of estimation used in practice is $B = 2 \times se(\hat{p}_X - \hat{p}_Y)$.

Example 5.17

In the article "Smoking in 6 diverse chicago communities: a population study" published in the *American Journal of Public Health* (Dell et al., 2005), the authors analyzed the smoking habits of the residents living in several communities in Chicago, Illinois. The authors estimated the smoking prevalence at 20% in South Lawndale based on a random sample of $n = 300$ individuals and 39% in North Lawndale based on a random sample of $n = 303$ individuals. Using this information, determine

a. the estimated standard errors of the smoking prevalence proportions for both North and South Lawndale.

b. the estimated standard error of the difference between the smoking prevalence proportions for North and South Lawndale.

c. whether 0 is a reasonable estimate of the difference between the smoking prevalence proportions for North and South Lawndale.

Solutions Let $\hat{p}_N$ and $\hat{p}_S$ be the estimated prevalence proportions for North and South Lawndale.

a. Because the number of units in these two populations is unknown, the estimated standard errors of the smoking prevalence proportions for both North and South Lawndale are

$$se(\hat{p}_S) = \sqrt{\frac{0.20 \times 0.80}{300}} = 0.023$$

$$se(\hat{p}_N) = \sqrt{\frac{0.39 \times 0.61}{303}} = 0.028$$

b. The estimated standard error of the difference between the smoking prevalence proportions for North and South Lawndale is

$$se(\hat{p}_N - \hat{p}_S) = \sqrt{se_N^2 + se_S^2} = \sqrt{0.023^2 + 0.028^2} = 0.036$$

and the bound on the error of estimation is $B = 2 \times se = 0.072$.

c. Based on these samples, the reasonable estimates of the difference between the smoking prevalence proportions for North and South Lawndale fall in the interval $\hat{p}_N - \hat{p}_S \pm 2 \times se$ that yields an interval of reasonable estimates of 0.118–0.262. Thus, based on the observed sample data 0 is not a reasonable estimate of the difference between the smoking prevalence for North and South Lawndale. In fact, on the basis of this data it appears that the smoking prevalence in North Lawndale is at least 11% higher than in South Lawndale and possibly as much as 26% higher.

Determining the sample size to be used in comparative study is a critical step in the planning stages of study. The key factors in the determination of the sample sizes used in comparing two proportions are the desired accuracy of the estimates (i.e., *B*) and the costs associated with sampling. In determining the sample sizes to be used when estimating the difference between two population proportions, special consideration must be given to the desired prespecified accuracy, the cost of sampling a unit from each population, and whether there are reasonable prior guesses of p_X and p_Y available before sampling. Formulas for the individual sample sizes n_X and n_Y will be given for the following four cases:

1. The overall number of observations, $n = n_X + n_Y$, is fixed and the goal is to minimize the bound on the error of estimation for estimating $p_X - p_Y$.

2. The value of B is fixed and the goal is to minimize the overall sample size $n = n_X + n_Y$.

3. The total cost of sampling the X and Y populations is fixed and the goal is to minimize the bound on the error of estimation for estimating $p_X - p_Y$.

4. The value of B is fixed and the goal is to minimize the total cost of sampling the X and Y populations.

Also, in each case formulas for the sample sizes n_X and n_Y will be given (1) when there are reasonable prior guesses of p_X and p_Y available before sampling and (2) when there are no reasonable prior guesses of p_X and p_Y available before sampling.

CASE 1: MINIMIZING THE VALUE OF B FOR A FIXED SAMPLE SIZE

Suppose the overall number of observations $n = n_X + n_Y$ is fixed and the goal is to minimize the bound on the error of estimation for estimating $p_X - p_Y$. When reasonable prior guesses of p_X and p_Y are available, say $\hat{p}_X$ and $\hat{p}_Y$, then the minimum bound on the error of estimation occurs when

$$n_X = \frac{n}{1 + \sqrt{\frac{\hat{p}_Y(1-\hat{p}_Y)}{\hat{p}_X(1-\hat{p}_X)}}}$$

$$n_Y = n_X \times \sqrt{\frac{\hat{p}_Y(1-\hat{p}_Y)}{\hat{p}_X(1-\hat{p}_X)}}$$

When no reasonable estimates of p_X and p_Y are available prior to sampling, conservative estimates of n_X and n_Y can be found using $\hat{p}_X = \hat{p}_Y = 0.5$. In this case, $n_X = n_Y = n/2$.

Note that the formulas given above often do not yield whole number answers and must be rounded off so that n_X and n_Y are whole numbers with $n_X + n_Y = n$. In this case, the general rule of rounding can be used when determining the values of n_X and n_Y.

Example 5.18

Determine the sample sizes n_x and n_y for an overall sample size of $n = 250$ that minimizes the bound on the error of estimation for estimating $p_X - p_Y$ when

a. $\hat{p}_X = 0.4$, $\hat{p}_Y = 0.3$.

b. $\hat{p}_X = \hat{p}_Y = 0.5$.

Solutions

a. $n_X = \dfrac{250}{1 + \sqrt{\frac{0.3 \times 0.7}{0.4 \times 0.6}}} = 129.2$ and

$$n_Y = n_X \times \sqrt{\frac{0.3 \times 0.7}{0.4 \times 0.6}} = 129.2 \times 0.94 = 120.8$$

Thus, take $n_X = 129$ and $n_Y = 121$.

b. Since $\hat{p}_X = \hat{p}_Y = 0.5$, the conservative values of n_X and n_Y are

$$n_X = n_Y = \frac{250}{2} = 125$$

Note that the values of n_X and n_Y are fairly similar in Example 5.18 parts (a) and (b). In general, the values of n_X and n_Y will be relatively close to $n/2$ unless one of the values of $\dot{p}_X$ and $\dot{p}_Y$ is close to 0 or 1 and the other is not relatively close to 0 or 1. For example, if $n = 250$ and $\dot{p}_X = 0.1$ and $\dot{p}_Y = 0.6$, then the rounded values of n_X and n_Y are $n_X = 155$ and $n_Y = 95$. Furthermore, when $\dot{p}_X \approx \dot{p}_Y$ the values of n_X and n_Y will be approximately equal to $n/2$, regardless of the values of $\dot{p}_X$ and $\dot{p}_Y$.

CASE 2: MINIMIZING THE SAMPLE SIZE FOR A FIXED VALUE OF B

Suppose the value of B, the bound on the error of estimation for estimating $p_X - p_Y$, is fixed and the goal is to minimize the overall sample size $n = n_X + n_Y$. When reasonable prior guesses of p_X and p_Y are available, say $\dot{p}_X$ and $\dot{p}_Y$, then the minimum sample size and allocation of the overall sample size is

$$n_Y = n_x \times \sqrt{\frac{\dot{p}_Y(1 - \dot{p}_Y)}{\dot{p}_X(1 - \dot{p}_X)}}$$

When no reasonable estimates of p_X and p_Y are available prior to sampling, conservative estimates of n_X and n_Y can be found using $\dot{p}_X = \dot{p}_Y = 0.5$. Then, $n_X = n/2$ and $n_Y = n/2$.

$$n = \frac{4\left[\dot{p}_X(1 - \dot{p}_X) + \sqrt{\dot{p}_X(1 - \dot{p}_X)\dot{p}_Y(1 - \dot{p}_Y)}\right]\left[1 + \sqrt{\frac{\dot{p}_Y(1-\dot{p}_Y)}{\dot{p}_X(1-\dot{p}_X)}}\right]}{B^2}$$

$$n_X = \frac{4\left[\dot{p}_X(1 - \dot{p}_X) + \sqrt{\dot{p}_X(1 - \dot{p}_X)\dot{p}_Y(1 - \dot{p}_Y)}\right]}{B^2}$$

Example 5.19

For a prespecified value of $B = 0.05$, determine the values of n_X and n_Y that minimize the overall sample size n when

a. $\dot{p}_X = 0.2$, $\dot{p}_Y = 0.6$.

b. $\dot{p}_X = \dot{p}_Y = 0.5$.

Solutions

a. $$n_X = \frac{4\left[0.2 \times 0.8 + \sqrt{0.2 \times 0.8 \times 0.6 \times 0.4}\right]}{0.05^2} = 569.5 \text{ and}$$

$$n_Y = n_X \times \sqrt{\frac{0.6 \times 0.4}{0.2 \times 0.8}} = 697.5$$

Thus, take $n_X = 570$, $n_Y = 698$, and $n = 1268$.

b. Since $\dot{p}_X = \dot{p}_Y = 0.5$, the conservative values of n_X, n_Y, and n are

$$n_X = n_Y = \frac{2}{0.05^2} = 800$$

and $n = 1600$. Also, because these are conservative estimates the bound on the error of estimation should be less than 0.05.

CASE 3: MINIMIZING THE VALUE OF B FOR A FIXED COST

Suppose the total cost of sampling the X and Y populations is fixed and the goal is to minimize the bound on the error of estimation for estimating $p_X - p_Y$. Suppose the total cost of sampling is $C = n_x C_x + n_y C_Y$, where the cost of sampling from population X is C_X and the cost of sampling from population Y is C_Y. When reasonable prior guesses of p_X and p_Y are available, say $\hat{p}_X$ and $\hat{p}_Y$, the minimum bound on the error of estimation occurs when

$$n = \frac{C\left[1 + \sqrt{\frac{\hat{p}_Y(1-\hat{p}_Y)C_X}{\hat{p}_X(1-\hat{p}_X))C_Y}}\right]}{\left[C_X + C_Y\sqrt{\frac{\hat{p}_Y(1-\hat{p}_Y)C_X}{\hat{p}_X(1-\hat{p}_X))C_Y}}\right]}$$

$$n_X = \frac{C}{C_X + C_Y\sqrt{\frac{\hat{p}_Y(1-\hat{p}_Y)C_X}{\hat{p}_X(1-\hat{p}_X))C_Y}}}$$

$$n_Y = n_X \times \sqrt{\frac{\hat{p}_Y(1 - \hat{p}_Y)C_X}{\hat{p}_X(1 - \hat{p}_X)C_Y}}$$

When no reasonable estimates of p_X and p_Y are available prior to sampling, conservative estimates of n_X and n_Y can be found using $\hat{p}_X = \hat{p}_Y = 0.5$. In this case,

$$n = \frac{C\left[1 + \sqrt{\frac{C_X}{C_Y}}\right]}{C_X + C_Y\sqrt{\frac{C_X}{C_Y}}}$$

$$n_X = \frac{C}{C_X + C_Y\sqrt{\frac{C_X}{C_Y}}}$$

$$n_Y = n_X \times \sqrt{\frac{C_X}{C_Y}}$$

Example 5.20

For a fixed cost of sampling $C = \$1000$ and individual costs of sampling the X and Y populations of $C_X = \$5$ and $C_Y = \$10$, respectively, determine the values of n, n_X, and n_Y that minimize the bound on the error of estimation when

a. $\hat{p}_X = 0.2$, $\hat{p}_Y = 0.3$.

b. $\hat{p}_X = \hat{p}_Y = 0.5$.

Solutions

a. The overall sample size is

$$n = \frac{1000\left[1 + \sqrt{\frac{0.3 \times 0.7 \times 5}{0.2 \times 0.8 \times 10}}\right]}{\left[5 + 10\sqrt{\frac{0.3 \times 0.7 \times 5}{0.2 \times 0.8 \times 10}}\right]} = 138.2$$

and because the cost is fixed, use $n = 138$. The values of n_X and n_Y are

$$n_X = \frac{1000}{5 + 10\sqrt{\frac{0.3 \times 0.7 \times 5}{0.2 \times 0.8 \times 10}}} = 76.3$$

$$n_Y = n_X \times \sqrt{\frac{0.3 \times 0.7 \times 5}{0.2 \times 0.8 \times 10}} = 61.8$$

Thus, take $n_X = 76$ and $n_Y = 62$ to minimize the bound on the error of estimation for a total cost of $C = 1000$.

b. Since $\hat{p}_X = \hat{p}_Y = 0.5$, the conservative value of n is

$$n = \frac{1000\left[1 + \sqrt{\frac{5}{10}}\right]}{\left[5 + 10\sqrt{\frac{5}{10}}\right]} = 141.4$$

and because the cost is fixed, use $n = 141$. The conservative values of n_X and n_Y are

$$n_X = \frac{1000}{5 + 10\sqrt{\frac{5}{10}}} = 82.8$$

$$n_Y = n_X \times \sqrt{\frac{5}{10}} = 58.5$$

Thus, take $n_X = 82$ and $n_Y = 59$ to minimize the bound on the error of estimation for a total cost of $C = 82 \times \$5 + 59 \times \$10 = 1000$.

CASE 4: MINIMIZING THE COST FOR A FIXED VALUE OF B

Suppose the value of B is fixed and the goal is to minimize the total cost of sampling the X and Y populations. Suppose the total cost of sampling is $C = n_X C_X + n_Y C_Y$, where the cost of sampling from population X is C_X and the cost of sampling from population Y is C_Y. When reasonable prior guesses of p_X and p_Y are available, say $\hat{p}_X$ and $\hat{p}_Y$, the minimum cost occurs when

When no reasonable estimates of p_X and p_Y are available prior to sampling, conservative estimates of n_X and n_Y can be found using $\hat{p}_X = \hat{p}_Y = 0.5$. In this case,

$$n_X = \frac{1 + \sqrt{\frac{C_X}{C_Y}}}{B^2}$$

$$n_Y = n_X \times \sqrt{\frac{C_X}{C_Y}}$$

$$n_X = \frac{4\left[\hat{p}_X(1 - \hat{p}_X) + \sqrt{\hat{p}_Y(1 - \hat{p}_Y)\hat{p}_X(1 - \hat{p}_X)} \times \sqrt{\frac{C_X}{C_Y}}\right]}{B^2}$$

$$n_Y = n_X \times \sqrt{\frac{\hat{p}_Y(1 - \hat{p}_Y)C_X}{\hat{p}_X(1 - \hat{p}_X)C_Y}}$$

Example 5.21

For a prespecified value of $B = 0.04$, determine the values of n_x and n_y that minimize the overall cost C for sampling costs of $C_X = 15$ and $C_Y = 6$ when

a. $\hat{p}_X = 0.4$, $\hat{p}_Y = 0.75$.

b. $\hat{p}_X = \hat{p}_Y = 0.5$.

Solutions

a. The sample sizes that minimize the overall cost are

$$n_X = \frac{4\left[0.4 \times 0.6 + \sqrt{0.75 \times 0.25 \times 0.4 \times 0.6} \times \sqrt{\frac{15}{6}}\right]}{0.04^2} = 1438.5$$

$$n_Y = n_X \times \sqrt{\frac{0.75 \times 0.25 \times 15}{0.4 \times 0.6 \times 6}} = 2010.4$$

Thus, take $n_X = 1439$ and $n_Y = 2011$ and then bound on the error of estimation will be $B = 0.04$ and the total cost of sampling will be

$$C = 1439 \times \$15 + 2011 \times \$6 = \$33,651$$

b. Since $\hat{p}_X = \hat{p}_Y = 0.5$, the conservative values of n_X and n_Y are

$$n_X = \frac{1 + \sqrt{\frac{15}{6}}}{0.04^2} = 1613.2$$

$$n_Y = n_X \times \sqrt{\frac{15}{6}} = 2550.7$$

Thus, use the conservative values $n_X = 1613$ and $n_Y = 2551$ and then bound on the error of estimation no larger than $B = 0.04$. The total cost of sampling will be $C = 1613 \times \$15 + 2551 \times \$6 = \$39{,}501$.

Note that in practice, prior estimates of the population proportions are often not available. In this case, the conservative sample sizes should be used. One drawback of using the conservative sample sizes is that the cost of sampling will be higher than it would be when good prior guesses of the proportions are available. Note that in some cases reasonable prior values for p_X and p_Y can be obtained from a literature search, prior research experiences, or prior studies that are normally considered in the planning stages of a research study.

5.4.2 Comparing Two Population Means

In comparative studies where the response variable is a quantitative variable, the questions of interest often involve comparing the means of population X and population Y. The comparison of means is usually made by looking at the difference between the two means, $\mu_X - \mu_Y$. Then, inferences as to whether $\mu_X > \mu_Y$, $\mu_X < \mu_Y$, or $\mu_X = \mu_Y$ are based on whether the sample data suggest $\mu_X - \mu_Y$ is greater than 0, less than 0, or roughly equal to 0. The point estimate of $\mu_X - \mu_Y$ is $\bar{x} - \bar{y}$, where $\bar{x}$ and $\bar{y}$ are the sample means for the samples selected from the X and Y populations.

When independent random samples from the X and Y populations are collected, the summary statistics that will be used in comparing the means of these two populations are the sample means and the sample standard deviations. Let $\bar{x}$ and s_X be the sample mean and sample standard deviation computed from the sample drawn from the X population, and let $\bar{y}$ and s_Y be the sample mean and sample standard deviation computed from the sample drawn from the Y population. The summary statistics that will be used in estimating $\mu_X - \mu_Y$ are summarized in Table 5.6.

The point estimate of $\mu_X - \mu_Y$ is $\bar{x} - \bar{y}$ and because $\bar{x}$ and $\bar{y}$ are unbiased estimators of μ_X and μ_Y, it follows that $\bar{x} - \bar{y}$ is an unbiased estimator of $\mu_X - \mu_Y$. Furthermore, because $\bar{x} - \bar{y}$ is an unbiased estimator, the accuracy of $\bar{x} - \bar{y}$ is measured by the standard error of the sampling distribution of $\bar{x} - \bar{y}$. The standard error of $\bar{x} - \bar{y}$ is given by

$$\text{SE}(\bar{x} - \bar{y}) = \sqrt{\text{SE}(\bar{x})^2 + \text{SE}(\bar{y})^2}$$

TABLE 5.6   The Summary Statistics Used in Estimating $\mu_X - \mu_Y$

Population	Sample Size	Sample Mean	Sample Standard Deviation
X	n_X	$\bar{x}$	s_X
Y	n_Y	$\bar{y}$	s_y

As was the case with the standard error of $\widehat{p}_X - \widehat{p}_Y$, the finite population correction factor is usually ignored and the conservative standard error is used. In this case,

$$\text{SE}(\bar{x} - \bar{y}) = \sqrt{\frac{\sigma_X^2}{n_X} + \frac{\sigma_Y^2}{n_Y}}$$

where σ_X and σ_Y are the standard deviation of the X and Y populations, respectively. The bound on the error of estimation of $\bar{x} - \bar{y}$ is

$$B = 2 \times \text{SE}(\bar{x} - \bar{y})$$

and it is unlikely for $\bar{x} - \bar{y}$ to be more than B from the unknown value of $\mu_X - \mu_Y$.

Note that the standard error of $\bar{x} - \bar{y}$ depends on the values of σ_X and σ_Y that are usually unknown to the researcher. Thus, in practice the estimated standard error is used that is computed using the plug-in rule with s_X and s_Y in place of σ_X and σ_Y. Thus, the estimated standard error of $\bar{x} - \bar{y}$ is

$$\text{se}(\bar{x} - \bar{y}) = \sqrt{\frac{s_X^2}{n_X} + \frac{s_Y^2}{n_Y}}$$

and the observed bound on the error of estimation is $B = 2 \times \text{se}(\bar{x} - \bar{y})$.

Example 5.22
In the article " Relationship of axial length and retinal vascular caliber in children" published in the *American Journal of Ophthalmology* (Cheung et al., 2007), the authors reported the results of a study on the axial length and retinal vascular caliber of children. The summary statistics listed in Table 5.7 were reported on the systolic blood pressure and the weights of children with and without myopia (nearsightedness) in this article. Use the summary statistics given in Table 5.7 to determine

    a. the estimated standard error of the difference between the mean systolic blood pressures for children with and without myopia.

    b. the estimated standard error of the difference between the mean weights for children with and without myopia.

Solutions The estimated standard error of the difference between the

    a. mean systolic blood pressures for children with and without myopia is

$$\text{se} = \sqrt{\frac{15.4^2}{620} + \frac{13.0^2}{147}} = 1.24$$

    b. mean weights for children with and without myopia is

$$\text{se} = \sqrt{\frac{8.21^2}{620} + \frac{10.42^2}{147}} = 0.92$$

Note that the difference in the sample mean weights for individuals with and without myopia is $30.86 - 34.62 = -3.76$, which is more than $B = 2 \times 0.92 = 1.84$ from 0. In fact, based on the summary statistics in Table 5.7 the reasonable estimates of the difference in the mean weights are

TABLE 5.7   Summary Statistics for Systolic Blood Pressure and Weight of Children With and Without Myopia

Variable	Myopia ($n = 620$)		No Myopia ($n = 147$)	
	Mean	Stand. Deviation	Mean	Stand. Deviation
Systolic blood pressure	110.1	15.4	110.0	13.0
Weight (kg)	30.86	8.21	34.62	10.42

-3.76 ± 1.84 that yields the interval of reasonable estimates -5.86 to -1.92. Thus, it appears from this sample data that children with myopia have a mean weight of at least 1.92 kg less than children without myopia and possibly as much as 5.86 lb less.

In determining the sample sizes to be used when estimating the difference between two population means, there are several facets of the sampling plan to consider. In particular, special consideration must be given to the prespecified level of reliability, the cost of sampling a unit from each population, and obtaining reasonable prior guesses of σ_X and σ_y before sampling. Formulas for the individual sample sizes n_X and n_Y will be given for four cases. In particular, the sample sizes can be determined when

1. the overall number of observations, $n = n_X + n_Y$, is fixed and the goal is to minimize the bound on the error of estimation for estimating $\mu_X - \mu_Y$.

2. the value of B is fixed and the goal is to minimize the overall sample size n.

3. the total cost of sampling the X and Y populations is fixed and the goal is to minimize the bound on the error of estimation for estimating $\mu_X - \mu_Y$.

4. the value of B is fixed and the goal is to minimize the total cost of sampling the X and Y populations.

Note that in each case it will be necessary to have reasonable prior guesses of the values of σ_X and σ_y before sampling. Reasonable guesses of the standard deviations of the populations are usually based on a prior research, a pilot study, or a solid understanding of the populations being compared.

CASE 1: MINIMIZING B WHEN n IS FIXED

Suppose the overall number of observations $n = n_X + n_Y$ is fixed and the goal is to minimize the bound on the error of estimation of $\bar{x} - \bar{y}$. When the reasonable prior guesses of σ_X and σ_Y are $\dot{\sigma}_X$ and $\dot{\sigma}_Y$, the minimum bound on the error of estimation occurs when

$$n_X = n \times \frac{\dot{\sigma}_X}{\dot{\sigma}_Y + \dot{\sigma}_X}$$

$$n_Y = n_x \times \frac{\dot{\sigma}_Y}{\dot{\sigma}_X}$$

Example 5.23
Determine the values of n_X and n_Y that minimize the bound on the error of estimation for estimating $\mu_X - \mu_Y$ when

a. $n = 250, \dot{\sigma}_X = 12$, and $\dot{\sigma}_Y = 20$.

b. $n = 500, \dot{\sigma}_X = 50$, and $\dot{\sigma}_Y = 50$.

Solutions The values of n_X and n_Y that minimize the bound on the error of estimation for estimating $\mu_X - \mu_Y$ when

a. $n = 250, \dot{\sigma}_X = 12$, and $\dot{\sigma}_Y = 20$ are

$$n_X = 250 \times \frac{12}{20 + 12} = 93.75$$

$$n_Y = 93.75 \times \frac{20}{12} = 156.25$$

Thus, the sample sizes are $n_X = 94$ and $n_Y = 156$.

b. $n = 500, \acute{\sigma}_X = 50$, and $\acute{\sigma}_Y = 80$.

$$n_X = 500 \times \frac{50}{50 + 80} = 192.31$$

$$n_Y = 192.31 \times \frac{50}{80} = 307.69$$

Thus, the sample sizes are $n_X = 192$ and $n_Y = 308$.

Note that in Case 1 the values of n_X and n_Y will be equal when the prior guesses of σ_X and σ_Y are equal. Thus, when the overall sample size n is fixed and the prior guesses of σ_X and σ_Y are equal, the bound on the error of estimation will be minimized by taking samples of size $n_X = n_Y = n/2$ from the X and Y populations.

CASE 2: MINIMIZING n WHEN B IS FIXED

Suppose the value of B is fixed and the goal is to minimize the overall sample size $n = n_X + n_Y$. When $\acute{\sigma}_X$ and $\acute{\sigma}_Y$ are the prior guesses of σ_X and σ_Y the minimum sample size and the allocation of the sample size is

$$n = \frac{4\left[\acute{\sigma}_X^2 + \acute{\sigma}_X\acute{\sigma}_Y\right]\left[\acute{\sigma}_X + \acute{\sigma}_Y\right]}{B^2 \times \acute{\sigma}_X}$$

$$n_X = \frac{4\left[\acute{\sigma}_X^2 + \acute{\sigma}_X\acute{\sigma}_Y\right]}{B^2}$$

$$n_Y = n_x \times \frac{\acute{\sigma}_Y}{\acute{\sigma}_X}$$

Example 5.24

Determine the values of n, n_X, and n_Y that minimize the overall sample size n when

a. $B = 2.5, \acute{\sigma}_X = 10$, and $\acute{\sigma}_Y = 25$.

b. $B = 5, \acute{\sigma}_X = 50$, and $\acute{\sigma}_Y = 60$.

c. $B = 2.5$ and $\acute{\sigma}_X = \acute{\sigma}_Y = 25$.

Solutions The values of n, n_X, and n_Y that minimize the overall sample size n when

a. $B = 2.5, \acute{\sigma}_X = 10$, and $\acute{\sigma}_Y = 25$ are

$$n = \frac{4\left[10^2 + 10 \times 25\right][10 + 25]}{2.5^2 \times 10} = 784$$

$$n_X = \frac{4\left[10^2 + 10 \times 25\right]}{2.5^2} = 224$$

$$n_Y = 166.4 \times \frac{25}{10} = 560$$

Thus, use $n = 784, n_X = 224$, and $n_Y = 560$ to minimize the bound on the error of estimation for estimating $\mu_X - \mu_Y$.

b. $B = 5, \acute{\sigma}_X = 50$, and $\acute{\sigma}_Y = 60$.

$$n = \frac{4\left[50^2 + 50 \times 60\right][50 + 60]}{5^2 \times 50} = 1936$$

$$n_X = \frac{4\left[50^2 + 50 \times 60\right]}{5^2} = 880$$

$$n_Y = 880 \times \frac{60}{50} = 1056$$

Thus, use $n = 1936$, $n_X = 880$, and $n_Y = 1056$ to minimize the bound on the error of estimation for estimating $\mu_X - \mu_Y$.

c. $B = 2.5$ and $\dot{\sigma}_X = \dot{\sigma}_Y = 25$.

$$n = \frac{4\left[25^2 + 25 \times 25\right][25 + 25]}{2.5^2 \times 25} = 1600$$

$$n_X = \frac{4\left[25^2 + 25 \times 25\right]}{2.5^2} = 800$$

$$n_Y = 800 \times \frac{25}{25} = 800$$

Thus, use $n = 1600$, $n_X = 800$, and $n_Y = 800$ to minimize the bound on the error of estimation for estimating $\mu_X - \mu_Y$.

Note that in part (c) of Example 5.24 $\dot{\sigma}_X = \dot{\sigma}_Y$, and therefore, $n_X = n_Y$. Thus, when $\dot{\sigma}_X = \dot{\sigma}_Y$, in Case 2 it also turns out that the values of n_X and n_Y will be equal with $n_X = n_Y = n/2$.

CASE 3: MINIMIZING B WHEN THE COST IS FIXED

Suppose the total cost of sampling the X and Y populations is fixed and the goal is to minimize the bound on the error of estimation for estimating $\mu_X - \mu_Y$. When the total cost of sampling is C, the cost of sampling from population X is C_X, the cost of sampling from population Y is C_Y, and the prior guesses of σ_X and σ_Y are $\dot{\sigma}_X$ and $\dot{\sigma}_Y$, the minimum bound on the error of estimation when

$$n = \frac{C\left[\dot{\sigma}_X\sqrt{C_Y} + \dot{\sigma}_Y\sqrt{C_X}\right]}{C_X\dot{\sigma}_X\sqrt{C_Y} + C_Y\dot{\sigma}_Y\sqrt{C_X}}$$

$$n_X = \frac{C \times \dot{\sigma}_X \times \sqrt{C_Y}}{C_X\dot{\sigma}_X\sqrt{C_Y} + C_Y\dot{\sigma}_Y\sqrt{C_X}}$$

$$n_Y = n_x \times \frac{\dot{\sigma}_Y}{\dot{\sigma}_X} \times \sqrt{\frac{C_X}{C_Y}}$$

Example 5.25
Determine the values of n, n_X, and n_Y that minimize the bound on the error of estimation when

a. $\dot{\sigma}_X = 10$, $\dot{\sigma}_Y = 25$, $C = \$5000$, $C_X = 10$, and $C_Y = 5$.
b. $\dot{\sigma}_X = 10$, $\dot{\sigma}_Y = 5$, $C = \$15,000$, $C_X = 25$, and $C_Y = 25$.
c. $\dot{\sigma}_X = 50$, $\dot{\sigma}_Y = 80$, $C = \$5000$, $C_X = 8$, and $C_Y = 6$.

Solutions The values of n, n_X, and n_Y that minimize the bound on the error of estimation when

a. $\dot{\sigma}_X = 10$, $\dot{\sigma}_Y = 25$, $C = \$5000$, $C_X = 10$, and $C_Y = 5$ are

$$n = \frac{5000\left[10\sqrt{5} + 25\sqrt{10}\right]}{10(10)\sqrt{5} + 25(5)\sqrt{10}} = 819.3$$

$$n_X = \frac{5000(10)\sqrt{5}}{10(10)\sqrt{5} + 25(5)\sqrt{10}} = 180.7$$

$$n_Y = 180.7 \times \frac{25}{10} \times \sqrt{\frac{10}{5}} = 638.9$$

Thus, use $n = 819$, $n_X = 180$, and $n_Y = 638$ to minimize the bound on the error of estimation for estimating $\mu_X - \mu_Y$. Note that in this case the rounding off n_X would cause the total cost to exceed \$5000 and thus, n_X was truncated rather than rounded off.

b. $\acute{\sigma}_X = 10$, $\acute{\sigma}_Y = 5$, $C = \$15{,}000$, $C_X = 25$, and $C_Y = 25$ are

$$n = \frac{15{,}000 \left[10\sqrt{25} + 5\sqrt{25} \right]}{25(10)\sqrt{25} + 25(5)\sqrt{25}} = 600$$

$$n_X = \frac{15{,}000(10)\sqrt{25}}{25(10)\sqrt{25} + 25(5)\sqrt{25}} = 400$$

$$n_Y = 400 \times \frac{5}{10} \times \sqrt{\frac{25}{25}} = 200$$

Thus, use $n = 600$, $n_X = 400$, and $n_Y = 200$ to minimize the bound on the error of estimation for estimating $\mu_X - \mu_Y$ for a total cost of $C = \$15{,}000$.

c. $\acute{\sigma}_X = 50$, $\acute{\sigma}_Y = 80$, $C = \$5000$, $C_X = 8$, and $C_Y = 6$ are

$$n = \frac{5000 \left[50\sqrt{6} + 80\sqrt{8} \right]}{8(50)\sqrt{6} + 6(80)\sqrt{8}} = 746$$

$$n_X = \frac{5000(50)\sqrt{6}}{25(10)\sqrt{25} + 25(5)\sqrt{25}} = 261.9$$

$$n_Y = 261.9 \times \frac{80}{50} \times \sqrt{\frac{8}{6}} = 484.0$$

Thus, use $n = 746$, $n_X = 262$, and $n_Y = 484$ to minimize the bound on the error of estimation for estimating $\mu_X - \mu_Y$ for a total cost of $C = \$5000$.

In case 3, the only time the individual sample sizes will be same (i.e., $n_X = n_Y$) is when $\acute{\sigma}_X = \acute{\sigma}_Y$ and $C_X = C_Y$.

CASE 4: MINIMIZING THE COST WHEN B IS FIXED

Suppose the value of B is fixed and the goal is to minimize the total cost of sampling the X and Y populations. When the total cost of sampling is C, the cost of sampling from population X is C_X, the cost of sampling from population Y is C_Y, and the prior guesses of σ_X and σ_Y are $\acute{\sigma}_X$ and $\acute{\sigma}_Y$, the minimum cost occurs when

$$n_X = \frac{4 \left[\acute{\sigma}_X \sqrt{C_X} + \acute{\sigma}_Y \acute{\sigma}_X \sqrt{C_Y} \right]}{B^2 \times \sqrt{C_X}}$$

$$n_Y = n_x \times \frac{\acute{\sigma}_Y}{\acute{\sigma}_X} \times \sqrt{\frac{C_X}{C_Y}}$$

Example 5.26

Determine the values of n_X and n_Y that minimize the total cost of sampling when

a. $B = 2.5$, $\acute{\sigma}_X = 20$, $\acute{\sigma}_Y = 40$, $C_X = 5$, and $C_Y = 10$.

b. $B = 0.5$, $\acute{\sigma}_X = 10$, $\acute{\sigma}_Y = 5$, $C_X = 2$, and $C_Y = 5$.

Solutions The values of n_X and n_Y that minimize the total cost of sampling when

a. $B = 2.5$, $\dot\sigma_X = 20$, $\dot\sigma_Y = 40$, $C_X = 5$, and $C_Y = 10$ are

$$n_X = \frac{4\left[20\sqrt{5} + 40(20)\sqrt{10}\right]}{2.5^2 \times \sqrt{5}} = 736.9$$

$$n_Y = 85.2 \times \frac{40}{20} \times \sqrt{\frac{5}{10}} = 1042.1$$

Thus, take $n_X = 737$ and $n_Y = 1043$ to minimize the total cost of sampling when $B = 2.5$. In this case, the total cost of sampling is

$$C = 737 \times \$5 + 1043 \times \$10 = \$15{,}115$$

b. $B = 0.5$, $\dot\sigma_X = 10$, $\dot\sigma_Y = 5$, $C_X = 2$, and $C_Y = 5$ are

$$n_X = \frac{4\left[10\sqrt{2} + 5(10)\sqrt{5}\right]}{0.5^2 \times \sqrt{2}} = 1424.9$$

$$n_Y = 1053.0 \times \frac{5}{10} \times \sqrt{\frac{2}{5}} = 450.6$$

Thus, take $n_X = 1425$ and $n_Y = 451$ to minimize the total cost of sampling when $B = 0.5$. In this case, the total cost of sampling is

$$C = 1425 \times \$2 + 451 \times \$5 = \$5105$$

Because the sample sizes n_X and n_Y will influence the accuracy of the comparison of two means, it is critical to design the sampling plan so that a reasonable level of accuracy is attained. The worst case scenario occurs when there is a significant difference between the two means, but the sample sizes are not large enough to provide the accuracy necessary to detect the difference between the means. In most research studies, the correct approach to use for determining the sample sizes is to predetermine a reasonable value of B, and then determine the sample sizes that minimize the cost (i.e., Case 4); when the resulting sample sizes cause a significant cost overrun, the only two choices are (1) find more money for sampling or (2) do not carry out the study. Carrying out the study with a budget that does not provide the predetermined accuracy for comparing μ_X and μ_Y is generally a waste of resources and should be avoided.

5.5 BOOTSTRAPPING THE SAMPLING DISTRIBUTION OF A STATISTIC

For many statistics, the sampling distribution is quite difficult to determine because the sampling distributions differ dramatically from one underlying distribution to another. Also, because the standard error measures the reliability of an unbiased estimator, it is important to be able to estimate the standard error of every unbiased estimator. Unfortunately, there are estimators that do not have simple formulas that can be used for estimating their standard errors. For example, the sample median, sample standard deviation, sample interquartile range, sample percentiles, and the coefficient of variation are commonly used estimators that do not have convenient formulas for computing their standard errors. Efron and Tibshirani (1993) introduced a computer-based method for estimating the standard error of an estimator that is called *bootstrapping*.

The idea behind bootstrapping is to use the observed data to simulate the sampling distribution of the estimator for which the standard error is desired. The simulated sampling distribution is found by resampling the observed data a large number of times with replacement using a computer to create a large number, say M, of bootstrap samples. Then for each of the bootstrap samples, the estimate is computed and the simulated sampling distribution of the estimator is determined from the M values of the estimate. The *bootstrap standard error* is found by computing the standard deviation of the simulated sampling distribution. In most problems, a value of $M \geq 200$ will be suitable for determining the value of the bootstrap standard error. The algorithm for computing the bootstrap standard error of a statistic T is outlined below.

THE BOOSTRAP ALGORITHM FOR se (T)

To find the bootstrap standard error of the estimator T from a random sample of n observations,

1. select a random sample of n observations from the observed sample by sampling with replacement.

2. compute the value of T for this bootstrap sample.

3. repeat steps 1 and 2 until M values of T have been computed.

4. compute the standard deviation of the M simulated values of the estimator T using

$$s_T = \sqrt{\frac{1}{M-1}\sum(T - \bar{T})^2}$$

where $\bar{T}$ is the mean of the M simulated values of the estimator T.

5. the bootstrap standard error of T is $\text{se}(T) = s_T$.

Efron and Tibshirani (1993) suggest that rarely are needed more than $M = 200$ simulated samples for determining the value of the bootstrap standard error; however, with the speed of modern computers, it is better to base the estimated standard error on $M = 500$ or $M = 1000$ bootstrap samples. Also, note that the resampling of the observed data is done with replacement. That is, in selecting each bootstrap sample once a sample observation is selected, the observation is returned to the data set and is available for selection again when the next observation in the bootstrap sample is selected.

Example 5.27
The sample median and sample 95th percentile for the variables body density (Density) and percent body fat (PCTBF) for the $n = 252$ observations in the Body Fat data set are summarized in Table 5.8. Using the observed sample values of the variables Density and PCTBF and $M = 500$ bootstrap samples, the bootstrap standard errors of the estimates of the sample medians and sample 95th percentiles were computed and are summarized in Table 5.9.

The bound on the error of estimation B of an unbiased estimator can be computed from the bootstrap standard error using $B = 2 \times \text{se}$, where se is the bootstrap estimate of the standard error. Furthermore, it is still unlikely that an unbiased estimator will be more than B from the value of the unknown value of the parameter being estimated even when the bootstrap standard error is used in computing the value of B.

TABLE 5.8   Estimates of the Median and 95th Percentile for the Variables Body Density and Percent Body Fat Based on the Body Fat Dataset

Variable	Sample Median	95th Percentile
Body density	1.0549	1.0853
Percent body fat	19.2	32.6

TABLE 5.9 Estimates of the Median and 95th Percentile and Their Bootstrap Standard Errors for the Variables Body Density and Percent Body Fat Based on the Body Fat Dataset

Variable	Sample Median	se	95th Percentile	se
Body density	1.0549	0.00186	1.0853	0.0021
Percent body fat	19.2	0.776	32.6	0.704

Suppose that a parameter, say θ, is to be compared for two different populations, say population X and population Y, and T is an estimator of θ that does not have a convenient form for its standard error. When independent samples are collected from the X and Y populations and $T_X - T_Y$ is used to estimate the difference between the values of the parameter θ (i.e., $\theta_X - \theta_Y$), bootstrapping can again be used for estimating the standard error of $T_X - T_Y$ as outlined below.

BOOSTRAPPING se $(T_X - T_Y)$

To find the bootstrap standard error of the estimator $T_X - T_Y$ from independent samples consisting of n_X and n_Y observations,

1. draw a random sample of n_X observations from the observed sample from population X by sampling with replacement.

2. draw a random sample of n_Y observations from the observed sample from population Y by sampling with replacement.

3. compute the values of T_X and T_Y for these simulated samples.

4. compute the value of $T_X - T_Y$.

5. repeat steps 1 and 2 until M values of $T_X - T_Y$ have been computed.

6. compute the standard deviation of the M simulated values of the estimator $T_X - T_Y$ using

$$s_{T_X - T_Y} = \sqrt{\frac{1}{M-1} \sum \left[(T_X - T_Y) - (\bar{T}_X - \bar{T}_Y) \right]^2}$$

where $\bar{T}_X$ and $\bar{T}_Y$ are the means of the M simulated values of the estimators T_X and T_Y.

7. the bootstrap standard error of $T_X - T_Y$ is

$$se(T_X - T_Y) = s_{T_X - T_Y}.$$

Example 5.28

The Birth Weight data set will be used to compare the median birth weights of babies born to mothers who smoked during pregnancy and babies born to mothers who did not smoke during pregnancy. The median estimates of the birth weights (BWT) are given in Table 5.10.

Thus, the estimated difference between the median birth weights of babies born to mothers who smoked during pregnancy versus mothers who did not smoke is -324.5. Using the observed sample data for mothers who smoked during pregnancy and mothers who did not smoke during pregnancy and $M = 500$ bootstrap samples, the bootstrap standard error of the estimated difference of sample medians is se $= 167.6$. Therefore, the bound on the error of estimation is $B = 2 \times 167.6 = 335.2$.

TABLE 5.10 Estimates of the Median Birth Weight of Babies in the Birth Weight Data Set by Mother's Smoking Status

Mother's Smoking Status	n	Sample Median
Smoked	74	2775.5
Did not smoke	115	3100.0

Based on the estimated difference of -324.5 and its bound on the error of estimation $B = 335.2$, it appears that the reasonable estimates of the difference in the median birth weights ranges from a low of -659.7 g to a high of 10.7 g. Thus, on the basis of the observed data it appears that the median weight of babies born to mothers who smoked during pregnancy could be as much as 660 g less than that of the median weight of babies born to mothers who did not smoke during pregnancy; however, on the basis of this data, the median weight of babies born to mothers who smoked during pregnancy could also be as much as 11 g more than that of the median weight of babies born to mothers who did not smoke during pregnancy.

GLOSSARY

Bias The bias of an estimator T of a parameter θ is

$$\text{Bias}(T, \theta) = \mu_T - \theta$$

where μ_T is the mean of the sampling distribution of the statistic T.

Biased Estimator A biased estimator is an estimator for which the mean of the sampling distribution is not equal to the parameter of being estimated.

Bootstrapping Bootstrapping is a computer-based method for estimating the sampling distribution of an estimator from the observed data.

Bootstrap Standard Error The bootstrap standard error of an estimator is the standard deviation of the bootstrapped sampling distribution of the estimator.

Bound on the Error of Estimation The bound on the error of estimation of an unbiased or low-bias estimator is two times the standard error of the estimator (i.e., $B = 2 \times \text{SE}$).

Estimated Standard Error The estimated standard error is computed by replacing the values of unknown parameters in the formula for the standard error with data-based estimates of their values.

Finite Population Correction Factor The finite population correction factor is $\sqrt{\frac{N-n}{N-1}}$ and should always be used when the sampling proportion is at least 5%.

Mean Squared Error The mean squared error (MSE) of an estimator T of a parameter θ is

$$\text{MSE}(T, \theta) = \text{Bias}(T, \theta)^2 + \text{SE}(T)^2$$

Sampling Distribution The sampling distribution of an estimator is the probability distribution formed by computing the value of the estimator over all possible samples for a fixed sample size.

Simple Random Sample A simple random sample is a sample of n units drawn from a population of N units chosen in a fashion so that each possible sample of size n has the same chance of being selected.

Square Root Law The Square Root Law states that the accuracy of an estimator is inversely proportional to the square root of the sample size n.

Standard Error The standard error of an estimator is the standard deviation of the sampling distribution of the estimator.

Unbiased Estimator An unbiased estimator is an estimator for which the mean of the sampling distribution is equal to the parameter being estimated.

EXERCISES

5.1   What is the sampling distribution of a statistic?

5.2   Does the sampling distribution of a statistic depend on the size of the sample that the statistic is based on?

5.3   What are the advantages of using a simple random sample in place of a sample of convenience?

5.4   What information do the mean and the standard deviation of a sampling distribution provide about the accuracy of an estimator?

5.5   What does it mean when a statistic T is said to be an unbiased estimator of a parameter θ?

5.6   Name three unbiased estimators and the parameters they estimate.

5.7   How is the bias of an estimator T of a parameter θ computed?

5.8   What does it mean when the bias of an estimator T of a parameter θ is

(a) positive?   (b) equal to 0?

5.9   What is the standard error of a statistic?

5.10   How is the standard error of a statistic different from the standard deviation of the target population?

5.11   How is the accuracy of an estimator measured?

5.12   What is the mean squared error of a statistic?

5.13   How is the mean squared error of an estimator different from the standard error of the estimator?

5.14   What is the relationship between the mean squared error of an unbiased estimator and the standard error of the estimator?

5.15   Use the sampling distributions of the estimators T_1 and T_2 that are used for estimating the parameter η shown in Figure 5.5 to answer the following:

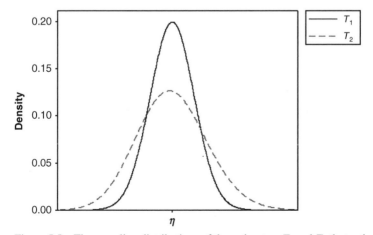

Figure 5.5   The sampling distributions of the estimators T_1 and T_2 that estimate η.

TABLE 5.11   The Means and Standard Deviations of the Sampling Distribution of T_1 and T_2

Estimator	Mean	Standard Deviation
T_1	0.98θ	5θ
T_2	θ	5.5θ

(a) Is T_1 an unbiased estimator of η? Explain.

(b) Is T_2 an unbiased estimator of η? Explain.

(c) Which estimator has the smaller standard error? Explain.

5.16   Use the information in Table 5.11 on the sampling distributions of the estimators of T_1 and T_2 that are used to estimate θ to answer the following:

(a) Determine the bias of the estimator T_1.

(b) Determine the bias of the estimator T_2.

(c) Is one of the estimators an unbiased estimator of θ? Explain.

(d) Compute the value of the mean squared error for the estimator T_1.

(e) Compute the value of the mean squared error for the estimator T_2.

(f) Which estimator of θ is more accurate, T_1 or T_2? Explain.

5.17   Explain how a biased estimator T can still be an accurate estimator of θ.

5.18   What is the formula for computing the bound on the error of estimation of an unbiased estimator T?

5.19   Why is it important to know the bound on the error of estimation of an unbiased estimator?

5.20   Many researchers report their results in the form estimate $\pm$ standard error. Assuming the sampling distribution of the estimator is roughly mound shaped, how likely is it for an unbiased estimator to fall within

(a) one standard error of the value of the parameter being estimated?

(b) two standard errors of the value of the parameter being estimated?

(c) B of the value of the parameter being estimated?

5.21   How do the true standard error (SE) and the estimated standard error (se) of an estimator differ?

5.22   What is the finite population correction factor and when should it be used?

5.23   What are the mean and standard deviation of the sampling distribution of $\widehat{p}$?

5.24   Is the sample proportion $\widehat{p}$ an unbiased estimator of the population proportion p? Explain.

5.25   What is the difference between $\mathrm{SE}(\widehat{p})$ and $\mathrm{se}(\widehat{p})$?

5.26   How does increasing the sample size n affect the standard error of $\widehat{p}$?

5.27   Compute the standard error and bound on the error of estimation associated with $\widehat{p}$ using the finite population correction factor when

(a) $N = 1000$, $n = 150$, and $p = 0.25$.

(b) $N = 5000$, $n = 200$, and $p = 0.65$.

(c) $N = 8000$, $n = 1000$, and $p = 0.13$.

(d) $N = 10{,}000$, $n = 2500$, and $p = 0.88$.

(e) $N = 100{,}000$, $n = 2500$, and $p = 0.70$.

5.28 For each part in Exercise 5.27 compute the standard error of $\widehat{p}$ without using the finite population correction factor where appropriate.

5.29 For a random sample of $n = 100$ is standard error of $\widehat{p}$ larger when $p = 0.8$ or $p = 0.4$? Explain.

5.30 Compute the estimated standard error of $\widehat{p}$ when

(a) $N = 1000$, $n = 100$, and $\widehat{p} = 0.58$.

(b) $N = 5000$, $n = 400$, and $\widehat{p} = 0.17$.

(c) $N = 5000$, $n = 900$, and $\widehat{p} = 0.46$.

(d) N is unknown, $n = 500$, and $\widehat{p} = 0.81$.

(e) N is unknown, $n = 2500$, and $\widehat{p} = 0.65$.

5.31 If the population proportion p is expected to lie between 0.4 and 0.6, what is the most you would expect the sample proportion $\widehat{p}$ to be from the true value of p when the population consists of $N = 5000$ units and the sample size is $n = 300$?

5.32 In the article "The impact of obesity on illness absence and productivity in an industrial population of petrochemical workers" published in the journal *Annals of Epidemiology* (Tsai et al., 2008), the authors studied the relationship between body mass index (BMI) and illness and absence from work. Table 5.12 was extracted from this article and contains a summary of the 3612 males and 541 females in the study according to the BMI categories $18.5 \leq \text{BMI} \leq 24.9$, $25 \leq \text{BMI} \leq 29.9$, and $\text{BMI} \geq 30$. Use the information in Table 5.12 to answer the following:

(a) Estimate the proportion of males having BMI greater than or equal to 30.

(b) Compute the estimated standard error for the estimate of the proportion of males having BMI greater than or equal to 30.

(c) Based on the observed data what are the most likely values of the proportion of males having BMI greater than or equal to 30.

(d) Does the observed sample provide any evidence that the proportion of males having BMI greater than or equal to 30 is at least 0.40? Explain.

TABLE 5.12 Summarized Data on the BMI Values of 3612 Males and 541 Females

Gender	Body Mass Index		
	18.5–24.9	25–25.9	≥ 30
Male	833	1695	1084
Female	262	159	120

TABLE 5.13   Summarized Data on the Cure Rates of the Treatments Pristinamycin and Penicillin for Treating Erysipelas

Treatment	Cured	Not Cured
Pristinamycin	83	19
Penicillin	68	34

5.33   Use the data in Table 5.12 for females to answer the following:
(a) Estimate the proportion of females having BMI greater than or equal to 30.
(b) Compute the estimated standard error for the estimate of the proportion of females having BMI greater than or equal to 30.
(c) Based on the observed data what are the most likely values of the proportion of females having BMI greater than or equal to 30.
(d) Does the observed sample provide any evidence that the proportion of females having BMI greater than or equal to 30 is at least 0.40? Explain.

5.34   In the article "Oral pristinamycin versus standard penicillin regimen to treat erysipelas in adults: randomized, non-inferiority, open trial" published in British Medical Journal (Bernard et al., 2002), the authors reported the data in Table 5.13 for the cure rates of the treatments pristinamycin and penicillin for treating erysipelas, a dermal–hypodermal infection. Use the data in Table 5.13 to answer the following:

(a) Estimate proportion of patients with erysipelas that were cured with pristinamycin.
(b) Compute the bound on the error of estimation for estimating the proportion of patients with erysipelas that were cured with pristinamycin.
(c) Estimate the proportion of patients with erysipelas that were cured with penicillin.
(d) Compute the bound on the error of estimation for the estimate of the proportion of patients with erysipelas that were cured with penicillin.
(e) Does there appear to be a difference in the cure rates of erysipelas for the treatments pristinamycin and penicillin? Explain.

5.35   Determine the conservative value of n required to achieve the bound on the error of estimation of $\hat{p}$ when
(a) $N = 1000$ and $B = 0.05$.
(b) $N = 5000$ and $B = 0.025$.
(c) $N = 5000$ and $B = 0.035$.
(d) N is unknown and $B = 0.04$.
(e) N is unknown and $B = 0.03$.

5.36   Determine the cost of sampling for each of the scenarios in Exercise 5.35 when the initial cost of sampling is $C_0 = \$2500$ and the cost per unit sampled is $C = \$5$.

5.37   What does the Central Limit Theorem say about the sampling distribution of $\hat{p}$?

5.38   Under what conditions does the Central Limit Theorem apply to the sampling distribution of $\hat{p}$?

5.39   Use the Central Limit Theorem to approximate the probability that $0.47 \leq \hat{p} \leq 0.53$ when

(a) $n = 25$ and $p = 0.5$.
(b) $n = 50$ and $p = 0.5$.
(c) $n = 400$ and $p = 0.5$.

5.40 Assuming that the Central Limit Theorem applies to the sampling distribution of $\widehat{p}$, approximate the probability that $\widehat{p}$ is within

(a) 1.5 standard errors of p (b) 2.5 standard errors of p

5.41 What are the mean and standard deviation of the sampling distribution of $\bar{x}$?

5.42 Is the sample mean an unbiased estimator of the population mean? Explain.

5.43 What is the difference between $SE(\bar{x})$ and $se(\bar{x})$?

5.44 How does increasing the sample size n affect the standard error of $\bar{x}$?

5.45 Compute the standard error and bound on the error of estimation for $\bar{x}$, using the finite population correction factor, when

(a) $N = 5000$, $n = 400$, and $\sigma = 10$.
(b) $N = 15{,}000$, $n = 2000$, and $\sigma = 100$.
(c) $N = 8000$, $n = 1000$, and $\sigma = 40$.
(d) $N = 10{,}000$, $n = 1500$, and $\sigma = 500$.
(e) $N = 100{,}000$, $n = 6000$, and $\sigma = 4$.

5.46 For each part in Exercise 5.45, compute the standard error of $\bar{x}$ without using the finite population correction factor.

5.47 Suppose that $SE(\bar{x}) = 5$ for a random sample of $n = 25$ observations and $n/N < 0.05$. How large would n have to be for the standard error to be

(a) 2.5?   (b) 1?

5.48 Compute the estimated standard error of $\bar{x}$ when

(a) $N = 1000$, $n = 100$, and $s = 25$.
(b) $N = 5000$, $n = 400$, and $s = 55$.
(c) $N = 5000$, $n = 900$, and $s = 2.8$.
(d) N is unknown, $n = 500$, and $s = 118$.
(e) N is unknown, $n = 2500$, and $s = 12$.

5.49 In the article "A study of a pathway to reduce pressure ulcers for patients with a hip fracture" published in the *Journal of Orthopaedic Nursing* (Hommel et al., 2007), the authors reported the information given in Table 5.14 on the variable body mass index (BMI) for a control group and an intervention group. Use the summary statistics in Table 5.14 to answer the following:

TABLE 5.14   **Summary Statistics for the Variable BMI for the Control and Intervention Groups**

Group	n	$\bar{x}$	s
Control	201	24.7	4.6
Intervention	197	23.8	4.1

TABLE 5.15 Summary Statistics for Beck Depression Inventory (BDI) Score for the Diet-as-Usual and the Nondieting Groups

Group	n	$\bar{x}$	s
Diet-as-usual	84	8.98	6.73
Nondieting	73	8.88	6.09

(a) Compute the estimated standard error of the sample mean for the control group.

(b) Compute the bound on the error of estimation for the sample mean of the control group.

(c) Compute the estimated standard error of the sample mean for the intervention group.

(d) Compute the bound on the error of estimation for the sample mean of the intervention group.

5.50 In the article "Experimental investigation of the effects of naturalistic dieting on bulimic symptoms: moderating effects of depressive symptoms" published in *Appetite* (Presnell et al., 2008), the summary statistics given in Table 5.15 on the variable Beck Depression Inventory (BDI) were reported for 84 participants in a diet-as-usual group and 73 participants in a nondieting group. Use the summary statistics in Table 5.15 to answer the following:

(a) Compute the estimated standard error of the sample mean for the diet-as-usual group.

(b) Compute the bound on the error of estimation of the sample mean of the diet-as-usual group.

(c) Compute the estimated standard error of the sample mean of the nondieting group.

(d) Compute the bound on the error of estimation for the sample mean of the nondieting group.

5.51 Determine the value of n required to achieve the desired bound on the error of estimation of $\bar{x}$ when

(a) $N = 1000$, $\sigma = 25$, and $B = 2$.

(b) $N = 5000$, $\sigma = 60$, and $B = 4$.

(c) $N = 5000$, $\sigma = 210$, and $B = 5$.

(d) N is unknown, $\sigma = 3.5$, and $B = 0.5$.

(e) N is unknown, $\sigma = 0.90$, and $B = 0.05$.

5.52 Determine the cost of sampling for each of the parts in Exercise 5.51 when the initial cost of sampling is $C_0 = \$5300$ and the cost per unit sampled is $C = \$22$.

5.53 What does the Central Limit Theorem say about the sampling distribution of $\bar{x}$?

5.54 Under what conditions does the Central Limit Theorem apply to the sampling distribution of $\bar{x}$?

5.55 For a population with $\mu = 10$ and $\sigma = 1.5$, use the Central Limit Theorem to approximate the probability that $9.8 \leq \bar{x} \leq 10.2$ when

(a) $n = 100$. **(b)** $n = 200$.

5.56 Many researchers report the estimate of the mean in the form of sample mean plus and minus the standard error. Assuming that the Central Limit Theorem applies, what is the approximate probability that $\mu - SE(\bar{x}) \leq \bar{x} \leq \mu + SE(\bar{x})$?

5.57 Assuming that the Central Limit Theorem applies to the sampling distribution of $\bar{x}$, approximate the probability that $\bar{x}$ is within

(a) 1 standard error of μ (b) 1.65 standard errors of μ
(c) 2 standard errors of μ (d) 3 standard errors of μ

5.58 Under what conditions does the distribution of $\frac{\bar{x}-\mu}{s/\sqrt{n}}$ follow a t distribution?

5.59 When sampling from a normal population, what is the distribution of $\frac{\bar{x}-\mu}{s/\sqrt{n}}$ for a sample of size n?

5.60 What happens to a t distribution as the degrees of freedom become extremely large?

5.61 For independent random samples selected from the X and Y populations, what are the mean and standard deviation of the sampling distribution of $\hat{p}_X - \hat{p}_Y$?

5.62 For independent random samples selected from the X and Y populations what is the formula for computing the

(a) $\text{SE}(\hat{p}_X - \hat{p}_Y)$?   (b) $\text{se}(\hat{p}_X - \hat{p}_Y)$?

5.63 Under what conditions is the sampling distribution of $\hat{p}_X - \hat{p}_Y$ approximately normally distributed?

5.64 Suppose independent random samples from the X and Y populations have been drawn. Determine the estimated standard error of $\hat{p}_X - \hat{p}_Y$ when
(a) $n_X = 100, n_Y = 80, \hat{p}_X = 0.56$, and $\hat{p}_Y = 0.63$.
(b) $n_X = 50, n_Y = 40, \hat{p}_X = 0.16$, and $\hat{p}_Y = 0.31$.
(c) $n_X = 75, n_Y = 75, \hat{p}_X = 0.76$, and $\hat{p}_Y = 0.82$.

5.65 Determine the bound on the error of estimation for each part in Exercise 5.64.

5.66 In the article "Experimental investigation of the effects of naturalistic dieting on bulimic symptoms: moderating effects of depressive symptoms" published in *Appetite* (Presnell et al., 2008), the summary counts in Table 5.16 were reported for the number of participants increasing their level of exercise for the 84 participants in the diet as-usual-group and 73 participants in the nondieting group. Use the summary counts in Table 5.16 to answer the following:
(a) Estimate the proportion of the diet-as-usual population who will increase their exercise level.
(b) Estimate the proportion of the nondieting population who will increase their exercise level.
(c) Estimate the difference in the proportion of individuals who will increase their exercise level for the diet-as-usual and nondieting populations.
(d) Compute the estimated standard error of the difference of these proportions.
(e) Compute the bound on the error of estimation for estimating the difference of these proportions.

TABLE 5.16 **Summary Statistics for Beck Depression Inventory (BDI) Score for the Diet-as-usual and the Nondieting Groups**

Group	n	No. of people Increasing Exercise
Diet as usual	84	31
Nondieting	73	10

5.67 In developing the sampling plan for estimating the difference between the proportions p_X and p_Y (i.e., $p_X - p_Y$), suppose that the goal is to minimize the bound on the error of estimation for a overall sample size fixed at $n = 100$. Determine the population sample sizes, n_X and n_Y, when
(a) $\hat{p}_X = 0.40$ and $\hat{p}_Y = 0.50$.
(b) $\hat{p}_X = 0.80$ and $\hat{p}_Y = 0.60$.
(c) no reasonable prior guesses $\hat{p}_X$ and $\hat{p}_Y$ are available.

5.68 Determine the total cost of sampling for the resulting sampling plan in Exercise 5.67 when the initial cost of sampling is $C_0 = \$1500$ and the costs of sampling a unit from populations X and Y are $C_X = \$5$ and $C_Y = \$8$.

5.69 In developing a sampling plan for estimating the difference between the proportions p_X and p_Y (i.e., $p_X - p_Y$), suppose the goal is to minimize the overall sample size n. Determine the overall sample size and population sample sizes, n_X and n_Y, when $B = 0.04$ and
(a) $\hat{p}_X = 0.25$ and $\hat{p}_Y = 0.35$.
(b) $\hat{p}_X = 0.75$ and $\hat{p}_Y = 0.80$.
(c) no reasonable prior guesses $\hat{p}_X$ and $\hat{p}_Y$ are available.

5.70 Determine the total cost of sampling for the resulting sampling plan in Exercise 5.69 when the initial cost of sampling is $C_0 = \$800$ and the costs of sampling a unit from populations X and Y are $C_X = \$15$ and $C_Y = \$10$, respectively.

5.71 In developing a sampling plan for estimating the difference between the proportions p_X and p_Y (i.e., $p_X - p_Y$), suppose the goal is to minimize the bound on the error of estimation when the total cost of sampling is fixed at $C = \$2500$. Determine the overall sample size and population sample sizes, n_X and n_Y, when
(a) $\hat{p}_X = 0.25$, $\hat{p}_Y = 0.35$, and $C_X = \$10$, $C_Y = \$15$.
(b) $\hat{p}_X = 0.75$, $\hat{p}_Y = 0.80$, and $C_X = \$40$, $C_Y = \$25$.
(c) no reasonable prior guesses $\hat{p}_X$ and $\hat{p}_Y$ are available and $C_X = C_Y = \$10$.

5.72 In developing a sampling plan for estimating the difference between the proportions p_X and p_Y (i.e., $p_X - p_Y$), suppose the goal is to minimize the total cost of sampling for a fixed value of the bound on the error of estimation. Determine the overall sample size and population sample sizes, n_X and n_Y, when
(a) $\hat{p}_X = 0.25$, $\hat{p}_Y = 0.35$, $B = 0.04$, and $C_X = \$10$, $C_Y = \$12$.
(b) $\hat{p}_X = 0.75$, $\hat{p}_Y = 0.80$, $B = 0.05$, and $C_X = \$20$, $C_Y = \$30$.
(c) no reasonable prior guesses $\hat{p}_X$ and $\hat{p}_Y$ are available, $B = 0.03$, and $C_X = \$25$ and $C_Y = \$15$.

5.73 For independent random samples from the X and Y populations, what are the mean and standard deviation of the sampling distribution of $\bar{x} - \bar{y}$?

5.74 For independent random samples from the X and Y populations, what is the formula for computing the
(a) $SE(\bar{x} - \bar{y})$? (b) $se(\bar{x} - \bar{y})$?

5.75 Under what conditions is the sampling distribution of $\bar{x} - \bar{y}$ approximately normally distributed?

5.76 Suppose independent random samples from the X and Y populations have been drawn. Determine the estimated standard error of $\bar{x} - \bar{y}$ when

TABLE 5.17 Summary Statistics for the Variable Total Cholesterol (TC) for 69 Boys in the Control Group and 29 Boys in the Obese Group

Group	n	Sample Mean	se Mean
Control	69	4.30	0.07
Obese	29	4.91	0.19

(a) $n_X = 100, n_Y = 80, s_X = 5.6$, and $s_Y = 6.9$.
(b) $n_X = 50, n_Y = 40, s_X = 21.3$, and $s_Y = 12.1$.
(c) $n_X = 75, n_Y = 75, s_X = 500.6$, and $s_Y = 450.8$.

5.77 Determine the bound on the error of estimation for each part in Exercise 5.76.

5.78 In the article "Increase serum cholesterol ester transfer protein in obese children" published in the journal *Obesity Research* (Asayama et al., 2002), the authors reported the summary statistics given in Table 5.17 for the variable total cholesterol for 69 boys in a control group and 29 boys in the obese group. Use the summary statistics in Table 5.17 to answer the following:
(a) Estimate the difference between the mean total cholesterol for the control and obese groups.
(b) Compute the standard error for the difference of the sample means.
(c) Compute the bound on the error of estimation for the difference of the sample means.

5.79 In developing a sampling plan for estimating the difference between the means μ_X and μ_Y (i.e., $\mu_X - \mu_Y$), suppose the goal is to minimize the bound on the error of estimation for a overall sample size fixed at $n = 250$. Determine the population sample sizes, n_X and n_Y, when
(a) $\dot{\sigma}_X = 24$ and $\dot{\sigma}_Y = 18$.
(b) $\dot{\sigma}_X = 100$ and $\dot{\sigma}_Y = 120$.

5.80 Determine the total cost of sampling for the resulting sampling plan in Exercise 5.79 when the initial cost of sampling is $C_0 = \$3500$ and the costs of sampling a unit from populations X and Y are $C_X = \$12$ and $C_Y = \$8$, respectively.

5.81 In developing a sampling plan for estimating the difference between the means μ_X and μ_Y (i.e., $\mu_X - \mu_Y$), suppose the goal is to minimize the overall sample size n. Determine the overall sample size and population sample sizes, n_X and n_Y, when
(a) $B = 2, \dot{\sigma}_X = 6$, and $\dot{\sigma}_Y = 15$.
(b) $B = 0.25, \dot{\sigma}_X = 1$, and $\dot{\sigma}_Y = 1.8$.

5.82 Determine the total cost of sampling for the resulting sampling plan in Exercise 5.81 when the initial cost of sampling is $C_0 = \$900$ and the costs of sampling a unit from populations X and Y are $C_X = \$5$ and $C_Y = \$12$, respectively.

5.83 In developing a sampling plan for estimating the difference between the means μ_X and μ_Y (i.e., $\mu_X - \mu_Y$), suppose the goal is to minimize the bound on the error of estimation when the total cost of sampling is fixed at $C = \$5000$. Determine the overall sample size and population sample sizes, n_X and n_Y, when
(a) $\dot{\sigma}_X = 5, \dot{\sigma}_Y = 3$, and $C_X = \$20, C_Y = \$10$.
(b) $\dot{\sigma}_X = 50, \dot{\sigma}_Y = 80$, and $C_X = \$50, C_Y = \$25$.

5.84   In developing a sampling plan for estimating the difference between the means μ_X and μ_Y (i.e., $\mu_X - \mu_Y$), suppose the goal is to minimize the total cost of sampling for a fixed value of the bound on the error of estimation. Determine the overall sample size and population sample sizes, n_X and n_Y, when

(a) $\acute{\sigma}_X = 12$, $\acute{\sigma}_Y = 15$, $B = 2$, and $C_X = \$8$, $C_Y = \$12$, respectively.

(b) $\acute{\sigma}_X = 25$, $\acute{\sigma}_Y = 40$, $B = 8$, and $C_X = \$20$, $C_Y = \$30$.

5.85   How can a computer be used to estimate the standard error of a statistic?

5.86   What is the bootstrap algorithm for estimating the standard error of a statistic T?

5.87   Explain how the bootstrap algorithm would be used to estimate the standard error of the

(a) sample median.

(b) sample interquartile range.

(c) Q1.

(d) s.

5.88   Suppose independent random samples are drawn from populations X and Y. Explain how the bootstrap algorithm would be used to estimate the standard error of $\tilde{x} - \tilde{y}$.

5.89   Using the data on the variable abdomen circumference in the Body Fat data set and a statistical computing package,

(a) estimate the median abdomen circumference.

(b) bootstrap the standard error of the sample median of abdomen circumference.

CONFIDENCE INTERVALS

6.1 INTERVAL ESTIMATION

In Chapter 4, point estimation was introduced and in Chapter 5 measures of reliability for point estimators were discussed. In Chapter 6, point estimators and their measures of reliability are combined to create data-based intervals of plausible estimates of an unknown parameter. Recall that a point estimator produces a single number that is used for estimating the value of an unknown parameter, and it is unlikely for an unbiased estimator to be farther than the bound on the error of estimation from the true value of the parameter. Thus, in practice a researcher will often report an interval in plausible estimates of the form

$$\text{estimate} \pm \text{bound on the error of estimation}$$

A statistical procedure that produces an interval of estimates of an unknown parameter is called an *interval estimator*. Interval estimators are simply rules that tell a researcher how to use the observed sample data to generate an interval of reasonable estimates of the parameter of interest. In general, interval estimators are based on the sampling distribution of a point estimator. For example, an interval estimator that incorporates the value of the point estimate and its bound on the error of estimation is given by

$$\text{point estimate} \pm B$$

which produces the interval of plausible estimates

$$\text{point estimate} - B \text{ to point estimate} + B$$

AN INTERVAL ESTIMATOR BASED ON B

When T is an unbiased estimator of a parameter θ, the interval of plausible estimates of θ based on T and its bound on the error of estimation is

$$T \pm B$$

which yields an interval of estimates $T - B$ to $T + B$.

Example 6.1

Based on the Birth Weight data set, the point estimate of the median birth weight of a baby born to a mother who smoked during pregnancy is $\tilde{x} = 2775.5$. The bootstrap standard error of $\tilde{x}$ is se $= 135.8$, and thus, an interval of reasonable estimates of the median birth weight of a baby born to a mother who smoked during pregnancy is

$$2775.5 \pm 2 \times 135.8$$

Thus, based on the observed data, the plausible estimates of the median birth weight of a baby born to a mother who smoked during pregnancy ranges from a low of 2775.5 to a high of 3047.1.

One advantage of using an interval estimator based on the bound on the error of estimation is that it can be used for any parameter that can be estimated. The large sample interval estimators based on the bound on the error of estimation for estimating proportions, means, variances, or standard deviations are listed below.

LARGE SAMPLE INTERVAL ESTIMATORS BASED ON B

For $n > 100$, the interval estimator based on the bound of estimation for a

1. population proportion p is

$$\widehat{p} \pm 2\sqrt{\frac{\widehat{p}(1 - \widehat{p})}{n}}$$

2. population mean μ is

$$\bar{x} \pm 2\frac{s}{\sqrt{n}}$$

3. population variance σ^2 is

$$s^2 \pm 2s^2\sqrt{\frac{2}{n}}$$

4. population standard deviation σ is

$$s \pm 2\frac{s}{\sqrt{2n}}$$

Example 6.2

The estimate of the variance (σ^2) of the variable percent body fat (PCTBF) for the $n = 252$ observations in the Body Fat data set is $s^2 = 70.06$. The large sample interval of estimates of σ^2 based on the observed data is

$$70.06 \pm 2 \times 70.06\sqrt{\frac{2}{252}}$$

Thus, the interval of reasonable estimates of σ^2 is 57.58–82.54.

Although using point estimate $\pm B$ is a convenient method of determining an interval of reasonable estimates of an unknown parameter, the disadvantage of using this procedure is that there is no measure of the procedure's reliability. That is, the interval based on the point estimate and its bound on the error of estimation is based on the idea that it will be unlikely for an observed value of the point estimator to be more than B from the true value of the parameter being estimated. Because the likelihood of being within B of the true value is actually unknown, the reliability of this procedure is also unknown.

6.2 CONFIDENCE INTERVALS

An interval estimator that has a prespecified measure of reliability is called a *confidence interval*. A confidence interval is an interval estimator that is designed to produce an interval of estimates that captures the unknown value of the parameter being estimated with a prespecified probability. The prespecified probability of capturing the true value of the parameter being estimated is called the *confidence level*, and the confidence level is the measure of reliability for a confidence interval. The generic form of the confidence level is given by

$$\text{confidence level} = (1 - \alpha) \times 100\%$$

where α is the probability that the procedure will not capture the true value of the parameter being estimated. Usually a high confidence level, such as 90%, 95%, or 99%, is used in practice; however, it seems that 95% confidence intervals are generally used by researchers in most studies. One reason that 95% confidence intervals are so frequently used is that for a point estimator having a mound-shaped sampling distribution, the interval

$$\text{point estimate} \pm B$$

is approximately a 95% confidence interval.

It is important to note that the confidence level measures the reliability of the confidence interval procedure, not the resulting interval produced by applying the confidence interval estimator to the observed sample. That is, a 95% confidence interval will capture the true value of the parameter being estimated for 95% of all of the possible samples of size n that can be drawn from the target population. Thus, 5% of the possible samples will result in confidence intervals that do not capture the true value of the parameter. In other words, 95% of all of the possible random samples from a target population will produce 95% confidence intervals that will capture the value of the parameter being estimated.

In practice, an observed confidence interval may or may not capture the value of the parameter; however, because the procedure does capture the value of the unknown parameter with a high prespecified probability (i.e., the confidence level), the resulting interval of estimates will most likely capture the true value of the parameter. In fact, even when the true value is not in the resulting interval, it will almost certainly be close to one of the ends of a confidence interval. Thus, the observed confidence interval can safely be used as a plausible set of estimates of the unknown parameter. Hence, a confidence interval procedure produces a set of reasonable estimates of the unknown parameter based upon the observed sample data, and when the sample is truly representative of the population it is likely that the confidence interval will contain the value of the parameter of interest.

It is often helpful to envision the confidence interval process as follows.

CONFIDENCE INTERVAL BOX MODEL

First, a box containing all of the possible confidence intervals for random samples of size n for estimating a parameter θ exists. That is, the box consists of all of the confidence intervals computed from all of the possible random samples of size n. Furthermore, $(1 - \alpha) \times 100\%$ of the intervals in the box contain the true value of θ and $\alpha \times 100\%$ of the intervals in the box do not contain θ.

Second, the researcher reaches the box of confidence intervals and selects a confidence interval at random that results in the interval L to U. The confidence interval the researcher selected may or may not contain θ; however, there was a 95% chance of selecting a confidence interval from the box that did contain the true value of θ. Thus, the researcher can be confident in the observed confidence interval L to U.

Example 6.3

Suppose that a researcher computes a 95% confidence interval for the mean of a population, which results in the interval 23.2–28.9. Note that there is no information in the observed confidence interval that can convey whether or not the true value of the population mean is between 23.2 and 28.9; however, because the procedure produces a confidence interval that does capture the value of the population mean 95% of the time, the researcher can be confident that the interval 23.2–28.9 does capture the true value of μ. It is important to keep in mind that the confidence level refers to the reliability of

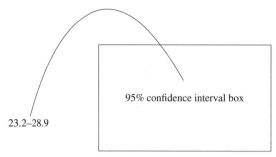

23.2–28.9

Figure 6.1   The 95% confidence interval box model and an observed confidence interval of 23.2–28.9.

the procedure, not the observed confidence interval computed from the sample data. Also, a common misconception is that there is a 95% chance that the population mean will be in the interval 23.2–28.9 (Figure 6.1). This is an incorrect interpretation of the observed confidence interval since the population mean is either between 23.2 and 28.9 or it is not. Thus, the chance that $23.2 \le \mu \le 28.9$ is either 0 or 100%, not 95%. Again, the 95% chance of capturing the mean refers to the reliability of the confidence interval procedure and not the particular interval produced by applying the procedure to an observed sample.

The most common form of a confidence interval is

$$\text{point estimate} \pm \text{margin of error}$$

where the margin of error (ME) takes into account the accuracy of the point estimator and the reliability of the confidence interval (i.e., the confidence level). In this case, the width of a confidence interval is $W = 2 \times \text{ME}$. In general, the width of confidence interval depends on the variability of the population sampled, the confidence level, and the sample size. The larger the sample size is, the narrower the confidence interval will be, and the more variability there is in the target population, the wider the confidence interval will be, also. Larger confidence levels also produce the wider confidence intervals. For example, a 95% confidence interval will be wider than a 90% confidence interval since a wider interval will be required to achieve the higher level of reliability.

Finally, when a confidence interval is used for estimating the difference between the values of a parameter for two distinct populations or subpopulations whether or not 0 is in the resulting interval is an important consideration. When 0 is in a comparative confidence interval, the interval is suggesting that there is no statistical evidence of a difference between the values of the parameter for the two populations. On the other hand, when the values in the confidence interval for the difference are all larger than 0, the interval is suggesting that the parameter of interest in one of the populations is significantly larger than the value of the parameter in the other population; similarly, when the values in the confidence interval for the difference are all less than 0, the interval is suggesting that the parameter of interest of one of the populations is significantly smaller than the value of the parameter in the other population.

6.3   SINGLE SAMPLE CONFIDENCE INTERVALS

In this section, confidence intervals for the parameters of a single population X will be discussed. In particular, the confidence interval procedure for estimating population

TABLE 6.1   The z_{crit} Values Used in the Large Sample 90%, 95%, and 95% Confidence Intervals for a Proportion

	90%	95%	99%
z_{crit}	1.645	1.96	2.576

proportions, the population mean, and the *bootstrap confidence interval* procedure will be discussed.

6.3.1 Confidence Intervals for Proportions

Suppose that the parameter of interest is the proportion of the population X having a certain characteristic. Let p be the unknown value of this proportion and $\widehat{p}$ the point estimator of p based on a random sample. The formula for a large sample $(1 - \alpha) \times 100\%$ confidence interval for p is given below.

LARGE SAMPLE CONFIDENCE INTERVALS FOR P

When both np and $n(1 - p)$ are greater than 5, a $(1 - \alpha) \times 100\%$ confidence interval for p is

$$\widehat{p} \pm \underbrace{z_{crit} \times \sqrt{\frac{\widehat{p}(1 - \widehat{p})}{n}}}_{ME}$$

where z_{crit} is the value in a standard normal distribution such that $P(-z_{crit} \leq Z \leq z_{crit}) = 1 - \alpha$.

The values of z_{crit} can be found in Table A.4. The values of z_{crit} used in 90%, 95%, and 99% confidence intervals are given in Table 6.1.

The large sample confidence interval procedure for estimating a proportion p is appropriate when both np and $n(1 - p)$ are greater than 5 because the sampling distribution of $\widehat{p}$ will be approximately normal under these conditions according to the Central Limit Theorem. However, since the value of p is unknown, this procedure can be safely used in practice when both $n\widehat{p}$ and $n(1 - \widehat{p})$ are greater than 5. Also, this procedure may produce a confidence interval with a lower end point that is negative or an upper end point that is greater than 1. In these cases, since the true value of p is always between 0 and 1, the resulting interval must be adjusted appropriately. Thus, when the lower end point of the confidence interval is negative, replace the lower end point with 0, and when the upper end point of the confidence interval is greater than 1, replace the upper end point with 1.

Confidence intervals for proportions are often reported as confidence intervals in terms of percentages. To convert a confidence interval for a proportion into a confidence interval in terms of percentages, simply multiply the lower and upper boundaries of the confidence interval for the proportion by 100.

Example 6.4

In the article "The impact of obesity on illness absence and productivity in an industrial population of petrochemical workers" published in *Annals of Epidemiology* (Tsai et al., 2008), the authors reported that 32.3% of the workers in the study who had a body mass indexes (BMI) of greater than 30 also had at least three of the risk factors current smoking, high cholesterol, hypertension, elevated glucose, and elevated triglycerides. If the number of individuals having body mass index greater than 30 was $n = 1130$, compute a 95% confidence interval for the percentage of individuals with a body mass index greater than 30 who have at least three of the risk factors.

Solution Converting 32.3% to a proportion yields $\widehat{p} = 0.323$, and since $1130(0.323) = 365$ and $1130(1 - 0.323) = 765$, the large sample confidence interval procedure for proportions can be used for estimating the proportion of individuals having a body mass index greater than 30 who have at least three of the risk factors.

The value of z_{crit} for a large sample 95% confidence interval for a proportion is $z_{crit} = 1.96$, and thus, the 95% confidence interval for the proportion of individuals with a body mass index greater than 30 who have at least three of the risk factors is

$$0.323 \pm 1.96 \times \sqrt{\frac{0.323(1 - 0.323)}{1130}}$$

Thus, the resulting confidence interval for the proportion individuals with a body mass index greater than 30 who have at least three of the risk factors is 0.296–0.350, and in terms of percentages the confidence interval is 29.6%–35.0%. Thus, it appears that the percentage of individuals having body mass index greater than 30 that have at least three of the risk factors is at least 29.6% and possibly as high as 35.0%.

A one-sided confidence interval for a proportion can also be computed when a lower or upper bound for the value of the proportion is needed. That is, when a researcher is interested in making inferences such as $p \geq p_L$ or $p \leq p_U$ a one-sided confidence interval for the proportion is called for. For example, a researcher might want to estimate the upper bound on the prevalence of a disease or the lower bound on the specificity of a diagnostic test. The formulas for the one-sided large sample confidence intervals for a proportion are given below.

LARGE SAMPLE ONE-SIDED CONFIDENCE INTERVALS FOR P

When both np and $n(1 - p)$ are greater than 5, then a $(1 - \alpha) \times 100\%$

1. upper bound confidence interval for p is

$$p \leq \widehat{p} + z_{crit} \times \underbrace{\sqrt{\frac{\widehat{p}(1 - \widehat{p})}{n}}}_{ME}$$

where z_{crit} is the value in a standard normal distribution such that $P(Z \geq z_{crit}) = \alpha$.

2. lower bound confidence interval for p is

$$p \geq \widehat{p} - z_{crit} \times \underbrace{\sqrt{\frac{\widehat{p}(1 - \widehat{p})}{n}}}_{ME}$$

where z_{crit} is the value in a standard normal distribution such that $P(Z \geq z_{crit}) = \alpha$.

The values of z_{crit} used in one-sided 90%, 95%, and 99% confidence intervals are given in Tables 6.2 and A.4.

Example 6.5

In the article "Oral pristinamycin versus standard penicillin regimen to treat erysipelas in adults: randomized, non-inferiority, open trial" published in *British Medical Journal* (Bernard et al., 2002), the cure rate for erysipelas using pristinamycin was reported to be 81% for a sample of 102 individuals.

TABLE 6.2   The z_{crit} Values Used in the Large Sample 90%, 95%, and 99% One-Sided Confidence Intervals for a Proportion

	90%	95%	99%
z_{crit}	1.282	1.645	2.326

Use this information to compute a 95% lower bound confidence interval for the cure rate for patients treated with pristinamycin.

Solution Since $102(0.81) = 82.6$ and $102(1 - 0.81) = 19.4$ are both greater than 5, the large sample 95% lower bound confidence interval for the cure rate using pristinamycin is

$$0.81 - 1.645 \times \sqrt{\frac{0.81(1 - 0.81)}{102}}$$

which yields an interval of 0.75–1.00. Thus, on the basis of the observed sample and the lower bound 95% confidence interval, it appears that the cure rate for erysipelas using pristinamycin is 75%.

When the proportion p or $1 - p$ is expected to be small, as is often the case with proportions such as the prevalence, specificity, and sensitivity, the large sample confidence interval formulas for proportions should not be used. In the case of a small proportion (i.e., p or $1 - p$ is small), where it is unlikely that np and $n(1 - p)$ will both be greater than 5, there are other methods available for computing a confidence interval for a proportion and one of these methods should be used. As a matter of fact, many of the commonly used statistical computing packages used in biostatistical analyses do provide methods for computing exact confidence intervals for proportions when either p or $1 - p$ is small.

Finally, in planning a research study where the statistical analysis will include a confidence interval, it is possible to determine the sample size required to produce a $(1 - \alpha) \times 100\%$ confidence interval that will have a prespecified margin of error. The formulas for determining the sample size n needed for a prespecified margin of error in a $(1 - \alpha) \times 100\%$ confidence interval are given below.

DETERMINING n FOR A CONFIDENCE INTERVAL FOR A PROPORTION

The sample size required for producing a margin of error of ME for a large sample $(1 - \alpha) \times 100\%$ confidence interval for a proportion is

1. $n = \hat{p}(1 - \hat{p}) \times \left[\dfrac{z_{crit}}{ME}\right]^2$, where $\hat{p}$ is a reasonable prior guess of the value of p.

2. $n = \left[\dfrac{z_{crit}}{2 \times ME}\right]^2$, when no reasonable prior guess of the value of p is available.

Note that when there is no reasonable prior estimate of the value of p, the value of n will be a conservative value. That is, $n = [\frac{z_{crit}}{2 \times ME}]^2$ is equal to the largest value of n that would be obtained using any value of $\hat{p}$. Also, both of the formulas for determining the value of n for a prespecified margin of error apply to both the one-sided and the two-sided confidence interval procedures.

Example 6.6

Determine the sample size required to produce a margin of error equal to ME = 0.03 with a large sample confidence interval

    a. for a two-sided 95% confidence interval with $\hat{p} = 0.25$.

    b. for a two-sided 95% confidence interval when no reasonable prior estimate of the value of p is available.

    c. for a one-sided 95% confidence interval with $\hat{p} = 0.80$.

    d. for a one-sided 99% confidence interval with $\hat{p} = 0.25$.

    e. for a two-sided 90% confidence interval when no reasonable prior estimate of the value of p is available.

Solutions   Using the z_{crit} values from Tables 6.1 and 6.2, the sample size required to produce a margin of error of ME = 0.03

    a. for a two-sided 95% confidence interval with $\hat{p} = 0.25$ is

$$n = 0.25(1 - 0.25) \times \left[\frac{1.96}{0.03}\right]^2 = 800.3$$

Thus, the sample size is $n = 801$.

    b. for a two-sided 95% confidence interval when no reasonable prior estimate of the value of p is available is

$$n = \left[\frac{1.96}{2 \times 0.03}\right]^2 = 1067.1$$

Thus, the sample size is $n = 1068$.

    c. for a one-sided 95% confidence interval with $\hat{p} = 0.80$ is

$$n = 0.80(1 - 0.80) \times \left[\frac{1.645}{0.03}\right]^2 = 481.1$$

Thus, the sample size is $n = 482$.

    d. for a one-sided 99% confidence interval with $\hat{p} = 0.25$ is

$$n = 0.25(1 - 0.25) \times \left[\frac{2.576}{0.03}\right]^2 = 1382.5$$

Thus, the sample size is $n = 1383$.

    e. for a two-sided 90% confidence interval when no reasonable prior estimate of the value of p is available is

$$n = \left[\frac{1.282}{2 \times 0.03}\right]^2 = 456.5$$

Thus, the sample size is $n = 457$.

    Note that in part (b) of Example 6.6, the conservative value of n is roughly 33% larger than the value of n found in part (a). Thus, whenever a reasonable prior estimate of the value of p is available, it should be used to reduce the number of observations needed, and hence, the cost of the research project.

6.3.2 Confidence Intervals for a Mean

For large samples where the Central Limit Theorem applies to the sampling distribution of $\bar{x}$, it turns out that the interval $\bar{x} \pm B$ is approximately a 95% confidence interval for

μ. However, the exact confidence level of the interval formed from $\bar{x} \pm B$ is unknown in practice, even with large samples. Thus, a more reliable approach for determining a confidence interval for estimating the mean of a population is needed.

The general form of a confidence interval for estimating the mean of a population is

$$\text{point estimate} \pm \text{margin of error}$$

where the margin of error takes into account the accuracy of $\bar{x}$ and the confidence level. Since the estimated standard error of $\bar{x}$ is se $= s/\sqrt{n}$, the general form of a confidence interval for a population mean μ will be

$$\bar{x} \pm \text{critical value} \times \frac{s}{\sqrt{n}},$$

where the critical value depends on the confidence level, and more importantly, which confidence interval procedure is appropriate for estimating the mean.

The three different confidence interval procedures that will be discussed are based on the following scenarios:

1. The sample size n is sufficiently large and the Central Limit Theorem applies to the sampling distribution of $\bar{x}$. In this scenario, the *large sample Z confidence interval* procedure will be appropriate for computing confidence intervals for estimating μ.

2. The underlying distribution being sampled is approximately normally distributed. In this scenario, the *t confidence interval* procedure will be appropriate for computing confidence intervals for estimating μ.

3. Neither the large sample nor the small sample procedures for estimating the mean apply. In this scenario, a bootstrap confidence interval procedure will be appropriate for estimating μ with a confidence interval.

The confidence interval procedure associated with the first scenario is often referred to as the *Large Sample Confidence Interval for the Mean*, and the confidence interval procedure associated with the second scenario is often referred to as the *Small Sample Confidence Interval for the Mean*. Also, note that the appropriate procedure to use for computing a $(1 - \alpha) \times 100\%$ confidence interval for the mean of a population depends on the sample size and the shape of the underlying distribution. In particular,

1. a sample size of $n \geq 100$ is considered sufficient for using the large sample Z confidence interval procedure for estimating μ.

2. when the histogram or a normal probability plot indicates the underlying distribution is roughly mound shaped and the $n < 100$, then the small sample t confidence interval procedure for estimating μ should be used.

3. when the histogram indicates the underlying distribution is not roughly mound shaped and $n < 100$, a bootstrap confidence interval can be used for estimating μ.

6.3.3 Large Sample Confidence Intervals for μ

When $n \geq 100$, the sampling distribution of $\bar{x}$ is approximately normal and the large sample confidence interval procedures can be used for estimating a population mean μ. The large sample formulas for the two-sided and both of the one-sided confidence intervals for μ are listed below.

LARGE SAMPLE CONFIDENCE INTERVALS FOR A MEAN

When $n \geq 100$

1. a two-sided confidence interval for μ is given by

$$\bar{x} \pm z_{\text{crit}} \times \frac{s}{\sqrt{n}}$$

2. a one-sided upper bound confidence interval for μ is given by

$$\mu \leq \bar{x} + z_{\text{crit}} \times \frac{s}{\sqrt{n}}$$

3. a one-sided lower bound confidence interval for μ is given by

$$\mu \geq \bar{x} - z_{\text{crit}} \times \frac{s}{\sqrt{n}}$$

The z_{crit} values can be found in Table A.4.

Note that the confidence levels for the large sample confidence intervals are approximate confidence levels, and the larger the sample size is the better the approximation will be.

Example 6.7
In the article "Birthsize and accelerated growth during infancy are associated with increased odds of childhood overweight in Mexican children" published in the *Journal of the American Dietetic Association* (Jones-Smith et al., 2007), the mean and standard deviation of the gestation time (in weeks) of $n = 163$ Mexican children are $\bar{x} = 40.17$ and $s = 4.74$. Use this information to compute

a. the estimated standard error of $\bar{x}$.

b. a 98% confidence interval for the mean gestation time of a Mexican child.

Solutions Using $n = 163, \bar{x} = 40.17$, and $s = 4.74$

a. the estimated standard error of $\bar{x}$ is

$$\text{se} = \frac{s}{\sqrt{n}} = \frac{4.74}{\sqrt{163}} = 0.37$$

b. and since $n = 163 \geq 100$, a large sample 98% confidence interval for the mean gestation time of a Mexican child is

$$40.17 \pm 2.326(0.37)$$

which yields a confidence interval for the mean gestation time of 39.31–41.03 weeks.

6.3.4 Small Sample Confidence Intervals for μ

When the sample size is smaller than 100 and the underlying distribution is approximately normal, confidence intervals for μ can be computed using a confidence interval based on the t distribution. Recall that when the underlying distribution is normally distributed

$$t = \frac{\bar{x} - \mu}{s/\sqrt{n}}$$

follows a t distribution with $n - 1$ degrees of freedom. Thus, the small sample confidence interval procedure for μ is based on the t distribution rather than the Z distribution. The small sample formulas for the two-sided and both one-sided confidence intervals for μ are listed below.

SMALL SAMPLE CONFIDENCE INTERVALS FOR A MEAN

When underlying distribution is approximately normally distributed

1. a two-sided confidence interval for μ is given by

$$\bar{x} \pm t_{\text{crit}} \times \frac{s}{\sqrt{n}}$$

2. a one-sided upper bound confidence interval for μ is given by

$$\mu \leq \bar{x} + t_{\text{crit}} \times \frac{s}{\sqrt{n}}$$

3. a one-sided lower bound confidence interval for μ is given by

$$\mu \geq \bar{x} - t_{\text{crit}} \times \frac{s}{\sqrt{n}}$$

where the t_{crit} values have $n - 1$ degrees of freedom and can be found in Table A.7.

Note that the only difference between the large sample Z confidence interval and the small sample t confidence interval formulas for estimating a mean is that they used different critical values (i.e., z_{crit} and t_{crit}). The value of t_{crit} depends on the confidence level and the degrees of freedom of s and approaches the value of z_{crit} as the degrees of freedom become large. For example, in a 95% confidence interval the z_{crit} value is always 1.96, whereas the t_{crit} values for 10, 20, 30, and 60 degrees of freedom are 2.228, 2.086, 2.042, and 2.000, respectively.

Example 6.8

In the article "Low ghrelin level affects bone biomarkers in childhood obesity" published in the journal *Nutrition Research* (Nassar, 2007), the variable bone age was studied for samples of 20 obese children and 12 normal weight children. The summary statistics given in Table 6.3 were reported in this article. Use this data to

a. compute a 95% confidence interval for the mean bone age of an obese child.

b. compute a 95% confidence interval for the mean bone age of an normal weight child.

c. determine whether there appears to be a difference between the mean bone ages of obese and normal weight children.

Solutions Based on the summary statistics in Table 6.3 and assuming that each of the subpopulations for bone age is approximately normal,

a. a 95% confidence interval for the mean bone age of an obese child is

$$10.75 \pm 2.093 \times \frac{3.51}{\sqrt{20}}$$

TABLE 6.3 Summary Statistics on Bone Age for 20 Obese and 12 Normal Weight Children

Weight Classification	Sample Size	Mean	Standard Deviation
Obese	20	10.75	3.51
Normal	12	8.83	2.86

where 2.093 is the value of t_{crit} for a 95% confidence interval with $20 - 1 = 19$ degrees of freedom. Thus, a 95% confidence interval for the mean bone age of an obese child is 9.11–12.39 years.

b. a 95% confidence interval for the mean bone age of a normal weight child is

$$8.83 \pm 2.201 \times \frac{2.86}{\sqrt{12}}$$

where 2.201 is the value of t_{crit} for a 95% confidence interval with $12 - 1 = 11$ degrees of freedom. Thus, a 95% confidence interval for the mean bone age of an obese child is 7.01–10.65 years.

c. because the confidence intervals in parts (a) and (b) overlap, there is no evidence based on the observed data that there is a difference between the mean bone ages for obese and normal weight children.

In Example 6.8, it was assumed that both the populations sampled were approximately normally distributed. In practice, the assumption of normality must be checked and verified before a small sample t confidence interval for the mean is computed. The normality assumption can be investigated with a normal probability plot or a histogram of the sampled data. Thus, when the assumption of normality is not satisfied, the actual confidence level may be substantially lower than claimed. When the normality assumption fails to be met and $n < 100$, a bootstrap confidence interval for the mean should be computed instead of a small sample confidence interval (see Section 6.3).

Example 6.9
The summary statistics in Table 6.4 and the normal probability plot given in Figure 6.2 were computed from the Birth Weight data set for the birth weights (BWT) of babies born to Caucasian mothers who smoked during pregnancy.
Use this data to

a. assess the normality assumption.

b. compute a 95% confidence interval for the mean birth weight of a baby born to a Caucasian mother who smoked during pregnancy.

Solutions Based on the summary statistics given in Table 6.4 and the normal probability plot in Figure 6.2,

a. since the normal probability plot passes the fat pencil test, it appears reasonable to assume the underlying distribution of birth weights of babies born to a Caucasian mother who smoked during pregnancy is approximately normal.

TABLE 6.4 Summary Statistics on the Birth Weights of $n = 52$ Babies Born to Caucasian Mothers Who Smoked During Pregnancy

Sample Size	Mean	Standard Deviation
52	2828.7	627

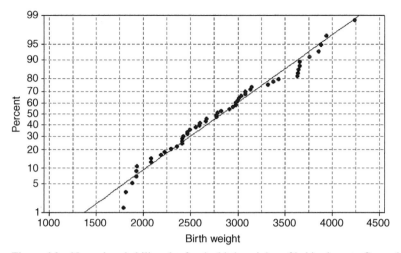

Figure 6.2   Normal probability plot for the birth weights of babies born to Caucasian mothers who smoked during pregnancy.

b. a 95% confidence interval for the mean birth weight of a baby born to a Caucasian mother who smoked during pregnancy will be based on the small sample t procedure with $52 - 1 = 51$ degrees of freedom. Because the t-values for 51 degrees of freedom are not listed in Table A.7, the degrees of freedom closest to 51 in Table A.7 will be used. Thus, the t_{crit} value for a 95% confidence interval with 60 degrees of freedom will be used, and the 95% confidence interval for the mean birth weight of a baby born to a Caucasian mother is

$$2828.7 \pm 2.000 \times \frac{627}{\sqrt{52}}$$

which yields the interval 2654.8–3002.6.

Thus, based on the observed sample it appears that the mean birth weight of a baby born to a Caucasian mother is at least 2655 g and possibly as much as 3003 g.

6.3.5 Determining the Sample Size for a Confidence Interval for the Mean

As was the case with confidence intervals for a population proportion, it is also possible to determine the sample size required to attain a prespecified margin of error in a $(1 - \alpha) \times 100\%$ confidence interval for the mean. Note that the margin of error in a confidence interval for the mean depends on the value of n through the standard error of $\bar{x}$ and the value of z_{crit} or t_{crit}. Since the value of t_{crit} cannot be determined without knowing the value of n, the formula used for determining the sample size n needed for a prespecified margin of error for a $(1 - \alpha) \times 100\%$ confidence interval will be based on the large sample procedure that uses z_{crit} instead of t_{crit} since z_{crit} is independent of n. The formula used to determine the value of n that will provide a margin of error of approximately equal to the prespecified value ME in a $(1 - \alpha) \times 100\%$ confidence interval for a mean is given below.

DETERMINING THE SAMPLE SIZE FOR A CONFIDENCE INTERVAL μ

The sample size required to produce a $(1 - \alpha) \times$ 100% confidence interval for estimating a mean having a prespecified margin of error equal to ME is

where $\dot{\sigma}$ is a reasonable prior estimate of the value of population standard deviation σ.

$$n = \left(\frac{z_{\text{crit}} \times \dot{\sigma}}{\text{ME}} \right)^2$$

Note that a reasonable prior estimate of the value of σ is required for determining the appropriate sample size. Thus, the researcher must come up with an educated guess of the approximate value of σ in order to determine the sample size needed for the study. The prior guess of σ can often be based on a pilot study, prior research, or in a worst case scenario $\dot{\sigma}$ can be based on the maximum and minimum values in target population using

$$\dot{\sigma} = \frac{\text{maximum value} - \text{minimum value}}{4}$$

Example 6.10

Determine the sample size needed to produce the prespecified margin of error when

    a. ME $= 5$ and $\dot{\sigma} = 50$ in a 98% confidence interval for the mean.

    b. ME $= 50$ and $\dot{\sigma} = 250$ in a 90% confidence interval for the mean.

    c. ME $= 5$ and $\dot{\sigma} = 10$ in a 99% confidence interval for the mean.

    d. ME $= 50$ and the population is believed to range from a minimum value of 100 to a maximum value of 1500 in a 95% confidence interval for the mean.

Solutions The sample size needed to produce the prespecified margin of error when

    a. ME $= 5$ and $\dot{\sigma} = 50$ in a 98% confidence interval for the mean is

$$n = \left[\frac{2.326 \times 50}{5} \right]^2 = 541.03$$

    Thus, use a sample size of $n = 542$ to attain a margin of error of roughly ME $= 5$ in a 98% confidence interval for the mean.

    b. ME $= 50$ and $\dot{\sigma} = 250$ in a 90% confidence interval for the mean is

$$n = \left[\frac{1.645 \times 250}{50} \right]^2 = 67.7$$

    Thus, use a sample size of $n = 68$ to attain a margin of error of roughly ME $= 50$ in a 90% confidence interval for the mean.

    c. ME $= 5$ and $\dot{\sigma} = 10$ in a 99% confidence interval for the mean is

$$n = \left[\frac{2.576 \times 10}{5} \right]^2 = 26.5$$

    Thus, use a sample size of $n = 27$ to attain a margin of error of roughly ME $= 5$ in a 99% confidence interval for the mean.

    d. ME $= 50$ and the population is believed to range from a minimum value of 100 to a maximum value of 1500 in a 95% confidence interval for the mean is

$$n = \left[\frac{2.326 \times \frac{1500 - 100}{4}}{50} \right]^2 = 188.3$$

Thus, use a sample size of $n = 189$ to attain a margin of error of roughly ME $= 50$ in a 95% confidence interval for the mean.

6.4 BOOTSTRAP CONFIDENCE INTERVALS

While the sampling distribution of $\bar{x}$ can usually be approximated by a normal distribution or a t distribution, the sampling distributions of many of the commonly used estimators are not so easily modeled. For example, the sampling distribution of the estimate of a percentile is generally hard to determine as is the sampling distribution of the sample standard deviation. Because a confidence interval for an unknown parameter is based on the sampling distribution of the estimator used to estimate the parameter, it is very important to know the sampling distribution of the estimator.

When the sampling distribution of an unbiased or a low-bias estimator of a parameter θ is unknown and cannot be approximated with a normal distribution, a *bootstrap confidence interval* can be used for estimating θ. The bootstrapping procedure actually produces a simulated sampling distribution for the estimator that can then be used to compute an approximate $(1 - \alpha) \times 100\%$ confidence interval for the unknown parameter being estimated. The bootstrap confidence interval procedure is outlined below.

THE BOOTSTRAP CONFIDENCE INTERVAL PROCEDURE

A $(1 - \alpha) \times 100\%$ bootstrap confidence interval for a parameter θ based on an estimator T and a random sample of n observations is computed as follows:

1. Draw a random sample of n observations from the observed sample drawing with replacement.

2. Compute the value of T for this simulated sample.

3. Repeat steps 1 and 2 until M values of T have been computed.

4. The M values of T form the approximate sampling distribution of T.

5. Determine the $100 \times \frac{\alpha}{2}$th and the $100 \times (1 - \frac{\alpha}{2})$th percentiles of the approximate sampling distribution of T.

6. The $(1 - \alpha) \times 100\%$ bootstrap confidence interval is L to U where L is the $100 \times \frac{\alpha}{2}$th percentile and U is the $100 \times (1 - \frac{\alpha}{2})$th percentile of the bootstrapped sampling distribution of T.

Note that the percentage of values trapped between the $100 \times \frac{\alpha}{2}$th and $100 \times (1 - \frac{\alpha}{2})$th percentiles of any distribution is $(1 - \alpha) \times 100\%$. Thus, the values falling between the $100 \times \frac{\alpha}{2}$th and $100 \times (1 - \frac{\alpha}{2})$th percentiles of the bootstrapped sampling distribution of T constitute an approximate $(1 - \alpha) \times 100\%$ confidence interval for θ. In particular, when T is an unbiased or has small bias for estimating a parameter θ

- the 5th and 95th percentiles of the bootstrap distribution of T form a 90% bootstrap confidence interval for θ;
- the 2.5th and 97.5th percentiles of the bootstrap distribution of T form a 95% bootstrap confidence interval for θ;
- the 1st and 99th percentiles of the bootstrap distribution of T form a 98% bootstrap confidence interval for θ;
- the 0.5th and 99.5th percentiles of the bootstrap distribution of T form a 99% bootstrap confidence interval for θ.

Example 6.11

Suppose a 95% confidence interval is desired for the median birth weight of babies born to mothers who smoked during pregnancy. Based on the Birth Weight data set the estimate of median birth weight of babies born to mothers who smoked during pregnancy is $\tilde{x} = 2775.5$ g. Now, because the sampling distribution of the estimator of the median is unknown, the bootstrap confidence interval procedure will be used to compute an approximate 95% confidence interval for median birth weight of babies born to mothers who smoked during pregnancy.

Now, $M = 1000$ bootstrap samples will be used to approximate the sampling distribution of the sample median. From the bootstrapped sampling distribution, an approximate 95% bootstrap confidence interval for the median is found by determining the 2.5th and 97.5th percentiles of the bootstrap sampling distribution of the sample median. The resulting 95% bootstrap confidence interval for the median birth weight of babies born to mothers who smoked during pregnancy is 2495–2998.5 g.

The bootstrap confidence interval procedure is easily implemented and works for most estimators. In particular, bootstrap confidence intervals can be used for estimating the median, percentiles, the coefficient of variation, and many other commonly used estimators. In fact, the bootstrap confidence interval procedure can be used for computing a small sample confidence interval for the mean when the underlying distribution is not approximately normally distributed. More information on bootstrap confidence intervals and their limitations can be found in *An Introduction to the Bootstrap* by Efron and Tibshirani (Efron and Tibshirani, 1993).

6.5 TWO SAMPLE COMPARATIVE CONFIDENCE INTERVALS

In comparative studies with two distinct populations, say X and Y, the goal is often to estimate and compare the values of the parameter of interest in each of the populations. In particular, proportions or means are typically compared by looking at the difference between their sample estimates based on the X and Y samples. In this section, confidence intervals for the difference of two proportions and confidence intervals for the relative risk will be considered. Due to special considerations that involve the sampling distribution of the difference of two sample means, the confidence intervals for the difference of two means will be discussed in Chapter 7 along with hypothesis tests for comparing two means.

6.5.1 Confidence Intervals for Comparing Two Proportions

Suppose independent random samples are collected from the X and Y populations, and n_X is the number of observations sampled from population X and n_Y the number sampled from population Y. A confidence interval based on the difference of the sample proportions can be used for making statistical inferences about the difference between the values of the X and Y population proportions.

Let p_X and p_Y be the unknown proportions associated with the X and Y populations, and let $\hat{p}_X$ and $\hat{p}_Y$ be the sample estimates of p_X and p_Y. The sampling distribution of $\hat{p}_X - \hat{p}_Y$ will be approximately normally distributed when each of

$$n_X p_X, \ n_Y p_Y, \ n_X(1 - p_X), \ \text{and} \ n_Y(1 - p_Y)$$

is greater than 5. The formula for a large sample $(1 - \alpha) \times 100\%$ confidence interval for the difference of two proportions is given below.

LARGE SAMPLE CONFIDENCE INTERVALS FOR $p_X - p_Y$

When $n_X p_X$, $n_Y p_Y$, $n_X(1 - p_X)$, and $n_Y(1 - p_Y)$ are all greater than 5, a $(1 - \alpha) \times$ 100% confidence interval for $p_X - p_Y$ is

$$\hat{p}_X - \hat{p}_Y \pm z_{\text{crit}} \times \sqrt{\frac{\hat{p}_X(1 - \hat{p}_X)}{n_X} + \frac{\hat{p}_Y(1 - \hat{p}_Y)}{n_Y}}$$

where z_{crit} can be found in Table A.4.

Note that the formula for a large sample confidence interval for the difference of two proportions follows the general formula for a large sample confidence interval that is given by

$$\text{estimate} \pm z_{\text{crit}} \times \text{se}$$

In this case, the estimate of the difference is $\hat{p}_X - \hat{p}_Y$ and the estimated standard error of $\hat{p}_X - \hat{p}_Y$ is

$$\text{se}(\hat{p}_X - \hat{p}_Y) = \sqrt{\frac{\hat{p}_X(1 - \hat{p}_X)}{n_X} + \frac{\hat{p}_Y(1 - \hat{p}_Y)}{n_Y}}$$

Also, because p_X and p_Y will be unknown, a large sample confidence interval for the difference of two proportions can be safely used when

$$n_X \hat{p}_X, \ n_Y \hat{p}_Y, \ n_X(1 - \hat{p}_X), \ \text{and} \ n_Y(1 - \hat{p}_Y)$$

are all greater than 5.

A confidence interval for the difference of two proportions produces a plausible set of estimates of the difference based on the observed data. Furthermore, when 0 is included in the confidence interval the sample data is suggesting that 0 is a reasonable estimate of the difference in the proportions. In this case, the data are suggesting it is plausible for the two population proportions to be equal. On the other hand, when 0 is not in the confidence interval the sample data provides some evidence that the two population proportions are not equal (i.e., $p_X \neq p_Y$). When a confidence interval for the difference of two proportions does not contain the value 0, the population proportions are said to be *statistically significantly different*. That is, when 0 is not in the confidence interval for the difference, there is enough statistical evidence to conclude that the two proportions are different. A more detailed discussion of statistical significance is given in Chapter 7.

Example 6.12

Central retinal vein occlusion (CRVO) is a serious eye problem affecting approximately 60,000 people per year. CRVO is caused by a blood clot in the central retinal vein and can lead to retinal detachment or glaucoma. In the retrospective case–control study, "Central Retinal Vein Occlusion Case–Control Study," investigating the risk factors for CRVO, published in the *American Journal of Ophthalmology* (Koizumi et al., 2007), the authors reported the summary statistics given in Table 6.5. Use this data to compute a 95% confidence interval for the difference in the proportion of the CRVO population and the control population having

a. the hypertension risk factor.

b. the diabetes risk factor.

Solutions Table 6.6 contains the sample proportions corresponding to the counts given in Table 6.5 that will be used in computing the confidence intervals for the difference of the proportions.

TABLE 6.5   Summary Counts for a Study on the CRVO Risk Factors for Individuals in the CRVO Group ($n = 144$) and Control Group ($n = 144$)

Risk Factor	CRVO Group	Control Group
Hypertension	90	59
Diabetes	23	12
Glaucoma	44	13
Atrial fibrillation	18	8

The 95% confidence interval for the difference in the proportion of the CRVO population and the control population having

a. the hypertension risk factor is

$$0.625 - 0.410 \pm 1.96\sqrt{\frac{0.625(1 - 0.625)}{144} + \frac{0.410(1 - 0.410)}{144}}$$

which results in the interval 0.215 ± 0.114. Thus, a 95% confidence interval for the difference in the CRVO and control proportions having the hypertension risk factor is 0.101–0.329. Hence, it appears that the proportion of the CRVO population having hypertension is at least 10% more than that of the control population and possibly as much as 36% more. Thus, because 0 is not included in the confidence interval there is a statistically significant difference between the proportion of CRVO and the control populations having the hypertension risk factor.

b. the diabetes risk factor is

$$0.160 - 0.083 \pm \sqrt{\frac{0.160(1 - 0.160)}{144} + \frac{0.083(1 - 0.083)}{144}}$$

which results in the interval 0.077 ± 0.075. Thus, a 95% confidence interval for the difference in the proportion of CRVO and the control individuals having the diabetes risk factor is 0.002–0.152. Hence, it appears that the proportion of the CRVO population having diabetes is at least 0.2% more than that of a control population and possibly as much as 15% more. Thus, because 0 is not included in the confidence interval there is a statistically significant difference between the proportion of CRVO and the control populations having the diabetes risk factor.

A one-sided confidence interval for the difference of two proportions is sometimes preferable to a two-sided confidence interval. For example, suppose the goal of a research project is to show that a new drug is better than the drug that has been used previously.

TABLE 6.6   Sample Proportions for the CRVO Risk Factors for Individuals in the CRVO Group ($n = 144$) and Control Group ($n = 144$)

Risk Factor	CRVO Group	Control Group
Hypertension	0.625	0.410
Diabetes	0.160	0.083
Glaucoma	0.306	0.090
Atrial fibrillation	0.125	0.056

Let p_N and p_O be the proportions of individuals whose condition is improved after being administered the new and old drugs, respectively. Because the researcher believes that the new drug is better than the old drug, it is reasonable to assume that p_N will be larger than p_O. Thus, a lower bound confidence interval for $p_N - p_O$ would be useful in determining how much better the new drug is. The formulas for the large sample one-sided confidence intervals for the difference of two proportions are given below.

LARGE SAMPLE ONE-SIDED CONFIDENCE INTERVALS FOR $p_X - p_Y$

When $n_X p_X$, $n_Y p_Y$, $n_X(1 - p_X)$, and $n_Y(1 - p_Y)$ are all greater than 5, a $(1 - \alpha) \times 100\%$

1. lower bound confidence interval for $p_X - p_Y$ is $p_X - p_Y \geq$

$$\widehat{p}_X - \widehat{p}_Y - z_{\text{crit}} \times \text{se}(\widehat{p}_X - \widehat{p}_Y)$$

2. upper bound confidence interval for $p_X - p_Y$ is $p_X - p_Y \leq$

$$\widehat{p}_X - \widehat{p}_Y + z_{\text{crit}} \times \text{se}(\widehat{p}_X - \widehat{p}_Y)$$

where z_{crit} can be found in Table A.4.

Note that when 0 is not included in a one-sided confidence interval for the difference $p_X - p_Y$, there is a statistically significant difference between the proportions p_X and p_Y.

Example 6.13
For the CRVO study in Example 6.12, suppose the researchers believe that individuals in the CRVO population are more likely to have the hypertension risk factor than are individuals in the control population. In this case, it would be reasonable to consider a lower bound confidence interval to determine how much larger the proportion is for the CRVO group.

Using the CRVO data in Table 6.6, a 95% lower bound confidence interval for the difference in the proportion of CRVO and the control individuals having the hypertension risk factor is

$$0.625 - 0.410 \pm 1.645 \sqrt{\frac{0.625(1 - 0.625)}{144} + \frac{0.410(1 - 0.410)}{144}}$$

which results in the interval $p_X - p_Y \geq 0.120$. Thus, based on the observed data it appears that the proportion of the CRVO population having hypertension is at least 12% more than that of the control population. Furthermore, because 0 is not in the lower bound confidence interval for the difference of the proportions, there the proportion of the CRVO population having the hypertension risk factor is statistically significantly larger than that of the control population.

The sample size required for a prespecified margin of error for a large sample $(1 - \alpha) \times 100\%$ confidence interval for the difference of two proportions can be determined by solving the equation

$$\text{ME} = z_{\text{crit}} \times \sqrt{\frac{\widehat{p}_X(1 - \widehat{p}_X)}{n} + \frac{\widehat{p}_Y(1 - \widehat{p}_Y)}{n}}$$

for n. In this case, n is the common sample size n that will be used for the samples drawn from the X and Y populations (i.e., $n_X = n_Y = n$). The formulas that produce the common value of n_X and n_Y for a prespecified margin of error for a $(1 - \alpha) \times 100\%$ confidence interval for the difference $p_X - p_Y$ are given below.

DETERMINING THE SAMPLE SIZE FOR A CONFIDENCE INTERVAL FOR $p_X - p_Y$

---

1. When $\hat{p}_X$ and $\hat{p}_Y$ are prior estimates of the unknown values of p_X and p_Y, the overall sample size required for a margin of error equal to ME for a $(1 - \alpha) \times 100\%$ confidence interval for estimating $p_X - p_Y$ is

$$n = \left(\frac{z_{\text{crit}}}{\text{ME}}\right)^2 \times (\hat{p}_X(1 - \hat{p}_X) + \hat{p}_Y(1 - \hat{p}_Y))$$

2. When no prior estimates of the values of p_X and p_Y are available, a conservative estimate of the common sample size n is

$$n = \frac{1}{2}\left(\frac{z_{\text{crit}}}{\text{ME}}\right)^2$$

In both cases, $n_X = n_Y = \frac{n}{2}$.

When a common value of n_X and n_Y is undesirable, more information, such as cost restrictions or total sample size restrictions, must be supplied along with the prespecified margin of error. Also, the conservative values of n_X and n_Y are found by using $\hat{p}_X = \hat{p}_Y = 0.5$. In order to reduce the cost of sampling, it is always preferable to use reasonable estimates of the proportions p_X and p_Y whenever available. The conservative value of n should only be used in cases where no reasonable prior estimates of the values of the proportions p_X and p_Y can be obtained.

Example 6.14
Determine the common value of the sample sizes n_X and n_Y when

a. ME = 0.04, $\hat{p}_X = 0.30$, and $\hat{p}_Y = 0.40$ in a 90% two-sided confidence interval for $p_X - p_Y$.

b. ME = 0.05, $\hat{p}_X = 0.60$, and $\hat{p}_Y = 0.80$ in a 95% two-sided confidence interval for $p_X - p_Y$.

c. Prior guesses of p_X and p_Y are unavailable and ME = 0.08 in a 99% two-sided confidence interval for $p_X - p_Y$.

d. Prior guesses of p_X and p_Y are unavailable and ME = 0.05 in a 95% two-sided confidence interval for $p_X - p_Y$.

Solutions The common value of the sample sizes n_X and n_Y when

a. ME = 0.04, $\hat{p}_X = 0.30$, and $\hat{p}_Y = 0.40$ in a 90% two-sided confidence interval for $p_X - p_Y$ is

$$n = \left(\frac{1.282}{0.04}\right)^2 \times (0.30(1 - 0.30) + 0.40(1 - 0.40)) = 462.24$$

Thus, by using $n_X = n_Y = 463$ for the common sample size, the margin of error in a 90% two-sided confidence interval for $p_X - p_Y$ will be roughly ME = 0.04.

b. ME = 0.05, $\hat{p}_X = 0.60$, and $\hat{p}_Y = 0.80$ in a 95% two-sided confidence interval for $p_X - p_Y$ is

$$n = \left(\frac{1.96}{0.05}\right)^2 \times (0.60(1 - 0.60) + 0.80(1 - 0.80)) = 614.66$$

Thus, by using $n_X = n_Y = 615$ for the common sample size, the margin of error in a 95% two-sided confidence interval for $p_X - p_Y$ will be roughly ME = 0.05.

c. prior guesses of p_X and p_Y are unavailable and ME = 0.08 in a 99% two-sided confidence interval for $p_X - p_Y$ is

$$n = \frac{1}{2}\left(\frac{2.576}{0.08}\right)^2 = 518.42$$

Thus, by using $n_X = n_Y = 519$ for the conservative value of the common sample size, the margin of error in a 99% two-sided confidence interval for $p_X - p_Y$ will be roughly ME = 0.08.

d. prior guesses of p_X and p_Y are unavailable and ME = 0.05 in a 95% two-sided confidence interval for $p_X - p_Y$ is

$$n = \frac{1}{2}\left(\frac{1.96}{0.05}\right)^2 = 768.32$$

Thus, by using $n_X = n_Y = 519$ for the conservative value of the common sample size, the margin of error in a 99% two-sided confidence interval for $p_X - p_Y$ will be roughly ME = 0.05.

6.5.2 Confidence Intervals for the Relative Risk

While the comparison of two proportions is often based on their difference, the ratio of two proportions can also be used for comparing proportions and is often used in biomedical research. For example, the relative risk is a parameter that is commonly studied in epidemiology, and the relative risk is formed by taking the ratio of two risk proportions. In particular, the relative risk is defined to be a proportion of diseased individuals who were exposed to a particular risk factor divided by the proportion of diseased individuals who were not exposed to the risk factor. That is,

$$\text{Relative risk} = \text{RR} = \frac{P(\text{disease}|\text{exposure to the risk factor})}{P(\text{disease}|\text{no exposure to the risk factor})}$$

and takes on values between 0 and ∞ and is used as a measure of the strength of association between the risk factor and the disease.

The relative risk is a parameter that is often estimated in a prospective cohort study where individuals with and without a particular disease or condition are studied in regard to a particular set of risk factors. It is also important to note that the relative risk cannot be estimated in a case–control study because a case–control study is a retrospective study. That is, the individuals in a case–control study are selected on the basis of the outcome variable, diseased or not, rather than the exposure to the risk factors.

The relative risk for a particular risk factor provides a simple comparison of the risk of the disease for an individual exposed to the risk factor and the risk of the disease for an individual who is not exposed to the risk factor. In particular, when the relative risk is

- RR = 1 then there is no difference in the risk of contracting the disease for individuals exposed to the risk factor and those who were not exposed to the risk factor.
- RR < 1 then the risk of contracting the disease is actually less for an individual exposed to the risk factor than it is for an individual not exposed to the risk factor.
- RR > 1 means the risk of contracting the disease is higher for an individual exposed to the risk factor than it is for an individual not exposed to the risk factor.

Thus, when the relative risk is less than 1 the risk factor appears to be a protective factor, and when the relative risk is greater than 1 the risk factor appears to increases the risk of contracting the disease. For example, a relative risk of 2.5 indicates that an individual exposed to the risk factor is 2.5 times as likely to contract the disease as is an

TABLE 6.7 A 2 × 2 Contingency Table Summary of the Data Used in Estimating the Relative Risk

		Disease Present	Disease not Present	Total
Risk factor	Present	a	b	$a + b$
	Absent	c	d	$c + d$

individual who is not exposed to the risk factor, and a risk factor of 0.5 would indicate an individual exposed to the risk factor is only half as likely to contract the disease as is an individual who is not exposed to the risk factor.

Using the sample data that result from a clinical trial or prospective study, it is possible to estimate the relative risk of a disease or particular condition for exposure to a risk factor. When the sample consists of $a + b$ individuals exposed to the risk factor of which a have the disease, and $c + d$ individuals in the study were not exposed to the risk factor of which c have the disease, the sample data are often summarized in a 2 × 2 contingency table as shown in Table 6.7,

Based on the 2 × 2 contingency table given in Table 6.7, the estimated risk for the exposure group is

$$\widehat{P}(\text{disease}|\text{exposure to the risk factor}) = \widehat{p}_{\text{E}} = \frac{a}{a + b}$$

and the estimated risk for the nonexposure group is

$$\widehat{P}(\text{disease}|\text{no exposure to the risk factor}) = \widehat{p}_{\text{U}} = \frac{c}{c + d}$$

The point estimator of the relative risk is based on the ratio of the estimates of the risk associated with the disease for the exposure group and the unexposed group. That is,

$$\widehat{RR} = \frac{\widehat{p}_{\text{E}}}{\widehat{p}_{\text{U}}} = \frac{\frac{a}{a+b}}{\frac{c}{c+d}}$$

The sampling distribution of $\widehat{RR}$ is not generally approximately normally distributed for even large samples; however, the sampling distribution of the natural logarithm of $\widehat{RR}$ is approximately normally distributed for large samples. In fact, $\ln(\widehat{RR})$ is approximately normally distributed with mean $\ln(RR)$ and standard distribution is approximately equal to the estimated standard error of $\ln(\widehat{RR})$, which is

$$\text{se}(\ln(\widehat{RR})) = \sqrt{\frac{b}{a(a + b)} + \frac{d}{c(c + d)}}$$

A large sample confidence interval for the relative risk can be based on the estimator $\ln(\widehat{RR})$. The procedure for computing a large sample $(1 - \alpha) \times 100\%$ confidence for the relative risk is outlined below.

A LARGE SAMPLE CONFIDENCE INTERVAL FOR THE RELATIVE RISK

Using the 2×2 contingency table given in Table 6.7, a large sample $(1 - \alpha) \times 100\%$ confidence interval for the relative risk, L to U, is found by performing the following steps:

1. Compute the value of the estimate of the relative risk (i.e., $\widehat{RR}$).

2. Take the natural logarithm of $\widehat{RR}$ (i.e., $\ln(\widehat{RR})$).

3. Compute the value of the estimated standard error of $\ln(\widehat{RR})$.

$$se = \sqrt{\frac{b}{a(a+b)} + \frac{d}{c(c+d)}}$$

4. Determine a $(1 - \alpha) \times 100\%$ confidence for the natural logarithm of the relative risk using

$$\ln(\widehat{RR}) \pm z_{\text{crit}} \times se$$

5. A $(1 - \alpha) \times 100\%$ confidence interval for the relative risk is found by exponentiating the lower and upper end points of the confidence interval for $\ln(RR)$ that results in.

$$L = e^{\ln(\widehat{RR}) - z_{\text{crit}} \times se}$$

and

$$U = e^{\ln(\widehat{RR}) + z_{\text{crit}} \times se}$$

The value of z_{crit} can be found in Table A.4.

Because the relative risk is the ratio of two proportions, a ratio having the value 1 is the key value in determining whether the risk factor is statistically significant or not. That is, when 1 is a reasonable estimate of the relative risk, the data are suggesting that exposure to the risk factor does not significantly increase or decrease the risk associated with contracting the disease. On the other hand, when 1 is not a reasonable estimate of the relative risk, the data are suggesting that the risk factor does significantly increase or decrease the risk associated with contracting the disease. Thus, when a confidence interval for the relative risk contains the value 1 there is no statistical evidence that the risk factor is significant; when a confidence interval for the relative risk does not contain the value 1, then there is sufficient statistical evidence to conclude that the risk is significant.

Example 6.15

A prospective study on the association between skin color and cardiovascular disease (CVD) mortality is reported in the article "Skin color and mortality risk among men: The Puerto Rico Health Program" published in the *Annals of Epidemiology* (Borrell et al., 2007). One of the goals of the study was to investigate the relative risk of CVD death for light and dark skinned males. The authors reported the summary data given in Table 6.8.

One of the research hypotheses put forth in this study was that dark skinned males have a higher risk of death due to CVD than do light skinned males. Use the summary data in Table 6.8 to

a. estimate the relative risk of death due to CVD for dark skinned males compared to light skinned males.

b. compute the estimated standard error of $\ln(\widehat{RR})$.

c. compute a 95% confidence interval for the relative risk of death due to CVD for dark skinned males compared to light skinned males.

d. determine whether the sample data provide any evidence suggesting that dark skinned males have a higher risk of death due to CVD than do light skinned males.

TABLE 6.8 A 2 × 2 Contingency Table of Mortality Counts Due to CVD and Other Causes According to Skin Color

		Death due to CVD	Death not due to CVD	Total
Skin Color	Dark skin	37	590	· 627
	Light skin	209	4162	4371

Solutions Using the mortality data given in Table 6.8

a. the estimated relative risk of death due to CVD for dark skinned males compared to light skinned males is

$$\widehat{RR} = \frac{\frac{37}{627}}{\frac{590}{4371}} = 1.23$$

b. the estimated standard error of $\ln(\widehat{RR})$ is

$$se = \sqrt{\frac{590}{37(627)} + \frac{4162}{209(4371)}} = 0.173$$

c. a 95% confidence interval for the relative risk of death due to CVD for dark skinned males compared to light skinned males is

$$e^{\ln(1.23)-1.96\times0.173} \text{ to } e^{\ln(1.23)+1.96\times0.173}$$

which yields an interval of estimates of the relative risk of 0.88–1.73.

d. the sample data do not provide statistically significant evidence suggesting that dark skinned males have a higher risk of death due to CVD than do light skinned males since the value 1 is in the confidence interval for the relative risk.

GLOSSARY

Bootstrap Confidence Interval A bootstrap confidence interval of a parameter θ is formed from the $100 \times \frac{\alpha}{2}$th and $100 \times (1 - \frac{\alpha}{2})$th percentiles of the bootstrapped sampling distribution of an unbiased estimator T of a parameter θ.

Confidence Interval A confidence interval is an interval estimator that produces an interval of estimates that captures the true value of an unknown parameter with a prespecified probability.

Confidence Level The confidence level is the prespecified probability for which a confidence interval procedure will capture the true value of the parameter being estimated.

Interval Estimator An interval estimator is a rule that produces an interval of estimates of an unknown parameter.

Large Sample Confidence Interval for μ A large sample $(1 - \alpha) \times 100\%$ confidence interval for a mean μ is

$$\bar{x} \pm z_{crit} \times \frac{s}{\sqrt{n}}$$

Large Sample Confidence Interval for p A large sample $(1 - \alpha) \times 100\%$ confidence interval for a proportion p is

$$\widehat{p} \pm z_{\text{crit}} \times \sqrt{\frac{\widehat{p}(1 - \widehat{p})}{n}}$$

Large Sample Confidence Interval for $p_X - p_Y$ A large sample $(1 - \alpha) \times 100\%$ confidence interval for the difference of two proportions, $p_X - p_Y$, is

$$\widehat{p}_X - \widehat{p}_Y \pm z_{\text{crit}} \times \sqrt{\frac{\widehat{p}_X(1 - \widehat{p}_X)}{n_X} + \frac{\widehat{p}_Y(1 - \widehat{p}_Y)}{n_Y}}$$

Large Sample Confidence Interval for Relative Risk A large sample $(1 - \alpha) \times 100\%$ confidence interval for the relative risk is

$$e^{\ln(\widehat{RR}) - z_{\text{crit}} \times \text{se}} \quad \text{to} \quad e^{\ln(\widehat{RR}) + z_{\text{crit}} \times \text{se}}$$

Relative Risk The relative risk of contracting a disease or a having a particular condition for a risk factor is

$$RR = \frac{P(\text{disease}|\text{exposure to the risk factor})}{P(\text{disease}|\text{no exposure to the risk factor})}$$

Small Sample Confidence Interval for μ A small sample $(1 - \alpha) \times 100\%$ confidence interval for a mean μ is

$$\bar{x} \pm t_{\text{crit}} \times \frac{s}{\sqrt{n}}$$

provided the underlying distribution is approximately normal.

EXERCISES

6.1 What is an interval estimator?

6.2 What is the general form of the large sample interval estimator based on an estimator T and its bound on the error of estimation?

6.3 What is a confidence interval?

6.4 What is the confidence level associated with a confidence interval?

6.5 What is the measure of reliability of a confidence interval?

6.6 How does a confidence interval differ from the large sample interval estimator?

6.7 What is the probability that a 95% confidence interval for μ will contain the true value of μ
  (a) before the sample is drawn?   (b) after the sample is drawn?

6.8 A 95% confidence interval for σ computed from the information in a random sample of $n = 100$ observations is 4.8–8.7.
  (a) Interpret this confidence interval.
  (b) Would a 99% confidence interval for σ be wider or narrower than the 95% confidence interval? Explain.

6.9   For a random sample of size n, which confidence level, 90% or 95%, will produce a wider confidence interval? Explain.

6.10 For a 95% confidence interval, which sample size, 50 or 100, will produce a wider confidence interval? Explain.

6.11 Suppose a 90% and a 95% confidence interval for the population median were computed from a random sample resulting in the two intervals 114–134 and 118–129. Determine which of the intervals is the 90% confidence interval? Explain.

6.12 Suppose a 95% confidence interval for the variance of a population resulting from a random sample of $n = 56$ observations is 84–137. Explain why this confidence interval does or does not provide evidence that
(a) $\sigma^2 \approx 100$. 　　　　　　　　　　　　　　(b) $\sigma^2 \geq 150$.

6.13 Under what conditions can a large sample confidence interval be used for estimating a population proportion?

6.14 What is the form of the large sample confidence interval for estimating a population proportion?

6.15 What is the value of z_{crit} used in a two-sided large sample confidence interval for a proportion when the confidence level is
(a) 90%? 　　　　　　　　　　　　　　　　　　(b) 99%?

6.16 What would happen to the margin of error in a large sample 95% confidence interval for a proportion when the sample size is
(a) doubled? 　　　　　　　　　　　　　　　　(b) halved?

6.17 Use the large sample confidence interval formula to compute a
(a) 95% confidence interval for p when $n = 100$ and $\hat{p} = 0.56$.
(b) 90% confidence interval for p when $n = 60$ and $\hat{p} = 0.21$.
(c) 99% confidence interval for p when $n = 144$ and $\hat{p} = 0.88$.
(d) 95% confidence interval for p when $n = 1000$ and $\hat{p} = 0.96$.

6.18 Determine the sample size for a large sample
(a) 90% confidence interval for a population proportion when $p = 0.4$ and the desired margin of error is 0.04.
(b) 95% confidence interval for a population proportion when $p = 0.75$ and the desired margin of error is 0.03.
(c) 99% confidence interval for a population proportion when the desired margin of error is 0.04 and no prior guess of p is available.
(d) 95% confidence interval for a population proportion when the desired margin of error is 0.025 and no prior guess of p is available.

6.19 Determine the cost of sampling for each part in Exercise 6.18 when the initial cost of sampling is $C_0 = \$800$ and the cost of sampling a unit from this population is $5.

6.20 How is a one-sided confidence interval different from a two-sided confidence interval?

6.21 What is the value of z_{crit} used in a one-sided large sample confidence interval for a proportion when the confidence level is
(a) 90%? 　　　　　　　　　　　　　　　　　　(b) 95%?

6.22 Use the large sample confidence interval formula to compute
(a) a 95% lower bound confidence interval for p when $n = 100$ and $\hat{p} = 0.63$.

(b) a 99% lower bound confidence interval for p when $n = 144$ and $\widehat{p} = 0.87$.

(c) a 95% upper bound confidence interval for p when $n = 1000$ and $\widehat{p} = 0.11$.

(d) a 90% upper bound confidence interval for p when $n = 60$ and $\widehat{p} = 0.19$.

6.23 Determine the sample size for a large sample

(a) 90% upper bound confidence interval for a population proportion when $\dot{p} = 0.3$ and the desired margin of error is 0.05.

(b) 95% lower bound confidence interval for a population proportion when $\dot{p} = 0.25$ and the desired margin of error is 0.035.

(c) 99% lower bound confidence interval for a population proportion when the desired margin of error is 0.03 and no prior guess of p is available.

(d) 95% upper bound confidence interval for a population proportion when the desired margin of error is 0.025 and no prior guess of p is available.

6.24 Determine the cost of sampling for each part in Exercise 6.23 when the initial cost of sampling is $C_0 = \$2100$ and the cost of sampling a unit from this population is $7.50.

6.25 In the article "Paroxetine controlled release in the treatment of menopausal hot flashes: a randomized controlled trial" published in the *Journal of the American Medical Association* (Stearns et al., 2003), the authors reported that 12 of the $n = 58$ patients taking the treatment 25 mg/day paroxetine to control menopausal hot flashes experienced the adverse events dizziness and nausea. On the basis of this data, compute a 95% confidence interval for the proportion of women taking the treatment 25 mg/day paroxetine to control menopausal hot flashes who experience the adverse events dizziness and nausea.

6.26 In the article "Effects of tezosentan on symptoms and clinical outcomes in patients with acute heart failure: the VERITAS randomized controlled trials" published in the *Journal of the American Medical Association* (McMurray et al., 2007), the authors reported that 191 of the $n = 727$ patients in the study using tezosentan died or experienced worsening heart failure by day 7 of the trial. Using this data, compute a 95% confidence interval for the proportion of individuals who would die or experience worsening heart failure within 7 days of a tezosentan treatment.

6.27 For estimating a mean, when it is appropriate to use a

(a) large sample Z confidence interval?

(b) small sample t confidence interval?

6.28 For a confidence interval for a mean, what is the formula for the margin of error in a

(a) small sample t confidence interval?

(b) large sample Z confidence interval?

6.29 How does the estimated standard error of $\bar{x}$ affect the width of a confidence interval for the mean?

6.30 What happens to the margin of error in a confidence interval for the mean when the sample size is

(a) doubled? **(b)** quadrupled?

6.31 What is the value of z_{crit} in a

(a) 90% large sample confidence interval for the mean?

      (b) 95% large sample confidence interval for the mean?

      (c) 99% large sample confidence interval for the mean?

6.32 Using the large sample confidence interval formula, compute a 90% confidence interval for the mean when

      (a) $n = 125$, $\bar{x} = 27.3$, and $s = 8.1$.

      (b) $n = 225$, $\bar{x} = 121.9$, and $s = 21.5$.

      (c) $n = 185$, $\bar{x} = 4.3$, and $s = 0.51$.

6.33 Using the large sample confidence interval formula, compute a 95% confidence interval for the mean when

      (a) $n = 100$, $\bar{x} = 17.2$, and $s = 3.1$.

      (b) $n = 150$, $\bar{x} = 498.1$, and $s = 129.6$.

      (c) $n = 200$, $\bar{x} = 104.3$, and $s = 10.45$.

6.34 Using the large sample confidence interval formula, compute a 99% confidence interval for the mean when

      (a) $n = 120$, $\bar{x} = 33.8$, and $s = 11.4$.

      (b) $n = 250$, $\bar{x} = 1051.2$, and $s = 318.3$.

      (c) $n = 200$, $\bar{x} = 0.34$, and $s = 0.11$.

6.35 Using the large sample confidence interval formula, compute a 95% lower bound confidence interval for the mean when

      (a) $n = 100$, $\bar{x} = 107.2$, and $s = 13.1$.

      (b) $n = 150$, $\bar{x} = 49.8$, and $s = 12.9$.

6.36 Using the large sample confidence interval formula, compute a 95% upper bound confidence interval for the mean when

      (a) $n = 100$, $\bar{x} = 74.8$, and $s = 23.3$.

      (b) $n = 150$, $\bar{x} = 88.7$, and $s = 19.2$.

6.37 What is the value of t_{crit} used in a

      (a) 90% small sample confidence interval for the mean based on a sample of $n = 30$ observations?

      (b) 95% small sample confidence interval for the mean based on a sample of $n = 20$ observations?

      (c) 95% small sample confidence interval for the mean based on a sample of $n = 25$ observations?

      (d) 99% small sample confidence interval for the mean based on a sample of $n = 16$ observations?

6.38 What is the value of t_{crit} used in a

      (a) 90% small sample confidence interval for the mean based on a sample of $n = 60$ observations?

      (b) 95% small sample confidence interval for the mean based on a sample of $n = 80$ observations?

      (c) 95% small sample confidence interval for the mean based on a sample of $n = 115$ observations?

6.39 Which graphical method is best for checking the validity of the normality assumption required of the small sample t confidence interval procedure for estimating a mean?

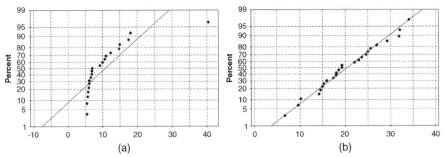

Figure 6.3   Normal probability plots for Exercise 6.40.

6.40 The normal probability plot given in Figure 6.3a contains normal probability plot for a random sample of $n = 121$ observations, and the normal probability plot in Figure 6.3b contains normal probability plot for a random sample of $n = 125$ observations. Determine whether the normal probability plot in

  (a) Figure 6.3a supports the use of the small sample confidence interval procedure for estimating a mean?
  (b) Figure 6.3b supports the use of the small sample confidence interval procedure for estimating a mean?

6.41 Assuming that the distribution being sampled is approximately normally distributed, use the small sample confidence interval formula to compute a 90% two-sided confidence interval for the mean when

  (a) $n = 12, \bar{x} = 77.8$, and $s = 18.4$.
  (b) $n = 22, \bar{x} = 21.9$, and $s = 5.5$.
  (c) $n = 18, \bar{x} = 204.3$, and $s = 29.7$.

6.42 Assuming that the distribution being sampled is approximately normally distributed, use the small sample confidence interval formula to compute a 95% two-sided confidence interval for the mean when

  (a) $n = 20, \bar{x} = 127.0$, and $s = 32.1$.
  (b) $n = 30, \bar{x} = 51.4$, and $s = 8.5$.
  (c) $n = 61, \bar{x} = 2.3$, and $s = 0.7$.

6.43 Assuming that the distribution being sampled is approximately normally distributed, use the small sample confidence interval formula to compute a
  (a) 90% lower bound confidence interval for the mean when $n = 16, \bar{x} = 22.1$, and $s = 1.4$.
  (b) 95% lower bound confidence interval for the mean when $n = 25, \bar{x} = 239.0$, and $s = 55.9$.
  (c) 90% upper bound confidence interval for the mean when $n = 12, \bar{x} = 1204.3$, and $s = 329.7$.
  (d) 95% upper bound confidence interval for the mean when $n = 41, \bar{x} = 24.7$, and $s = 9.1$.

6.44 Assuming that the distribution being sampled is approximately normally distributed, use the small sample confidence interval formula to compute a 95% lower bound confidence interval for the mean when

TABLE 6.9   Raw Data on Free Cortisol Levels at Time 0 and 60 min After Stimulation with Synacthen

Patient	Free Cortisol		Patient	Free Cortisol	
	0 min	60 min		0 min	60 min
1	33	84	6	4	67
2	50	138	7	8	33
3	21	66	8	27	81
4	17	82	9	7	45
5	20	82	10	15	60

(a) $n = 15$, $\bar{x} = 53.1$, and $s = 15.6$.
(b) $n = 25$, $\bar{x} = 849.0$, and $s = 188.5$.
(c) $n = 15$, $\bar{x} = 14.3$, and $s = 2.5$.

6.45 Assuming that the distribution being sampled is approximately normally distributed, use the small sample confidence interval formula to compute a 95% upper bound confidence interval for the mean when
(a) $n = 25$, $\bar{x} = 2.73$, and $s = 0.81$.
(b) $n = 53$, $\bar{x} = 95.4$, and $s = 13.8$.
(c) $n = 58$, $\bar{x} = 1.3$, and $s = 0.2$.

6.46 Using the Benign Breast Disease data set and the appropriate confidence interval formula, compute a 95% confidence interval for the mean weight of
(a) the case group ($n = 50$).
(b) the control group ($n = 150$).

6.47 In the article "Dialyzable free cortisol after stimulation with synacthen" published in the journal *Clinical Biochemistry* (Vogeser et al., 2002), the authors reported the raw data given in Table 6.9 on the free cortisol in 10 patients at time 0 and 60 min following stimulation with synacthen. Use the data given in Table 6.9 to answer the following:
(a) Compute the differences in free cortisol after stimulation with synacthen for the 10 patients in the study.
(b) Compute an estimate of the mean difference in free cortisol after stimulation with synacthen.
(c) Compute the estimated standard error of the mean difference in free cortisol after stimulation with synacthen.
(d) Create a normal probability plot of the differences and assess the assumption of normality required for a small sample confidence interval for the mean.
(e) Compute a 95% confidence interval for the mean difference in free cortisol after stimulation with synacthen.

6.48 In the article "Treatment of piriformis syndrome with Botox" published in *The Internet Journal of Anesthesiology* (Hernandez et al., 2003), the authors reported the summary statistics given in Table 6.10 on the decrease in pain as measured by VAS Score for a paired comparison study based on $n = 50$ subjects. Assuming the distribution of decrease in the visual analogue scale (VAS) pain score is approximately normally

TABLE 6.10   Summary Statistics on the Decrease in Pain as Measured by VAS Score

n	$\bar{x}$	s
50	4.34	1.80

distributed, use the summary statistics in Table 6.10 to compute a 90% confidence interval for the decrease in mean VAS score.

6.49 Using the Body Fat data set compute a 95% confidence interval for the mean percent body fat (PCTBF) of an adult male.

6.50 Determine sample size required for a 95% confidence interval for the mean when
(a) $\acute{\sigma} = 10$ and the desired margin of error is ME = 1.5.
(b) $\acute{\sigma} = 25$ and the desired margin of error is ME = 5.
(c) $\acute{\sigma} = 2.5$ and the desired margin of error is ME = 0.25.
(d) $\acute{\sigma} = 50$ and the desired margin of error is ME = 15.

6.51 Determine sample size required for a 90% confidence interval for the mean when
(a) $\acute{\sigma} = 100$ and the desired margin of error is ME = 15.
(b) $\acute{\sigma} = 50$ and the desired margin of error is ME = 10.
(c) $\acute{\sigma} = 0.5$ and the desired margin of error is ME = 0.04.
(d) $\acute{\sigma} = 60$ and the desired margin of error is ME = 18.

6.52 Determine sample size required for a 95% lower bound confidence interval for the mean when
(a) $\acute{\sigma} = 10$ and the desired margin of error is ME = 1.5.
(b) $\acute{\sigma} = 25$ and the desired margin of error is ME = 5.

6.53 Determine sample size required for a 95% upper bound confidence interval for the mean when
(a) $\acute{\sigma} = 2.5$ and the desired margin of error is ME = 0.4.
(b) $\acute{\sigma} = 50$ and the desired margin of error is ME = 10.

6.54 What is the bootstrap algorithm for computing a 95% bootstrap confidence interval for a parameter θ based on estimator T?

6.55 What are the percentiles of the bootstrap sampling distribution of an estimator T used in computing a
(a) 90% bootstrap confidence interval?
(b) 95% bootstrap confidence interval?
(c) 98% bootstrap confidence interval?

6.56 Explain how bootstrapping can be used to compute a 95%
(a) lower bound confidence interval?   (b) upper bound confidence interval?

6.57 The normal probability plot given in Figure 6.4 is based on the bootstrapped sampling distribution of the sample median. Use the normal probability plot in Figure 6.4 to determine a 95% bootstrap confidence interval for the population median.

6.58 Using the variable thigh circumference (Thigh) in the Body Fat data set
(a) estimate the median thigh circumference of an adult male.

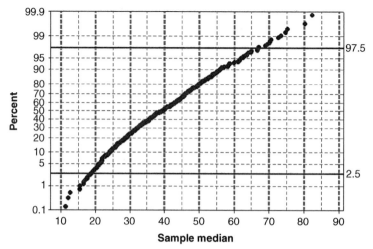

Figure 6.4   Normal probability plot for bootstrapped sampling distribution of the sample median.

(b) compute a bootstrap estimate of the standard error of the sample median.

(c) compute a 95% bootstrap confidence interval for the median thigh circumference of an adult male.

6.59 Under what conditions can the large sample confidence interval formula be used for estimating the difference between two proportions?

6.60 Determine whether or not it is appropriate to use the large sample confidence interval formula for estimating the difference between two proportions when

(a) $n_X = 25$, $n_Y = 20$, $\widehat{p}_X = 0.14$, and $\widehat{p}_Y = 0.20$.

(b) $n_X = 52$, $n_Y = 45$, $\widehat{p}_X = 0.23$, and $\widehat{p}_Y = 0.18$.

(c) $n_X = 121$, $n_Y = 135$, $\widehat{p}_X = 0.92$, and $\widehat{p}_Y = 0.89$.

6.61 After computing a confidence interval for the difference of two proportions, why is it important to determine whether or not 0 falls in the confidence interval?

6.62 What does it mean when two proportions are said to be statistically significantly different?

6.63 Using the large sample confidence interval formula, compute a

(a) 90% confidence interval for $p_X - p_Y$ when $n_X = 40$, $n_Y = 48$, $\widehat{p}_X = 0.24$, and $\widehat{p}_Y = 0.31$.

(b) 95% confidence interval for $p_X - p_Y$ when $n_X = 83$, $n_Y = 78$, $\widehat{p}_X = 0.84$, and $\widehat{p}_Y = 0.77$.

(c) 95% confidence interval for $p_X - p_Y$ when $n_X = 112$, $n_Y = 91$, $\widehat{p}_X = 0.73$, and $\widehat{p}_Y = 0.76$.

(d) 99% confidence interval for $p_X - p_Y$ when $n_X = 224$, $n_Y = 187$, $\widehat{p}_X = 0.04$, and $\widehat{p}_Y = 0.13$.

6.64 Determine whether or not there is a statistically significant difference in p_X and p_Y suggested by each of the confidence intervals in Exercise 6.63.

6.65 Using the large sample confidence interval formula, compute a 95%

(a) lower bound confidence interval for $p_X - p_Y$ when $n_X = 50, n_Y = 52, \widehat{p}_X = 0.35$, and $\widehat{p}_Y = 0.42$.

(b) lower bound confidence interval for $p_X - p_Y$ when $n_X = 67, n_Y = 67, \widehat{p}_X = 0.72$, and $\widehat{p}_Y = 0.55$.

(c) upper bound confidence interval for $p_X - p_Y$ when $n_X = 143, n_Y = 139, \widehat{p}_X = 0.70$, and $\widehat{p}_Y = 0.75$.

(d) upper bound confidence interval for $p_X - p_Y$ when $n_X = 354, n_Y = 387, \widehat{p}_X = 0.05$, and $\widehat{p}_Y = 0.10$.

6.66 Determine the overall sample size required so that a 90% confidence interval for the difference of two proportions will have a margin of error of ME $= 0.04$ when

(a) $\dot{p}_X = 0.4$ and $\dot{p}_Y = 0.5$.

(b) $\dot{p}_X = 0.25$ and $\dot{p}_Y = 0.20$.

(c) no prior guesses of the proportions are available.

6.67 Determine the overall sample size required so that a 95% confidence interval for the difference of two proportions will have a margin of error of ME $= 0.04$ when

(a) $\dot{p}_X = 0.8$ and $\dot{p}_Y = 0.6$.

(b) $\dot{p}_X = 0.5$ and $\dot{p}_Y = 0.30$.

(c) no prior guesses of the proportions are available.

6.68 Determine the overall sample size required so that a 95% lower bound confidence interval for the difference of two proportions will have a margin of error of ME $= 0.04$ when

(a) $\dot{p}_X = 0.7$ and $\dot{p}_Y = 0.6$.

(b) $\dot{p}_X = 0.25$ and $\dot{p}_Y = 0.30$.

(c) no prior guesses of the proportions are available.

6.69 Determine the overall sample size required so that a 95% upper bound confidence interval for the difference of two proportions will have a margin of error of ME $= 0.04$ when

(a) $\dot{p}_X = 0.75$ and $\dot{p}_Y = 0.6$.

(b) $\dot{p}_X = 0.4$ and $\dot{p}_Y = 0.25$.

(c) no prior guesses of the proportions are available.

6.70 In the article "Adjuvant chemotherapy in older and younger women with lymph node—positive breast cancer" published in the *Journal of the American Medical Association* (Muss et al., 2005), the authors reported the summarized data given in Table 6.11 on the clinical characteristics of progesterone receptor status and tamoxifen use for 3506 women aged 50 or less and 2981 women older than 50. Use the data in Table 6.11 to answer the following.

(a) Compute a 95% confidence interval for the difference in the proportions of women aged 50 or less and women older than 50 who have a positive progesterone receptor.

(b) Does the confidence interval in part (a) support the hypothesis of a significant difference in the proportion of women who have a positive progesterone receptor for these two age groups? Explain.

(c) Compute a 95% confidence interval for the difference in proportions of women aged 50 or less and women older than 50 who have used tamoxifen.

TABLE 6.11 Summarized Data for 3506 Women Aged 50 or Less and 2981 Women Older than 50 for a Breast Cancer Study

Characteristic	Age	
	≤ 50	> 50
Progesterone receptor positive	1532	1034
Tamoxifen use yes	1417	1250

    (d) Does the confidence interval in part (c) support the hypothesis of a significant difference in the proportion of women who use tamoxifen for these two age groups? Explain.

6.71 In the article "Screening for bipolar disorder in a primary care practice" published in the *Journal of the American Medical Association* (Das et al., 2005), the authors reported the summary data given in Table 6.12 on the work loss in the past month for 81 subjects screening positive for bipolar disorder and 664 screening negative for bipolar disorder. Use the data in Table 6.12 to compute a 95% confidence interval for the difference of the proportion of individuals having a work loss of more than 7 days in a month for the populations of individuals testing positive and negative for bipolar disorder.

6.72 Using the Birth Weight data set
    (a) estimate the proportion of low weight babies for mothers who smoked during pregnancy.
    (b) estimate the standard error of the estimate of the proportion of low weight babies for mothers who smoked during pregnancy.
    (c) estimate the proportion of low weight babies for mothers who did not smoke during pregnancy.
    (d) estimate the standard error of the estimate of the proportion of low weight babies for mothers who did not smoke during pregnancy.
    (e) compute a 95% confidence interval for the difference of the proportion of low weight babies for mothers who smoked during pregnancy and mothers who did not smoke during pregnancy.

6.73 What is the relative risk of a disease/condition for exposure to a particular risk factor?

6.74 What are the largest and smallest values that the relative risk can take on?

TABLE 6.12 Summary Counts on Extensive Work Loss for Subjects Screening Positive and Negative for Bipolar Disorder

Bipolar Screen	n	Work Loss (≥ 7 Days)
Positive	81	42
Negative	664	181

TABLE 6.13   2 × 2 Contingency Table Summarizing the Number of Myocardial Infarctions by Smoking Status

Uses Smokeless Tobacco	Dental Caries	
	Yes	No
Yes	218	581
No	35	489

6.75 After computing a confidence interval for the relative risk why is it important to determine whether or not the value 1 is in the confidence interval?

6.76 Why is the confidence interval for the relative risk based on the large sample sampling distribution of $\ln(\widehat{RR})$ rather than the sampling distribution of $\widehat{RR}$?

6.77 The use of smokeless tobacco is known to be associated with increased risk of gingivitis (gum disease) and dental caries (tooth decay). Suppose the data given in Table 6.13 was collected in a study on smokeless tobacco use and dental caries.

(a) Compute an estimate of the relative risk of developing tooth caries due to the risk factor uses smokeless tobacco.

(b) Compute the value of the estimated standard error of $\ln(\widehat{RR})$.

(c) Compute an approximate 95% confidence interval for the relative risk of developing tooth caries due to the risk factor uses smokeless tobacco.

6.78 In the article "Smoking and risk of myocardial infarction in women and men: longitudinal population study" published in the *British Medical Journal* (Prescott et al., 1998), the authors reported the results of a longitudinal study investigating the health problems associated with smoking among women. The summary data given in Table 6.14 shows the number of myocardial infarctions by smoking status for the women in this study. Use Table 6.14 to compute

(a) an estimate of the relative risk of a myocardial infarction due to the risk factor smokes.

(b) the estimated standard error of $\ln(\widehat{RR})$.

(c) an approximate 95% confidence interval for the relative risk of a myocardial infarction due to the risk factor smokes.

TABLE 6.14   2 × 2 Contingency Table Summarizing the Number of Myocardial Infarctions by Smoking Status

Smokes	Myocardial Infarction	
	Yes	No
Yes	380	6081
No	132	4879

6.79 Using the Birth Weight data set

(a) create a 2×2 contingency table summarizing the number of low weight babies by mother's smoking status.

(b) estimate the relative risk of having a low weight baby associated with the risk factor smokes during pregnancy.

(c) compute a 95% confidence interval for the relative risk of having a low weight baby associated with risk factor smokes during pregnancy.

CHAPTER 7

TESTING STATISTICAL HYPOTHESES

7.1 HYPOTHESIS TESTING

In the previous chapter the specialized use of a confidence intervals for determining statistical significance was introduced. In particular, a confidence interval suggests that the true value of the parameter is statistically significantly different than the hypothesized value of a parameter when the hypothesized value is not in the confidence interval for the parameter. The reason why a parameter is said to be statistically significantly different from the hypothesized value of the parameter when the hypothesized value is not in a confidence interval is that the difference between the hypothesized value and the observed estimate of the parameter is most likely not due to chance (i.e., sampling variability). That is, because a confidence interval captures the true value of the parameter with a prespecified probability close to 1, the chance that an observed confidence interval does not contain the true value of the parameter is small. Thus, a hypothesized value outside of a confidence interval is unlikely to be the true value of the parameter.

Example 7.1
Suppose a 95% confidence interval for the relative risk is 1.2–5. Then, based on the observed sample, the relative risk is statistically significantly different than the value 1. However, an important question that the confidence interval cannot answer is "how significantly different from the value 1 is the relative risk?" In particular, the confidence interval of 1.2–5 suggests that the relative risk is also significantly different from any value of the relative risk less than 1.2 or greater than 5. Thus, the sample data suggest that relative risk is significantly different than the values 1 and 1.19, however, since the value 1.19 is closer to the lower end point of the confidence interval, the relative risk should be less significantly different from 1 than it is from 1.19.

A confidence interval can be used to identify statistical significance, but on the other hand, a confidence interval cannot be used to assess the strength of the statistical significance. In this chapter, an alternative method for identifying statistical significance known as *hypothesis testing* will be discussed. In particular, a hypothesis test is a statistical procedure that can be used to determine whether or not the information contained in an observed sample supports a particular research hypothesis. The research hypothesis in a hypothesis test is simply a statement about the distribution of the population being studied, and in many cases, the research hypothesis will be a statement about a particular parameter of the population such as a proportion or a mean.

7.1.1 The Components of a Hypothesis Test

The goal of a hypothesis test is to decide whether or not the observed data supports a particular research hypothesis. In general, the research hypothesis should suggest a new finding or a deviation from the status quo. In a hypothesis test, the status quo hypothesis is referred to as the *null hypothesis* and is denoted by H_0. The research hypothesis in a hypothesis test is called the *alternative hypothesis* and is denoted by H_A. For example, in clinical study involving two different treatments, the null hypothesis is usually a statement such

H_0 : There is no difference between the effects of the two treatments being studied.

and in this case, the alternative hypothesis is

H_A : There is a difference between the effects of the two treatments being studied.

Every hypothesis test will have a null hypothesis H_0 and an alternative hypothesis H_A, and the goal of a hypothesis test is to evaluate whether or not the sample data supports the research hypothesis H_A. Thus, in a hypothesis test the null hypothesis is being tested against the alternative hypothesis and the test is said to be a test of H_0 versus H_A. Furthermore, the result of a hypothesis test is a decision concerning the null hypothesis, and the two possible decisions that can be made in a hypothesis test are to *reject H_0* or to *fail to reject H_0*. The null hypothesis will only be rejected in favor of the alternative hypothesis when the sample contains strong evidence against the null hypothesis; when the sample does not contain sufficiently strong evidence against H_0, the decision of the test will be to fail to reject H_0. Note that it is inappropriate to use the term "accept H_0" when there is insufficient evidence for rejecting the null hypothesis. The reasons for using the terms "reject H_0" and "fail to reject H_0" for the decisions in a hypothesis test are based on the measures of reliability of a hypothesis test, which will be discussed later in this section. Examples of the null and alternative hypotheses that will be discussed in this chapter and in later chapters are given in Example 7.2.

Example 7.2
The following null and alternative hypotheses are often tested in biomedical research.

   a. When comparing the proportions p_X and p_Y, a test of $H_0 : p_X = p_Y$ versus $H_A : p_X \neq p_Y$ is often performed.

   b. When comparing the means μ_X and μ_Y, a test of $H_0 : \mu_X = \mu_Y$ and $H_A : \mu_X \neq \mu_Y$ is often performed.

   c. When modeling a response variable Y as a linear function of an explanatory variable X, a test of the slope of the line, which is represented by the parameter β_1, is often performed by testing $H_0 : \beta_1 = 0$ versus $H_A : \beta_1 \neq 0$.

   d. When investigating association between a risk factor and a disease, a test of

H_0 : The disease outcome is independent of exposure to the risk factor.

versus

H_A : The disease outcome is associated with exposure to the risk factor.

is often performed.

For a parameter θ, the three most commonly tested pairs of null and alternative hypotheses are listed below.

HYPOTHESIS TESTS FOR θ

The three most common tests for a parameter θ are

1. $H_0 : \theta = \theta_0$ versus $H_A : \theta \neq \theta_0$

2. $H_0 : \theta \leq \theta_0$ versus $H_A : \theta > \theta_0$

3. $H_0 : \theta \geq \theta_0$ versus $H_A : \theta < \theta_0$

where θ_0 is a hypothesized value of θ.

A hypothesis test of $H_0 : \theta = \theta_0$ versus $H_A : \theta \neq \theta_0$ is called a *two-tailed test* because the alternative can be written as $H_A : \theta < \theta_0$ or $\theta > \theta_0$, the test of $H_0 : \theta \leq \theta_0$ versus $H_A : \theta > \theta_0$ is called an *upper-tail test*, and the test of $H_0 : \theta \geq \theta_0$ versus $H_A : \theta < \theta_0$ is called a *lower-tail test*. Note that the tail of a test is determined from the form of the alternative hypothesis, not the null hypothesis. In practice, the null and alternative hypotheses will be based on the goals of the research study.

Example 7.3

One of the research phases in the development of a new drug is designed for investigating the side effects of the drug. In particular, the side effects of a new drug are usually compared with the side effects for a placebo treatment. A new drug is usually expected to have higher rates of side effects than the placebo, and therefore, it is common in a drug trial to test the $H_0 : p_{\text{drug}} \leq p_{\text{placebo}}$ versus $H_A : p_{\text{drug}} > p_{\text{placebo}}$ where p_{drug} and p_{placebo} are the proportions of individuals who will experience adverse side effects.

Once a researcher has determined the null and alternative hypotheses that will be tested, a mechanism for weighing the evidence contained in the sample for or against the null hypothesis is needed. The statistic that is used to determine whether or not the observed sample provides evidence against a null hypothesis is called the *test statistic*. A test statistic is usually based on a point estimator of the parameter being tested and its sampling distribution is determined assuming that the null hypothesis is true. In particular, a test statistic compares the estimated value of a parameter with a hypothesized value of the parameter specified in the null hypothesis. For example, the test statistic that is used with large samples for testing $H_0 : \mu = 10$ versus $H_A : \mu \neq 10$ is

$$z = \frac{\bar{x} - 10}{\text{se}(\bar{x})}$$

The sampling distribution of a test statistic, assuming that H_0 is true, is used to determine the values of the test statistic for which H_0 is to be rejected, and the set of values of the test statistic for which H_0 is to be rejected is called the *rejection region*. When the observed value of the test statistic falls in the rejection region there is sufficient statistical evidence to *reject H_0*; when the value of the test statistic does not fall in the rejection region there is not sufficient statistical evidence to reject H_0, and therefore, H_0 is *failed to be rejected*.

The general form of the rejection region is given by

Reject H_0 when the observed value of the test statistic falls in the region R

where the region R depends on the sampling distribution of the test statistic when H_0 is true and the alternative hypothesis. In particular, the rejection region R is determined so that H_0 is only rejected when the sample data provides strong evidence against H_0.

It is important to note that rejecting H_0 does not mean that H_0 is necessarily false. Similarly, failing to reject H_0 does not mean H_0 is the true state of nature. That is, the decisions made up H_0 are based on a sample, and therefore, provide statistical inferences and not scientific proof about the true state of nature.

Example 7.4

For testing $H_0 : \mu = 10$ versus $H_A : \mu \neq 10$ with a sample $n \geq 100$ observations, there is approximately a 95% chance under H_0 (i.e., $\mu = 10$) that the test statistic

$$z = \frac{\bar{x} - 10}{\text{se}(\bar{x})}$$

will fall between -2 and 2. Consider the following decision rules for testing $H_0 : \mu = 10$ versus $H_A : \mu \neq 10$.

Reject H_0 if the observed value of $z < -2$ to $z > 2$.

Fail to reject H_0 if the observed value of z falls between -2 and 2.

Under these decision rules, the test statistic is $z = \frac{\bar{x}-10}{\text{se}}$ and the rejection region is $z < -2$ or $z > 2$. Furthermore, if H_0 is true, then there is roughly a 5% chance of observing a value of z in the rejection region. Thus, when H_0 is the true state of nature there is only a 5% chance of obtaining sample data that would result in a false rejection of H_0.

Since a hypothesis test is based on a sample and not a census, the decision concerning H_0 in a hypothesis test can result in a incorrect conclusion about the true state of nature. In fact, the three possible outcomes of a hypothesis test are (1) a correct decision about H_0 is made, (2) H_0 is rejected when in fact it is actually true, and (3) H_0 is failed to be rejected when it is actually false. Note that two of these three decisions are incorrect conclusions about the true state of nature, and in these cases the conclusion drawn from the hypothesis test results in a *testing error*. The two types of testing errors that can be made in a hypothesis test are

---

TESTING ERRORS

A *Type I error* is made by rejecting the null hypothesis when it is the true state of nature. That is, a Type I error results from a false rejection of H_0.

A *Type II error* is made by failing to reject the null hypothesis when the alternative is the true state of nature. That is, a Type II error results from a failing to reject H_0 when H_A is true.

The four possible outcomes of a hypothesis test are summarized in Table 7.1.

TABLE 7.1   The Possible Outcomes of a Hypothesis Test

	True State of Nature	
Decision	H_0	H_A
Reject H_0	Type I error	No error
Fail to reject H_0	No error	Type II error

Note that the only error that can be made when H_0 has been rejected is a Type I error and only a Type II error can be made when H_0 has been failed to be rejected. The Type I and Type II errors are made when the sample data that has been collected does not support the true state of nature, which can be due to sampling variability. To control for errors in a hypothesis test there should be only a small chance of making either a Type I error or a Type II error. The probability of making a Type I error in a hypothesis test is called the *significance level* or simply the *level* of the test and is denoted by α, and the probability of making a Type II error in a hypothesis test is denoted by β. The values of α and β are the measures of reliability for a hypothesis test, and in a well-designed hypothesis test the values of both α and β will be relatively small. Furthermore, because the values of α and β play an important role in determining the sample size required to have valid hypothesis tests they should be chosen prior to collecting the sample data.

Since α is the probability of rejecting H_0 when it is true, the value of α must be chosen by the researcher in determining the rejection region for a test. In fact, a researcher has complete control over the probability of making a Type I error and can choose α to be any small probability. In practice, the choice of the significance level α that will be used in a hypothesis test should be based on the consequences of making a Type I error. That is, when the consequences of making a Type I error are serious, a small value of α should be used, and when the consequences of making a Type I error are not too serious, a larger value of α can be used. In all cases, it is strongly recommended that $\alpha \leq 0.10$.

On the other hand, computing the probability of making a Type II error requires knowledge of the true value of the parameter being tested, which of course is unknown to the researcher. In fact, because the value of β depends on the parameter being tested, it is actually a function of the parameter being tested. That is, for a hypothesis test about a parameter θ, the probability of a Type II error is

$$\beta(\theta) = P(\text{Type II error}|\theta)$$

Unlike the value of α, the value of β depends on the true value of θ, and therefore, is harder to control for.

A third measure of reliability of a hypothesis test that is based on $\beta(\theta)$ is the *power of a test*. The power function associated with a hypothesis test is defined as

$$\text{Power}(\theta) = 1 - \beta(\theta)$$

The value of the power function for a test measures the ability of the test to a distinguish value of θ in the alternative hypothesis from the value θ_0 specified in the null hypothesis. Moreover, the power function of a test measures the ability of the test to correctly reject H_0, and the farther a value of θ is from θ_0, the more powerful the test will be. Also, the larger the power of a test is at a particular value θ, the smaller the probability of a Type II error will be at this value of θ.

Because the power of a test measures the ability of a test to distinguish values of θ in the alternative hypothesis from the value of θ_0, a good test will have power of at least 0.8 at a critical value of θ, say θ_{crit}. The value of θ_{crit} is the value of θ closest to θ_0 that a researcher considers different in a practical sense from the value of θ_0. Thus, to use the power as a measure of correctly rejecting H_0, a researcher must determine the value of θ_{crit} that has practical implications (i.e., scientific significance) different from those attributed to the value of θ_0.

The power function associated with a hypothesis test depends on several factors including the sample size, the significance level α, the value of θ_{crit}, and the amount of variability in the underlying distribution. However, the only factors that a researcher can control are the significance level α and the sample size. Therefore, an important step in the sampling plan is to determine the sample size that will produce a prespecified level of power for the particular value of α being used, the value of θ_{crit} determined by the researcher to have practical implications, and the amount of variability in the underlying distribution. An example of a power function is given in Example 7.5.

Example 7.5

The power function for a large sample test of $H_0 : \mu = 100$ versus $H_A : \mu \neq 100$ using the test statistic

$$z = \frac{\bar{x} - \mu}{\sigma/\sqrt{n}}$$

for $n = 100$, $\sigma = 25$, and $\alpha = 0.05$ is given in Figure 7.1.

The three points identified in Figure 7.1 represent the power at the values $\mu = 102.5$, 105, and 110. Note how the power increases as the value of μ moves away from $\mu_0 = 100$. The test is not very powerful at $\mu = 102.5$ having Power(102.5) = 0.17. The test has better power for detecting the difference between $\mu = 105$ and $\mu_0 = 100$ with Power(105) = 0.52, and the test is even better for detecting the difference between $\mu = 110$ and $\mu_0 = 100$ with Power(110) = 0.98. Furthermore, note that the power function for this test is symmetric about $\mu = 100$, and the power of the test exceeds 0.80 for values of μ greater than 107 or less than 93.

By determining the sample size that produces a prespecified power of at least 0.8 in the planning stages of the study, the reliability of the reject H_0 and the fail to reject H_0 decisions will be ensured. That is, because α is the probability of falsely rejecting H_0 and the value of α is known and is small (i.e., $\alpha \leq 0.10$), and when the power is at least 0.8 it will be unlikely to make either a Type I or a Type II error in a hypothesis test. Thus, the measures of reliability for a hypothesis test are α, $\beta(\theta)$, and the power function. Furthermore, because the researcher has a complete control over the value of α, and α is small, it turns out that rejecting the null hypothesis is always a reliable decision. On the other hand, failing to reject H_0 is only a reliable decision when $\beta(\theta) \leq 0.2$ or Power(θ) ≥ 0.8. When neither the power nor probability of a Type II error was taken into account in planning a hypothesis test, failing to reject H_0 becomes an unreliable decision because the researcher has no way of knowing how likely it was to make a Type II error.

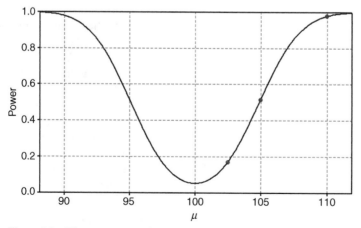

Figure 7.1   The power curve for a large sample test of $H_0 : \mu = 100$ versus $H_A : \mu \neq 100$ when $n = 100$, $\sigma = 25$, and $\alpha = 0.05$.

It is important to note that the value of α does not depend on the sample size, however, the value of β depends heavily on the sample size. In particular, the power of a test increases as n increases. Thus, when a researcher determines that a particular value of θ has real scientific significance but the power at this value of θ_{crit} is less than 0.80 for the planned sample size, the researcher needs to adjust the sampling plan so that a larger sample size is used. In particular, a sample size that will produce power of greater than 0.80 at the value of θ_{crit} should always be used. Example 7.6 illustrates that the power function of a large sample Z-test changes with the sample size.

Example 7.6
The power function for a large sample test of $H_0 : \mu = 100$ versus $H_A : \mu \neq 100$ using the test statistic

$$z = \frac{\bar{x} - \mu}{\sigma/\sqrt{n}}$$

for $n = 100$, 150, and $n = 200$ when $\sigma = 25$ and $\alpha = 0.05$ is given in Figure 7.2.
    Based on Figure 7.2, the power function is largest at each value of $\theta \neq 100$ for $n = 200$. For example, the power at either $\mu = 105$ or $\mu = 95$ is 0.52 for $n = 100$, 0.69 for $n = 150$, and 0.80 for $n = 200$. Also, a power of 0.80 is attained for $\theta = 107$ when $n = 100$, $\theta = 195.7$ when $n = 150$, and $\theta = 105$ when $n = 200$. Thus, the larger the sample is in a large sample Z-test the larger the power will be.

    In a well-designed hypothesis test, a researcher must provide several important pieces of information in the planning of the hypothesis test. In particular, a researcher must provide the values of α, θ_0, θ_{crit}, and the value of desired value of the power or β at θ_{crit}. These values will be used in determining the sample size necessary to produce accurate and reliable statistical inferences about the parameter θ that are based on the results of the hypothesis test.
    With a well-designed hypothesis test in hand, all that is left for the researcher to do is to collect a random sample and perform the hypothesis test. Note that a hypothesis test results in only a decision about whether or not the data supports the null hypothesis, and therefore, a confidence interval for parameter of interest should be reported along with the

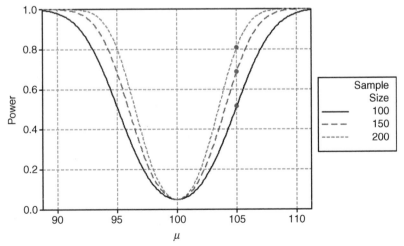

Figure 7.2   The power curves for a large sample test of $H_0 : \mu = 100$ versus $H_A : \mu \neq 100$ for $n = 100$, 150, and $n = 200$ when $\sigma = 25$ and $\alpha = 0.05$.

results of the test. An important reason for including a confidence interval along with the results of the test is to address the practical or scientific significance of the result of the hypothesis test. There are four possible outcomes concerning the statistical and scientific significance of a hypothesis test. In particular,

1. the value of $\widehat{\theta}$ can be both statistically and scientifically significantly different from θ_0.

2. the value of $\widehat{\theta}$ can be statistically but not scientifically significantly different from θ_0.

3. the value of $\widehat{\theta}$ can be neither statistically nor scientifically significantly different from θ_0.

4. the value of $\widehat{\theta}$ can be scientifically significantly but not statistically different from θ_0.

In Cases 1 and 3, there is no problem since the statistical and scientific significance are in agreement, however, in Cases 2 and 4 there is a problem since the statistical and scientific significance do not agree. Case 2, where $\widehat{\theta}$ is statistically significant but not scientifically significant, often occurs when a very large samples are used. Case 4 often occurs when the sample is to small to produce an estimate that is accurate enough to be distinguished from θ_0, but is sufficiently different from θ_0 to have practical implications. By determining the value of θ_{crit} and the value of n to achieve a prespecified power of at least 0.80 at θ_{crit}, it will be unlikely for either Case 2 or Case 4 to occur.

7.1.2 *P*-Values and Significance Testing

Another component of a hypothesis test that is often reported along with the decision concerning H_0 is the *p-value* that was first suggested by Fisher (1925) as a measure of the evidence contained in a sample against the null hypothesis.

P-VALUES

The *p*-value associated with an observed value of the test statistic is the probability of observing a sample that will produce a value of the test statistic as or more extreme than the observed value of the test statistic when the null hypothe-sis is true. That is, the *p*-value, which also called the *observed significance level* of the test, is

$$p = P(\text{ A more extreme value of the test statistic is observed} | H_0 \text{ is true})$$

The *p*-value is simply a measure how strongly the sample data agrees with the null hypothesis, and thus, the important question a researcher must answer when examining a *p*-value is whether or not to believe H_0 is the true state of nature. When the *p*-value associated with a test statistic is small, a researcher can conclude that it would be unlikely to have observed data as or more extreme than the observed data if H_0 were actually true. Thus, a small *p*-value suggests it is unlikely that H_0 is the true state of nature because if H_0 were true, sample data more consistent with H_0 should have been collected.

Fisher actually introduced the idea of a *p*-value along with an alternative approach to testing a null hypothesis called *significance testing*. The idea behind significance testing is to use the *p*-value to determine whether or not the observed sample supports the null hypothesis. Fisher (1925) suggested that

- for *p*-values between 0.1 and 0.9 there is no reason to suspect the null hypothesis being tested is false.

- for p-values less than 0.02 there is sufficiently strong evidence to conclude that the null hypothesis does not reflect the true state of nature, and hence, it is unlikely that the null hypothesis being tested is true.

Thus, for Fisher values above 0.9 or below 0.1 indicate that there is some evidence contained in the sample that is contradictory to the null hypothesis. Moreover, according to Fisher, a small p-value suggests that either the null hypothesis is untrue or the reason the test statistic is an unusually extreme value is due purely to chance; Fisher also concluded that extremely large p-values, such as 0.999, should be rare when the null hypothesis is true, and thus, large p-values also provide evidence against the null hypothesis.

Fisher's significance test for a null hypothesis is based entirely on interpreting the p-value associated with the observed value of the test statistic and does not consider Type I or Type II errors. The result of a significance test is decision about the apparent truth of a null hypothesis, and thus, a significance test results in one of the following conclusions:

- Reject the null hypothesis when the p-value is sufficiently small or sufficiently large.
- There is no reason to suspect the null hypothesis is false when the p-value is not small.

For Fisher, the question of what is a small or a large p-value must be answered subjectively by the researcher. Of course, two different researchers may interpret the size of a p-value differently with one saying $p = 0.056$ is small enough to reject H_0 and the other saying it is not sufficiently small for the rejection of H_0. While this might seem like a disadvantage to using a significance test, it really is not. That is, when there is substantial evidence against H_0, the p-value will be close to 0, and two researchers may disagree about the strength of the evidence against H_0 when the p-value is less than 0.1 but not when the p-value is close to 0. Of course, close to 0 is also subjectively determined, however, most researchers believe $p < 0.001$ is fairly convincing evidence against a null hypothesis. In fact, according to Fisher (1947)

> It is usual and convenient for experimenters to take 5 per cent as a standard level of significance, in the sense that they are prepared to ignore all results which fail to reach this standard, and, by this means, to eliminate from further discussion the greater part of the fluctuations which chance causes have introduced into their experimental results.

Thus, Fisher recommends rejecting the null hypothesis for p-values less than 0.05, and clearly, the closer the p-value is to 0 the stronger the evidence is for supporting the rejection of the null hypothesis.

Example 7.7

A large sample significance test of $H_0 : \mu = 100$ normal test can be performed by computing the value of the p-value associated with the observed value of the test statistic

$$z = \frac{\bar{x} - 100}{s/\sqrt{n}}$$

In particular, because the sampling distribution of z, is approximately distributed as a standard normal distribution for large samples when H_0 is true, the p-value is the probability of observing a Z-value farther from 0 than the observed Z-value. For example, suppose the observed value of the test statistic

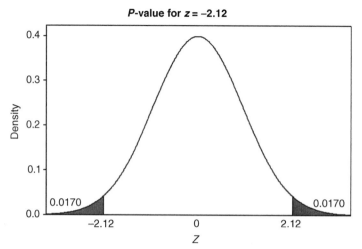

Figure 7.3   The area representing the p-value for $z_{obs} = -2.12$ in a large sample Z-test of $H_0 : \mu = 100$.

is $z_{obs} = 2.12$. Then the Z-values that are as or more extreme than z_{obs} are $Z < -2.12$ or $Z > 2.12$. Therefore, the p-value is

$$P(Z \leq -2.12 \text{ or } Z \geq 2.12) = 0.034$$

which is illustrated in Figure 7.3.

Thus, the chance of observing a value of the test statistic as or more extreme than $z_{obs} = -2.12$ is 0.034, about a 1 in 33 chance, which according to Fisher's general rules is a small enough p-value for the rejecting H_0.

The advantage a significance test has over a hypothesis test is that when the null hypothesis is rejected, a significance test supports the decision with the p-value measuring the strength of the evidence against the null hypothesis, while a hypothesis test has no such measure. On the other hand, a significance test has several weaknesses when compared to a hypothesis test. In particular,

1. the research hypothesis (H_A) is not explicitly stated in a significance test.
2. Type II errors are not controlled for in a significance test.
3. there is no clearly defined method for determining the sample size that should be used in a significance test.
4. significance tests are not designed to detect the difference between θ_0 and θ_{crit}.

Because the p-value is part of the standard computer output for a hypothesis test, the modern approach to testing a null hypothesis versus an alternative hypothesis utilizes the ideas of both hypothesis and significance testing. In particular, the modern approach to testing H_0 versus H_A is designed as a hypothesis test, and once the value of the test statistic is computed the p-value is used to measure the strength of the evidence against the null hypothesis. Furthermore, the p-value can be used in place of the rejection region for testing H_0 versus H_A by following the decision rules.

The modern approach to hypothesis testing controls for both types of testing errors, allows the test to be designed to detect values of θ scientifically different from θ_0, and when H_0 is rejected, provides a measure of how strong the evidence actually is against H_0. In summarizing the results of a hypothesis test, a researcher will usually report the p-value along with their decision about H_0.

Example 7.8
For testing $H_0 : \sigma = 5$ versus $H_A : \sigma \neq 5$ in a well-designed hypothesis test, determine whether the sample data provides sufficient evidence for rejecting H_0 when

    a. $\alpha = 0.01$ and the p-value is $p = 0.003$.

    b. $\alpha = 0.01$ and the p-value is $p = 0.038$.

    c. $\alpha = 0.05$ and the p-value is $p = 0.049$.

    d. $\alpha = 0.05$ and the p-value is $p = 0.051$.

Solutions The decision that should be made about $H_0 : \sigma = 5$ when

    a. $\alpha = 0.01$ and the p-value is $p = 0.003$ is to reject H_0 since the p-value is less than α. In this case, there is sufficient evidence in the sample to conclude that the σ significantly differs from 5.

    b. $\alpha = 0.01$ and the p-value is $p = 0.038$ is to fail to reject H_0 since the p-value is less than α. In this case, there is not sufficient evidence in the sample to conclude that the σ significantly differs from 5.

    c. $\alpha = 0.05$ and the p-value is $p = 0.049$ is to reject H_0 since the p-value is less than α. In this case, there is sufficient evidence in the sample to conclude that the σ significantly differs from 5.

    d. $\alpha = 0.05$ and the p-value is $p = 0.051$ is to fail to reject H_0 since the p-value is less than α. In this case, there is not sufficient evidence in the sample to conclude that the σ significantly differs from 5.

While the decision a researcher makes about the null hypothesis can be based entirely on the value of the p-value, it is important to give special care to the interpretation of p-values that are close to α. For example, in parts (c) and (d) of Example 7.8, the p-values are 0.049 and 0.051 were both compared with a significance level of $\alpha = 0.05$. In part (c) H_0 is rejected because $p < 0.05$, while in part (d) H_0 is not rejected since $p \geq 0.05$. Since these p-values are borderline significant and essentially contain the same information about H_0, the researcher should report in both cases that there is only weak evidence against the null hypothesis. Therefore, in borderline cases where the p-value is either slightly more or slightly less than the value of α, the decision concerning the rejection or failure to reject the null hypothesis should be taken lightly, and the p-value should be reported along with the decision concerning the null hypothesis.

Clearly, a p-value of $p = 0.001$ provides much more convincing evidence that H_0 is false than does a p-value of $p = 0.04$, and in fact, some statisticians have suggested the following guidelines for interpreting the value of a p-value.

GENERAL GUIDELINES FOR INTERPRETING P-VALUES

When the *p*-value associated with an observed value of a test statistics is

1. greater than 0.10, a researcher can conclude that the observed sample contains no evidence against the null hypothesis.

2. between 0.05 and 0.10, a researcher can conclude that the observed sample contains only weak evidence against the null hypothesis.

3. between 0.01 and 0.05, a researcher can conclude that the observed sample contains moderate evidence against null hypothesis.

4. between 0 and 0.01, a researcher can conclude that the observed sample contains convincing evidence against the null hypothesis.

While it is convenient to have firm rules for interpreting *p*-values it should be kept in mind that the guidelines above are very general, and it is the researcher's responsibility to interpret *p*-values with regards to the particular problem being studied and the consequences of making an error. Moderate or weak evidence usually suggests that further research is needed to determine whether H_0 or H_A is the true state of nature. Moderate and weak evidence against H_0 often occur in poorly designed studies where the sample size was insufficient for distinguishing between the null and alternative hypotheses. Moreover, it is critical that a researcher interpret a *p*-value, the results of a hypothesis test, and a confidence interval for the parameter of interest in terms of the statistical and the scientific significance of the results.

Finally, since the *p*-value does not measure whether the estimated value of θ is scientifically different from the value of θ_0 it is also common practice to include a confidence interval for θ in the summary of the test results. At the minimum, an estimate of θ and the estimated standard error of the estimate should be reported along with the results of the hypothesis test. In either case, the scientific and practical implications of the decision concerning the null hypothesis should be addressed when a researcher summarizes the results of a hypothesis test.

7.2 TESTING HYPOTHESES ABOUT PROPORTIONS

In many biomedical studies the parameters being studied are population proportions. For example, in the development of a new diagnostic test for a disease the sensitivity and specificity proportions are often the parameters of interest. In this section, hypothesis tests for proportions that are commonly encountered in biomedical research will be discussed. In particular, the large sample hypothesis tests for testing a single population proportion, for comparing proportions in two populations, and a test of independence will be discussed. While small sample tests exist for each of these tests, only the large sample tests are discussed in this section.

7.2.1 Single Sample Tests of a Population Proportion

Let *p* be the proportion of the population having a particular characteristic or property and let p_0 be the hypothesized value of *p*. Then, there are three possible research hypotheses concerning the value of *p*, namely, $p > p_0$, $p < p_0$, and $p \neq p_0$. Since the research hypothesis is used as the alternative hypothesis in a hypothesis test, there are three possible hypothesis tests that can be carried out in testing claims about a proportion p. The three possible hypothesis tests for a population proportion are listed below.

HYPOTHESIS TESTS FOR PROPORTIONS

---

1. $H_0 : p \leq p_0$ versus $H_A : p > p_0$ **3.** $H_0 : p = p_0$ versus $H_A : p \neq p_0$

2. $H_0 : p \geq p_0$ versus $H_A : p < p_0$

A test of $H_0 : p \leq p_0$ versus $H_A : p > p_0$ is referred to as an *upper-tail test*, the test of $H_0 : p \geq p_0$ versus $H_A : p < p_0$ is referred to as a *lower-tail test*, and the test of $H_0 : p = p_0$ versus $H_A : p \neq p_0$ is referred to as a *two-tailed test*. The tail of the test is determined by the alternative hypothesis. In general, hypothesis tests with greater than alternatives are upper-tail tests, tests with less than alternatives are lower-tail tests, and tests with a not equals alternative are two-tailed tests. The particular null and alternative hypotheses that will be tested in a hypothesis test must be chosen by the researcher and will be based on the research question of interest. For example, when an existing diagnostic test has specificity known to be 0.95, in the development of a new diagnostic test the research hypothesis should be that the specificity of the new test is greater than 0.95. In this case, the null and alternative hypotheses tested against each would be

$$H_0 : \text{specificity} \leq 0.95$$

versus

$$H_0 : \text{specificity} > 0.95$$

Recall that the estimator of the proportion of the population having a particular characteristic is

$$\widehat{p} = \frac{\text{number sampled with the characteristic}}{n}$$

and the standard error of $\widehat{p}$ is

$$SE(\widehat{p}) = \sqrt{\frac{p(1-p)}{n}}$$

Furthermore, when n is sufficiently large, the sampling distribution of

$$Z = \frac{\widehat{p} - p}{\sqrt{\frac{p(1-p)}{n}}}$$

is approximately distributed as a standard normal. Thus, when H_0 is true and n is sufficiently large the sampling distribution of

$$Z = \frac{\widehat{p} - p_0}{\sqrt{\frac{p_0(1-p_0)}{n}}}$$

is approximately a standard normal. Thus, Z is a statistic that can be used for testing claims comparing p with the hypothesized value p_0. That is, when H_0 is true the value of Z will almost certainly be between -3 and 3, however, when H_A is true the value of Z would be expected to fall outside of the normal range of a standard normal variable.

TABLE 7.2 The Rejection Regions for Hypothesis Tests Concerning a Proportion

Test	H_0	H_A	Rejection Region
Upper-tail	$H_0 : p \leq p_0$	$H_A : p > p_0$	$z_{obs} > z_{crit,\alpha}$
Lower-tail	$H_0 : p \geq p_0$	$H_A : p < p_0$	$z_{obs} < z_{crit,\alpha}$
Two-tail	$H_0 : p = p_0$	$H_A : p \neq p_0$	$|z_{obs}| > z_{crit,\alpha}$

Thus, $Z = (\widehat{p} - p_0)/\sqrt{p_0(1 - p_0)/n}$ is a large sample test statistic that can be used for testing claims about a proportion $np_0 \geq 5$ and $n(1 - p_0) \geq 5$. The rejection regions for the large sample Z for the upper, lower, and two-tailed tests for a population proportion are given in Table 7.2.

The value of z_{obs} is computed by plugging the value of $\widehat{p}$ into the test statistic, and H_0 is rejected only when the value of z_{obs} falls in the rejection region; when the value of z_{obs} is not in the rejection region H_0 will be failed to be rejected. The value of $z_{crit,\alpha}$ ensures that the probability of a Type I error is α and can be found in Table 7.3 or Table A.5. Also, note that the inequality sign in the rejection region is the same as the inequality sign in the alternative hypothesis. For example, in the lower-tail test the alternative is $H_A : p < p_0$ and the rejection region is "Reject H_0 when $z_{obs} < z_{crit,\alpha}$." In the two-tailed test, the alternative is $p \neq p_0$ that can also be stated as $H_A : p < p_0$ or $p > p_0$, and $|z_{obs}| > z_{crit,\alpha}$ is equivalent to $z_{obs} < z_{crit,\alpha}$ or $z_{obs} > z_{crit,\alpha}$.

Regardless of the outcome of the hypothesis test, it is always a good idea to report a confidence interval for p along with the results of the hypothesis test. The large sample confidence interval for a proportion p is

$$\widehat{p} \pm z_{crit} \times \sqrt{\frac{\widehat{p}(1 - \widehat{p})}{n}}$$

where the value of z_{crit} depends on the confidence level and can be found in Table A.4.

Example 7.9

Suppose that $H_0 : p \leq 0.30$ versus $H_A : p > 0.30$ will be tested using the information in a random sample of $n = 50$ observations. Determine

  a. whether or not the large sample Z-test is appropriate.
  b. the exact form of the test statistic.
  c. the rejection region for a test with probability of Type I error $\alpha = 0.01$.
  d. the value of z_{obs} when $\widehat{p} = 0.40$.
  e. the decision concerning H_0 that would be made based on parts (c) and (d).
  f. a 95% confidence interval for the value of p.

TABLE 7.3 The $z_{crit,\alpha}$ Values for the Upper, Lower, and Two-tailed Z-Tests

α	Upper-tail $z_{crit,\alpha}$	Lower-tail $z_{crit,\alpha}$	Two-tail $z_{crit,\alpha}$
0.10	1.282	−1.282	1.645
0.05	1.645	−1.645	1.96
0.01	2.326	−2.326	2.576

Solutions For testing $H_0 : p \leq 0.30$ versus $H_A : p > 0.30$ with a random sample of $n = 50$ observations

    a. the large sample Z-test is appropriate for testing $H_0 : p \leq 0.30$ versus $H_A : p > 0.30$ since both $50(0.30) = 15$ and $50(1 - 0.30) = 35$ are greater than 5.

    b. the exact form of the test statistic is

$$z = \frac{\widehat{p} - 0.30}{\sqrt{\frac{0.30(1-0.30)}{50}}} = \frac{\widehat{p} - 0.30}{0.065}$$

    c. the rejection region for a test with probability of Type I error $\alpha = 0.01$ is

$$\text{Reject } H_0 \text{ when } z > 2.326$$

    d. the value of z_{obs} when $\widehat{p} = 0.40$ is $z_{obs} = \dfrac{0.40 - 0.30}{0.065} = 1.538$.

    e. the decision based on parts (c) and (d) is to fail to reject H_0 since $z_{obs} = 1.538$ does not fall in the rejection region.

    f. a 95% confidence interval for the value of p is

$$0.40 \pm 1.96 \times \sqrt{\frac{0.40(1 - 0.40)}{50}}$$

which results in the interval of estimates 0.26–0.54.

The p-value for the large sample Z-tests for a proportion are computed using the standard normal distribution Z. The rules for computing the p-values associated with the large sample test of a proportion are given below.

P-VALUES FOR THE LARGE SAMPLE Z-TEST

The p-value for a large sample Z-test is
  1. p-value $= P(Z \geq z_{obs})$ in an upper-tail test.

  2. p-value $= P(Z \leq z_{obs})$ in a lower-tail test.

  3. p-value $= P(Z \geq |z_{obs}|)$ in a two-tailed test.

Example 7.10
In Example 7.9, the value of $z_{obs} = 1.538$, and since test was an *upper-tail test the* p-value associated with z_{obs} is $p = P(Z \geq 1.538)$, which is represented by the shaded area in Figure 7.4. Using the standard normal table, Table A.2, the p-value associated with $z_{obs} = 1.538$ is 0.062. Thus, based on this p-value there is only weak and inconclusive evidence against the null hypothesis contained in the observed sample.

Note that the p-value in Example 7.10 is larger than $\alpha = 0.05$ because z_{obs} did not fall in the rejection region. That is, the p-value will only be less than α when the value of z_{obs} is in the rejection region.

Example 7.11
Suppose that the existing diagnostic test for a particular disease has specificity of 0.90, and a new diagnostic test is being developed for this disease. Suppose in studying the effectiveness of the new diagnostic test, the summary data given in Table 7.4 resulted from a well-planned experiment. Use the data in Table 7.4 to test $H_0 :$ specificity ≤ 0.90 versus $H_A :$ specificity > 0.90 at the $\alpha = 0.05$ level.

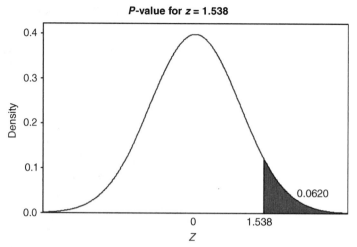

P-value for z = 1.538

Figure 7.4 The p-value for $z_{obs} = 1.538$ in an upper-tail test.

Solution Recall that the specificity of a diagnostic test is the conditional probability of a negative test for the subpopulation of individuals who do not have the disease (i.e., P(Negative|Disease Absent)). Thus, based on the sample data given in Table 7.4, the estimate of the specificity is

$$\widehat{\text{specificity}} = \frac{164}{6 + 164} = 0.965$$

Because $n = 170$ and $170(0.90) = 153$ and $170(1 - 0.90) = 17$ are both greater than 5, the large sample Z-test of H_0 : specificity ≤ 0.90 versus H_A : specificity > 0.90 is appropriate. Thus, the test statistic for testing H_0 versus H_A is

$$z = \frac{\widehat{\text{specificity}} - 0.90}{\sqrt{\frac{0.90(1-0.90)}{170}}}$$

and the rejection region for testing H_0 versus H_A at a significance level of $\alpha = 0.05$ is

$$\text{Reject } H_0 \text{ when } z_{obs} > z_{crit,0.05} = 1.645$$

The value of z_{obs} is found by plugging the estimated value of the specificity into the test statistic that results in

$$z_{obs} = \frac{0.965 - 0.90}{\sqrt{\frac{0.90(1-0.90)}{170}}} = 2.82$$

Therefore, because $z_{obs} = 2.82$ does fall in the rejection region there is sufficient evidence to reject H_0 : specificity ≤ 0.90. Thus, it appears that the new diagnostic test has specificity exceeding

TABLE 7.4 The Summary Data for a Diagnostic Test for a Disease

Test Result	Disease	
	Present	Absent
Positive	98	6
Negative	8	164

0.90, the specificity of the previously used diagnostic test. Furthermore, the p-value associated with $z_{obs} = 2.82$ is $p = P(Z \geq 2.82) = 0.0024$ indicating that the sample data provides strong evidence against H_0.

Finally, in the planning of a hypothesis test, which should be part of the sampling plan, the sample size needed to produce a reliable hypothesis test must be determined. In order to determine the sample size required to have a reliable test of H_0 versus H_A, the values of p_0, α, p_{crit}, which is the value of p in the alternative hypothesis that is considered scientifically different from p_0, and the value of β p_{crit} must be specified. The formula that determines the sample size for an upper-, lower-, or two-tailed test having probability of Type I error equal to α and probability of Type II error equal to β at $p = p_{crit}$ is

$$ n = \left(\frac{z_\alpha \sqrt{p_0(1 - p_0)} + z_\beta \sqrt{p_{crit}(1 - p_{crit})}}{p_{crit} - p_0} \right)^2 $$

where $z_\alpha = |z_{crit,\alpha}|$ and the value of z_β can be found in Table A.6 for the values $\beta = 0.15, 0.10, 0.05,$ and $0.01.$ Note that only the positive values of $z_{crit,\alpha}$ are used in determining the sample size. For convenience, Table A.6 is reproduced below in Table 7.5.

Because using a value of $\beta > 0.15$ can rarely be justified, the largest value of β given in Table A.6 is $\beta = 0.15.$ Also, for values of β that are not given in Table A.6, the value of z_β can be found using the table of the standard normal percentiles, Table A.3, with z_β equal to the $(1 - \beta) \times 100$ percentile of the standard normal. For example, if the desired value of β is 0.03, then the value of z_β is the 97th percentile of the standard normal that is $z_{0.03} = 1.88.$

Example 7.12
Determine the sample size required to have a reliable large sample hypothesis test when testing

    a. $H_0 : p = 0.25$ versus $H_A : p \neq 0.25$ with $\alpha = 0.05$, $p_{crit} = 0.30$, and $\beta = 0.10.$
    b. $H_0 : p \geq 0.60$ versus $H_A : p < 0.60$ with $\alpha = 0.05$, $p_{crit} = 0.50$, and $\beta = 0.15.$
    c. $H_0 : p \leq 0.75$ versus $H_A : p > 0.75$ with $\alpha = 0.01$, $p_{crit} = 0.85$, and $\beta = 0.05$.

Solutions The sample size required when testing

    a. $H_0 : p = 0.25$ versus $H_A : p \neq 0.25$ with $\alpha = 0.05$, $p_{crit} = 0.30$, and $\beta = 0.10$ is

$$ n = \left(\frac{1.96\sqrt{0.25(1 - 0.25)} + 1.282\sqrt{0.30(1 - 0.30)}}{0.30 - 0.25} \right)^2 = 825.1 $$

Thus, use a sample of $n = 826$ observations to ensure the value of β is 0.10.

TABLE 7.5 **The Values of z_β for $\beta = 0.15, 0.10, 0.05,$ and 0.01 that are Used in Determining the Sample Size n in the One- and Two-tailed Z-Tests for Prespecified Values of α and β**

β	z_β
0.15	1.036
0.10	1.282
0.05	1.645
0.01	2.326

b. $H_0 : p \geq 0.60$ versus $H_A : p < 0.60$ with $\alpha = 0.05$, $p_{crit} = 0.50$, and $\beta = 0.15$ at $p_{crit} = 0.50$ is

$$n = \left(\frac{1.645\sqrt{0.60(1 - 0.60)} + 1.036\sqrt{0.50(1 - 0.50)}}{0.50 - 0.60} \right)^2 = 175.3$$

Thus, use a sample of $n = 176$ observations to ensure the value of β is 0.15.

c. $H_0 : p \leq 0.75$ versus $H_A : p > 0.75$ with $\alpha = 0.01$, $p_{crit} = 0.85$, and $\beta = 0.05$ at $p_{crit} = 0.85$ is

$$n = \left(\frac{2.326\sqrt{0.75(1 - 0.75)} + 1.645\sqrt{0.85(1 - 0.85)}}{0.85 - 0.75} \right)^2 = 254.3$$

Thus, use a sample of $n = 255$ observations to ensure the value of β is 0.05.

It is important to note that the smaller the α and β are, the larger the sample size will be. For example, in Example 7.12 part (a) the sample size needed when $\alpha = 0.05$ and $\beta = 0.10$ was $n = 826$, however, if $\beta = 0.15$ was used instead of $\beta = 0.10$, the value of n would have been $n = 911$. Also, when the value of p_{crit} is close to p_0, it will be harder to distinguish the null hypothesis from the alternative hypothesis, and hence, larger samples will be required for detecting a small difference between the values p_{crit} and p_0.

Example 7.13
In a test of $H_0 : p \geq 0.5$ versus $H_A : p < 0.5$ with $\alpha = 0.05$ and $\beta = 0.10$, determine the values of n required when $p_{crit} = 0.55$ and $p_{crit} = 0.52$.

Solution The value of n when $p_{crit} = 0.55$ is

$$n = \left(\frac{1.645\sqrt{0.5(1 - 0.5)} + 1.282\sqrt{0.55(1 - 0.55)}}{0.55 - 0.5} \right)^2 = 853$$

and the value of n when $p_{crit} = 0.52$ is

$$n = \left(\frac{1.645\sqrt{0.5(1 - 0.5)} + 1.282\sqrt{0.52(1 - 0.52)}}{0.52 - 0.5} \right)^2 = 5351$$

Thus, more than six times as many observations are required when $p_{crit} = 0.52$ than are required for $p_{crit} = 0.55$ when $\beta = 0.10$.

7.2.2 Comparing Two Population Proportions

In many biomedical research studies the goal of the research is to study and compare the proportions of individuals having a particular characteristic in two different populations, say X and Y. For example, in the article "A randomized, controlled trial of aspirin in persons recovered from myocardial infarction" published in the *Journal of the American Medical Association* (1980), the Aspirin Myocardial Infarction Research Study Group sponsored by the National Heart, Lung and Blood Institute studied 4524 individuals who were given either 1 g of aspirin per day ($n = 2267$) or a placebo ($n = 2257$). One of the goals of this study was to compare the proportions of fatalities in the aspirin group with that of the placebo group. Clearly, the researchers were interested in testing the following research hypothesis.

The proportion of individuals having fatal myocardial infarctions is less for the individuals taking 1 g of aspirin per day than it is for individuals taking the placebo.

In this section the large sample test for comparing the proportions in two populations, say X and Y, having a particular characteristic will be discussed. Let p_X and p_Y be the proportions of the X and Y populations having the characteristic of interest. Then, there are three possible research hypotheses concerning the values of p_X and p_Y, namely, $p_X > p_Y$, $p_X < p_Y$, and $p_X \neq p_Y$. For example, in the Aspirin Myocardial Infarction Study, the research hypothesis would have been $p_{\text{aspirin}} < p_{\text{placebo}}$, where p_{aspirin} is the proportion of individuals taking 1 g of aspirin a day that would have fatal myocardial infarctions and p_{placebo} is the proportion of individuals taking the placebo each day that would have fatal myocardial infarctions. Since the research hypothesis is the alternative hypothesis in a hypothesis test, there are three hypothesis tests that can be carried out in testing claims about the difference between two proportions that are listed below.

HYPOTHESIS TESTS FOR COMPARING TWO PROPORTIONS

1. $H_0 : p_X \leq p_Y$ versus $H_A : p_X > p_Y$ **3.** $H_0 : p_X = p_Y$ versus $H_A : p_X \neq p_Y$

2. $H_0 : p_X \geq p_Y$ versus $H_A : p_X < p_Y$

As was the case with tests concerning a single proportion, the three tests comparing two proportions are also referred to as upper-, lower-, and two-tailed tests. That is, $H_0 : p_X \leq p_Y$ versus $H_A : p_X > p_Y$ is the upper-tail test, the test of $H_0 : p_X \geq p_Y$ versus $H_A : p_X < p_Y$ is the lower-tail test, and the test of $H_0 : p_X = p_Y$ versus $H_A : p_X \neq p_Y$ is the two-tailed test. The particular null and alternative hypotheses used in a test comparing two proportions should be chosen by the researcher and will be based on the research question being studied.

Recall that two proportions are usually compared by looking at their difference, and based on independent random samples from the X population and the Y population, the estimator of $p_X - p_Y$ is $\hat{p}_X - \hat{p}_Y$. Also, the estimated standard error of $\hat{p}_X - \hat{p}_Y$ is

$$\text{se}(\hat{p}_X - \hat{p}_Y) = \sqrt{\frac{\hat{p}_X(1 - \hat{p}_X)}{n_X} + \frac{\hat{p}_Y(1 - \hat{p}_Y)}{n_Y}}$$

where n_X and n_Y are the number of observations sampled from the X and Y populations. When n_X and n_Y are sufficiently large the sampling distribution of

$$z = \frac{(\hat{p}_X - \hat{p}_Y) - (p_X - p_Y)}{\text{se}(\hat{p}_X - \hat{p}_Y)}$$

is approximately distributed as a standard normal and can be used for testing claims about p_X and p_Y. The null value of $p_X - p_Y$ in each of the three possible hypothesis tests for comparing p_X with p_Y will be 0 because when $p_X - p_Y = 0$ it follows that $p_X = p_Y$. Thus, the large sample Z statistic for comparing p_X and p_Y is

$$Z = \frac{\hat{p}_X - \hat{p}_Y}{\text{se}(\hat{p}_X - \hat{p}_Y)}$$

Furthermore, when $p_X = p_Y$, a *pooled estimate* of their common value, say p, will be used in computing the estimated standard error of $\hat{p}_X - \hat{p}_Y$. In particular, the value of $\hat{p}$ is

$$\hat{p} = \frac{n_X \hat{p}_X + n_Y \hat{p}_Y}{n_X + n_Y}$$

TABLE 7.6 **The Rejection Regions for Hypothesis Tests Comparing Two Proportions**

Test	H_0	H_A	Rejection Region
Upper-tail	$H_0 : p_X \leq p_Y$	$H_A : p_X > p_Y$	$z_{\text{obs}} > z_{\text{crit},\alpha}$
Lower-tail	$H_0 : p_X \geq p_Y$	$H_A : p_X < p_Y$	$z_{\text{obs}} < z_{\text{crit},\alpha}$
Two-tail	$H_0 : p_X = p_Y$	$H_A : p_X \neq p_Y$	$|z_{\text{obs}}| > z_{\text{crit},\alpha}$

and the estimated standard error used in the Z statistic is

$$\text{se}_0 = \sqrt{\widehat{p}(1 - \widehat{p})\left(\frac{1}{n_X} + \frac{1}{n_Y}\right)}$$

Thus, the large sample test statistic for testing claims comparing p_X and p_Y is given by

$$Z = \frac{\widehat{p}_X - \widehat{p}_Y}{\sqrt{\widehat{p}(1 - \widehat{p})\left(\frac{1}{n_X} + \frac{1}{n_Y}\right)}}$$

and it is appropriate to use Z as the test statistic for comparing two proportions when each of the quantities $n_X \widehat{p}_X$, $n_Y \widehat{p}_Y$, $n_X(1 - \widehat{p}_X)$, and $n_Y(1 - \widehat{p}_Y)$ is greater than 5. The rejection regions for upper-, lower-, and two-tailed tests are given in Table 7.6.

Note that these are exactly the same rejection regions that are used in testing the upper-, lower-, and two-tailed tests for a single proportion given in Table 7.2. As a matter of fact, the rejection regions listed in Tables 7.2 and 7.6 are the rejection regions for all hypothesis tests that are based on a Z-test statistic.

The observed value of the test statistic z_{obs} is computed from the observed data by plugging the values of $\widehat{p}_X$ and $\widehat{p}_Y$ into the test statistic; the pooled estimate $\widehat{p}$ of p must also be computed and plugged into the formula for Z. Once the value of z_{obs} has been computed, H_0 is rejected when the value of z_{obs} is in the rejection region, and when the value of z_{obs} is not in the rejection region then H_0 is failed to be rejected. Again, the value of $z_{\text{crit},\alpha}$ ensures that the probability of a Type I error is α and can be found in Table A.5.

Because the distribution of the test statistic Z is approximately distributed as a standard normal and the rejection regions are the same for all Z-tests, it turns out that the p-values associated with the observed value of the Z statistic are computed in the same fashion for every Z-test. The p-values for a Z-test are always computed as outlined below.

P-VALUES FOR A Z-TEST

The p-values for the Z-tests are

1. p-value $= P(Z \geq z_{\text{obs}})$ in an upper-tail test.

2. p-value $= P(Z \leq z_{\text{obs}})$ in a lower-tail test.

3. p-value $= P(Z \geq |z_{\text{obs}}|)$ in a two-tailed test.

After performing a test comparing p_X and p_Y, a confidence interval for the difference $p_X - p_Y$ should be computed and reported along with the test decision and its p-value. The formula for a large sample confidence interval for $p_X - p_Y$ is

$$\widehat{p}_X - \widehat{p}_Y \pm z_{\text{crit}} \times \sqrt{\frac{\widehat{p}_X(1 - \widehat{p}_X)}{n_X} + \frac{\widehat{p}_Y(1 - \widehat{p}_Y)}{n_Y}}$$

where the value of z_{crit} depends on the confidence level being used.

Example 7.14

In the article "Risk factors for insomnia in a rural population" published in the *Annals of Epidemiology* (Hartz et al., 2007), data on 1588 individuals living in rural areas of the United States were analyzed. One of the insomnia risk factors that was studied dealt with whether or not an individual had previous thoughts of taking their own life (i.e., suicidal thoughts). Let p_N be the proportion of individuals living in rural areas of the United States who experience insomnia and have not had suicidal thoughts, and let p_Y be the proportion of individuals living in rural areas of the United States who experience insomnia and have had suicidal thoughts. Use the summary data in Table 7.7 to test $H_0 : p_N \geq p_Y$ versus $H_A : p_N < p_Y$ at the $\alpha = 0.01$ significance level.

Solution Since $n_Y \widehat{p}_Y = 122(0.58) > 5$, $n_Y(1 - \widehat{p}_Y) = 122(1 - 0.58) > 5$, $n_N \widehat{p}_N = 1457(0.36) > 5$, and $n_N(1 - \widehat{p}_N) = 1457(1 - 0.36) > 5$, the large sample Z-test is an appropriate test for comparing the proportions p_Y and p_N. The large sample test statistic is

$$Z = \frac{\widehat{p}_N - \widehat{p}_Y}{\sqrt{\widehat{p}(1 - \widehat{p})\left(\frac{1}{n_N} + \frac{1}{n_Y}\right)}}$$

and because this is a lower-tail test and $\alpha = 0.01$ the rejection region is

$$\text{Reject } H_0 \text{ when } z < z_{\text{crit}, 0.01} = -2.326$$

Now, the pooled estimate $\widehat{p}$ is

$$\widehat{p} = \frac{1457(0.36) + 122(0.58)}{1457 + 122} = 0.38$$

and plugging $\widehat{p}_N$, $\widehat{p}_Y$, and $\widehat{p}$ into the z statistic produces

$$z_{\text{obs}} = \frac{0.36 - 0.58}{\sqrt{0.38(1 - 0.38)\left(\frac{1}{1457} + \frac{1}{122}\right)}} = -4.81$$

Since $z_{\text{obs}} = -4.81$ does fall in the rejection region, $H_0 : p_N \geq p_Y$ is to rejected in favor of $H_A : p_N < p_Y$. The p-value associated with $z_{\text{obs}} = -4.81$ is $p = P(Z \leq -4.81) = 0.0000$. Thus, since the p-value is 0.0000 the sample data provides very strong evidence supporting $p_N < p_Y$.

A 95% confidence interval for the difference $p_N - p_Y$ is

$$(0.36 - 0.58) \pm 1.96 \times \sqrt{\frac{0.36(1 - 0.36)}{1457} + \frac{0.58(1 - 0.58)}{122}}$$

TABLE 7.7 Summary Statistics for Insomnia Risk Factor "Previous Suicidal Thoughts"

Suicidal Thoughts	Sample Size	Proportion
Yes	$n_Y = 122$	$\widehat{p}_Y = 0.58$
No	$n_N = 1457$	$\widehat{p}_N = 0.36$

which yields the interval of estimates -0.31 to -0.13. Thus, based on the observed data there is a statistically significant difference between p_N and p_Y (p-value = 0.0000), and it appears that p_Y is at least 0.13 larger than p_N and possibly as much as 0.31 larger.

Note that the estimated standard error used in the test statistic for comparing p_X and p_Y uses the pooled estimate $\widehat{p}$, however, the estimated standard error used in the confidence interval for $p_X - p_Y$ uses the estimates $\widehat{p}_X$ and $\widehat{p}_Y$ rather than $\widehat{p}$. The reason why the estimated standard error in testing H_0 is computed using $\widehat{p}$ rather than $\widehat{p}_X$ and $\widehat{p}_Y$ is that $p_X = p_Y$ under H_0. On the other hand, a confidence interval for $p_X - p_Y$ is independent of H_0, and therefore uses $\widehat{p}_X$ and $\widehat{p}_Y$. Most statistical computing packages have programs that can be used for testing the equality of two proportions that will compute the pooled estimate $\widehat{p}$, z_{obs}, and the p-value associated with the value of z_{obs}. For example, the statistical computing package MINITAB was used to analyze the data in Example 7.14, and the MINITAB output for the data in Example 7.14 analysis is given in Example 7.15.

Example 7.15
The MINITAB output for testing $H_0 : p_N \geq p_Y$ versus $H_A : p_N < p_Y$ for the summary data given in Table 7.7 is given in Figure 7.5. Note that MINITAB provides a table of the sample data, the observed difference in the sample proportions, an upper bound confidence interval for the difference in proportions, z_{obs}, and the p-value associated with z_{obs}. Also, because MINITAB computes the proportions with more accuracy than was used in the analysis in Example 7.14, the value of z_{obs} is slightly different in the MINITAB output (i.e., -4.81 versus -4.85).

Several pieces of information are required for determining a common sample size (i.e., $n_X = n_Y$) that is needed to produce a reliable hypothesis test for comparing the values of p_X and p_Y. In particular, the values of α, β, and the critical difference between p_X and p_Y, say p_{crit}, must be specified. A conservative estimate of the overall sample size is usually determined, and the formula for determining a conservative estimate of the overall sample size for an upper-, lower-, or two-tailed test having probability of Type I error equal to α and probability of Type II error equal to β at $p_X - p_Y = p_{crit}$ is

$$n = \frac{1}{2}\left(\frac{z_\alpha + z_\beta}{p_{crit}}\right)^2$$

where $z_\alpha = |z_{crit,\alpha}|$ and the value of z_β can be found in Table A.6. Then, the conservative individual population sample sizes are $n_X = n_Y = \frac{n}{2}$.

```
Test and CI for Two Proportions

Sample    X     N  Sample p
1        525  1457  0.360329
2         71   122  0.581967


Difference = p (1) - p (2)
Estimate for difference:  -0.221638
95% upper bound for difference:  -0.145328
Test for difference = 0 (vs < 0):  Z = -4.85  P-Value = 0.000
```
Figure 7.5 The MINITAB output for testing $H_0 : p_N \geq p_Y$ versus $H_A : p_N < p_Y$ in Example 7.14.

It is important to note that the conservative estimate of the common sample size is the largest possible sample size needed to obtain the prespecified value of β at p_{crit}. In particular, when the proportions p_X and p_Y are close to 0 or 1 the conservative estimate will be much larger than the exact sample size needed to attain the value of β. For example, for a test of $H_0 : p_X = p_Y$ with $\alpha = 0.05$, $\beta = 0.10$, $p_{\text{crit}} = 0.10$ when the value of p_X is around 0.40 and the value of p_Y is around 0.30 the conservative estimate of n is 526, while the actual value of n is 477.

Example 7.16
Determine a conservative estimate of the common sample size required to have a reliable large sample hypothesis test when testing

  a. $H_0 : p_X = p_Y$ versus $H_A : p_X \neq p_Y$ with $\alpha = 0.05$, $p_{\text{crit}} = 0.10$, and $\beta = 0.10$.
  b. $H_0 : p_X \geq p_Y$ versus $H_A : p_X < p_Y$ with $\alpha = 0.05$, $p_{\text{crit}} = 0.05$, and $\beta = 0.15$.
  c. $H_0 : p_X \leq p_Y$ versus $H_A : p_X > p_Y$ with $\alpha = 0.01$, $p_{\text{crit}} = 0.10$, and $\beta = 0.15$.

Solutions The conservative estimate of the common sample size, $n = n_X = n_Y$, required when testing

  a. $H_0 : p_X = p_Y$ versus $H_A : p_X \neq p_Y$ with $\alpha = 0.05$, $p_{\text{crit}} = 0.10$, and $\beta = 0.10$ is

$$n = \frac{1}{2} \left(\frac{1.96 + 1.282}{0.10} \right)^2 = 525.5$$

Thus, use a sample $n = 526$ observations from each population to ensure the value of $\beta = 0.10$.

  b. $H_0 : p_X \geq p_Y$ versus $H_A : p_X < p_Y$ with $\alpha = 0.05$, $p_{\text{crit}} = 0.05$, and $\beta = 0.15$ is

$$n = \frac{1}{2} \left(\frac{1.645 + 1.036}{0.05} \right)^2 = 1437.5$$

Thus, use a sample $n = 1438$ observations from each population to ensure the value of $\beta = 0.15$.

  c. $H_0 : p_X \leq p_Y$ versus $H_A : p_X > p_Y$ with $\alpha = 0.01$, $p_{\text{crit}} = 0.10$, and $\beta = 0.15$ is

$$n = \frac{1}{2} \left(\frac{2.326 + 1.036}{0.10} \right)^2 = 565.2$$

Thus, use a sample $n = 566$ observations from each population to ensure the value of $\beta = 0.15$.

7.2.3 Tests of Independence

When the response and explanatory variables are both qualitative variables a commonly tested research question is whether or not the response variable is independent of the explanatory variable. For example, epidemiological studies often investigate the relationship between a disease and a particular risk factor, and when the disease is independent of the risk factor the presence of the risk factor does not actually affect the chance of an individual contracting the disease.

The question of whether or not the response variable is independent of an explanatory variable is based on the joint probability distribution of the two variables and the definition of independent events. In Chapter 2, two events A and B were defined to *independent events* when

$$P(A \text{ and } B) = P(A) \times P(B)$$

Thus, two qualitative variables, say X and Y, are *independent variables* when

$$P(X = a \text{ and } Y = b) = P(X = a) \times P(Y = b)$$

for every pair of possible values of the variables X and Y. Furthermore, when X and Y are independent it turns out that

$$P(Y = b | X = a) = P(Y = b)$$

which means knowing the value of the X variable does not change the probability of the Y variable. Qualitative variables that are not independent variables are said to be *associated* or *dependent* variables.

Example 7.17
In many epidemiological studies the research goal is to determine whether or not the presence of a disease is independent of a particular risk factor. For example, in the Framingham Heart Study one of the research goals was to determine the major risk factors for cardiovascular disease. In particular, the researchers studied the independence of cardiovascular disease and serum cholesterol level, and the results obtained in the Framingham Heart Study provided strong evidence of an association between cardiovascular disease and serum cholesterol levels.

Let Y be the response variable and X the explanatory variable and suppose that Y and X are dichotomous variables. In a hypothesis test of the independence of Y and X, the null hypothesis is

H_0: The response variable Y is independent of the explanatory variable X

and the alternative hypothesis is

H_A: The response variable Y and the explanatory variable X are associated

Before proceeding with the details of a test of independence some new notation will be introduced. In particular, because a test of the independence of two variables is based on their joint probability distribution, specialized notation for the probability that X is in category i and Y is in category j will be introduced. Let

$$p_{ij} = P(X \text{ is in category } i \text{ and } Y \text{ is in category } j)$$

$$p_{i\bullet} = P(X \text{ is in category } i)$$

and

$$p_{\bullet j} = P(Y \text{ is in category } j)$$

where $i = 1, 2$ and $j = 1, 2$. The probabilities $p_{i\bullet}$ and $p_{\bullet j}$ are called the *marginal probabilities* associated with X and Y. The marginal probabilities associated with the X variable are found by summing all of the probabilities having a particular X value. Thus, for a dichotomous variable X, the marginal probability $p_{1\bullet}$ is found by summing p_{11} and p_{12}, and the marginal probability $p_{2\bullet}$ is found by summing p_{21} and p_{22}. That is,

$$p_{1\bullet} = p_{11} + p_{12}$$

and

$$p_{2\bullet} = p_{21} + p_{22}$$

TABLE 7.8   A 2 × 2 Table of the Probabilities for Two Dichotomous Variables

X	Y		
	Category 1	Category 2	X Marginals
Category 1	p_{11}	p_{12}	$p_{1\bullet}$
Category 2	p_{21}	p_{12}	$p_{2\bullet}$
Y Marginals	$p_{\bullet 1}$	$p_{\bullet 2}$	

Similarly, the marginal probabilities associated with the Y variable are found by summing all of the probabilities having a particular Y value, and therefore, the Y marginal probabilities are

$$p_{\bullet 1} = p_{11} + p_{21}$$

and

$$p_{\bullet 2} = p_{12} + p_{22}$$

The joint and marginal probabilities associated two dichotomous variables can be summarized in the 2×2 table of the form given in Table 7.8.

When the response variable Y is independent of the explanatory variable X it follows that

$$p_{ij} = p_{i\bullet} \times p_{\bullet j}$$

for the four possible set of values i, j. In this case, the joint probabilities are summarized in Table 7.9. Using the probabilities in Tables 7.8 and 7.9, the null and alternative hypotheses in a test of independence for two dichotomous variables can be restated as

$$H_0 : p_{ij} = p_{i\bullet} \times p_{\bullet j} \quad \text{for } i = 1, 2 \text{ and } j = 1, 2$$

and

$$H_A : p_{ij} \neq p_{i\bullet} \times p_{\bullet j} \quad \text{for } i = 1, 2 \text{ and } j = 1, 2$$

That is, when the null hypothesis is true there is a specific model, namely the independence model, for the joint probabilities associated with the values of the X and Y variables, while under the alternative hypothesis no particular model is specified for the joint probabilities.

The data for testing the independence of two dichotomous variables is based on a simple random sample from the joint population of X and Y values, and the n observations

TABLE 7.9   A 2 × 2 Table of the Probabilities for Two Independent Dichotomous Variables

X	Y		
	Category 1	Category 2	X Marginals
Category 1	$p_{1\bullet} \times p_{\bullet 1}$	$p_{1\bullet} \times p_{\bullet 2}$	$p_{1\bullet}$
Category 2	$p_{2\bullet} \times p_{\bullet 1}$	$p_{2\bullet} \times p_{\bullet 2}$	$p_{2\bullet}$
Y marginals	$p_{\bullet 1}$	$p_{\bullet 2}$	

TABLE 7.10   The General Form of a 2 × 2 Contingency Table Summarizing the Observed Frequencies from a Simple Random Sample that has been Cross-Classified According to the Dichotomous Variables X and Y

X	Y		
	Category 1	Category 2	Row Total
Category 1	a	b	$a + b$
Category 2	c	d	$c + d$
Column total	$a + c$	$b + d$	n

in the simple random sample are cross-classified according to the variables X and Y and summarized in a 2×2 contingency table as shown in Table 7.10.

The test of the independence of X and Y is based on comparing the observed frequencies in Table 7.10 with the expected frequencies computed assuming that the variables X and Y are independent (i.e., under H_0). The expected frequencies, under the null hypothesis, are computed assuming that X and Y are independent and the expected frequency for $X = i$ and $Y = j$ is denoted by E_{ij}. The values of the four expected frequencies E_{11}, E_{12}, E_{21}, and E_{22} are computed using

$$E_{ij} = \frac{\text{row } i \text{ total} \times \text{column } j \text{ total}}{n}$$

For example, the expected frequency when $X = 1$ and $Y = 1$ is given by

$$E_{11} = \frac{\text{row 1 total} \times \text{column 1 total}}{n} = \frac{(a + b) \times (a + c)}{n}$$

Moreover, when the observed cell counts are not close to the expected frequencies there will be evidence that the variables are not independent. The test statistic for testing the independence of the variables X and Y is denoted by X^2 and is given by

$$X^2 = \sum_{\text{all 4 cells}} \frac{(\text{observed frequency} - \text{expected frequency})^2}{\text{expected frequency}}$$

Thus, for the 2×2 contingency table given in Table 7.10 the value of X^2 is

$$X^2 = \frac{(a - E_{11})^2}{E_{11}} + \frac{(b - E_{12})^2}{E_{13}} + \frac{(c - E_{21})^2}{E_{21}} + \frac{(d - E_{22})^2}{E_{22}}$$

The value of X^2 can also be computed using the following simpler form of X^2.

$$X^2 = \frac{n(ad - bc)^2}{(a + b) \times (c + d) \times (a + c) \times (b + d)}$$

Now, when all of the expected frequencies are at least 5 and when the null hypothesis is true, the sampling distribution of X^2 can be approximated by a chi-squared distribution with 1 degree of freedom (χ_1^2). Thus, the rejection region for a large sample test of independence will be based on the chi-squared distribution with 1 degree of freedom, and the critical values of a chi-squared distribution can be found in Table A.10. The rejection for a chi-squared test of independence is given below.

REJECTION REGION FOR A TEST OF INDEPENDENCE FOR DICHOTOMOUS VARIABLES

For testing

H_0 : The variables X and Y are independent

versus

H_A : The variables X and Y are associated

when all of the expected cell frequencies are at least 5, the rejection region is

Reject H_0: X and Y are independent when

$$X_{obs}^2 > \chi_{1,\alpha,crit}^2$$

where the value of $\chi_{1,\alpha,crit}^2$ can be found in Table A.10.

The p-value for the large sample test of independence is given by

$$p\text{-value} = P(\chi_1^2 \geq X_{obs}^2)$$

which cannot be determined from the table of chi-squared values given in Table A.10, however, the p-value for a test of independence is provided along with the value of the test statistic when a statistical computing package is used to carry out the test of independence.

Example 7.18

In the article "Aspirin and risk of hemorrhagic stroke" published in the *Journal of American Medical Association* (He et al., 1998), the authors studied the relationship between strokes and the use of aspirin in a meta-analysis of previous studies. In particular, the incidence of two types of strokes, hemorrhagic and ischemic strokes, was compared for two treatment groups, aspirin and control. The mean dose of aspirin was 237 mg/day for a mean treatment duration of 37 months; the control group was either given a placebo or no treatment at all. The data given in the 2×2 contingency table in Table 7.11 were reported in this article and summarizes the two types of stroke for the two treatment groups for $n = 1164$ individuals. Use this data to test the independence of type of stroke and treatment at the $\alpha = 0.01$ significance level.

Solution The expected frequencies for testing

$$H_0 : \text{Stroke type is independent of treatment}$$

versus

$$H_A : \text{Stroke type and treatment are associated}$$

are given in Table 7.12 Since, all of the expected frequencies are at least 5, the large sample test of independence is appropriate and the rejection region is

$$\text{Reject } H_0 \text{ when } X_{obs}^2 > \chi_{1,0.01,crit}^2 = 6.63$$

TABLE 7.11 A 2×2 Contingency Table Summarizing $n = 1164$ Individuals Cross-classified by Type of Stroke and Treatment Group

Treatment Group	Stroke Subtype		Row Total
	Hemorrhagic	Ischemic	
Aspirin	75	480	555
Control	33	576	609
Column total	108	1056	1164

TABLE 7.12   The Expected Frequencies Computed under H_0

Treatment Group	Stroke Subtype		Row Total
	Hemorrhagic	Ischemic	
Aspirin	51.49	503.51	555
Control	56.51	552.49	609
Column total	108	1056	1164

The observed value of the test statistic computed from the observed data in Table 7.11 and the expected frequencies in Table 7.12 is

$$X^2_{obs} = \frac{(75 - 51.49)^2}{51.49} + \frac{(480 - 503.51)^2}{503.51} + \frac{(33 - 56.51)^2}{56.51} + \frac{(576 - 552.49)^2}{552.49}$$

$$= 10.739 + 1.097 + 9.778 + 1.000 = 22.604$$

Thus, because $X^2_{obs} = 22.604$ falls in the rejection region there is sufficient evidence to reject the null hypothesis. Furthermore, since the p-value associated with $X^2_{obs} = 22.604$ is $P(\chi^2_1 \geq 22.604) = 0.000002$ there is very strong evidence that type of stroke is associated with the treatment received.

Note that the value of X^2_{obs} could also have been computed using the shortcut formula, and in this case, the value of X^2_{obs} is computed as

$$X^2_{obs} = \frac{1164(75 \times 576 - 480 \times 33)^2}{555 \times 609 \times 108 \times 1056} = 22.604$$

Because a test of independence yields only a decision on whether the sample data provides evidence for or against the independence of two variables, when the null hypothesis is rejected there is no measure of the strength of the association between the two variables. The relative risk is a commonly used measure of the association between a disease and a risk factor that can be used in prospective studies, however, the relative risk cannot be used to measure the association in case–control or retrospective studies. Furthermore, the relative risk is 1 when a disease is independent of the factor, and therefore, the farther the relative risk is from 1, the stronger the association will be between the disease and the risk factor.

Example 7.19

Using the data from Example 7.18 for the study on the association between hemorrhagic strokes and the use of aspirin, the estimated relative risk of a hemorrhagic stroke for the risk factor aspirin user is

$$\widehat{RR} = \frac{75/555}{33/609} = 2.49$$

A 95% confidence for the relative risk is

$$e^{\ln(2.49) \pm 1.96 \times 0.200}$$

which yields an interval of estimates of the relative risk ranging from 1.68 to 3.68. Thus, it appears that the type of stroke is associated with treatment type, and the relative risk of hemorrhagic stroke for aspirin users is at least 1.68 times the risk of the control group and possibly as much as 3.68 times greater risk.

While it is always important to design a hypothesis test with an appropriate sample size that will control for the probability of a Type II error, the computational aspects of determining the value of n for a test of independence are beyond the scope of this book and will not be discussed here.

Finally, when the variable X has r categories and the variable Y has c categories, a test of the independence of X and Y can also be performed using an approach that is similar to that used with two dichotomous variables. A qualitative variable taking on values in two or more categories is called a *polytomous* variable, and two polytomous variables are independent when

$$P(X = i \text{ and } Y = j) = P(X \text{ is in category } i) \times P(Y \text{ is in category } j)$$

Thus, the null hypothesis in a test of independence for two polytomous variables can be stated as either

$$H_0 : X \text{ and } Y \text{ are independent}$$

or

$$H_0 : p_{ij} = p_{i\bullet} \times p_{\bullet j}$$

where $p_{i\bullet}$ and $p_{\bullet j}$ are the X and Y marginal probabilities.

When a simple random sample of n observations is collected and cross-classified according to two polytomous variables X and Y, the data are usually summarized in a $r \times c$ contingency table as shown in Table 7.13. The value of n_{ij} in Table 7.13 represents the number of observations in the sample classified as category i of the X variable and category j of the Y variable.

When X and Y are independent polytomous variables, the expected frequencies for a random sample of n observations are

$$E_{ij} = \frac{n_{i\bullet} \times n_{\bullet j}}{n}$$

and the test statistic for testing the independence of the variables X and Y compares the observed cell frequencies with the expected cell frequencies computed under H_0. Thus, the

TABLE 7.13   The General Form of a $r \times c$ Contingency Table Summarizing the Observed Frequencies from a Simple Random Sample that has been Cross-Classified According to Polytomous Variables X and Y

X	Y				Row Total
	Category 1	Category 2	$\cdots$	Category c	
Category 1	n_{11}	n_{12}	$\cdots$	n_{1c}	$n_{1\bullet}$
Category 2	n_{21}	n_{22}	$\cdots$	n_{2c}	$n_{2\bullet}$
$\vdots$	$\vdots$	$\vdots$	$\vdots$	$\vdots$	
Category r	n_{r1}		$\cdots$	n_{rc}	$n_{r\bullet}$
Column total	$n_{\bullet 1}$	$n_{\bullet 2}$	$\cdots$	$n_{\bullet c}$	

test statistic for testing the independence of two polytomous variables is

$$X^2 = \sum_{\text{all } r \times c \text{ cells}} \frac{(\text{observed frequency} - \text{expected frequency})^2}{\text{expected frequency}}$$

$$= \sum_{\text{all } r \times c \text{ cells}} \frac{(n_{ij} - E_{ij})^2}{E_{ij}}$$

When all of the expected cell frequencies are at least 5, the sampling distribution of X^2 is approximately a chi-squared distribution with $(r-1) \times (c-1)$ degrees of freedom. Thus, the rejection region for a large sample test of independence will be based on the chi-squared distribution with $(r-1) \times (c-1)$ degrees of freedom.

REJECTION REGION FOR A TEST OF INDEPENDENCE OF POLYTOMOUS VARIABLES

Reject H_0: X and Y are independent when   where the value of $\chi^2_{(r-1)(c-1),\alpha,\text{crit}}$ is found in Table A.10.

$$X^2_{\text{obs}} > \chi^2_{(r-1)(c-1),\alpha,\text{crit}}$$

The p-value for the large sample test of independence is given by

$$p\text{-value} = P(\chi^2_{(r-1)(c-1)} \geq X^2_{\text{obs}})$$

The p-value for a test of independence cannot be determined from the table of chi-squared values given in Table A.10, however, the p-value is provided along with the value of the test statistic when a statistical computing package is used to carry out a test of independence.

Example 7.20
In the article "Financial barriers to health care and outcomes after acute myocardial infarction" published in the *Journal of American Medical Association* (Rahimi et al., 2007), one of the research questions the authors investigated was whether or not an individual's quality of life after suffering a myocardial infarction was independent of financial barriers to obtaining healthcare services. The sample data for $n = 2439$ individuals is summarized in a 2×4 contingency table given in Table 7.14. Use this data to test

$$H_0 : \text{Quality of life is independent of financial status}$$

at the $\alpha = 0.01$ significance level.

TABLE 7.14   The Summarized Data for $n = 2439$ Individuals for a Study on the Quality of Life After Suffering a Myocardial Infarction

Quality of Life	Financial Status		
	N. Financial Barriers	Financial Barriers	
Severely diminished	70	57	127
Moderately diminished	319	107	426
Mildly diminished	899	179	1078
Good to excellent	709	99	808
Column total	1997	442	2439

TABLE 7.15 The Expected Frequencies Based on Table 7.14 and Assuming that Quality of Life and Financial Status are Independent

Quality of Life	Financial Status	
	N. Financial Barriers	Financial Barriers
Severely diminished	104.50	22.50
Moderately diminished	350.52	75.48
Mildly diminished	887.01	190.99
Good to excellent	654.97	141.03

Solution First, the expected cell frequencies are given in Table 7.15 and since they are all at least 5, the rejection region for testing the independence of quality of life and financial status at the $\alpha = 0.01$ significance level will be based on a chi-squared distribution with $(4-1) \times (2-1) = 3$ degrees of freedom. The rejection region for this test of independence is

$$\text{Reject } H_0 \text{ when } X_{obs}^2 > \chi_{3,0.01,\text{crit}} = 11.34$$

The expected frequencies under the independence model are given in Table 7.15, and the value of X_{obs}^2 is

$$X_{obs}^2 = \frac{(70 - 104.50)^2}{104.50} + \frac{(57 - 22.50)^2}{22.50} + \cdots + \frac{(99 - 141.03)^2}{141.03} = 106.36$$

The p-value associated with $X_{obs}^2 = 106.36$ is $p = 0.000$, and thus, based on the observed data it appears that quality of life and financial status are associated. Further analysis shows that the observed percentage of individuals having no financial barriers to healthcare services who had some level of diminished quality of life was 64%, while among the individuals having financial barriers the percentage was 78%; the percentage of individuals having a good or excellent quality of life was 36% for the individuals having no financial barriers and only 22% for those having financial barriers. Clearly, the financial status of an individual is affecting the quality of their life post-myocardial infarction.

7.3 TESTING HYPOTHESES ABOUT MEANS

When the research question being investigated involves a quantitative variable it is often the case that the research hypothesis will involve a statement about the mean of the population being studied. In many research studies, the research hypothesis is a statement comparing the means of two populations. For example, in a study investigating the effects of a drug designed to lower the LDL cholesterol level of an individual, the research hypothesis might be a statement about the mean LDL cholesterol level before treatment and the mean LDL cholesterol level after the treatment.

In this section each of the hypothesis tests concerning the mean of a population will be based on a test statistic that has a t distribution, and hence, will referred to as a t-test. Because every t-tests is similar in nature, the procedural details of performing a t-test will be discussed before considering the t tests that are used for testing claims about population means.

7.3.1 t-Tests

The t-test is one of the most commonly used hypothesis tests and is used for testing claims about means, claims about the correlation coefficient, and claims about the slope of a line. Furthermore, the procedure used in a t-test is independent of the parameter being tested. That is, every t-test has the same rejection regions and the p-values associated with t_{obs} are computed in the same way in every t-test. The general form of a t statistic is given by

$$t = \frac{\text{estimate} - \text{parameter}}{\text{estimated standard error}}$$

Thus, when the parameter being estimated is θ and $\widehat{\theta}$ is the estimator that is used to estimate θ, the t statistic is

$$t = \frac{\widehat{\theta} - \theta}{\text{se}}$$

where se is the estimated standard error of $\widehat{\theta}$. The t statistic is actually a measures of the *statistical distance* between the estimate and a particular value of the parameter, and for many commonly used estimators, the sampling distribution of the t statistic will follow a t distribution when the underlying population being sampled is approximately normally distributed.

The three most commonly tested null and alternative hypotheses about a parameter θ are

1. $H_0 : \theta \leq \theta_0$ versus $H_A : \theta > \theta_0$, which is the upper-tail test.
2. $H_0 : \theta \geq \theta_0$ versus $H_A : \theta < \theta_0$, which is the lower-tail test.
3. $H_0 : \theta = \theta_0$ versus $H_A : \theta \neq \theta_0$, which is the two-tailed test.

When θ_0 is the true value of θ the sampling distribution of

$$t = \frac{\widehat{\theta} - \theta_0}{\text{se}}$$

will often follow a t distribution with the degrees of freedom associated with se. In this case, the rejection regions for the upper, lower, and two-tailed t-tests are given in Table 7.16. The value of $t_{\alpha, \nu, \text{crit}}$ can be found in Table A.7, however, the critical values of the t distribution are given in Table A.7 for only $\nu = 1, 2, \ldots, 30, 40, 60, 120, \infty$ degrees of freedom. In practice, when the degrees of freedom ν for a t-test are not listed in Table A.7, it is acceptable to use the critical value associated with the degrees of freedom in the table that are closest to ν. For example, when a t-test has $\nu = 43$ degrees of freedom, the critical value in Table A.7 with 40 degrees of freedom should be used. When the degrees of freedom for the t-test are much greater than 120 the critical values associated with $\nu = \infty$ degrees of freedom should be used.

TABLE 7.16 The Rejections for the Upper-, Lower-, and Two-tailed t-Tests

Test	H_0	H_A	Rejection Region
Upper-tail	$H_0 : \theta \leq \theta_0$	$H_A : \theta > \theta_0$	$t_{obs} > t_{\alpha, \nu, \text{crit}}$
Lower-tail	$H_0 : \theta \geq \theta_0$	$H_A : \theta < \theta_0$	$t_{obs} < -t_{\alpha, \nu, \text{crit}}$
Two-tailed	$H_0 : \theta = \theta_0$	$H_A : \theta \neq \theta_0$	$|t_{obs}| > t_{\alpha, \nu, \text{crit}}$

Example 7.21

Determine the rejection regions for a t-test when

    a. an upper-tail test is being performed at the $\alpha = 0.05$ significance level and the sampling distribution of the test statistic has $\nu = 12$ degrees of freedom.

    b. a lower-tail test is being performed at the $\alpha = 0.01$ significance level and the sampling distribution of the test statistic has $\nu = 29$ degrees of freedom.

    c. a two-tailed test is being performed at the $\alpha = 0.02$ significance level and the sampling distribution of the test statistic has $\nu = 18$ degrees of freedom.

    d. a two-tailed test is being performed at the $\alpha = 0.01$ significance level and the sampling distribution of the test statistic has $\nu = 128$ degrees of freedom.

Solutions The rejection region for

    a. an upper-tail test with $\alpha = 0.05$ and $\nu = 12$ degrees of freedom is

$$\text{Reject } H_0 \text{ when } t_{\text{obs}} > t_{0.05, 12, \text{crit}} = 1.782$$

    b. a lower-tail test with $\alpha = 0.01$ and $\nu = 29$ degrees of freedom is

$$\text{Reject } H_0 \text{ when } t_{\text{obs}} < -t_{0.01, 29, \text{crit}} = -2.462$$

    c. a two-tailed test with $\alpha = 0.02$ and $\nu = 18$ degrees of freedom is

$$\text{Reject } H_0 \text{ when } |t_{\text{obs}}| > t_{0.02, 18, \text{crit}} = 2.552$$

    d. a two-tailed test with $\alpha = 0.01$ and $\nu = 128$ degrees of freedom is

$$\text{Reject } H_0 \text{ when } |t_{\text{obs}}| > t_{0.01, 128, \text{crit}} = 2.576$$

The formulas for computing the p-values in a t-test are summarized below.

P-VALUES FOR A t-TEST

The p-value for a t-test with ν degrees of freedom is

    1. $p\text{-value} = P(t_\nu \geq t_{\text{obs}})$ in an upper-tail t-test.

    2. $p\text{-value} = P(t_\nu \leq t_{\text{obs}})$ in a lower-tail t-test.

    3. $p\text{-value} = P(t_\nu \geq |t_{\text{obs}}|)$ in a two-tailed t-test.

In general, the p-value for a t-test must be determined by a computer, however, it is possible to approximate the p-value of a t-test using Tables A.8 and A.9. Tables A.8 and A.9 provide the upper tail probabilities for a t-distribution with ν degrees of freedom for observed values of t-close to $t = 1.7, 1.8, 1.9, \ldots, 3.4$. The procedure that can be used for approximating the p-value associated with t_{obs} in a t-test using Tables A.8 and A.9 is outlined below.

    1. Locate the row corresponding the degrees of freedom, say ν, of the test statistic.

    2. Locate the value of t in the t column that is closest to t_{obs} or $|t_{\text{obs}}|$ when t_{obs} is negative.

    3. The approximate p-value for an upper- or lower-tail t-test is the value inside the table in the row having ν degrees of freedom and under the column of the t-value closest to t_{obs}. The approximate p-value for a two-tailed t-test is twice the value inside the table in the row having ν degrees of freedom and under the column of the t-value closest to t_{obs}.

Note that when the value of t that is closest to t_{obs} is also less than t_{obs}, the p-value is guaranteed to be no larger than the approximate value. Also, for a two-tailed test the value from the table must be doubled since the test is a two-tailed test, and when the value of t_{obs} is larger than 3.4 then the p-value should be reported as being less than the p-value listed for $t_{obs} = 3.4$. For example, if $t_{obs} = 4.81$ and the test has 22 degrees of freedom the p-value is less than the value listed under $t = 3.4$ that is 0.001. In this case, the p-value should be reported as $p < 0.001$.

In tests where the null hypothesis has been failed to be rejected, then the p-value is larger than the significance level. Therefore, when there is insufficient evidence for the rejection of H_0, the p-value associated with t_{obs} only needs to be approximated when the value of t_{obs} is close to the boundary of the rejection region. For example, if $t_{obs} = 1.72$ and the rejection region for testing H_0 is $t > 1.782$, then there is insufficient evidence to reject H_0. Since t_{obs} is near the boundary of the rejection region the p-value should be approximated. and in this case, $p \approx 0.057$.

Example 7.22
Find the approximate value of the p-value when

- **a.** H_0 was rejected in an upper-tail test with $\nu = 21$ degrees of freedom and $t_{obs} = 3.36$.
- **b.** H_0 was rejected in a two-tailed test with $\nu = 25$ degrees of freedom and $t_{obs} = 2.33$.
- **c.** H_0 was failed to be rejected in a lower-tail test with $\nu = 20$ degrees of freedom and $t_{obs} = -1.87$.
- **d.** H_0 was rejected in a two-tailed test with $\nu = 40$ degrees of freedom and $t_{obs} = 5.31$.

Solutions   The approximate value of the p-value when

- **a.** H_0 is rejected in an upper-tail test with $\nu = 21$ degrees of freedom and $t_{obs} = 3.36$ is found by using $\nu = 21$ degrees of freedom and $t = 3.3$ in Table A.9. Thus, the approximate value of the p-value is 0.002.
- **b.** H_0 is rejected in a two-tailed test with $\nu = 25$ degrees of freedom and $t_{obs} = 2.33$ is twice the table value found in the $\nu = 25$ row and $t = 2.3$ column in Table A.8. Thus, the approximate value of the p-value is $2 \times 0.015 = 0.030$.
- **c.** H_0 is failed to be rejected in a lower-tail test with $\nu = 20$ degrees of freedom and $t_{obs} = -1.87$ is 0.043.
- **d.** H_0 is rejected in a two-tailed test with $\nu = 40$ degrees of freedom and $t_{obs} = 5.31$ is less than $2 \times 0.001 = 0.002$.

Finally, each t-test produces valid decisions and accurate p-values only when a specific set of assumptions is satisfied. The assumptions needed to have a valid t-test will vary from one test to another, but every t-test that the sample comes from population that has a normal distribution. In most research studies, the researcher will use a statistical computing package to analyze the data and perform the relevant hypothesis tests. The advantages of using a statistical computing package to perform a t-test are that it is easy to check the normality assumption and that the statistical computing package will report the exact value of the p-value along with the observed value t statistic.

7.3.2 *t*-Tests for the Mean of a Population

The first application of the t-test that will be discussed deals with testing claims about the mean of a population. If μ_0 is the hypothesized value of the mean, then research

TABLE 7.17   The Null and Alternative Hypotheses for Tests About the Mean of a Population

Test	H_0	H_A
Upper-tail	$H_0 : \mu \leq \mu_0$	$H_A : \mu > \mu_0$
Lower-tail	$H_0 : \mu \geq \mu_0$	$H_A : \mu < \mu_0$
Two-tailed	$H_0 : \mu = \mu_0$	$H_A : \mu \neq \mu_0$

question is investigated by testing one of the pairs of null and alternative hypotheses given in Table 7.17.

Suppose that a simple random sample of n observations is to be selected from the target population. Then, the estimator of μ is $\bar{x}$ and the estimated standard error of $\bar{x}$ is

$$\text{se}(\bar{x}) = \frac{s}{\sqrt{n}}$$

and the test statistic for testing claims about the mean is

$$t = \frac{\bar{x} - \mu_0}{s / \sqrt{n}}$$

When the population being studied is normally distributed the sampling distribution of the t statistic follows a t distribution with $n - 1$ degrees of freedom. Note that the degrees of freedom of the t-test are the same as the degrees of freedom of s, the estimate of the population standard deviation; in general, the degrees of freedom of a t-test are based on the degrees of freedom of the estimate of the population standard deviation. Thus, a t-test is only appropriate when the *normality assumption* is met or the degrees of freedom of the t-test are greater than 120. The normality assumption can be checked with a normal probability plot or a histogram of the sample data. In particular, the normality assumption will be supported by the observed data when either the normal probability plot passes the fat pencil test or the histogram is mound shaped. On the other hand, when the normal probability plot or the histogram suggest the normality assumption is not satisfied, a t-test should not be used for testing claims about a population mean when $n < 100$. In particular, when the normality assumption is violated, the decision and p-value resulting from a t-test cannot be trusted.

When the degrees of freedom of the t-test are greater than 100, then the normality assumption can be relaxed because the Central Limit Theorem applies and the t-test is essentially a Z-test. That is, the sampling distribution of the t statistic can be approximated a standard normal when the degrees of freedom of the test are greater than 100. Thus, for large samples the t-test will be an appropriate test for claims about the mean even when the target population is not normally distributed.

Now, the rejection regions that are used in every upper-, lower-, or two-tailed t-test were given in Table 7.16, and the rejections for testing claims about the mean of a population are given listed in Table 7.18.

TABLE 7.18   The Rejection Regions for a t-Test

Test	H_0	H_A	Rejection Region
Upper-tail	$H_0 : \mu \leq \mu_0$	$H_A : \mu > \mu_0$	$t_{\text{obs}} > t_{\text{crit}}$
Lower-tail	$H_0 : \mu \geq \mu_0$	$H_A : \mu < \mu_0$	$t_{\text{obs}} < -t_{\text{crit}}$
Two-tailed	$H_0 : \mu = \mu_0$	$H_A : \mu \neq \mu_0$	$|t_{\text{obs}}| > t_{\text{crit}}$

The value of t_{crit} can be found in Table A.7 and depends upon both α and the degrees of freedom of the test. The p-value associated with the observed value of the t statistic, t_{obs}, can be approximated using Tables A.8 and A.9 or will be computed by a computer when a statistical computing package is used for performing a t-test.

After performing a test about the mean of a population it is also standard procedure to report a confidence interval for the mean along with the decision concerning the null hypothesis. Thus, when the population sampled is approximately normal a $(1 - \alpha) \times 100\%$ confidence interval for μ is

$$\bar{x} \pm t_{crit} \frac{s}{\sqrt{n}}$$

where t_{crit} depends on the confidence level and the degrees of freedom of s. The confidence interval often allows a researcher to distinguish between the statistical and scientific significance of a result.

Example 7.23

In the article "A comparison of body fat determined by underwater weighing and volume displacement" published in the *American Journal of Physiology* (Ward et al., 1978), the authors found that the mean percent body fat for males aged 25–61 was 20%. Use the data in Table 7.19 compiled from the Body Fat data set for males aged 65 and older to test

$$H_0 : \text{The mean body fat percentage for males 65 and older is} \leq 20\%$$

versus

$$H_0 : \text{The mean body fat percentage for males 65 and older is} > 20\%$$

at the $\alpha = 0.01$ significance level.

Solution   First, the normal probability plot for the $n = 21$ observations in Table 7.19 is given in Figure 7.6. Since the normal probability plot passes the fat pencil test, the normality assumption appears to be satisfied. Thus, a t-test of H_0 versus H_A is appropriate, and the rejection region when $\alpha = 0.01$ is

$$\text{Reject } H_0 \text{ when } t_{obs} > t_{crit} = 2.528$$

Based on the data in Table 7.19, $\bar{x} = 25.74$ and $s = 6.90$. Thus,

$$t_{obs} = \frac{25.74 - 20}{6.90/\sqrt{21}} = 3.81$$

Since $t_{obs} = 3.81$ is in the rejection region H_0 is rejected, and the approximate value of the p-value is less than 0.001. Hence, there is strong evidence against

$$H_0 : \text{The mean body fat percentage for males 65 and older is} \leq 20\%$$

TABLE 7.19   The Percent Body Fat for $n = 21$ Males Age 65 or Older in the Body Fat Data Set

Observed Data						
22.2	21.5	18.8	31.4	27.0	27.0	26.6
14.9	29.9	17.0	35.0	30.4	32.6	29.0
15.2	30.2	11.0	33.6	29.3	26.0	31.9

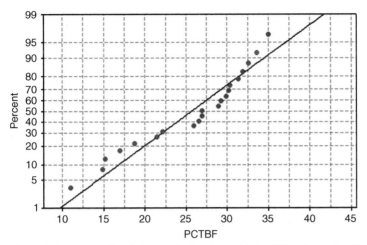

Figure 7.6   A normal probability plot for the variable PCTBF for males 65 or older in the Body Fat data set.

A 95% confidence interval for the mean body fat percentage for males 65 and older is

$$25.74 \pm 1.725 \frac{6.90}{\sqrt{21}}$$

which yields interval of 23.14–28.34. Thus, based on the observed sample it appears that the mean percent body fat for a male age 65 or older is significantly different than 20% and appears to be at least 23% and possibly as much as 28%.

In designing a t-test, the researcher must choose the significance level α of the test, the value of μ that is scientifically different from μ_0, say μ_{crit}, and the value of β at μ_{crit}. The researcher must also provide a prespecified guess of the value of σ that will be denoted by $\acute{\sigma}$. Once the researcher has determined these values the appropriate sample size for testing H_0 versus H_A can be determined. The approximate sample size required for a t-test will be prespecified values of α, β, μ_{crit}, and $\acute{\sigma}$ is

$$n = \acute{\sigma}^2 \left(\frac{z_\alpha + z_\beta}{\mu_0 - \mu_{\text{crit}}} \right)^2$$

where $z_\alpha = |z_{\alpha,\text{crit}}|$ and z_β can be found in Table A.6.

Example 7.24

Determine the approximate sample size needed for a t-test when

   a. $H_0 : \mu = 10$, $H_A : \mu \neq 10$, $\alpha = 0.05$, $\beta = 0.10$, $\mu_{\text{crit}} = 12$, and $\acute{\sigma} = 5$.
   b. $H_0 : \mu \geq 250$, $H_A : \mu < 250$, $\alpha = 0.01$, $\beta = 0.15$, $\mu_{\text{crit}} = 225$, and $\acute{\sigma} = 50$.
   c. $H_0 : \mu \leq 1.0$, $H_A : \mu > 1.0$, $\alpha = 0.05$, $\beta = 0.01$, $\mu_{\text{crit}} = 1.1$, and $\acute{\sigma} = 0.15$.

Solutions   The approximate sample size needed in a t-test when

   a. $H_0 : \mu = 10$, $H_A : \mu \neq 10$, $\alpha = 0.05$, $\beta = 0.10$, $\mu_{\text{crit}} = 12$, and $\acute{\sigma} = 5$ is

$$n = 5^2 \left(\frac{1.96 + 1.282}{10 - 12} \right)^2 = 65.69$$

Thus, use a sample of $n = 66$ observations.

b. $H_0 : \mu \geq 250$, $H_A : \mu < 250$, $\alpha = 0.01$, $\beta = 0.15$, $\mu_{\text{crit}} = 225$, and $\acute{\sigma} = 50$ is

$$n = n = 50^2 \left(\frac{2.326 + 1.04}{250 - 225} \right)^2 = 45.3$$

Thus, use a sample of $n = 46$ observations.

c. $H_0 : \mu \leq 1.0$, $H_A : \mu > 1.0$, $\alpha = 0.05$, $\beta = 0.01$, $\mu_{\text{crit}} = 1.1$, and $\acute{\sigma} = 0.15$ is

$$n = 0.15^2 \left(\frac{1.645 + 2.326}{1.0 - 1.1} \right)^2 = 35.5$$

Thus, use a sample of $n = 36$ observations.

7.3.3 Paired Comparison *t*-Tests

A *t*-test can also be used for comparing the means of two populations, and the *paired comparison t*-test is a commonly used test in biomedical research. The goal in a paired comparison is to compare the means of two populations, say X and Y. Furthermore, the observations of the populations X and Y in a paired comparison are related (i.e., not independent) and are sampled in pairs of observations. That is, each observation in a paired comparison is a bivariate observation of the form (X, Y). Paired comparisons are often used when comparing two different treatments or for comparing the values of a response variable which will be measured before and after a treatment is applied.

The sampling plan used to collect data in a paired comparison must generate pairs of observations, and the two most commonly used sampling plans are the *within-subject* and *matched pairs* sampling plans. A within-subjects sampling plan is used when the set of subjects used in the study receive each treatment; a matched pairs sampling plan is used when the units in the study are matched according to a particular set of explanatory variables either before the treatment is applied or after the units have been sampled. Both sampling plans are designed to control for external variables by making the units, before treatment, as similar as possible. Paired comparisons are often used when the units of the population being treated are not homogeneous. That is, by pairing the observations and analyzing the difference within the pairs, the inherent differences between the units of the population can be controlled for.

Example 7.25
A paired comparison might be used in a study of the effects of a new drug designed to lower blood pressure because there are a wide variety of external factors influencing an individual's blood pressure (i.e., weight, diet, stress level, etc.). Thus, measuring an individual's blood pressure before administering the treatment and comparing it with the individual's blood pressure after the treatment period controls for inherent differences between individuals. Here a within-subjects sampling plan would be used.

Example 7.26
A paired comparison might be used in studying the efficacy of a new cancer treatment in comparison with the efficacy of an existing treatment. Because there are a wide variety of external factors that might affect how an individual responds to a cancer treatment (i.e., gender, age, cancer stage, race, etc.), individuals in the study might be paired according to a particular set of explanatory variables to control for the inherent differences in the individuals. That is, by matching individuals on a set of relevant variables the two treatment groups can be made as similar as possible before the treatments are applied. Here a matched pairs sampling plan would be used.

TABLE 7.20 The Null and Alternative Hypotheses for Paired Comparison Tests for the Means of Two Populations

Test	H_0	H_A
Upper-tail	$H_0 : \mu_X \leq \mu_Y$	$H_A : \mu_X > \mu_Y$
Lower-tail	$H_0 : \mu_X \geq \mu_Y$	$H_A : \mu_X < \mu_Y$
Two-tailed	$H_0 : \mu_X = \mu_Y$	$H_A : \mu_X \neq \mu_Y$

Let X and Y represent the populations being compared. The hypotheses concerning the means of these two populations that can be tested in a paired comparison are the upper-, lower-, and two-tailed hypotheses listed in Table 7.20.

A random sample of n pairs of observations is used for testing the null hypothesis comparing μ_X and μ_Y in a paired comparison. Let

$$(x_1, y_1), (x_2, y_2), \ldots, (x_n, y_n)$$

be the observed data. Note that while there are n observations from each of the populations, a total of $2n$ measurements, and a paired comparison is actually a one-sample problem since only n pairs of observations are sampled. Thus, the sample size in a paired comparison is the number of pairs observed, not the number of measurements recorded.

The parameter of interest in a paired comparison t-test is difference of the two means, $\mu_X - \mu_Y$. Note that when $\mu_X - \mu_Y = 0$ it follows that $\mu_X = \mu_Y$, when $\mu_X - \mu_Y > 0$ it follows that $\mu_X > \mu_Y$, and when $\mu_X - \mu_Y < 0$ it follows that $\mu_X < \mu_Y$. The point estimator of $\mu_X - \mu_Y$ is $\bar{d}$, which is the sample mean of the n differences formed by subtracting the Y value from the X value in each observed pair of observations. That is, the n differences in a paired comparison are

$$d_1 = x_1 - y_1, d_2 = x_2 - y_2, \ldots, d_n = x_n - y_n$$

and the estimate of $\mu_X - \mu_Y$ is formed averaging the n differences $d_1, d_2, \ldots, d_n$. Thus,

$$\bar{d} = \text{average of the } n \text{ differences} = \frac{\sum d}{n}$$

Also, the estimated standard error of $\bar{d}$ is

$$\text{se}(\bar{d}) = \frac{s_d}{\sqrt{n}}$$

where s_d is the sample standard deviation computed from the n observed differences.

The t statistic that is used for testing claims about μ_X and μ_Y in a paired comparison study is

$$t = \frac{\bar{d}}{s_d/\sqrt{n}}$$

which has a sampling distribution that follows a t distribution with $n - 1$ degrees of freedom when the population of differences, $X - Y$, is approximately normally distributed. Thus, provided a normal probability plot or a histogram of the n observed differences suggests no obvious departure from normality, a t-test will be appropriate for testing claims about μ_X and μ_Y in a paired comparison study. When a normal probability plot or a histogram do suggest that the differences may not be normally distributed, a t-test should not be used for comparing μ_X and μ_Y unless $n \geq 120$.

TABLE 7.21 The Rejection Regions for a *t*-Test

Test	H_0	H_A	Rejection Region
Upper-tail	$H_0 : \mu_X \leq \mu_Y$	$H_A : \mu_X > \mu_Y$	$t_{obs} > t_{crit}$
Lower-tail	$H_Y : \mu_X \geq \mu_Y$	$H_A : \mu_X < \mu_Y$	$t_{obs} < -t_{crit}$
Two-tailed	$H_Y : \mu_X = \mu_Y$	$H_A : \mu_X \neq \mu_Y$	$|t_{obs}| > t_{crit}$

The rejection regions for a paired *t*-test are given in Table 7.21. The value of t_{crit} used in a particular rejection region can be found in the Table A.7, and the value of t_{crit} will depend on the values of α and the degrees of freedom associated with the *t* statistic.

The *p*-value associated with the observed value of t_{obs} can be approximated using Tables A.8 and A.9, and the *p*-value will also provided in the standard output of *t*-test when a statistical computing package is used to carry out the test.

A $(1 - \alpha) \times 100\%$ confidence interval for the difference of the two means, $\mu_X - \mu_Y$, in a paired comparison can be computed, provided the normality assumption is satisfied, using

$$\bar{d} \pm t_{crit} \times \frac{s_d}{\sqrt{n}}$$

where t_{crit} depends on the confidence level and has $n - 1$ degrees of freedom.

Example 7.27
In the article "Xylocaine spray reduces patient discomfort during nasogastric tube insertion" published in *The Internet Journal of Surgery* (Power et al., 2006), the authors measured patient discomfort on a visual analogue scale (VAS) on 11 patients before (VAS1) and after (VAS2) a single spray of lignocaine 1%. The data for the 11 patients in this study are given in Table 7.22. Use the data given in Table 7.22 to test the null hypothesis that the mean VAS score before the lignocaine spray is no more than the mean VAS score after the lignocaine spray at a significance level of $\alpha = 0.01$.

Solution Note that the data in Table 7.22 is the result of a within-subject sampling plan because each patient's VAS score was measured before and after the lignocaine spray. Let μ_1 be the mean VAS score before the lignocaine spray and μ_2 the mean VAS score after the lignocaine spray. A paired comparison *t*-test can be used to test $H_0 \mu_1 \leq \mu_2$ versus $H_A : \mu_1 > \mu_2$ provided the $n = 11$ differences indicate that the population of differences is approximately normally distributed.

The $n = 11$ observed differences are 26, 21, 8, 29, 6, 32, 16, 36, 22, 14, 32, and based on these values $\bar{d} = 22$ and $s_d = 10.07$. A normal probability plot of the 11 observed differences is given in

TABLE 7.22 VAS Levels Before (VAS1) and After (VAS2) Lignocaine Spray Use for $n = 11$ Patients

Patient	VAS1	VAS2	Patient	VAS1	VAS2
1	83	57	7	61	45
2	92	71	8	82	46
3	50	42	9	78	56
4	64	35	10	68	54
5	88	82	11	84	52
6	70	38			

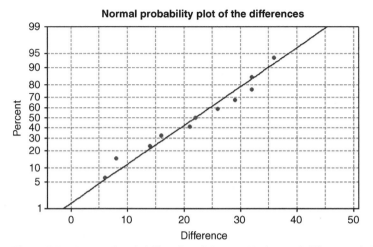

Figure 7.7 A normal probability plot of the $n = 11$ observed differences in VAS scores.

Figure 7.7. Since the normal probability supports the normality assumption, a paired t-test will be appropriate for testing H_0 versus H_A.

The rejection region for testing $H_0 : \mu_1 \le \mu_2$ versus $H_A : \mu_1 > \mu_2$ is based on a t distribution with 10 degrees of freedom and is

$$\text{Reject } H_0 \text{ when } t_{\text{obs}} > t_{\text{crit}} = 2.764$$

The observed value of the paired t statistic is

$$t_{\text{obs}} = \frac{22}{10.07/\sqrt{11}} = 7.25$$

and therefore, H_0 is rejected since $t_{\text{obs}} = 7.25$ does fall in the rejection region. Using Tables A.8 and A.9, the p-value associated with $t_{\text{obs}} = 7.25$ is less than 0.003, and thus, there is strong evidence supporting the hypothesis that the mean VAS score is higher before lignocaine spray than after the spray.

A 95% confidence interval for the mean difference, $\mu_1 - \mu_2$, is

$$22 \pm 1.812 \times \frac{10.07}{\sqrt{11}}$$

which yields 16.50–27.50. Therefore, based on the observed data it appears that the mean VAS score before the lignocaine spray is used in significantly larger than the mean VAS score after the spray. In particular, the mean VAS score before the spray is used appears to be at least 16.50 larger than the mean VAS score after the lignocaine is used and possibly as much as 27.50 larger.

It is highly recommended that a statistical computing package be used in performing a hypothesis test because a statistical computing package will perform the test accurately, provides methods for checking the assumptions of the test, and will compute the p-value associated with the observed value of the test statistic. The MINITAB output for the paired t-test using the data from Example 7.27 is given in Example 7.28.

Example 7.28
The MINITAB output for the paired t-test of $H_0\mu_1 \le \mu_2$ versus $H_A : \mu_1 > \mu_2$ in Example 7.27 is given in Figure 7.8. Note that the MINITAB output includes a table of the sample means, standard deviations, and the estimated standard errors of the sample means, along with a lower bound confidence interval for the difference in means, the value of t_{obs}, and the p-value associated with t_{obs}. As an option

```
Paired T-Test and CI: VAS1, VAS2

Paired T for VAS1 - VAS2

                N    Mean   StDev   SE Mean
VAS1           11   74.55   12.94     3.90
VAS2           11   52.55   14.05     4.23
Difference     11   22.00   10.07     3.04


95% lower bound for mean difference: 16.50
T-Test of mean difference = 0 (vs > 0):   T-Value = 7.25
P-Value = 0.000
```

Figure 7.8   The MINITAB output for the paired t-test of $H_0 \mu_1 \le \mu_2$ versus $H_A : \mu_1 > \mu_2$ in Example 7.27.

in the MINITAB paired t-test program, a researcher can ask for a histogram and/or a boxplot of the observed differences that can be used to check the normality assumption of the t-test.

In a well-designed paired comparison the sample size should be determined to produce a highly reliable testing procedure. In designing a paired t-test the necessary sample size n required to attain a prespecified probability of making a Type II error requires information on the significance level of the test, the value of $\mu_X - \mu_Y = \delta$ different from 0 that has scientific meaning, the probability of making a Type II error, and a reasonable guess of the standard deviation of $X - Y$. Once a researcher has determined the values of α, δ, β, and $\dot{\sigma}_d$, the approximate sample size required in a paired comparison t-test is

$$n = \dot{\sigma}_d^2 \left(\frac{z_\alpha + z_\beta}{\delta} \right)^2$$

where $z_\alpha = |z_{\alpha,\text{crit}}|$. In order for the value of approximate value of n to be useful, the researcher must also have evidence that the distribution of $X - Y$ is approximately normal. Similar to determining a reasonable guess of the standard deviation, prior research or experimental experiences should be used for supporting the normality assumption before the sample data are collected.

Example 7.29
Determine the approximate sample size needed in a paired t when

    a. $H_0 : \mu_X \le \mu_Y$, $H_A : \mu_X > \mu_Y$, $\alpha = 0.05$, $\beta = 0.15$, $\delta = 5$, and $\dot{\sigma}_d = 15$.
    b. $H_0 : \mu_X = \mu_Y$, $H_A : \mu_X \ne \mu_Y$, $\alpha = 0.01$, $\beta = 0.05$, $\delta = 25$, and $\dot{\sigma}_d = 40$.
    c. $H_0 : \mu_X \ge \mu_Y$, $H_A : \mu_X < \mu_Y$, $\alpha = 0.05$, $\beta = 0.10$, $\delta = 0.05$, and $\dot{\sigma} = 0.10$.

Solutions   The sample size needed for a t-test when

    a. $H_0 : \mu_X \le \mu_Y$, $H_A : \mu_X > \mu_Y$, $\alpha = 0.05$, $\beta = 0.15$, $\delta = 5$, and $\dot{\sigma}_d = 15$ is

$$n = 15^2 \left(\frac{1.645 + 1.04}{5} \right)^2 = 64.8$$

Thus, use a sample of $n = 65$ observations.

b. $H_0 : \mu_X = \mu_Y$, $H_A : \mu_X \neq \mu_Y$, $\alpha = 0.01$, $\beta = 0.05$, $\delta = 25$, and $\dot\sigma_d = 40$ is

$$n = n = 40^2 \left(\frac{2.576 + 1.282}{25} \right)^2 = 45.6$$

Thus, use a sample of $n = 46$ observations.

c. $H_0 : \mu_X \geq \mu_Y$, $H_A : \mu_X < \mu_Y$, $\alpha = 0.05$, $\beta = 0.10$, $\delta = 0.05$, and $\dot\sigma = 0.10$ is

$$n = 0.10^2 \left(\frac{1.645 + 1.282}{0.05} \right)^2 = 34.3$$

Thus, use a sample of $n = 35$ observations.

Again, most of the commonly used statistical computing packages have programs that can be used for determining the sample size required for a paired t-test and for performing the paired t-test once the sample data are observed. Moreover, it is strongly recommended that a statistical computing package be used for all t-tests since they perform the computations accurately, they provide the important and necessary graphical procedures required in data analyses, and they provide the p-values associated with any hypothesis tests that are performed.

7.3.4 Two Independent Sample t-Tests

When the research goal is to compare the means of two distinct populations, and pairing is not required to control for external factors, the comparison can be based on the data contained in random samples drawn from each of the two populations. When the samples from the two populations are selected independently they constitute a stratified random sample, and any comparisons based on the two samples are referred to as *two independent sample* comparisons. Furthermore, provided specific assumptions are met a t-test can be used to test hypotheses comparing the two means.

Let X and Y be the two populations being studied. Then, the parameters that are important for comparing the means of these two populations are μ_X, μ_Y, σ_X, and σ_Y, and given independently selected random samples of n_X and n_Y observations from the X and Y populations, the point estimators of the parameters μ_X, μ_Y, σ_X, and σ_Y are $\bar{x}$, $\bar{y}$, s_X, and s_Y. In particular,

$\bar{x}$ = average of the n_X sample observations from population X

$\bar{y}$ = average of the n_Y sample observations from population Y

s_X = sample standard deviation of the n_X sample observations from population X

s_Y = sample standard deviation of the n_Y sample observations from population Y

The values of $\bar{x}$, $\bar{y}$, s_X, and s_Y contain the important sample information that will be used in testing claims comparing μ_X and μ_Y.

The hypotheses concerning the two means, μ_X and μ_Y, that can be tested are similar to those in a paired comparison. In particular, the null and alternative hypotheses for the upper-, lower-, and two-tailed two sample mean comparisons are given in Table 7.23.

The test statistic that is used for testing claims about μ_X and μ_Y in two independent sample comparisons is the *two-sample t* statistic that is given by

$$t = \frac{\bar{x} - \bar{y}}{se}$$

TABLE 7.23   The Null and Alternative Hypotheses for Tests Comparing the Means of Two Populations

Test	H_0	H_A
Upper-tail	$H_0 : \mu_X \leq \mu_Y$	$H_A : \mu_X > \mu_Y$
Lower-tail	$H_0 : \mu_X \geq \mu_Y$	$H_A : \mu_X < \mu_Y$
Two-tailed	$H_0 : \mu_X = \mu_Y$	$H_A : \mu \neq \mu_Y$

where se is the estimated standard error of $\bar{x} - \bar{y}$. Also, because the samples are independent the estimated standard error of $\bar{x} - \bar{y}$ is

$$se(\bar{x} - \bar{y}) = \sqrt{\frac{s_X^2}{n_X} + \frac{s_Y^2}{n_Y}}$$

The two-sample t-test statistic measures the statistical distance between the two sample means. When the statistical distance is "large", then the sample data are suggesting the two population means are different. The size of the statistical distance can only be judged by considering the sampling distribution of the two-sample t statistic. The sampling distribution of the two-sample t statistic depends on the distributions of the populations X and Y as well as the standard deviations of these populations. In particular,

1. when both sample sizes, n_X and n_Y, are at least 60 the Central Limit Theorem applies and the sampling distribution of the two-sample t statistic is approximately distributed as a standard normal (i.e., a t distribution with ∞ degrees of freedom).

2. when each of the populations is normally distributed, the standard deviations of the two populations are not equal (i.e., $\sigma_X \neq \sigma_Y$), but $n_X \approx n_Y$, the sampling distribution of the two-sample t statistic follows a t distribution with $n_X + n_Y - 2$ degrees of freedom.

3. when each of the populations is normally distributed and the standard deviations of the two populations are equal (i.e., $\sigma_X = \sigma_Y$), the sampling distribution of the two-sample t statistic follows a t-distribution with $n_X + n_Y - 2$ degrees of freedom.

In each of these three cases the two-sample t statistic will follow a t distribution, and hence, a t-test can be used for testing hypotheses comparing μ_X and μ_Y. In all other cases, the sampling distribution of the two-sample t statistic is complicated and will not be discussed here. For example, when the populations are not approximately normal or the standard deviations are extremely different some form of the two-sample t statistic may or may not be appropriate for use in testing claims about the means of the two populations.

In order to have a valid two-sample t-test, one of the three cases listed above must be supported by the observed data. Normal probability plots or histograms can be used to check the assumption of the normality of each population, which is a critical requirement in a t-test except when both n_X and n_Y are large. When inspecting a normal probability plot or a histograms look for deviations from normality in these plots such as a long tail, outliers, or multiple modes.

In case 3, the standard deviations of the two populations are required to be equal, and as long as the ratio of the sample standard deviations does not differ by a factor of more than 2 it is reasonable to assume that $\sigma_X = \sigma_Y$. That is, as long as the populations sampled are approximately normal and

$$0.5 \leq \frac{s_X}{s_Y} \leq 2$$

it is reasonable to use a two-sample t-test for testing hypotheses comparing μ_X and μ_Y. Furthermore, when the standard deviations are equal and have common value $\sigma_x = \sigma_y = \sigma$, both s_X and s_Y are estimators of σ. In this case a more accurate estimator of σ can be found by pooling the information about σ contained in the estimators s_X and s_Y. The *pooled estimator of σ* is

$$S_p = \sqrt{\frac{(n_X - 1)s_x^2 + (n_Y - 1)s_y^2}{n_X + n_Y - 2}}$$

and has $n_X + n_Y - 2$ degrees of freedom. Note that S_p is the square-root of a weighted average of the two sample variances, s_X^2 and s_Y^2. Also, S_p^2 is an unbiased estimator of the common variance σ^2 of the X and Y populations when $\sigma_X = \sigma_Y$.

When the pooled estimate S_p of σ is used the estimated standard error of $\bar{x} - \bar{y}$ is given by

$$se = \sqrt{\frac{S_p^2}{n_X} + \frac{S_p^2}{n_Y}}$$

The pooled two-sample t statistic is

$$t = \frac{\bar{x} - \bar{y}}{\sqrt{\frac{S_p^2}{n_X} + \frac{S_p^2}{n_Y}}}$$

and has $n_X + n_Y - 2$ degrees of freedom.

THE TWO-SAMPLE t STATISTIC

The two-sample t statistic used for testing claims about μ_X and μ_Y is

$$t = \begin{cases} \dfrac{\bar{x} - \bar{y}}{\sqrt{\frac{S_p^2}{n_X} + \frac{S_p^2}{n_Y}}} & \text{when } \sigma_X = \sigma_Y \\[4ex] \dfrac{\bar{x} - \bar{y}}{\sqrt{\frac{s_X^2}{n_X} + \frac{s_Y^2}{n_Y}}} & \text{when } \sigma_X \neq \sigma_Y \text{ or } n_X \text{ and } n_Y \text{ are greater than } 60 \end{cases}$$

The rejection regions the upper-, lower-, and two-tailed tests for a two-sample t-test are given in Table 7.21, and the p-value associated with the observed value of the t-statistic can be approximated using Tables A.8 and A.9. Also, a $(1 - \alpha) \times 100\%$ confidence interval for the difference in the two means, $\mu_X - \mu_Y$, is

$$\bar{x} - \bar{y} \pm t_{crit} \times se$$

where the appropriate form of the estimated standard error is used.

Example 7.30

In the article "Relationship of axial length and retinal vascular caliber in children" published in the *American Journal of Ophthalmology* (Cheung et al., 2007), the authors investigated factors that they believed are related to myopia (near-sightedness). One of the factors the authors considered was the weight of a child. The summary statistics given in Table 7.24 were reported in this article for the weights (in kg) in a sample of 620 children diagnosed with myopia and a sample of 147 children without myopia.

TABLE 7.24 Summary Statistics for the Samples on the Weights of Children With and Without Myopia

Population	Sample Size	Mean Weight	SD
Myopia	620	30.86	8.21
No myopia	147	34.62	10.42

Let μ_M be the mean weight of the population of children with myopia and μ_N the mean weight of the population of children without myopia. Use the summary statistics in Table 7.24 to test $H_0 : \mu_M \geq \mu_N$ versus $H_A : \mu_M < \mu_N$ at the $\alpha = 0.05$ significance level.

Solution Since $n_M = 620$ and $n_N = 147$ are both greater than 60 the Central Limit Theorem applies, and therefore, the two-sample t statistic can be used with $\nu = \infty$ degrees of freedom for testing H_0 versus H_A. The rejection region for testing $H_0 : \mu_M \geq \mu_N$ versus $H_A : \mu_M < \mu_N$ at the $\alpha = 0.05$ significance level is

$$\text{Reject } H_0 \text{ when } t_{obs} < -t_{crit} = -1.645$$

The observed value of the two-sample t statistic is

$$t = \frac{30.86 - 34.62}{\sqrt{\frac{8.21^2}{620} + \frac{10.42^2}{147}}} = -4.08$$

and thus, since $t_{obs} = -4.08$ is in the rejection region $H_0 : \mu_M \geq \mu_N$ is rejected. Using Tables A.8 and A.9 the p-value is less than 0.000, and hence, there is very strong evidence that the mean weight of a child with myopia is less than that of a child without myopia.

A 95% confidence interval for the difference in the mean weights of children with and without myopia is

$$(30.86 - 34.62) \pm 1.96 \times \sqrt{\frac{8.21^2}{620} + \frac{10.42^2}{147}}$$

which yields an interval of -5.56 to -1.96 kg. Thus, based on the observed data there appears to be a significant difference between the mean weights of children with and without myopia, and it appears that the mean weight of children without myopia is at least 1.96 kg larger than the mean weight of children with myopia and possibly as much as 5.56 kg more.

Example 7.31
In the Birth Weight data set there are 16 African-American mothers who did not smoke during pregnancy and 10 who did smoke during pregnancy. The summary statistics for the birth weights (in grams) of babies born to African-American mothers broken down according to smoking status during pregnancy are given in Table 7.25, and normal probability plots of each sample are given in Figure 7.9.

Let μ_S be the mean weight of a baby born to an African-American mother who smoked during pregnancy, and let μ_{NS} be the mean weight of a baby born to an African-American mother who did not smoke during pregnancy. Use the summary statistics in Table 7.25 to test $H_0 : \mu_S \geq \mu_{NS}$ versus $H_A : \mu_S < \mu_{NS}$ at the $\alpha = 0.05$ significance level.

Solution First, the normal probability plots given in Figure 7.9 support the assumption that each population is normally distributed. Now, since both sample sizes are small (i.e., less than 60) and they are not equal, the two-sample t-test will only be appropriate when $\sigma_S = \sigma_{NS}$. The ratio of the two sample standard deviations which is $\frac{637}{621} = 1.03$, and since the ratio of the two sample standard

TABLE 7.25 Summary Statistics for the Samples on the Birth Weights of Babies Born to African-American Mothers by Smoking Status

Smoking Status	Sample Size	Birth Weight Mean	SD
Smoked	10	2504	637
Did not smoke	16	2855	621

deviations is between 0.5 and 2, it is reasonable to assume that $\sigma_S = \sigma_{NS}$. Thus, the pooled two-sample t statistic with $10 + 16 - 2 = 24$ degrees of freedom will be used for testing H_0 versus H_A. The rejection region for testing $H_0 : \mu_S \geq \mu_{NS}$ versus $H_A : \mu_S < \mu_{NS}$ at the $\alpha = 0.05$ significance level is

$$\text{Reject } H_0 \text{ when } t_{obs} < -t_{crit} = -1.711$$

The pooled estimate of the standard deviation is

$$S_p = \sqrt{\frac{(10 - 1) \times 637^2 + (16 - 1) \times 621^2}{10 + 16 - 2}} = 627.05$$

and the estimated standard error of the difference in the sample means is

$$se = \sqrt{\frac{627.05^2}{10} + \frac{627.05^2}{16}} = 252.77$$

Thus, the value of t_{obs} is

$$t_{obs} = \frac{2504 - 2855}{252.77} = -1.39$$

and since $t_{obs} = -1.39$ is not in the rejection region, H_0 is failed to be rejected. Thus, there is insufficient evidence in the observed sample to reject H_0.

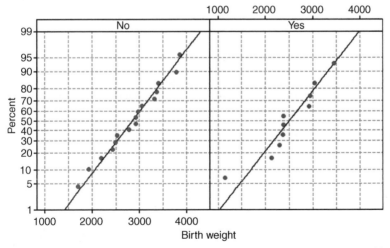

Figure 7.9 Normal probability plots for the birth weights of babies born to African-American mothers by smoking status.

```
Two-Sample T-Test and CI

Sample   N   Mean   StDev   SE Mean
1        10  2504   637        201
2        16  2855   621        155

Difference = mu (1) - mu (2)
Estimate for difference:  -351
95% upper bound for difference:  81
T-Test of difference = 0 (vs <): T-Value = -1.39
P-Value = 0.089   DF = 24
Both use Pooled StDev = 627.0478
```
Figure 7.10   The MINITAB output for the pooled two-sample t-test in Example 7.31.

A 95% confidence interval for the difference in the mean birth weights is

$$(2504 - 2855) \pm 2.064 \times 252.77$$

which yields an interval -872.7 to 170.7 g.

The MINITAB output for the pooled two-sample t-test is given in Figure 7.10. Note that MINITAB provides a table of the sample means, standard deviations, and the estimated standard errors for the sample means, along with an upper bound confidence interval for the difference in means, the value of t_{obs}, the p-value associated with t_{obs}, the degrees of freedom of the t statistic, and the pooled estimate of the common standard deviation. Also, as an option in the MINITAB two-sample t-test program, a researcher can ask for boxplots for each of the observed samples that can be used to check the normality assumption.

Determining the sample size required to have a reliable two-sample t-test will require a researcher to prespecify the values of α, β, $\delta = \mu_X - \mu_Y$, σ_X, and σ_Y. The sample sizes are generally determined so that equal sample sizes will be used for the X and Y samples (i.e., $n_X = n_Y$). Also, designing a t-test with common sample sizes, n_X and n_Y allows the two-sample t statistic to be used even when the standard deviations are different, however, the formula used to determine the approximate sample size $n = n_X = n_Y$ is based on the assumption that $\sigma_X = \sigma_Y$. The approximate sample size required to have a reliable hypothesis test with prespecified values of α, β, $\delta = \mu_X - \mu_Y$, and a prior guess of the common standard deviation, $\dot{\sigma}$, is

$$n = \dot{\sigma}^2 \left(\frac{z_\alpha + z_\beta}{\delta} \right)^2$$

$z_\alpha = |z_{\alpha,\text{crit}}|$ as before and z_β is found in Table A.6. Note that the formula for n gives the individual subpopulation sample sizes, n_X and n_Y, and not the total sample size $n_X + n_Y$. Thus, the overall sample size is $n_X + n_Y = 2n$.

Example 7.32
The approximate sample size needed to have a reliable lower-tail test when $\alpha = 0.01$, $\beta = 0.05$, $\delta = 15$, and $\dot{\sigma} = 25$ is

$$n = 25^2 \left(\frac{2.326 + 1.645}{15} \right)^2 = 43.8$$

Thus, the individual sample sizes are $n_X = 44$ and $n_Y = 44$, and the overall sample size is 88. Then, provided the sample data supports the normality of both the X and Y populations, the two-sample t-test statistic will have $44 + 44 - 2 = 86$ degrees of freedom regardless of whether or not the data supports $\sigma_X = \sigma_Y$ since $n_X = n_Y$.

7.4   SOME FINAL COMMENTS ON HYPOTHESIS TESTING

A hypothesis test is a powerful statistical tool when used correctly. In fact, hypothesis tests have been developed for testing any parameter of a population, and each of the remaining chapters in this book presents hypothesis tests for the relevant parameters being studied. For example, in Chapters 8, 9, 10, 12, and 13 hypothesis tests for the parameters in several different statistical models will be discussed.

Hypothesis testing is also one of the most commonly abused statistical procedures in practice. Some of the common abuses and misuses of hypothesis testing include:

1. Hypothesis tests that are poorly designed are often used. In particular, tests are often used with an insufficient sample size to detect a scientifically important difference or with data that was not selected according to a well-designed random sampling plan.

2. Hypothesis tests are often used even when the data clearly violates of the assumptions required to have a valid test.

3. Researchers sometimes force a hypothesis test to produce a statistically significant result by using an inflated significance level or by oversampling the population.

4. Researchers often incorrectly interpret a nonsignificant test as strong support for the null hypothesis without considering the probability of a Type II error.

5. Researchers often incorrectly interpret the p-value as the size of the treatment effect, difference between the observed and null value of the parameter, or the strength of relationship.

Abuses and misuses of a hypothesis test can be avoided by using a well-designed hypothesis test that is based on a well-designed sampling plan. In particular, in planning a hypothesis test special consideration must be given to the sampling plan, significance level, probability of making a Type II error, sample size, and the assumptions of the test. That is, the researcher must determine

1. a sampling plan that will produce representative data and will lead to a valid hypothesis test.

2. the appropriate significance level for testing the null hypothesis against the alternative.

3. the critical value of the parameter being tested, that is different from the null value, and that has scientific or practical importance.

4. the probability of making a Type II error or the power at the value of the parameter that is scientifically different from the null value.

5. the sample size required to have a prespecified probability of Type II error at the value of the parameter that is scientifically different from the null value.

6. the assumptions required to have a valid hypothesis test.

Even with well-planned hypothesis test the assumptions of the test must be checked and the test should only be carried out as planned when the observed data actually supports the validity of the assumptions. A confidence interval should also be reported along with the results of the hypothesis test. Finally, it is always best to use a statistical computing package in analyzing the observed data since nearly all of the commonly used statistical computing packages provide graphical methods for checking assumptions, the p-value associated with the test, and confidence intervals for the parameter being tested.

GLOSSARY

Alternative Hypothesis   In a hypothesis test the research hypothesis is referred to as the alternative hypothesis and is denoted by H_A.

Dependent Variables   Qualitative variables that are not independent are said to be dependent or associated variables.

Dichotomous Variable   A dichotomous variable is a qualitative variable that takes on only two possible values.

Hypothesis Test   A hypothesis test is a statistical procedure that is used to determine whether or not the data contained in an observed sample supports a particular research hypothesis.

Independent Events   Two events A and B are independent events when $P(A \text{ and } B) = P(A) \times (B)$.

Independent Variables   Two qualitative variables X and Y are independent variables when

$$P(X = a \text{ and } Y = b) = P(X = a) \times P(Y = b)$$

for every pair of possible values of X and Y.

Lower-tail Test   A lower-tail test of a parameter θ is a test of the null hypothesis $H_0 : \theta \geq \theta_0$ versus $H_A : \theta < \theta_0$, where θ_0 is the null value of θ.

Matched Pairs Study   A matched pairs sampling plan is used when the units in the study are matched according to a particular set of variables before the treatment is applied.

Null Hypothesis   In a hypothesis test the status quo hypothesis is referred to as the null hypothesis and is denoted by H_0.

P-value   The p-value associated with an observed value of the test statistic is the probability of observing a sample that will produce a value of the test statistic as or more extreme than the observed value of the test statistic when the null hypothesis is true.

Polytomous Variable   A polytomous variable is a qualitative variable taking on two or more values.

Power   The power of a test measures the ability of the test to distinguish values of θ in the alternative hypothesis from the null value θ_0 specified in the null hypothesis.

Probability of a Type II Error   The probability of making a Type II error is denoted by β.

Rejection Region   The rejection region is the set of values of the test statistic for which H_0 is rejected.

Significance Level   The significance level in a hypothesis test is the probability of making a Type I error in a hypothesis test and is denoted by α.

Statistical Distance   The statistical distance between an estimate T and a particular value of a parameter θ is

$$\text{statistical distance} = \frac{T - \theta}{\text{se}}$$

where se is the estimated standard error of the statistic T.

Test Statistic   The test statistic is the statistic used to determine whether the observed sample provides evidence for or against a null hypothesis.

Testing Decisions   In a hypothesis test the null hypothesis H_0 is either rejected or it is failed to be rejected.

Two-tailed Test   A two-tailed test of a parameter θ is a test of the null hypothesis $H_0 : \theta = \theta_0$ versus $H_A : \theta \neq \theta_0$, where θ_0 is the null value of θ.

Type I Error   A Type I error is made by rejecting the null hypothesis when it is the true state of nature.

Type II Error   A Type II error is made by failing to reject the null hypothesis when the alternative is the true state of nature.

Upper-tail Test   An upper-tail test of a parameter θ is a test of the null hypothesis $H_0 : \theta \leq \theta_0$ versus $H_A : \theta > \theta_0$, where θ_0 is the null value of θ.

Within-Subjects Study   A within-subjects sampling plan is used when the set of subjects used in the study receive each treatment.

EXERCISES

7.1   What are the two hypotheses that are tested in a hypothesis test? Which of these hypotheses is the research hypothesis?

7.2   In a hypothesis test of H_0 versus H_A what is
(a) the test statistic?   (b) the rejection region?
(c) a Type I error?   (d) a Type II error?
(e) the significance level?   (f) the p-value?

7.3   In a hypothesis test how is a
(a) Type I error made?   (b) Type II error made?

7.4   How should the significance level α be chosen in a hypothesis test?

7.5   Suppose in testing $H_0 : \sigma \leq 10$ versus $H_A : \sigma > 10$, the rejection region for a $\alpha = 0.05$ level test is "Reject H_0 when $s > 18.6$."
(a) What is the chance of making a Type I error before the sample is actually selected?
(b) If the sample yields an estimate of σ of $s = 21.6$, what is the testing decision about $H_0 : \sigma \leq 10$ that should be made?
(c) If standard deviation of the population is actually 8, was a testing error made in part (b)? If so, what type of testing error was made?

7.6   In each of the following scenarios determine whether or not a testing error was made, and if a testing error was made determine which type of error was made.
(a) H_0 was rejected and H_0 is actually false.
(b) H_0 was rejected and H_0 is actually true.
(c) H_0 was failed to be rejected and H_0 is actually false.
(d) H_0 was failed to be rejected and H_0 is actually true.

7.7   What are the symbols α and β used to represent in a hypothesis test? What are the acceptable values of α? What are the small values for β?

7.8   Under what conditions would using $\alpha = 0.01$ be preferable to using $\alpha = 0.05$ as the significance level of a hypothesis test?

7.9   Why is rejecting H_0 a reliable decision?

7.10   Why is failing to reject H_0 often an unreliable decision?

7.11 Under what conditions does the failure to reject H_0 become a reliable decision?

7.12 What is the power function in a hypothesis test?

7.13 What does the power of a test measure?

7.14 What is the relationship between the power of a test and the probability of making a Type II error?

7.15 What does it mean when the power is small at a particular value of the parameter being tested?

7.16 In each of the following scenarios determine whether the testing decisions reject H_0 and fail to reject H_0 are reliable decisions.
- **(a)** $\alpha = 0.01, \beta = 0.56$
- **(b)** $\alpha = 0.15, \beta = 0.06$
- **(c)** $\alpha = 0.05, \beta = 0.06$
- **(d)** $\alpha = 0.01, \beta = 0.26$
- **(e)** $\alpha = 0.30, \beta = 0.01$
- **(f)** $\alpha = 0.05, \beta = 0.10$

7.17 What happens to the value of
- **(a)** α when the sample size is increased?
- **(b)** β when the sample size is increased?
- **(c)** the power when the sample size is increased?

7.18 What information is needed before the sample is selected in order to have a well-planned and reliable hypothesis test?

7.19 What does it mean when the results of a hypothesis test are said to be
- **(a)** statistically significant?
- **(b)** scientifically significant?

7.20 What is the difference between statistical significance and practical/scientific significance?

7.21 Explain what it means when the results of a hypothesis test are
- **(a)** statistically significant but not scientifically significant?
- **(b)** not statistically significant but is scientifically significant?
- **(c)** both statistically and scientifically significant.

7.22 Why are small p-values taken as evidence against the null hypothesis?

7.23 What is the difference between the p-value and the significance level in a hypothesis test?

7.24 Why should a confidence interval for the parameter being tested be reported along with the results of the hypothesis test?

7.25 What is the difference between a significance test and a hypothesis test?

7.26 Explain why a rejection region is not necessary when using a statistical computing package to carry out a hypothesis test.

7.27 In each of the scenarios below, determine whether or not the observed sample provides sufficient evidence for rejecting the null hypothesis.
- **(a)** $p = 0.163, \alpha = 0.05$
- **(b)** $p = 0.043, \alpha = 0.10$
- **(c)** $p = 0.003, \alpha = 0.01$
- **(d)** $p = 0.231, \alpha = 0.05$
- **(e)** $p = 0.006, \alpha = 0.001$
- **(f)** $p = 0.032, \alpha = 0.01$

7.28 For each part in Exercise 7.27 use the guidelines for p-values to interpret the strength of evidence against H_0 provided by the observed p-value.

7.29 What are the three possible hypothesis tests that can be used when testing claims about a population proportion p?

7.30 In a hypothesis test for a population proportion what does p_0 represent?

7.31 Under what conditions can the large sample Z-test be used as the test statistic for a hypothesis test about a population proportion?

7.32 For each of the following hypothesis tests, determine whether or not it is appropriate to use a large sample Z-test.
(a) $H_0 : p \leq 0.25$ and $n = 25$.   (b) $H_0 : p \leq 0.10$ and $n = 25$.
(c) $H_0 : p \geq 0.8$ and $n = 40$.   (d) $H_0 : p = 0.05$ and $n = 80$.
(e) $H_0 : p = 0.90$ and $n = 100$.   (f) $H_0 : p \geq 0.98$ and $n = 200$.

7.33 What is the formula for the test statistic in a large sample Z-test for a hypothesis test about a population proportion?

7.34 Explain why
(a) p_0 is used in computing the standard error of $\widehat{p}$ in the large sample Z-test statistic for a hypothesis test about a population proportion?
(b) $\widehat{p}$ is used in computing the standard error of $\widehat{p}$ in the large sample confidence interval for a population proportion?

7.35 What is the general form of the rejection region for a Z-test that is
(a) a lower-tail test.
(b) an upper-tail test.
(c) a two-tailed test.

7.36 What is the value of z_{crit} used in a lower-tail Z-test when
(a) $\alpha = 0.05$?   (b) $\alpha = 0.01$?

7.37 What is the value of z_{crit} used in an upper-tail Z-test when
(a) $\alpha = 0.05$?   (b) $\alpha = 0.01$?

7.38 What is the value of z_{crit} used in a two-tailed Z-test when
(a) $\alpha = 0.05$?   (b) $\alpha = 0.01$?

7.39 Determine the rejection region for a large sample Z-test for a hypothesis test about a population proportion when
(a) $H_0 : p \leq 0.2$ and $\alpha = 0.05$.   (b) $H_0 : p \geq 0.6$ and $\alpha = 0.01$.
(c) $H_0 : p \geq 0.8$ and $\alpha = 0.01$.   (d) $H_0 : p = 0.4$ and $\alpha = 0.05$.
(e) $H_0 : p = 0.25$ and $\alpha = 0.05$.   (f) $H_0 : p \leq 0.95$ and $\alpha = 0.10$.

7.40 Compute the p-value associated with a large sample Z-test for a proportion when
(a) $H_0 : p = 0.5$ and $z_{\text{obs}} = 1.2$.
(b) $H_0 : p = 0.75$ and $z_{\text{obs}} = 3.2$.
(c) $H_0 : p \leq 0.25$ and $z_{\text{obs}} = 1.13$.
(d) $H_0 : p \leq 0.75$ and $z_{\text{obs}} = 2.59$.
(e) $H_0 : p \geq 0.15$ and $z_{\text{obs}} = -2.11$.
(f) $H_0 : p = 0.75$ and $z_{\text{obs}} = -3.01$.

7.41 For each p-value in Exercise 7.40 determine whether or not to reject H_0 when
(a) $\alpha = 0.05$.   (b) $\alpha = 0.01$.

7.42 In each of the following scenarios determine the rejection region, the value of z_{obs}, the p-value, and the appropriate testing decision for H_0.
(a) $H_0 : p = 0.25$, $\alpha = 0.05$, $n = 25$, and $\hat{p} = 0.20$.
(b) $H_0 : p \geq 0.60$, $\alpha = 0.05$, $n = 50$, and $\hat{p} = 0.48$.
(c) $H_0 : p \leq 0.20$, $\alpha = 0.05$, $n = 100$, and $\hat{p} = 0.24$.
(d) $H_0 : p = 0.90$, $\alpha = 0.01$, $n = 225$, and $\hat{p} = 0.80$.
(e) $H_0 : p \leq 0.40$, $\alpha = 0.05$, $n = 40$, and $\hat{p} = 0.50$.

7.43 For each of the tests in Exercise 7.42 compute a 95% confidence interval for the population proportion p.

7.44 Determine the sample size required to achieve the prespecified value of β in each of the following scenarios.
(a) $H_0 : p = 0.33$, $p_{crit} = 0.40$, $\alpha = 0.05$, and $\beta = 0.15$.
(b) $H_0 : p = 0.30$, $p_{crit} = 0.25$, $\alpha = 0.05$, and $\beta = 0.10$.
(c) $H_0 : p \leq 0.80$, $p_{crit} = 0.85$, $\alpha = 0.05$, and $\beta = 0.10$.
(d) $H_0 : p \leq 0.55$, $p_{crit} = 0.58$, $\alpha = 0.05$, and $\beta = 0.05$.
(e) $H_0 : p \geq 0.30$, $p_{crit} = 0.20$, $\alpha = 0.01$, and $\beta = 0.05$.
(f) $H_0 : p \geq 0.85$, $p_{crit} = 0.80$, $\alpha = 0.05$, and $\beta = 0.01$.

7.45 Using the Coronary Heart Disease data set
(a) estimate the proportion of the study population having evidence of coronary heart disease (p_C).
(b) test $H_0 : p_C = 0.50$ at the $\alpha = 0.05$ level.
(c) compute a confidence interval for the proportion of the study population having coronary heart disease.

7.46 Using the Body Fat data set
(a) estimate the proportion of adult males having at least 25% percent body fat (p_{25}).
(b) test $H_0 : p_{25} \leq 0.10$ at the $\alpha = 0.05$ level.
(c) compute a confidence interval for the proportion of male adults having at least 25% percent body fat.

7.47 Under what conditions can a large sample Z-test be used in a hypothesis test concerning the difference of two proportions?

7.48 What is the formula for the test statistic in a large sample Z-test for a hypothesis test about the difference between two population proportions?

7.49 Explain why
(a) $\hat{p} = \frac{n_X \hat{p}_X + n_Y \hat{p}_Y}{n_X + n_Y}$ is used in computing the standard error of $\hat{p}_X - \hat{p}_Y$ in the large sample Z-test statistic for a hypothesis test about the difference between two population proportions?
(b) $\hat{p}_X$ and $\hat{p}_Y$ are used in computing the standard error of $\hat{p}_X - \hat{p}_Y$ in the large sample confidence interval for the difference between two population proportions?

7.50 Determine the rejection region for a large sample Z-test for a hypothesis test about the difference between two population proportions when
(a) $H_0 : p_X \leq p_Y$ and $\alpha = 0.05$.
(b) $H_0 : p_X \leq p_Y$ and $\alpha = 0.01$.
(c) $H_0 : p_X \geq p_Y$ and $\alpha = 0.05$.
(d) $H_0 : p_X \geq p_Y$ and $\alpha = 0.01$.

(e) $H_0 : p_X = p_Y$ and $\alpha = 0.05$.   (f) $H_0 : p_X = p_Y$ and $\alpha = 0.01$.

7.51 Compute the value of the p-value for each of the following values of z_{obs} for a large sample Z-test for the difference between two proportions when

    (a) $H_0 : p_X = p_Y$ and $z_{\text{obs}} = 2.52$
    (b) $H_0 : p_X \geq p_Y$ and $z_{\text{obs}} = -2.97$
    (c) $H_0 : p_X \leq p_Y$ and $z_{\text{obs}} = 1.38$

7.52 For each p-value in Exercise 7.51 determine whether or not to reject H_0 when $\alpha = 0.01$.

7.53 Compute the pooled estimate of $p = p_X = p_Y$ used in the large sample Z-test of the difference of two proportions when

    (a) $\widehat{p}_X = 0.48$, $\widehat{p}_Y = 0.55$, $n_X = 25$, and $n_Y = 36$.
    (b) $\widehat{p}_X = 0.13$, $\widehat{p}_Y = 0.15$, $n_X = 50$, and $n_Y = 66$.
    (c) $\widehat{p}_X = 0.28$, $\widehat{p}_Y = 0.15$, $n_X = 150$, and $n_Y = 131$.

7.54 In each of the following scenarios determine the rejection region, the value of z_{obs}, the p-value, and the appropriate testing decision for H_0.

    (a) $H_0 : p_X = p_Y$, $\alpha = 0.05$, $n_X = 35$, $\widehat{p}_X = 0.26$, $n_Y = 43$, and $\widehat{p}_Y = 0.35$.
    (b) $H_0 : p_X \leq p_Y$, $\alpha = 0.01$, $n_X = 57$, $\widehat{p}_X = 0.78$, $n_Y = 63$, and $\widehat{p}_Y = 0.59$.
    (c) $H_0 : p_X \geq p_Y$, $\alpha = 0.05$, $n_X = 105$, $\widehat{p}_X = 0.07$, $n_Y = 143$, and $\widehat{p}_Y = 0.23$.
    (d) $H_0 : p_X = p_Y$, $\alpha = 0.01$, $n_X = 87$, $\widehat{p}_X = 0.11$, $n_Y = 90$, and $\widehat{p}_Y = 0.18$.
    (e) $H_0 : p_X \leq p_Y$, $\alpha = 0.05$, $n_X = 215$, $\widehat{p}_X = 0.93$, $n_Y = 167$, and $\widehat{p}_Y = 0.85$.

7.55 For each of the tests in Exercise 7.54, compute a 95% confidence interval for the difference in the population proportions.

7.56 Determine the conservative sample size required to achieve the prespecified value of β in each of the following scenarios.

    (a) $H_0 : p_X = p_Y$, $p_{\text{crit}} = 0.05$, $\alpha = 0.05$, and $\beta = 0.15$.
    (b) $H_0 : p_X = p_Y$, $p_{\text{crit}} = 0.10$, $\alpha = 0.05$, and $\beta = 0.05$.
    (c) $H_0 : p_X \leq p_Y$, $p_{\text{crit}} = 0.10$, $\alpha = 0.05$, and $\beta = 0.10$.
    (d) $H_0 : p_X \leq p_Y$, $p_{\text{crit}} = 0.10$, $\alpha = 0.05$, and $\beta = 0.05$.
    (e) $H_0 : p_X \geq p_Y$, $p_{\text{crit}} = 0.05$, $\alpha = 0.05$, and $\beta = 0.10$.
    (f) $H_0 : p_X \geq p_Y$, $p_{\text{crit}} = 0.02$, $\alpha = 0.05$, and $\beta = 0.10$.

7.57 In the article "Glycemic control in English- versus Spanish-speaking Hispanic patients with Type 2 diabetes mellitus" published in the *Archives of Internal Medicine* (Lasater et al., 2001), the authors reported the summary counts given in Table 7.26 for 183 Hispanic patients with diabetes mellitus on the use of insulin for 106 English speaking Hispanic patients and 77 Spanish speaking Hispanic patients. Use the data in Table 7.26 to answer the following:

    (a) Estimate the proportion of English speaking patients using insulin (p_E).
    (b) Estimate the proportion of Spanish speaking patients using insulin (p_S).
    (c) Test $H_0 : p_E = p_S$ at the $\alpha = 0.05$ level.
    (d) Compute the p-value associated with the test in part (c).
    (e) Compute a 95% confidence interval for $p_E - p_S$.

7.58 In the article "Tuberculin skin test screening practices among U.S. colleges and universities" published in the *Journal of the American Medical Association* (Hennessey

TABLE 7.26   Summary Counts on the Use of Insulin for 106 English Speaking Hispanic Patients and 77 Spanish Speaking Hispanic Patients

English Speaking ($n = 106$)	Spanish Speaking ($n = 77$)
42	29

TABLE 7.27   Sample Percentages of Schools Requiring Screening for Tuberculosis for Universities and Colleges that Belong and do not Belong to the ACHA

ACHA Member	n	Require Screening
Yes	195	82%
No	409	53%

et al., 1998), the authors reported the percentages of schools requiring screening for tuberculosis for universities and colleges that belong and do not belong to the American College Health Association (ACHA) given in Table 7.27. Use the data in Table 7.27 to answer the following:

(a) Let p_Y be the proportion of colleges and universities belonging to ACHA who require screening for tuberculosis and p_N the proportion of colleges and universities not belonging to ACHA who require screening for tuberculosis. Test $H_0 : p_Y \le p_N$ at the $\alpha = 0.05$ level.

(b) Compute the p-value associated with the test in part (a).

(c) Compute a lower bound 95% confidence interval for $p_Y - p_N$.

7.59   In the article "Brief physician- and nurse practitioner-delivered counseling for high-risk drinkers: does it work?" published in the *Archives of Internal Medicine* (Ockene et al., 1999), the authors reported the percentages in Table 7.28 on the prevalence of excessive weekly drinking and binge drinking for 233 patients under the usual care and 248 patients who received special intervention treatment. Use the information given in Table 7.28 to answer the following:

(a) Let p_U be the prevalence of patients under usual care who exhibit safe drinking weekly and nonbinge drinking after 6 months and p_S the prevalence of patients receiving special intervention who exhibit safe drinking weekly and nonbinge drinking after 6 months. Test $H_0 : p_U = p_S$ at the $\alpha = 0.01$ level.

(b) Compute the p-value associated with the test in part (a).

(c) Compute a 95% confidence interval for $p_U - p_S$.

TABLE 7.28   Prevalence of Excessive Weekly Drinking and Binge Drinking by Treatment Condition

Treatment	n	% Safe Weekly/Nonbinge Drinking at 6 Months
Usual care	233	28%
Special intervention	248	39%

TABLE 7.29   Percentage Experiencing Nausea for Students with Cold Symptoms During Treatment

Treatment	n	Percentage
Placebo	124	16.1%
ZGG	123	29.3%

7.60   In the article "Zinc gluconate lozenges for treating the common cold in children: A Randomized Controlled Trial" published in the *Journal of the American Medical Association* (Macknin et al., 1998), the authors reported the percentages given in Table 7.29 for students with cold symptoms during treatment with zinc gluconate glycine lozenges (ZGG) or a placebo who experienced nausea during the treatment period. Use the information in Table 7.29 to answer the following:

(a) Let p_P be the proportion of students taking the placebo that experienced nausea during the treatment period and p_Z the proportion of students taking the ZGG lozenges that experienced nausea during the treatment period. Test $H_0 : p_P = p_Z$ at the $\alpha = 0.05$ level.

(b) Compute the p-value associated with the test in part (a).

(c) Compute a 95% confidence interval for $p_P - p_Z$.

7.61   In the article "Effects of long-term vitamin E supplementation on cardiovascular events and cancer: a randomized controlled trial" published in the *Journal of the American Medical Association* (Lonn, 2005), the author reported the results of a 4.5 year longitudinal study on the number of deaths due to cancer. Table 7.30 shows the number of deaths for 4761 subjects taking vitamin E and 4780 subjects taking a placebo. Use the information in Table 7.30 to answer the following:

(a) Let p_P be the proportion of deaths due to cancer for subjects taking the placebo and p_E the proportion of deaths for subjects taking the vitamin E treatment. Test $H_0 : p_P = p_E$ at the $\alpha = 0.05$ level.

(b) Compute the p-value associated with the test in part (a).

7.62   Using the Birth Weight data set,

(a) estimate the percentage of low birth weight babies for mothers who smoked during pregnancy (p_S).

(b) estimate the percentage of low birth weight babies for mothers who did not smoke during pregnancy (P_N).

(c) test $H_0 : p_S \leq p_N$ at the $\alpha = 0.05$ level.

(d) compute a 95% confidence interval for $p_S - p_N$.

TABLE 7.30   The Number of Deaths due to Cancer for 4761 Subjects Taking Vitamin E and 4780 Subjects Taking a Placebo

Treatment	Deaths due to Cancer
Vitamin E	156
Placebo	178

7.63 Using the Birth Weight data set,

    (a) estimate the percentage of low birth weight babies for mothers who are white (Race = 1), say p_W.

    (b) estimate the percentage of low birth weight babies for mothers who are not white (Race = 2 or 3), say p_{NW}.

    (c) test $H_0 : p_W = p_{NW}$ at the $\alpha = 0.05$ level.

    (d) compute a 95% confidence interval for $p_W - p_{NW}$.

7.64 Under what conditions are two qualitative variables independent?

7.65 What are the null and alternative hypotheses in a test of independence involving two qualitative variables?

7.66 What is the formula for the test statistic used to test the independence of two dichotomous variables?

7.67 Under what conditions is the sampling distribution of the test statistic X^2 approximately distributed as a chi-squared distribution in a test of independence for two dichotomous variables?

7.68 What is the rejection region for a test of independence based on the chi-squared distribution?

7.69 If a sample of $n = 100$ observations is cross-classified into a 2×2 contingency table, how many degrees of freedom will the test statistic X^2 in a test of independence?

7.70 Determine the rejection region for a test of the independence of two dichotomous variables that is based on the chi-squared distribution when

    (a) $\alpha = 0.01$ **(b)** $\alpha = 0.05$

7.71 In the article "Aspirin and the treatment of heart failure in the elderly" published in *Archives of Internal Medicine* (Krumholz et al., 2001), the authors reported the summarized data given in Table 7.31 on the number of deaths after 1 year for 456 patients prescribed aspirin and 654 patients not prescribed aspirin at discharge after hospitalization for heart failure. Use the data in Table 7.31 to answer the following:

    (a) Does the data in Table 7.31 support the use of a chi-squared test of independence?

    (b) Test the hypothesis that survival status is independent whether or not aspirin is prescribed at discharge.

    (c) Compute a confidence interval for the percentage of patients who were prescribed aspirin at discharge that die within 1 year of discharge.

    (d) Compute a confidence interval for the percentage of patients who were not prescribed aspirin at discharge that die within 1 year of discharge.

TABLE 7.31   **Summary Data on the Number of Deaths After 1 Year for 456 Patients Prescribed Aspirin and 654 Patients not Prescribed Aspirin at Discharge After Hospitalization for Heart Failure**

Aspirin Prescribed	Survival Status	
	Dead	Alive
Yes	90	366
No	174	480

TABLE 7.32 Summary Counts on the Usage of Protective Helmets for Skiers and Snowboarders for Individuals Suffering Head Injuries and a Group of Uninjured Skiers and Snowboarders

Helmet Use	Group	
	Head Injury	Uninjured Control
Yes	96	656
No	480	2330

7.72 In the article "Helmet use and risk of head injuries in alpine skiers and snowboarders" published in the *Journal of the American Medical Association* (Sulheim et al., 2005), the authors reported the data given in Table 7.32 on the usage of protective helmets for skiers and snowboarders for individuals suffering head injuries and a group of uninjured skiers and snowboarders. Use the data in Table 7.32 to answer the following:

(a) Does the data in Table 7.32 support the use of a chi-squared test of independence?

(b) Test the hypothesis that helmet use is independent of group.

7.73 In the article "Limited family structure and BRCA gene mutation status in single cases of breast cancer" published in the *Journal of the American Medical Association* (Weitzel et al., 2007), the authors reported the 2×2 contingency table given in Table 7.33 for investigating the association between family structure and whether or not an individual was a BRCA carrier. Use the contingency table in Table 7.33 to answer the following:

(a) Does the data in Table 7.33 support the use of a chi-squared test of independence?

(b) Test the hypothesis that family structure is independent of carrier status.

7.74 What is a polytomous variable?

7.75 What is the formula for the test statistic used to test the independence of two qualitative variables where one variable has r categories and the other has c categories?

7.76 Under what conditions is the sampling distribution of the test statistic X^2 approximately distributed as a chi-squared distribution in a test of independence for two qualitative variables?

7.77 What is the rejection region for a chi-squared test of independence based on a $r \times c$ contingency table?

TABLE 7.33 Summary Data on Family Structure and BRCA

BRCA	Family Structure	
	Limited	Adequate
Carrier	21	8
Noncarrier	132	145

TABLE 7.34 Summary Data on Race and the Birth weights of the $n = 189$ Babies in the Birth Weight Data Set

Race	Birth Weight	
	Low	Normal
White	23	73
Black	11	15
Other	25	42

7.78 If a sample of $n = 100$ observations is cross-classified into a 3×2 contingency table, how many degrees of freedom will the test statistic X^2 in a test of independence?

7.79 If a sample of $n = 140$ observations is cross-classified into a 3×5 contingency table, how many degrees of freedom will the test statistic X^2 in a test of independence?

7.80 If a sample of $n = 412$ observations is cross-classified into a 5×4 contingency table, how many degrees of freedom will the test statistic X^2 in a test of independence?

7.81 Determine the rejection region for a chi-squared test of the independence for a 4×3 contingency table when

(a) $\alpha = 0.01$ (b) $\alpha = 0.05$

7.82 Determine the rejection region for a chi-squared test of the independence for a 5×2 contingency table when

(a) $\alpha = 0.01$ (b) $\alpha = 0.05$

7.83 Determine the rejection region for a chi-squared test of the independence for a 4×4 contingency table when

(a) $\alpha = 0.01$ (b) $\alpha = 0.05$

7.84 The data given in Table 7.34 is based on the Birth Weight data set. Use Table 7.34 to answer the following:

(a) Does the data in Table 7.34 support the use of a chi-squared test of independence?

(b) Test the hypothesis that whether or not a baby has a low birth weight is independent of race.

TABLE 7.35 Summary Data on Race and Whether or Not a Mother Smoked During Pregnancy for the $n = 189$ Observations in the Birth Weight Data Set

Race	Smoked During Pregnancy	
	Yes	No
White	52	44
Black	10	16
Other	12	55

TABLE 7.36 Summary Data on the Skiing Ability for Skiers and Snowboarders for Individuals Suffering Head Injuries and an Uninjured Control Group

Skiing Ability	Group	
	Head Injury	Uninjured Control
Expert	108	570
Good	186	1055
Intermediate	147	1005
Beginner	123	348

7.85 The data given in Table 7.35 is based on the Birth Weight data set. Use Table 7.35 to answer the following:

(a) Does the data in Table 7.35 support the use of a chi-squared test of independence?

(b) Test the hypothesis that whether or not a mother smoked during pregnancy is independent of race.

7.86 In the article "Helmet use and risk of head injuries in alpine skiers and snowboarders" published in the *Journal of the American Medical Association* (Sulheim et al., 2005), the authors reported the data given in Table 7.36 on the skiing ability for skiers and snowboarders for individuals suffering head injuries and an uninjured control group. Use the data in Table 7.36 to answer the following:

(a) Does the data in Table 7.36 support the use of a chi-squared test of independence?

(b) Test the hypothesis that a skier's ability is independent of group.

7.87 What is the general form of a t statistic?

7.88 What are the null and alternative hypotheses in

(a) a lower-tail test for a population mean?

(b) a two-tailed test for a population mean?

(c) an upper-tail test for a population mean?

7.89 What is the rejection region for

(a) a lower-tail t-test based on 20 degrees of freedom and $\alpha = 0.05$?

(b) an upper-tail t-test based on 25 degrees of freedom and $\alpha = 0.01$?

(c) a two-tailed t-test based on 12 degrees of freedom and $\alpha = 0.05$?

7.90 Using Tables A.8 and A.9 approximate the p-value in

(a) a two-tailed test with 21 degrees of freedom when $t_{obs} = 2.8$.

(b) an upper-tail test with 29 degrees of freedom when $t_{obs} = 2.5$.

(c) a two-tailed test with 60 degrees of freedom when $t_{obs} = -3.2$.

(d) a lower-tail test with 19 degrees of freedom when $t_{obs} = -3.4$.

(e) an upper-tail test with 24 degrees of freedom when $t_{obs} = 4.5$.

7.91 What is the form of the t statistic for testing hypotheses about the mean of a population?

7.92 For testing hypotheses about the mean of a population, under what conditions does the sampling distribution of the test statistic follow a t distribution?

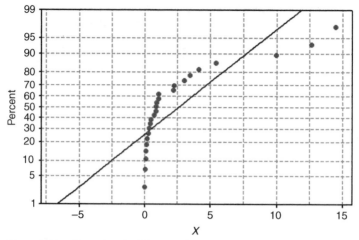

Figure 7.11 Normal probability plot for a random sample of $n = 25$ observations.

7.93 Determine the rejection region for a t-test when
(a) $H_0 : \mu \geq 100$, $\alpha = 0.05$, and $n = 29$.
(b) $H_0 : \mu \leq 100$, $\alpha = 0.01$, and $n = 22$.
(c) $H_0 : \mu = 100$, $\alpha = 0.05$, and $n = 61$.
(d) $H_0 : \mu = 100$, $\alpha = 0.05$, and $n = 200$.

7.94 Does the normal probability plot given in Figure 7.11 support the use of a t-test for testing a claim about a population mean? Explain.

7.95 What can be said about the validity of the p-value computed in a t-test when the normal probability plot clearly does not support the assumption of normality?

7.96 Assuming a random sample has been selected from a population that is approximately normal, use a t-test to perform each of the following hypothesis tests. In particular, include the rejection region, the value of t_{obs}, the decision concerning H_0, and the approximate value of the p-value associated with t_{obs}.
(a) Test $H_0 : \mu = 20$ when $\alpha = 0.05$, $n = 23$, $\bar{x} = 16.7$, and $s = 2.2$.
(b) Test $H_0 : \mu \leq 100$ when $\alpha = 0.05$, $n = 31$, $\bar{x} = 125.8$, and $s = 41.7$.
(c) Test $H_0 : \mu \geq 1.1$ when $\alpha = 0.01$, $n = 25$, $\bar{x} = 0.73$, and $s = 0.55$.
(d) Test $H_0 : \mu = 200$ when $\alpha = 0.01$, $n = 61$, $\bar{x} = 209.1$, and $s = 35.4$.

7.97 Determine the approximate sample size needed for a t-test about the mean of a population when
(a) $H_0 : \mu = 50$, $\mu_0 - \mu_{crit} = 2$, $\alpha = 0.05$, $\beta = 0.10$, and $\dot{\sigma} = 5$.
(b) $H_0 : \mu \geq 150$, $\mu_{crit} = 140$, $\alpha = 0.05$, $\beta = 0.01$, and $\dot{\sigma} = 40$.
(c) $H_0 : \mu \leq 5.0$, $\mu_{crit} = 5.3$, $\alpha = 0.05$, $\beta = 0.10$, and $\dot{\sigma} = 0.5$.
(d) $H_0 : \mu \leq 100$, $\mu_0 - \mu_{crit} = 5$, $\alpha = 0.05$, $\beta = 0.05$, and $\dot{\sigma} = 10$.

7.98 Using the Birth Weight data set, test the null hypothesis that the mean weight of a baby born to
(a) mothers who did not smoke during pregnancy is less than 3200 g. Be sure to check the assumption of normality!
(b) mothers who did smoke during pregnancy is less than 3200 g smokers is less than 3200 g. Be sure to check the assumption of normality!

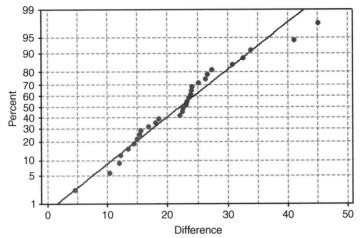

Figure 7.12   Normal probability plot for $n = 30$ differences resulting in a paired comparison study.

7.99   What are two commonly used sampling plans that are used in collecting data to be used in a paired comparison?

7.100   What is the formula for computing the value of the t-statistic in a paired comparison?

7.101   For a paired comparison t-test, under what conditions does the sampling distribution of the test statistic follow a t distribution?

7.102   Determine the rejection region for a paired comparison when
(a) $H_0 : \mu_X \geq \mu_Y$, $\alpha = 0.05$, and $n = 29$.
(b) $H_0 : \mu_X \leq \mu_Y$, $\alpha = 0.01$, and $n = 22$.
(c) $H_0 : \mu_x = \mu_Y$, $\alpha = 0.05$, and $n = 61$.
(d) $H_0 : \mu_X = \mu_Y$, $\alpha = 0.05$, and $n = 200$.

7.103   Does the normal probability plot given in Figure 7.12 support the use of a t-test for testing a claim about the difference of two means in a paired comparison study? Explain.

7.104   Assuming a random sample of n pairs has been selected and the distribution of the difference is approximately normal, use a t-test to perform each of the following hypothesis tests. In particular, include the rejection region, the value of t_{obs}, the decision concerning H_0, and the approximate value of the p-value associated with t_{obs}.
(a) Test $H_0 : \mu_X = \mu_Y$ when $\alpha = 0.05$, $n = 25$, $\bar{d} = 1.7$, and $s_d = 4.3$.
(b) Test $H_0 : \mu_X = \mu_Y$ when $\alpha = 0.01$, $n = 31$, $\bar{d} = 35.2$, and $s_d = 94.9$.
(c) Test $H_0 : \mu_X \leq \mu_Y$ when $\alpha = 0.05$, $n = 21$, $\bar{d} = 0.7$, and $s_d = 1.2$.
(d) Test $H_0 : \mu_X \geq \mu_Y$ when $\alpha = 0.05$, $n = 25$, $\bar{d} = -109.6$, and $s_d = 148.3$.

7.105   Compute a 95% confidence interval for $\mu_X - \mu_Y$ for each of the tests in Exercise 7.104.

7.106   Determine the approximate sample size needed for a paired comparison t-test when
(a) $H_0 : \mu_X = \mu_Y$, $\delta = 2.5$, $\alpha = 0.05$, $\beta = 0.05$, and $\acute{\sigma} = 5$.
(b) $H_0 : \mu_X \geq \mu_Y$, $\delta = 0.5$, $\alpha = 0.05$, $\beta = 0.15$, and $\acute{\sigma} = 2$.

(c) $H_0 : \mu_X = \mu_Y, \delta = 15, \alpha = 0.05, \beta = 0.05$, and $\dot\sigma = 30$.

(d) $H_0 : \mu_X \le \mu_Y, \delta = 25, \alpha = 0.05, \beta = 0.10$, and $\dot\sigma = 70$.

7.107 In the article "Effects of tonsillectomy on acoustic parameters" published in *The Internet Journal of Otorhinolaryngology* (Tolga et al., 2007) the authors reported the results of a paired comparison study on several acoustic parameters. The data analyzed in the study consists of F3 formant values before and after a tonsillectomy operation for $n = 20$ individuals. Based on the difference between pre- and postoperation F3 formant values (i.e., pre−post) $\bar d = 52$ and $s_d = 547$.

(a) What assumption must be valid in order to have a valid paired comparison t-test of $H_0 : \mu_{pre} \ge \mu_{post}$?

(b) What assumption must be valid in order to have a valid paired comparison t-test of $H_0 : \mu_{pre} \ge \mu_{post}$?

(c) Assuming the differences between pre- and postoperation F3 formant values are approximately normal, test $H_0 : \mu_{pre} \ge \mu_{post}$ at the $\alpha = 0.05$ level.

(d) Approximate the p-value associated with t_{obs}.

(e) Compute a 95% confidence interval for $\mu_{pre} - \mu_{post}$.

7.108 In the article "Evaluation of cerebral microembolic signals in patients with mechancial aortic valves" published in *The Internet Journal of Neuromonitoring* (Ghandehari and Izadimoud, 2007) the authors reported the results of a paired comparison study comparing microembolic signals (MES) for room air and breathing oxygen through a facial mask. The data analyzed in the study consists of MES for 30 minutes of either breathing room air (R) or oxygen (O) though a facial mask for $n = 12$ individuals. Based on the difference between R and O MES values (i.e., R−O) $\bar d = 56.3$ and $s_d = 67.9$.

(a) What assumption must be valid in order to have a valid paired comparison t-test of $H_0 : \mu_R \le \mu_O$?

(b) Assuming the differences between the R and O MES values are approximately normal, test $H_0 : \mu_R = \mu_O$ at the $\alpha = 0.05$ level.

(c) Approximate the p-value associated with t_{obs}.

(d) Compute a 95% confidence interval for $\mu_R - \mu_O$.

7.109 In the article "Melatonin improves sleep-wake patterns in psychomotor retarded children" published in *Pediatric Neurology* (Pillar et al., 2000) the authors reported the results of a paired comparison study on whether melatonin can increase the average sleep duration in psychomotor retarded children. The data analyzed in the study consists of the baseline sleep duration (B) and the sleep duration with melatonin (M) for $n = 5$ children. Based on the difference between B and M (i.e., B−M) $\bar d = -1.42$ and $s_d = 0.273$.

(a) What assumption must be valid in order to have a valid paired comparison t-test of $H_0 : \mu_B = \mu_M$?

(b) Assuming the differences between the B and M values are approximately normal, test $H_0 : \mu_B \ge \mu_M$ at the $\alpha = 0.05$ level.

(c) Approximate the p-value associated with t_{obs}.

(d) Compute a 95% confidence interval for $\mu_B - \mu_M$.

7.110 What is the general form of the t statistic for comparing the mean when two independent random samples have been collected?

7.111 How is the sampling plan for a two independent sample study different from the sampling plan for a paired comparison study?

7.112 What is the formula for computing the estimated standard error of $\bar{x} - \bar{y}$ when two independent samples have been collected?

7.113 Under what conditions is the sampling distribution of the two-sample t statistic approximated by a t distribution?

7.114 Under what conditions is the sampling distribution of the two-sample t statistic approximated by the Z distribution?

7.115 Under what conditions is it reasonable to assume that $\sigma_X = \sigma_Y$?

7.116 Suppose that σ_X and σ_Y can be assumed to be nearly equal. What is the formula for computing the
(a) pooled estimate of σ.
(b) estimated standard error of $\bar{x} - \bar{y}$?
(c) degrees of freedom associated with the t statistic?

7.117 Determine whether it is reasonable to assume that $\sigma_X \approx \sigma_Y$ when
(a) $n_X = 12, s_X = 143.9$ and $n_Y = 15, s_Y = 89.1$.
(b) $n_X = 23, s_X = 11.2$ and $n_Y = 43, s_Y = 9.7$.
(c) $n_X = 39, s_X = 67.6$ and $n_Y = 53, s_Y = 26.3$.
(d) $n_X = 66, s_X = 0.95$ and $n_Y = 73, s_Y = 0.28$.

7.118 For each of the parts of Exercise 7.117, compute the appropriate value of the estimated standard error of $\bar{x} - \bar{y}$.

7.119 How can the normality assumptions be checked prior to performing a two-sample t-test for comparing two means?

7.120 Assuming the normality assumptions are satisfied and $\sigma_X \approx \sigma_Y$, determine the rejection region for a two-sample t-test for comparing the means μ_X and μ_Y when
(a) $H_0 : \mu_X = \mu_Y, \alpha = 0.01, n_X = 12$, and $n_Y = 15$.
(b) $H_0 : \mu_X = \mu_Y, \alpha = 0.05, n_X = 72$, and $n_Y = 89$.
(c) $H_0 : \mu_X \geq \mu_Y, \alpha = 0.01, n_X = 21$, and $n_Y = 20$.
(d) $H_0 : \mu_X \leq \mu_Y, \alpha = 0.05, n_X = 28$, and $n_Y = 34$.

7.121 The summary statistics given in Table 7.37 were computed from the data in the Birth Weight data set for the weights of babies for white mothers by mother's smoking status. Use the summary statistics in Table 7.37 to answer the following:
(a) Based on the observed samples, is it reasonable to assume $\sigma_N \approx \sigma_Y$? Explain.
(b) Compute the estimated standard error of $\bar{N} - \bar{Y}$.

TABLE 7.37 Summary Statistics on the Weights of Babies for White Mothers by Mother's Smoking Status

Smoking Status	Sample Size	Mean	Standard Deviation
No (N)	44	3429	710
Yes (Y)	52	2828.7	627

TABLE 7.38 Summary Statistics on the Absolute Change in Fat Mass (kg) for 9 Individuals in the Control Group and 15 Individuals in the Treatment Group

Group	Sample Size	Mean	Standard Deviation
Control (C)	9	1.7	4.1
Treatment (T)	15	−6.6	3.4

(c) Assuming that each population sampled is approximately normally distributed, test $H_0 : \mu_N \le \mu_Y$ at the $\alpha = 0.01$ level.

(d) Compute the approximate p-value for the test in part (c).

(e) Compute a 95% confidence interval for the difference in mean birth weight of a baby born to a white mother according to smoking status (i.e., $\mu_N - \mu_Y$).

7.122 In the article "Effect of weight loss and exercise on frailty in obese older adults" published in *Archives of Internal Medicine* (Villareal et al., 2006), the authors reported the summary statistics given in Table 7.38 on the absolute change in fat mass (kg) after 6 months for 10 individuals in the control group and 17 individuals in the treatment group. Individuals in the treatment group received weekly behavioral therapy in conjunction with exercise training three times per week, and the individuals in the control group received no lifestyle changes. Use the summary statistics in Table 7.38 to answer the following:

(a) Based on the observed samples, is it reasonable to assume $\sigma_C \approx \sigma_T$? Explain.

(b) Compute the estimated standard error of $\bar{C} - \bar{T}$.

(c) Assuming that each population sampled is approximately normally distributed, test $H_0 : \mu_C \ge \mu_T$ at the $\alpha = 0.05$ level.

(d) Compute the approximate p-value for the test in part (c).

(e) Compute a 95% confidence interval for the difference in mean absolute change in fat mass (kg) for the control and treatment groups.

7.123 In the article "Laboratory tests to determine the cause of hypokalemia and paralysis" published in the *Archives of Internal Medicine* (Lin et al., 2004), the authors reported the summary statistics given in Table 7.39 for paralysis patients having hypokalemic periodic paralysis and nonhypokalemic periodic paralysis on the variable potassium level. Use the summary statistics in Table 7.39 to answer the following:

(a) Based on the observed samples, is it reasonable to assume $\sigma_{HK} \approx \sigma_{NHK}$? Explain.

(b) Compute the estimated standard error of $\bar{HK} - \bar{NHK}$.

TABLE 7.39 Summary Statistics on the Potassium Levels of 30 Patients with Hypokalemic Periodic Paralysis and 13 with Nonhypokalemic Periodic Paralysis

Type of Paralysis	Potassium Level (mmol/L)		
	Sample Size	Mean	Standard Deviation
Hypokalemic (HK)	30	9	3
Nonhypokalemic (NHK)	13	15	4

TABLE 7.40 **Summary Statistics on the Plasma Glucose Levels of 336 Low-Risk Subjects and 297 High-Risk Subjects**

Risk Group	Plasma Glucose Level (mmol/L)		
	Sample Size	Mean	Standard Deviation
Low-risk (L)	336	5.4	0.8
High-risk (H)	297	5.7	1.2

(c) Assuming that each population sampled is approximately normally distributed, test $H_0 : \mu_{HK} \geq \mu_{NHK}$ at the $\alpha = 0.05$ level.

(d) Compute the approximate p-value for the test in part (c).

(e) Compute a 95% confidence interval for the difference in mean potassium level for individuals having hypokalemic periodic paralysis and nonhypokalemic periodic paralysis.

7.124   In the article "Cardiovascular risk in midlife and psychological well-being among older men" published in the *Archives of Internal Medicine* (Strandberg et al., 2006), the authors reported the baseline summary statistics on plasma glucose given in Table 7.40 from a longitudinal study for 336 men in a low-risk group and 297 men in a high-risk group. Use the summary statistics in Table 7.40 to answer the following:

(a) Based on the observed samples, is it reasonable to assume $\sigma_L \approx \sigma_H$? Explain.

(b) Compute the estimated standard error of $\bar{L} - \bar{H}$.

(c) Assuming that each population sampled is approximately normally distributed, test $H_0 : \mu_L = \mu_H$ at the $\alpha = 0.01$ level.

(d) Compute the approximate p-value for the test in part (c).

(e) Compute a 95% confidence interval for the difference in mean plasma glucose level for individuals in the low- and high-risk groups.

7.125   In the article "Laboratory eating behavior in obesity" published in *Appetite* (Laessle et al., 2007), the authors reported the summary statistics on the total intake given in Table 7.41 for 23 normal weight males and 24 overweight males. Use the summary statistics in Table 7.41 to answer the following:

(a) Based on the observed samples, is it reasonable to assume $\sigma_N \approx \sigma_O$? Explain.

(b) Compute the estimated standard error of $\bar{O} - \bar{N}$.

(c) Assuming that each population sampled is approximately normally distributed, test $H_0 : \mu_O \leq \mu_N$ at the $\alpha = 0.01$ level.

(d) Compute the approximate p-value for the test in part (c).

(e) Compute a 95% confidence interval for the difference in mean total intake for normal weight and overweight males.

TABLE 7.41 **Summary Statistics on the Total Intake of 23 Normal Weight Males and 24 Overweight Males**

Weight Group	Total Intake (g)		
	Sample Size	Mean	Standard Deviation
Normal Weight (N)	23	389.8	175.0
Overweight (O)	24	481.3	266.7

7.126 Using the Coronary Heart Disease data set
   (a) estimate the mean age and the standard deviation for individuals with coronary heart disease (μ_P).
   (b) estimate the mean age and the standard deviation for individuals without coronary heart disease (μ_{crit}).
   (c) test $H_0 : \mu_P = \mu_{crit}$ at the $\alpha = 0.01$ level.

7.127 Determine the common sample size for a two-sample t-test when $\sigma_X \approx \sigma_Y$ and
   (a) $\acute{\sigma} = 10$, $\delta = 4$, $\alpha = 0.05$, $\beta = 0.05$ for an upper-tail test.
   (b) $\acute{\sigma} = 50$, $\delta = 30$, $\alpha = 0.05$, $\beta = 0.15$ for an upper-tail test.
   (c) $\acute{\sigma} = 35$, $\delta = 20$, $\alpha = 0.05$, $\beta = 0.01$ for a lower-tail test.
   (d) $\acute{\sigma} = 0.5$, $\delta = 0.2$, $\alpha = 0.05$, $\beta = 0.10$ for a lower-tail test.
   (e) $\acute{\sigma} = 2$, $\delta = 0.5$, $\alpha = 0.05$, $\beta = 0.05$ for a two-tailed test.
   (f) $\acute{\sigma} = 200$, $\delta = 125$, $\alpha = 0.05$, $\beta = 0.10$ for a two-tailed test.

CHAPTER 8

SIMPLE LINEAR REGRESSION

$\mathbf{O}$NE OF the primary uses of statistics in biomedical research is the building of a statistical model that can be used to understand how a response variable varies over a set of explanatory variables. In fact, statistical models are often useful in determining an approximate relationship between the mean of the response variable and the explanatory variables, and in a well-designed experiment a statistical model can provide strong evidence of a causal relationship between the response variable and the explanatory variable. In many research studies, the value of the response variable will depend on the values of a particular set of explanatory variables, and statistical models can be used to understand how a particular explanatory variable affects the response variable or to predict future values of the response variable. Thus, some statisticians refer to the response variable as the *dependent variable* and the explanatory variable as the *independent variable* or the *predictor variable*.

One of the simplest statistical models that can be used to model the relationship between a continuous response variable and a single quantitative explanatory variable is the *simple linear regression model*. In this chapter, the use of simple linear regression for modeling a response variable as a linear function of a single explanatory variable will be discussed. In particular, bivariate data summary statistics, components of a simple linear regression model, fitting a simple linear regression model, assessing the fit of a simple linear regression model, and the statistical inferences that can be made from a simple linear regression model will be discussed.

8.1 BIVARIATE DATA, SCATTERPLOTS, AND CORRELATION

A simple linear regression model is fit to two variables in either a bivariate or a multivariate data set. In particular, the sample data used to fit a simple linear regression model come from a random sample of n paired observations selected from the target population that contain measurements on the two variables X and Y for each unit sampled where the Y variable is the response variable and X is the explanatory variable.

8.1.1 Scatterplots

In a research study, where both the response variable and the explanatory variable are quantitative variables the relationship between X and Y can be investigated using a

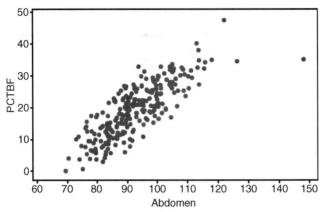

Figure 8.1   A scatterplot of percent body fat versus abdomen circumference for the Body Fat data set.

scatterplot as discussed in Chapter 4. Recall that a scatterplot based on a bivariate random sample of n observations is simply a two-dimensional plot of the observed data points $(x_1, y_1), (x_2, y_2), \ldots, (x_n, y_n)$. An example of a scatterplot is given in Figure 8.1 for the variables percent body fat (PCTBF) and abdomen circumference (Abdomen) for the $n = 252$ observations in the Body Fat data set.

Specifying a statistical model relating the response variable to the explanatory variable can be a difficult task; however, scatterplots are often useful in determining an approximate functional relationship between the response and the explanatory variables. The scatter of points in a scatterplot is called a *data cloud*, and the general shape of the data cloud is often suggestive of a model that can be used for relating a response to an explanatory variable. The analysis of a scatterplot is entirely visual and the typical patterns that a scatterplot might reveal include a data cloud sloping upward, downward, a curvilinear data cloud, or a data cloud exhibiting no obvious pattern.

When the data cloud in a scatterplot does reveal a pattern, the following characteristics of the scatterplot should be considered in specifying the functional form of the relationship between the response variable and the explanatory variable:

1. The shape of the data cloud. In particular, it is important to note whether the data cloud appears to exhibit a linear or a nonlinear pattern and whether the data cloud slopes upward or downward. If the data cloud appears to be sloping upward or downward linearly, then a straight line relationship might be an appropriate model for relating the response variable to the explanatory variable. On the other hand, when a nonlinear pattern is suggested by the data cloud, a straight line model will not be appropriate and a nonlinear model should be considered.

2. The strength of the pattern exhibited by the data cloud. When the data cloud is tightly grouped around a line or curve, some statistical model is likely to fit the observed data fairly well; however, when the data cloud is widely scattered about a line or a curve, then it is unlikely that a model will fit the observed data well.

3. Unusual or extreme points (i.e., bivariate outliers). Isolated points that do not appear to be consistent with the remaining points in the data cloud should be investigated. Bivariate outliers are often due to data errors and must be carefully investigated. A bivariate outlier can significantly affect the fit of the hypothesized model and left untreated may produce misleading inferences.

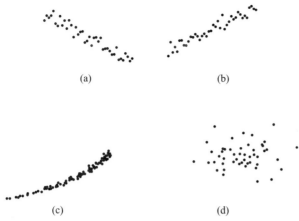

(a)   (b)

(c)   (d)

Figure 8.2   Examples of the common shapes seen in the data clouds in a scatterplot: (a) linear sloping upward; (b) linear sloping downward; (c) curvilinear; and (d) no obvious pattern.

When the data cloud exhibits no obvious pattern, the scatterplot is suggesting that the response variable does not depend on explanatory variable over the range of the observed values of the explanatory variable. Examples of the typical data clouds seen in a scatterplot are given in Figure 8.2.

Example 8.1

One of the response variables in the Body Fat data set that will be modeled later is body density (Density). The scatterplots given in Figure 8.3 are based on the $n = 252$ observations in the Body Fat data set and will be used to investigate the relationship between body density and the explanatory variables Age, Weight, Height, and Abdomen circumference.

Note that the scatterplot of body density versus age does not exhibit any strong pattern. The scatterplots of body density versus weight and body density versus abdomen circumference suggest a linear downward sloping relationship; the relationship appears to be stronger for abdomen circumference than for weight. The scatterplot of body density versus height reveals no obvious pattern but does suggest there is a bivariate outlier on the left side of the plot at a height of 29.5. In fact, in the article

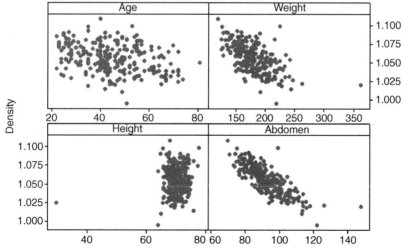

Figure 8.3   Scatterplots of body density versus the explanatory variables age, weight, height, and abdomen circumference for the Body Fat data set.

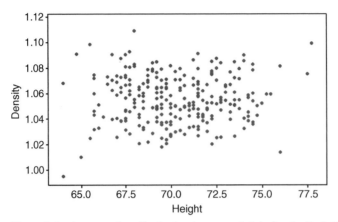

Figure 8.4   A scatterplot of body density versus height for the Body Fat data set with the corrected value for height.

"Fitting percentage of body fat to simple body measurements" published in the *Journal of Statistics Education* (Johnson, 1996), this point is identified as having been incorrectly recorded as a height of 29.5 instead of the correct value of 69.5. The scatterplot shown in Figure 8.4 is based on the Body Fat data set using the corrected value (i.e., Height = 69.5).

Note that the corrected scatterplot of body density versus height shown in Figure 8.4 suggests no obvious relationship between body density and height.

The interpretation of a scatterplot should be based on only obvious patterns suggested by the data cloud in the scatterplot. A good guideline to follow when interpreting a scatterplot is "If you do not see a clear pattern in the data cloud, then it probably does not exist."

8.1.2 Correlation

When the data cloud in a scatterplot suggests that there might be a linear relationship between the response variable and an explanatory variable, the *correlation* between the two variables can be used to measure the strength of the linear relationship. Recall from Chapter 2, the *population correlation coefficient* measures the strength of the *linear relationship* between the two quantitative variables. The population correlation is denoted by ρ and is defined as

$$\rho = \frac{1}{N} \sum \frac{[(X - \mu_x)(Y - \mu_y)]}{\sigma_x \sigma_y}$$

where μ_x, μ_y and σ_x, σ_y are the means and standard deviations of the X and Y variables. Properties of the correlation coefficient ρ include

1. ρ always between -1 and 1.

2. $\rho = \pm 1$ only when the two variables are perfectly correlated.

3. the closer ρ is to ± 1 the stronger the linear relationship between the two variables X and Y is.

4. $\rho \approx 0$ when there is no linear relationship between the two variables X and Y; however, there may be a curvilinear relationship between the variables X and Y when $\rho \approx 0$.

The statistic that is used to estimate ρ that can be computed from the information in a bivariate random sample of n observations is *Pearson's sample correlation coefficient* that is denoted by r. The formula for computing the value of r is

$$r = \frac{1}{n-1} \frac{\sum(x - \bar{x})(y - \bar{y})}{s_x \cdot s_y}$$

where s_x and s_y are the sample standard deviation of the X and Y sample values. Provided the data cloud in a scatterplot of Y versus X is suggestive of a linear relationship, the closer r is to ± 1 the stronger the linear relationship between X and Y is. Furthermore, the value of r

1. only measures the strength of the linear relationship between two variables X and Y.

2. is always between -1 and 1 (i.e., $-1 \leq r \leq 1$).

3. is equal to -1 or 1 only when all of the sample observations fall on a straight line.

4. is positive when the data cloud slopes upward. That is, a value of $r > 0$ indicates that the Y variable tends to increase as the X variable increases when $r > 0$.

5. is negative when the data cloud slopes downward. That is, a value of $r < 0$ indicates that the Y variable tends to decrease as the X variable increases when $r < 0$.

6. may be approximately 0 even when the data cloud suggests the variables are related in a nonlinear fashion.

It is important to keep in mind that the correlation coefficient only measures the linear relationship between two variables, and thus, the correlation coefficient is a meaningful measure only when the data cloud in a scatterplot suggests a linear relationship. Also, the sign of the correlation indicates whether the data cloud slopes upward or downward. Guidelines for interpreting the size of the sample correlation coefficient are given in Table 8.1.

Note that the above guidelines are guidelines only, and the actual importance of the magnitude of the sample correlation coefficient will depend on the particular problem being studied. That is, in some cases a researcher might believe a correlation of $r = 0.6$ does indicate an important relationship exists between the two variables, even though the guidelines suggest there is only a moderate linear relationship. Also, the cutoff values in these guidelines should not be used as absolute cutoffs since a data cloud with a correlation of $r = 0.81$ indicates about the same strength of linear relationship as a data cloud with a correlation of $r = 0.78$.

TABLE 8.1   Guidelines for Interpreting the Size of the Sample Correlation Coefficient

Value of r			Strength of the Linear Relationship
−1.0	to	−0.9	Very strong negative linear relationship
−0.9	to	−0.8	Strong negative linear relationship
−0.8	to	−0.5	Moderate negative linear relationship
−0.5	to	−0.3	Weak negative linear relationship
−0.3	to	0.3	No obvious linear relationship
0.3	to	0.5	Weak positive linear relationship
0.5	to	0.8	Moderate positive linear relationship
0.8	to	0.9	Strong positive linear relationship
0.9	to	1.0	Very strong positive linear relationship

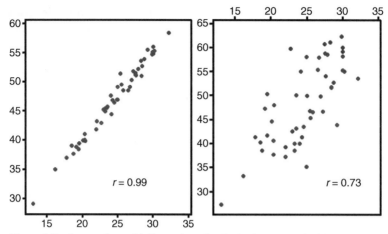

Figure 8.5   Scatterplots with linear data clouds sloping upward with $r = 0.99$ and $r = 0.73$.

Several examples of scatterplots and their corresponding sample correlation coefficients are given in Examples 8.2 and 8.3. In particular, the scatterplots in Example 8.2 all have upward sloping linear data clouds and the scatterplots in Example 8.3 all have downward sloping linear data clouds.

Example 8.2
The scatterplots showin in Figures 8.5 and 8.6 provide examples of scatterplots having linear data clouds sloping upward for $r = 0.99, 0.73, 0.50$, and 0.12. Note that the strength of the linear pattern in the data clouds decreases as the value of r decreases. Also, note that the variability within a data cloud increases as the value of r decreases.

Example 8.3
The scatterplots shown in Figures 8.7 and 8.8 provide examples of scatterplots having linear data clouds sloping downward for $r = -0.99, -0.72, -0.00$, and -0.16. As was the case with the upward sloping data clouds, the strength of the linear pattern in a downward sloping data cloud also decreases as the value of r decreases, and the variability in a data cloud increases as the value of r decreases.

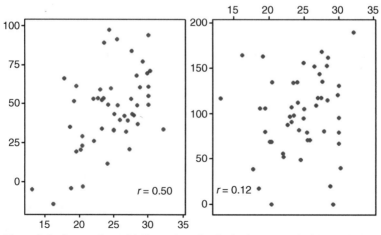

Figure 8.6   Scatterplots with linear data clouds sloping upward with $r = 0.50$ and $r = 0.12$.

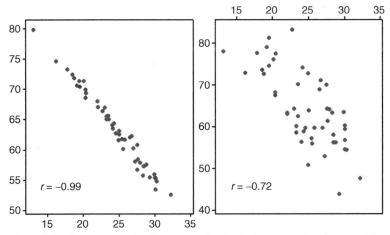

Figure 8.7   Scatterplots with linear data clouds sloping upward with $r = -0.99$ and $r = -0.72$.

Finally, it is important that the correlation is used only along with linear data clouds. It is possible for two variables to be strongly correlated even though the scatterplot has a data cloud that is nonlinear. It is also possible for two variables to have a strong nonlinear relationship when the correlation is approximately 0. For example, the scatterplot given in Figure 8.9 shows a data cloud that is suggesting that there is a strong nonlinear relationship between the variables X and Y. The sample correlation coefficient for this scatterplot is $r = 0.035$. Figure 8.10 also contains a scatterplot indicating there is a strong nonlinear relationship between the variables X and Y, but in this case the sample correlation coefficient is $r = 0.96$. Thus, Figures 8.9 and 8.10 show that the correlation coefficient alone cannot be used either to make the statistical inference that there is no relationship between the two variables when $r \approx 0$ or to infer that there is a strong linear relationship when r is close to ± 1. Thus, because the correlation coefficient only measures the strength of the linear relationship between two variables, the value of r is meaningful only when the scatterplot has a linear data cloud.

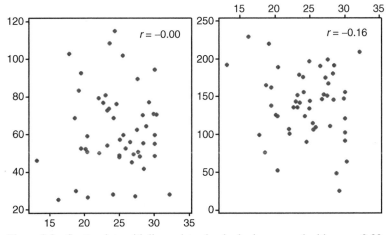

Figure 8.8   Scatterplots with linear data clouds sloping upward with $r = -0.00$ and $r = -0.16$.

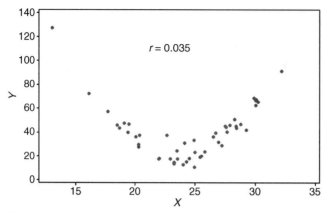

Figure 8.9   A scatterplot indicating a strong nonlinear relationship with $r = 0.035$.

8.2   THE SIMPLE LINEAR REGRESSION MODEL

When the data cloud in a scatterplot of the response variable versus the explanatory variable is linear, a plausible model for approximating the relationship between the response and explanatory variable is the *simple linear regression model*. A simple linear regression model uses a straight line relationship (i.e., linear) to approximate the relationship between the response variable and the explanatory variable. Thus, the closer the points in the data cloud are to a straight line, the better a simple linear regression model will fit the observed data. Therefore, when the data cloud exhibits a strong linear pattern and the sample correlation coefficient is large (i.e., $|r| \geq 0.8$), a simple linear regression model will be a plausible model for relating the response variable to the explanatory variable. The steps that must be carried out when fitting a simple linear regression model are outlined below.

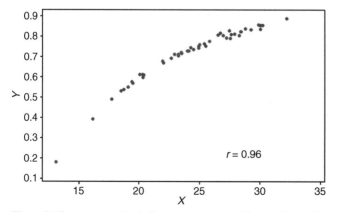

Figure 8.10   A scatterplot indicating a strong nonlinear relationship with $r = 0.96$.

THE SIMPLE LINEAR REGRESSION PROCEDURE

---

1. Develop a clear statement of the goals in a well-defined research problem.

2. Identify the response and the explanatory variables that are believed to have a strong linear relationship.

3. Develop a well-designed sampling plan that will provide data representative of the relationship between the response and the explanatory variables.

4. Collect the sample data according to the sampling plan.

5. Examine a scatterplot of the response variable versus the explanatory variable

and compute the value of r.

6. Fit the simple linear regression model to the data observed.

7. Assess the fit of the simple linear regression model.

8. Once the model has been assessed and is found to adequately fit the observed data, the model can be used to make statistical inferences about the relationship between the response variable and the explanatory variable.

One of the most important and often overlooked steps in building a simple linear regression model is assessing the adequacy of the fit of the model. Clearly, any model that will be used for making inferences about the relationship between the response and the explanatory variable should adequately fit the observed data and satisfy all of the assumptions required of the model.

Finally, it is important to keep in mind that statistical models are simply models that are used to approximate the true relationship between the response variable and the explanatory variable. As the famous statistician George Box states, "Essentially, all models are wrong, but some are useful," And "Remember that all models are wrong; the practical question is how wrong do they have to be to not be useful" (Box et al., 1987).

8.2.1 The Simple Linear Regression Model

Before formulating the simple linear regression model, recall the equation of a straight line relating a variable y to a variable x is

$$y = \beta_0 + \beta_1 x$$

where β_0 is the y-intercept and β_1 is the slope of the line. The y-intercept is the value of y that results when $x = 0$, and the slope of the line is the change in y for a one unit increase in x. When the slope is positive the line slopes upward, and when the slope is negative the line slopes downward.

The simple linear regression model is based on the equation of a straight line and can be used to model either the value of the response variable or the mean value of the response variable as a linear function of the explanatory variable. The simple linear regression model for a response variable Y and an explanatory variable X is

$$Y = \beta_0 + \beta_1 X + \epsilon$$

where β_0 is the y-intercept, β_1 is the slope of the linear relationship, and ϵ is a random error term that explains the disparity between observed points and the linear regression model. In the simple linear regression model

1. β_0 and β_1 are the unknown parameters that must be estimated from the data. The units of β_0 are the units of Y and the units of β_1 are the units of Y divided by the units of X.

2. $\beta_0 + \beta_1 X$ is the deterministic (i.e., not random) component of the model that models the mean value of the response variable Y for a given value of the explanatory variable X.

3. the slope, β_1, models the expected change in the response variable Y for a one unit increase in the explanatory variable X.

4. the error term, ϵ, is a random variable that explains the lack of fit of the straight line relationship for approximating the relationship between Y and X.

When the response and explanatory variables are perfectly correlated, the error term will be identically 0 and the relationship between Y and X would be perfectly linear. However, in most studies the response variable is not perfectly correlated with the explanatory variable so the error term is a random variable that accounts for the deviation from a perfect linear relationship. The error term ϵ is assumed to have mean 0 and standard deviation σ, and the weaker the linear relationship between the response and the explanatory variables, the more ϵ will vary. The standard deviation of the error term is also an unknown parameter of the simple linear regression model that will be estimated from the observed data.

Now, because the error term is assumed to have mean 0, the simple linear regression model can also be used to model the relationship between the mean of the response variable as a function of the explanatory variable. That is, because $\mu_\epsilon = 0$ it follows that the conditional mean of Y given X is described by the equation a straight line. In particular, the simple linear regression *line of means* is

$$\mu_{Y|X} = \beta_0 + \beta_1 X$$

Thus, a simple linear regression model can be used for both predicting future Y values and estimating the mean Y value for a given value of X.

Example 8.4
Figure 8.11 illustrates the relationship between the error term, the observed data points, and the simple linear regression line. In particular, the error terms ϵ_1, ϵ_2, ϵ_3, ϵ_4, and ϵ_5 explain the discrepancy between the actual points and the regression line, and the variability of the error terms is described by the standard deviation σ.

Furthermore, the mean value of Y for a particular X value lies on the simple linear regression line of means $\beta_0 + \beta_1 X$ that in this example is $\mu_{Y|X} = 7.1 + 1.9X$. For example, when $X = 12$ the mean value of Y is $\mu_{Y|X=12} = 7.1 + 1.9(12) = 29.9$. Also, the expected change in the mean value of Y for a one unit increase in X is $\beta_1 = 1.9$.

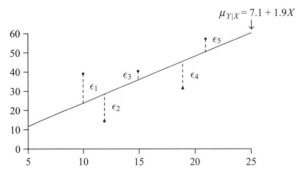

Figure 8.11 An example illustrating the relationship between the error term, the (X, Y) points, and the simple linear regression line.

8.2.2 Assumptions of the Simple Linear Regression Model

The simple linear regression model is an appropriate model for approximating the relationship between a response variable Y and an explanatory variable X only when certain model assumptions are satisfied. In particular, the error random variable ϵ must satisfy several key assumptions so that the use of a simple linear regression model will be appropriate. The assumptions of a linear regression model are listed below.

ASSUMPTIONS FOR A SIMPLE LINEAR REGRESSION MODEL

The assumptions required for using the simple linear regression model

$$Y = \beta_0 + \beta_1 X + \epsilon$$

to approximate the relationship between a response variable Y and an explanatory variable X are as follows:

A1 The observed values of the explanatory variable X are measured without error.

A2 Each observed value of the response variable Y is independent of the other values of the response variable.

A3 There is an approximate linear relationship between the response variable and the explanatory variable.

A4 The mean of the error random variable is 0 (i.e., $\mu_\epsilon = 0$).

A5 The standard deviation of the error random variable is exactly the same for each value of the explanatory variable.

A6 The probability distribution of the error random variable is normally distributed with mean zero and standard deviation σ.

Note that the first three assumptions (A1–A3) are assumptions that should be dealt with in the planning stages of the research project, and the last three assumptions (A4–A6) are assumptions about the error structure in the model. Assumption A5, the common standard deviation assumption, is also referred to as the *constant variance assumption* or the *homoscedasticity assumption* and assumption A6 is referred to as the *normality assumption*. Furthermore, when assumptions A4–A6 are valid the distribution of Y for any given value of X has the following properties.

THE DISTRIBUTION OF $Y = \beta_0 + \beta_1 X + \epsilon$

When ϵ is normally distributed with mean 0 and standard deviation σ, the conditional distribution of Y given X

1. has mean value $\mu_{Y|X} = \beta_0 + \beta_1 X$.

2. has standard deviation σ.

3. is normally distributed with mean $\beta_0 + \beta_1 X$ and standard deviation σ.

The distributional assumptions on ϵ and their impact on the distribution of Y for a given X value are illustrated in Figure 8.12. Note that when the simple linear regression model is correct or nearly correct model and assumptions A1–A6 are valid, the observed Y values for a given value of X represent a randomly selected observation from the normal distribution. Thus, some of the observed Y values will exceed their mean and some will be less than their mean, and hence, the observed data will most likely produce a scatterplot with a data cloud scattered about the line of means.

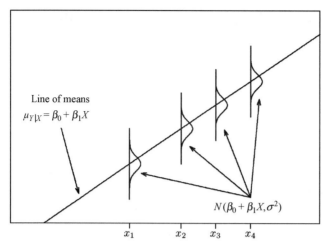

Figure 8.12 The simple linear regression model.

It is also important to note that the use of the simple linear regression model when any one of the assumptions is violated may produce incorrect or misleading statistical inferences about the relationship between the response and the explanatory variables. For example, when

1. there is a random error in measuring the value of the explanatory variable, the resulting fitted model may be severely biased.

2. the values of the response variable are not independent the estimates of β_0 and β_1 may be biased and any hypothesis test based on the model may be less reliable (i.e., reduced power) than expected.

3. there is a nonlinear relationship between the response and the explanatory variables, a simple linear regression model will often produce a poor or even misleading approximation for the relationship between the two variables.

4. the random error does not have mean equal to 0, there will be a systematic error in the model, and hence, the model will be biased.

5. the standard deviation is not constant over the range of the explanatory variable, the reliability of the model will vary from one value of the explanatory variable to another.

6. if the error random variable is not approximately normally distributed, small sample hypothesis tests and confidence intervals may provide unreliable results.

The proper use of the simple linear regression model for approximating the relationship between Y and X requires that (1) a well-designed research project and sampling plan be developed and (2) the sample data are used to assess the validity of the assumptions placed on the error structure of the model. Methods for checking of the error structure will be discussed in detail in Section 8.4.

8.3 FITTING A SIMPLE LINEAR REGRESSION MODEL

Once a random sample of n independent observations is collected on the response variable (Y) and the explanatory variable (X), and a scatterplot of the observed data suggests that a linear relationship exists between these two variables, the next step in building a simple linear regression model is to fit the model to the observed data. The method used to determine the equation of the simple linear regression model that best fits the observed data is the *method of least squares*. The method of least squares is used to determine the estimates of the model parameters β_0, β_1, and σ, and the resulting estimates of β_0, β_1, and σ produced by the method of least squares are called the *least squares estimates* of β_0, β_1, and σ. The least squares estimates of β_0, β_1, and σ are denoted by $\widehat{\beta}_0$, $\widehat{\beta}_1$, and s_e.

The method of least squares determines the values of β_0 and β_1 that minimize the sum of the squared distances from the observed points to the fitted line. That is, the method of least squares determines the line $\widehat{y} = \widehat{\beta}_0 + \widehat{\beta}_1 x$ that produces the smallest value of

$$\sum_{i=1}^{n}(y - \widehat{y})^2$$

where y is an observed value of the response variable and $\widehat{y} = \widehat{\beta}_0 + \widehat{\beta}_1 x$. The formulas for the least squares estimators of β_0 and β_1 are

$$\widehat{\beta}_1 = \frac{\sum (x - \bar{x})(y - \bar{y})}{\sum (x - \bar{x})^2}$$

$$\widehat{\beta}_0 = \bar{y} - \widehat{\beta}_1 \bar{x}$$

The equation of the *least squares regression line* is

$$\widehat{y} = \widehat{\beta}_0 + \widehat{\beta}_1 x$$

Note that the least squares estimate of β_1 can also be computed using

$$\widehat{\beta}_1 = r \times \frac{s_y}{s_x}$$

where s_x and s_y are the sample standard deviations of the observed X and Y values and r is the sample correlation coefficient.

The least squares method of fitting a simple linear regression model produces unbiased estimates of β_0 and β_1, and therefore, the least squares estimators $\widehat{\beta}_0$ and $\widehat{\beta}_1$ do not systematically under- or overestimate the parameters β_0 and β_1. The sampling distributions of $\widehat{\beta}_0$ and $\widehat{\beta}_1$ will be discussed in more detail in Section 8.5.

While the least squares estimates of β_0 and β_1 are relatively simple to compute by hand, they can be very sensitive to the number of significant digits used in computing the values of $\widehat{\beta}_0$ and $\widehat{\beta}_1$. Thus, it is always best to use a statistical computing package for fitting simple linear regression models and computing the values of $\widehat{\beta}_0$ and $\widehat{\beta}_1$. Furthermore, statistical computing packages generally have built-in methods for assessing the validity of the model assumptions and assessing the fit of the model.

Example 8.5

In studying the relationship between body density (i.e., weight/volume) of an adult male and certain body characteristics, there is a clear relationship between body density (Density) and the chest circumference (Chest). A scatterplot of body density versus chest circumference for the $n = 252$ observations in the Body Fat data set is given in Figure 8.13.

Note that the scatterplot of body density versus chest circumference suggests a linear downward sloping relationship with $r = -0.683$, and hence, the sample data suggests there is a moderate linear relationship between body density and chest circumference. Accordingly, the simple linear regression model

$$\text{Density} = \beta_0 + \beta_1 \text{Chest} + \epsilon$$

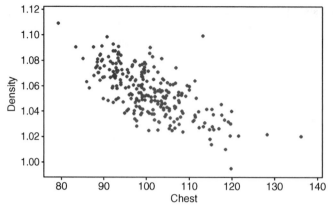

Figure 8.13   A scatterplot of body density versus chest circumference for the $n = 252$ adult males in the Body Fat data set.

will be fit to the observed data using the method of least squares and the statistical computing package MINITAB.

The resulting least squares estimates of β_0 and β_1 are $\widehat{\beta}_0 = 1.211$ and $\widehat{\beta}_1 = -0.001541$. Figure 8.14 contains a scatterplot of the observed data with the least squares regression line

$$\widehat{\text{Density}} = 1.211 - 0.001541\text{Chest}$$

drawn through the data cloud. A plot of the type given in Figure 8.14 is called a *fitted line plot* and can be useful in assessing the fit of the simple linear regression model to the observed data.

The fitted least squares regression line appears to fit the data cloud fairly well; however, there is one isolated observation (Chest ≈ 113) that does not appear to agree very well with the fitted model. Before using this fitted model to make statistical inferences about the relationship between body density and chest circumference, this point should be further investigated.

Finally, fitted models that do not satisfy the simple linear regression assumptions and poorly fitting models should not be used for making inferences about the relationship between the response and the explanatory variables. Thus, before using the fitted regression line for approximating the relationship between the response and the explanatory variables, the assumptions of the model and the fit of the model to the data must be assessed.

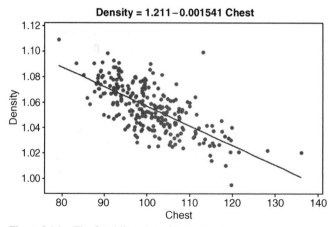

Figure 8.14   The fitted line plot of body density versus chest circumference.

8.4   ASSESSING THE ASSUMPTIONS AND FIT OF A SIMPLE LINEAR REGRESSION MODEL

A simple linear regression model should be used for approximating the relationship between the response variable and the explanatory variable only when the model assumptions are satisfied. Thus, it will be critical to assess the model assumptions before making any statistical inferences from a fitted simple linear regression model. The model assumptions for a simple linear regression model are as follows:

A1 The observed values of the explanatory variable X are measured without error.

A2 Each observed value of the response variable Y is independent of the other values of the response variable.

A3 There is an approximate linear relationship between the response variable and the explanatory variable.

A4 The mean of the error random variable is 0 (i.e., $\mu_\epsilon = 0$).

A5 The standard deviation of the error random variable is exactly the same for each value of the explanatory variable.

A6 The probability distribution of the error random variable is normally distributed with mean zero and standard deviation σ.

Assumptions A1 and A2 can be satisfied by using a well-designed sampling plan. That is, a researcher should have a clear understanding of the response and explanatory variables, and in particular, the researcher should design the study so that the explanatory variable is measured without error and the values of the response variable are independent. That being said, some research projects will involve explanatory variables that are measured with error. For example, in longitudinal studies where explanatory variables related to an individual's diet are used and the individual reports the value of these diet variables, there will almost certainly be a measurement error in these self-reported variables. An example where the explanatory variable would be expected to be measured with error is the self-reported variable percent fat in the diet that varies from day to day and is not easily measured. When the explanatory variable is suspected of being measured with error, a *measurement error modeling* approach should be used in building a model for approximating the relationship between the response and explanatory variables. For more information on measurement error modeling, see *Measurement Error in Nonlinear Models* (Carroll et al., 2006).

In the planning stages of the research study, the researcher should design the sampling plan around a well-planned random sample that will ensure that the observations on the response variable are independent. Thus, in a well-designed study the independence of the observations on the response variable should not be an issue; however, in a poorly planned study, this may be a problem. When the values of the response variable are not independent, the values are said to be *autocorrelated*. Because the readers of this book will only be using well-designed sampling plans, the problem of autocorrelated observations on the response variable will not be discussed any further; for more information on fitting models with correlated observations on the response variable, the reader is advised to see *Regression Analysis by Example* (Chatterjee et al., 2006) for methods of assessing and accounting for an autocorrelation problem.

The assumption of linearity, A3, is easily checked by inspecting a scatterplot of the observed responses versus their corresponding values of the explanatory variable. The scatterplot should suggest either (1) a linear relationship, (2) a nonlinear relationship, or (3) no obvious relationship between the response and explanatory variables. Clearly, a simple linear regression model should only be used to approximate the relationship between the response and the explanatory variables when the data cloud in a scatterplot is linear; regression models for nonlinear data clouds are discussed in Chapter 9.

The assumption A4 that the mean of the error variable ϵ is 0 cannot be easily assessed and is generally assumed to be true in a standard regression analysis; however, when the error term is a multiplicative error instead of an additive error, the mean of the error term will not be 0. The special case where the error term in a regression model is a multiplicative error is discussed in Section 8.4.2.

8.4.1 Residuals

The assumptions of constant variance and the normality of the error term, A5 and A6, are important assumptions placed on the error term in the model, and the validity of these assumptions is critical to having a fitted simple linear regression model that is meaningful. The validity of the assumption of constant variance and the assumption of the normality of the error term will be judged by the behavior of the *residuals* associated with the fitted model. The residuals associated with the fitted model contain information on how well the *fitted values* $\widehat{y}_1, \widehat{y}_2, \widehat{y}_3, \ldots, \widehat{y}_n$ fit their corresponding observed values $y_1, y_2, y_3, \ldots, y_n$. In particular, the ith residual is the difference between y_i and $\widehat{y}_i$ and is denoted by e_i. Thus, the ith residual e_i is

$$e_i = y_i - \widehat{y}_i$$

where $\widehat{y}_i = \widehat{\beta}_0 + \widehat{\beta}_i x_i$.

While the error term ϵ in the model describes the discrepancy of the observed Y values from the line of means, the residuals measure the distance from the observed value of Y to the fitted line. Thus,

$$\epsilon = Y - (\beta_0 + \beta_1 X),$$

the mean value of ϵ is 0, and the standard deviation of ϵ is σ, whereas

$$e = y - (\widehat{\beta}_1 + \widehat{\beta}_2 x),$$

$\bar{e} = 0$, and the residuals will be used to estimate the unknown value of σ.

Unlike the error term in the model, each residual will have a slightly different standard deviation, and thus it is common to use the *standardized residuals* that have the same standard deviation. The standardized residuals are also called *internally studentized residuals*, they will be denoted by e_s, and the standardized residuals are available in most of the commonly used statistical computing packages. The primary advantage of using the standardized residuals is that they all have standard deviation 1, and therefore, it is unlikely for a standardized residual to fall outside of the range -3 to 3 when assumptions A5 and A6 are valid. In fact, any observation having a standardized residual with $|e_s| > 3$ indicates the model is not fitting this point very well and should be carefully investigated.

8.4.2 Residual Diagnostics

The standardized residuals can be used to check the constant variance and the normality assumptions using graphical diagnostics such as scatterplots and normal probability plots. In particular, a scatterplot of the standardized residuals can be used to assess the validity of the assumptions of constant variance and linearity, and a normal probability plot of the standardized residuals will be used to assess the validity of the normality assumption.

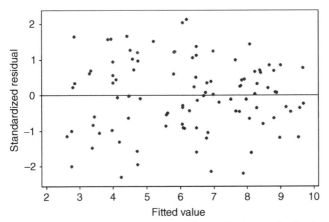

Figure 8.15 An example of a residual plot with the standardized residuals plotted against the fitted values.

The most commonly used residual diagnostic is the *residual plot* that is a scatterplot of the standardized residuals versus the fitted values or the X values. An example of a residual plot is given in Figure 8.15 with the standardized residuals plotted against the fitted values.

There are two commonly used forms of the residual plot. One form is a scatterplot of the standardized residuals versus the fitted values and the other is a scatterplot of the standardized residuals versus the observed X values. Both plots reveal exactly the same residual plot pattern when the slope of the fitted line is positive; however, when the slope of the fitted line is negative, they are mirror images. In either case, both forms of a residual plot can be used to assess the linearity and constant variance assumption as well as for identifying outliers.

Unlike a scatterplot of the response variable versus the explanatory variable, systematic patterns in a residual plot are undesirable and suggest a violation of one or more of the assumptions of the simple linear regression model. A "good" residual plot is a plot where (1) there are no systematic patterns, (2) there is equal vertical variation across the range of the fitted values (or X values), and (3) all of the standardized residuals fall between -3 and 3. In particular, a residual plot with no systematic patterns provides evidence supporting the assumption of linearity and the assumption of constant variance. A residual plot where all of the standardized residuals are between -3 and 3 suggests there are no obvious outliers in the data set.

On the other hand, any patterns in the residual plot are indicative of problems with the fitted model. The most commonly encountered patterns in a residual plot are curvilinear or funneling patterns. A curvilinear pattern in a residual plot indicates a nonlinear trend in the scatterplot of Y versus X. Thus, a curvilinear pattern in a residual plot suggests that the relationship between Y and X is not linear, and therefore, the simple linear regression model is not an inappropriate model for modeling the relationship between the response variable and the explanatory variable. Examples of curvilinear patterns in residual plots are given in Figure 8.16.

When a residual plot has a curvilinear pattern, one possible method of curing the curvilinear pattern in the residuals is to consider alternative statistical models that can be used when there is a curvilinear relationship between Y and X. More sophisticated models that allow curvilinear relationships between the response and the explanatory variables will be discussed in Chapter 9.

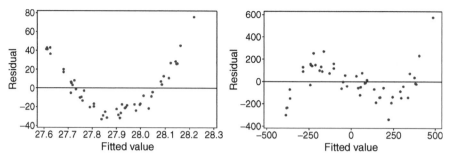

Figure 8.16   Examples of residual plots with curvilinear patterns.

A funnel-shaped pattern in a residual plot indicates that the variability of the residuals varies over the range of the fitted values. Thus, a funneling pattern in the residual plot suggests that the assumption of constant variance may not be valid and there is a potential *nonconstant variance* problem with the fitted model. Examples of the most common funneling shapes are given in Figure 8.17.

Nonconstant variation is often the consequence of having a multiplicative error instead of an additive error and sometimes can be cured by modeling the natural logarithm of Y as a linear function of X. The *log-Y model* is a simple linear regression model of the form

$$\ln(Y) = \beta_0 + \beta_1 X + \epsilon$$

where $\ln(Y)$ is the natural logarithm of Y. To fit this model, a researcher need only transform the Y values with the natural logarithm function, fit the log-Y model, and then check the residuals of the fitted log-Y model. If the residual plot for this new model still suggests problems with the fitted model, the model should be discarded and a new model must be tried.

When obvious patterns can be seen in a residual plot, they are also sometimes visible in the initial scatterplot of Y versus X. Examples 8.6 and 8.7 illustrate the relationship between patterns in the residual plot that can also be seen in the scatterplot of Y versus X; however, Example 8.8 illustrates how it can also be very difficult to anticipate a pattern in the residual plot from only a scatterplot of Y versus X.

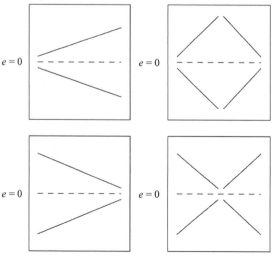

Figure 8.17   Possible funneling shapes in a residual plot.

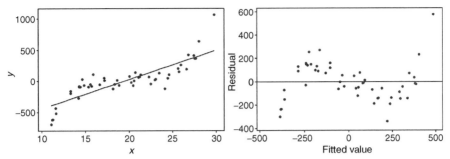

Figure 8.18 An example of scatterplot and residual plot that suggest a curvilinear relationship between Y and X.

Example 8.6
The scatterplot and residual plot in Figure 8.18 both indicate a curvilinear relationship between Y and X.

Example 8.7
The scatterplot and residual plot in Figure 8.19 both indicate a nonconstant variance problem with the fitted model.

Example 8.8
The scatterplot in Figure 8.20 appears to indicate a plausible linear relationship between Y and X. However, the residual plot for the fitted simple linear regression model given in Figure 8.21 reveals a curvilinear pattern in the residuals.

Examples 8.6–8.8 illustrate the importance of carefully inspecting both the scatterplot and the residual plot before blindly using a fitted simple linear regression model to make inferences about the relationship between Y and X. Also, because a fitted simple linear regression model can be somewhat sensitive to outliers, it is important to look for outliers in a residual plot. Outliers will show up in a residual plot as either points having standardized residuals falling below -3 or above 3, and the farther from ± 3 a standardized residual is the more extreme and possibly influential the outlier is. An example of a residual plot with a single outlier is given in Figure 8.22.

The influence that an outlier exerts on the fitted model depends on both the X and the Y values associated with the outlier and the number points used in fitting the model. The degree to which an outlier influences the fitted model decreases as the sample size increases. The location of the X value associated with an outlier also influences the fitted model. In particular, the farther the X value is from $\bar{x}$ the more leverage the outlier will have on the fitted model. Outliers with X values far from $\bar{x}$ influence both the intercept and the slope of

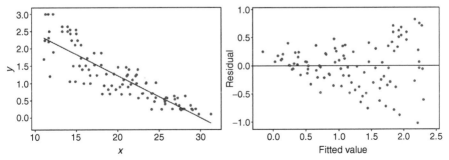

Figure 8.19 An example of scatterplot and residual plot that suggest a nonconstant variance problem with the fitted model.

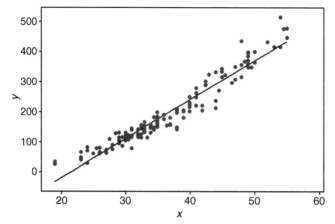

Figure 8.20   An example of scatterplot suggests a linear relationship between Y and X.

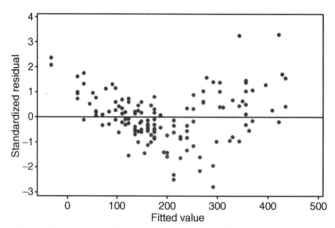

Figure 8.21   The residual plot for the simple linear regression model fit to the data shown in Figure 8.20.

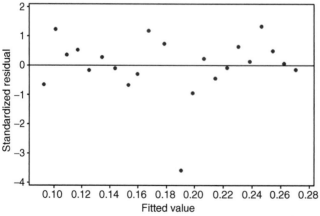

Figure 8.22   A residual plot with an outlier at the fitted value $\widehat{y} = 0.19$ with a standardized residual of -3.6.

the fitted model, and outliers near $\bar{x}$ generally will only influence the intercept of the fitted model.

When an outlier has been identified in a scatterplot or a residual plot, the outlier should first be investigated as an impossible value or a mistake in recording the data. Outliers that are impossible values should be eliminated from the data set and the model refit on the remaining sample observations; outliers that are clearly caused by recording errors should be corrected and the model refit on the corrected data set. When an outlier cannot be eliminated from a data set or its value corrected, the outlier should be temporarily removed from the data set and the model refit to the remaining sample data. If the estimates of the slope and intercept do not differ greatly for the model fit on the entire data set and the model fit on the data set without the outlier, then the outlier has little influence on the fitted model and does not merit further consideration. However, when the estimates of the slope and intercept are significantly different for the models fit on the full and reduced data sets, the outlier is influencing the fit of the model and more than the observed data is needed to resolve this problem.

A residual plot may indicate more than one problem with the fitted model. For example, a residual plot might suggest that the relationship is curvilinear, has nonconstant variance, and an outlier. Also, residual plots can be hard to interpret on small data sets with ambiguity arising over whether or not there is a problematic pattern in the residual plot. Thus, the best guideline to follow when looking at the residual plots is not to overanalyze the residual plot. That is, identify and cure only the obvious patterns in a residual plot and ignore any ambiguous patterns. Sometimes, it is helpful to cover up a isolated residual and examine the pattern in the remaining points in the residual plot.

A valid normality assumption is important to ensure the validity of any confidence intervals, hypothesis tests, or prediction intervals that are usually part of the statistical analysis associated with fitting a simple linear regression model. The normality assumption can easily be checked by creating a normal probability plot of standardized residuals and using the fat pencil test to assess the validity of this assumption. That is, a normal probability plot of the standardized residuals will support the assumption of the normality of the error term in the model when the points in the normal plot are roughly linear. When the points in the normal probability plot deviate strongly from a straight line, there is sufficient evidence to reject the normality assumption. For example, the normal probability plot given in Figure 8.23 supports the normality assumption, while the normal probability plot in Figure 8.24 suggests the normality assumption is not valid.

Example 8.9 illustrates the use of the residual diagnostics on the Body Fat data set for modeling percent body fat (PCTBF) as a linear function of chest circumference (Chest).

Example 8.9
The relationship between percent body fat (PCTBF) and chest circumference (Chest) will be investigated using the sample data in the Body Fat data set on $n = 252$ adult males. A scatterplot of percent body fat versus chest circumference is given in Figure 8.25.

Since the scatterplot in Figure 8.25 suggests there is a moderate linear relationship ($r = 0.703$) between percent body fat and chest circumference, the simple linear regression model

$$\text{PCTBF} = \beta_0 + \beta_1 \text{Chest} + \epsilon$$

was fit to this data set. The resulting residual plot and normal probability plot for the standardized residuals for the fitted model are given in Figure 8.26. Note that in the residual plot in Figure 8.26, all of the standardized residuals fall between -3 and 3, there is no evidence of curvilinear pattern in the residuals, and the variability of the residuals appears to be fairly constant over the range of fitted values. Also, the normal plot in Figure 8.26 clearly passes the fat pencil test, and thus, supports the assumption of normality.

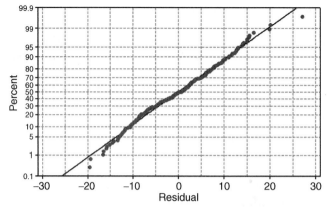

Figure 8.23   An example of a normal probability plot of the standardized residuals supporting the normal assumption.

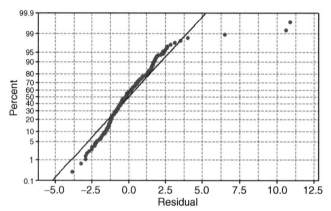

Figure 8.24   An example of a normal probability plot of the standardized residuals suggesting that the normality assumption is not valid.

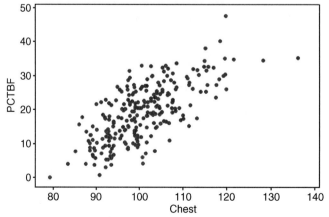

Figure 8.25   A scatterplot of percent body fat (PCTBF) versus chest circumference (Chest) for the $n = 252$ adult males in the Body Fat data set.

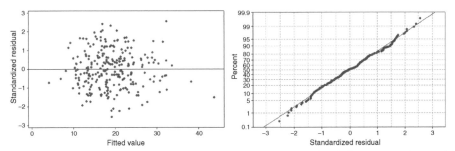

Figure 8.26   The residual plot and normal probability plot for a simple linear regression model relating percent body fat and chest circumference.

Since there are no apparent problems suggested by the residuals, the equation of the fitted model can now be reported and is

$$\widehat{\text{PCTBF}} = -51.17 + 0.6975 \text{ Chest}$$

8.4.3 Estimating σ and Assessing the Strength of the Linear Relationship

Once the model assumptions have been assessed and shown to be valid, the next step in a simple linear regression analysis is to estimate the standard deviation of the error term σ and assess the strength of the linear relationship suggested by the fitted regression model. Since σ is the standard deviation of the error term, the residuals contain all of the relevant sample information about the error random variable. Thus, the residuals will be used for estimating the value of σ, and the point estimator of σ is denoted by s_e. The value of s_e is

$$s_e = \sqrt{\frac{e_1^2 + e_2^2 + \cdots + e_n^2}{n-2}}$$

$$= \sqrt{\frac{(y_1 - \widehat{y}_1)^2 + (y_2 - \widehat{y}_2)^2 + \cdots + (y_n - \widehat{y}_n)^2}{n-2}}$$

$$= \frac{\sum e^2}{n-2}$$

where $e_1, e_2, e_3, \ldots, e_n$ are n residuals, $y_1, y_2, y_3, \ldots, y_n$ are n observed values, and $\widehat{y}_1, \widehat{y}_2, \widehat{y}_3, \ldots, \widehat{y}_n$ are n fitted values.

Note that the estimator s_e is based on the residuals and not the standardized residuals. Also, s_e has $n - 2$ degrees of freedom and s_e^2 is an unbiased estimator of σ^2. The degrees of freedom of s_e are $n - 2$ rather than $n - 1$ because the simple linear regression model has two parameters, β_0 and β_1, which must be estimated before σ can be estimated. In addition, the value of s_e provides a measure of the variability of the scatter of points about the fitted regression line and will be an important component in computing the estimated standard errors of $\widehat{\beta}_0$ and $\widehat{\beta}_1$.

Besides the variation about the fitted line, the other types of variation that are considered in a simple linear regression model are the total variation in the observed Y values and the variation explained by using the simple linear regression model. The total variation is denoted by SSTot and is defined to be

$$SSTot = (y_1 - \bar{y})^2 + (y_2 - \bar{y})^2 + \cdots + (y_2 - \bar{y})^2$$
$$= \sum (y - \bar{y})^2$$

Because $y = \widehat{y} + e$, it turns out that

$$(y - \bar{y}) = (\widehat{y} + e - \bar{y}) = (\widehat{y} - \bar{y}) + e$$

Replacing $y - \bar{y}$ with $(\widehat{y} - \bar{y}) + e$ in the formula for SSTot produces an algebraically equivalent form of SSTot that is given by

$$SSTot = \sum (y - \bar{y})^2 = \sum (\widehat{y} - \bar{y})^2 + \sum e^2$$

The sum of the n squared residuals, $\sum e^2$, is called the *sum of squares due to residual error* and will be denoted by SSE, and the sum of the squared deviations of the fitted values from $\bar{y}$ is called the *sum of squares due to the regression model* that is denoted by SSReg. Both SSE and SSReg are used to measure the degree to which the fitted model fits the observed data. In particular, SSE is used in the estimating σ since

$$s_e = \sqrt{\frac{\sum e^2}{n-2}} = \sqrt{\frac{SSE}{n-2}}$$

and SSReg is used in computing the *coefficient of determination* that measures the proportion of the total variation in the observed Y values that is explained by the fitted regression model. The coefficient of determination is denoted by R^2 and takes on values between 0 and 1. The formula for computing the value of R^2 is

$$R^2 = \frac{SSReg}{SSTot} = 1 - \frac{SSE}{SSTot}$$

The coefficient of determination associated with a fitted simple linear regression model is also the square of the sample correlation between the fitted values and the observed values, and for the simple linear regression model R^2 is the square of the correlation between the response and the explanatory variables (i.e., $R^2 = r^2$). The values of s_e and R^2 are part of the standard output reported by most statistical computing packages in a simple linear regression analysis.

In a good fitting simple linear regression model all of the model assumptions will be satisfied, the value of s_e will be small, and the value of R^2 will be large. Since $R^2 = 1 - SSE/SSTot$, when all of the residuals are 0 all of the observed Y values fall on the fitted line and $R^2 = 1$. Thus, the closer R^2 is to 1 the better the simple linear regression model fits the observed data. Furthermore, since $R^2 = r^2$ and values of r greater than 0.8 or less than -0.8 are considered evidence of strong linear relationships (see Table 8.1), values of R^2 greater than 0.64 are also considered evidence of strong linear relationships.

Example 8.10
For the simple linear regression analysis used in modeling percent body fat (PCTBF) as a linear function of chest circumference (Chest) in Example 8.5, the following summary output is reported by the statistical computing package MINITAB.

```
The regression equation is
PCTBF = - 51.17 + 0.6975 Chest

S = 5.96680    R-Sq = 49.4%    R-Sq(adj) = 49.2%
```

Note that MINITAB uses S for the estimate of σ instead of s_e and R-sq for the value of R^2. Also, MINITAB reports the value of R^2 as a percentage rather than as a proportion (i.e., $100\% \times R^2$). MINITAB also reports an adjusted value of R^2, R-Sq(adj), which will be discussed in Chapter 9.

Based on the MINITAB output, $s_e = 5.967$ and $R^2 = 0.494$ and the fitted model is

$$PCTBF = -51.17 + 0.6975 \text{ Chest}$$

Note that in Example 8.5 the sample correlation coefficient was $r = 0.703$ and $r^2 = 0.703^2 = 0.494 = R^2$. Thus, the simple linear regression model explains 49.4% of the total variation in the observed Y values.

Another component in the standard output provided by a statistical computing package along with the equation of the fitted simple linear regression model, s_e and R^2, is a table summarizing the sources of variation associated with the observed data and the fitted model. The table used to summarize SSTot, SSReg, and SSE is called an *analysis of variance table* or *ANOV table*. The standard form of an ANOV table summarizing the sources of variation in a simple linear regression analysis are shown in Table 8.2.

Note that along with the sum of squares for each source of variation, the degrees of freedom attributed to each source are listed. The other components in an ANOV table are

1. the *mean squares* (MS) that are the sum of squares divided by their corresponding degrees of freedom. The mean square for the error source of variation denoted by MSE is equal to s_e^2. Since MSE $= s_e^2$, s_e is also referred to as the *root mean square error* and is denoted by RMSE.

2. the F-ratio that is the ratio formed by dividing MSReg by MSE. The F-ratio is used for testing the utility of the simple linear regression model. In particular, the F-ratio is used for testing the $H_0 : \beta_1 = 0$ versus $H_A : \beta_1 \neq 0$.

3. the p-value associated with the F-ratio. The p-value associated with the observed F-ratio, say F_{obs}, is the probability that an F-ratio with 1 and $n - 2$ degrees of freedom is larger than F_{obs}. Small p-values are associated with large observed values of the F-ratio and suggest that $\beta_1 \neq 0$.

Because the F-ratio is used to test $H_0 : \beta_1 = 0$ versus $H_A : \beta_1 \neq 0$, it can also be thought of as a test of the utility of the simple linear regression model. That is, the null hypothesis $\beta_1 = 0$ is equivalent to the null hypothesis

$$H_0' : Y = \beta_0 + \epsilon$$

TABLE 8.2   The ANOV Table for a Simple Linear Regression Analysis

Source	df	SS	MS	F	P
Regression	1	SSReg	$MSReg = \dfrac{SSR}{1}$	$F_{obs} = \dfrac{MSReg}{MSE}$	p-value
Error	$n - 2$	SSE	$MSE = \dfrac{SSE}{n - 2}$		
Total	$n - 1$	SSTot			

```
Analysis of Variance

Source         DF       SS       MS       F       P
Regression      1    8678.3   8678.31  243.75  0.000
Error         250    8900.7    35.60
Total         251   17579.0
```
Figure 8.27   The MINITAB ANOV table for the model PCTBF $= \beta_0 + \beta_1$Chest $= \epsilon$ fit to the Body Fat data set.

and the alternative hypothesis $\beta_1 \neq 0$ is equivalent to

$$H'_A : Y = \beta_0 + \beta_1 X + \epsilon$$

Since $\mu_{Y|X}$ does not depend on X in H'_0, testing $\beta_1 = 0$ versus $\beta_1 \neq 0$ is actually a test whether or not there is a linear relationship between Y and X. The rejection region for the F-ratio test is

$$\text{Reject } H_0 : \beta_1 = 0 \text{ when the } p\text{-value is less than } \alpha$$

The p-value associated with the F-ratio in the ANOV table is a sensitive assumption of the simple linear regression model, especially the constant variance, independence, and normality assumptions, and hence, a hypothesis test of $\beta_1 = 0$ should be carried out only when the sampling plan and observed data support these assumptions. Also, a significant F-ratio does not necessarily mean that there is a practical difference between β_1 and 0. A confidence interval can be used to investigate the scientific/practical significance of β_1 when the F-ratio indicates that β_1 is statistically significantly different from 0.

Example 8.11
For the simple linear regression analysis used in modeling percent body fat (PCTBF) as a linear function of chest circumference (Chest) in Example 8.5, the MINITAB output also included the ANOV table given in Figure 8.27.
      The p-value for the observed F-ratio is 0.000 and thus there is sufficient evidence to reject $H_0 : \beta_1 = 0$. Therefore, it appears that there is a significant linear relationship between percent body fat (PCTBF) and chest circumference (Chest).

8.5 STATISTICAL INFERENCES BASED ON A FITTED MODEL

Once a simple linear regression model has been fit, the assumptions have been checked, problems with the fitted model that are suggested by the residual diagnostics have been cured, and the regression relationship is found to be significant, the fitted model can be used for making more detailed statistical inferences about the regression coefficients and the relationship between the response and the explanatory variables. In particular, when the normality assumption is plausible or the sample size is sufficiently large, (1) confidence intervals for the parameters of the simple linear regression model can be computed, (2) hypothesis tests of claims concerning the intercept and slope can be performed, (3) confidence intervals for the mean value of the response for a particular value of the explanatory variable can be computed, and (4) prediction intervals for the value of the response variable for a given value of the explanatory variable can be computed.

8.5.1 Inferences about β_0

Recall that β_0 is the y-intercept in the simple linear regression model and the least squares estimator of β_0 is $\widehat{\beta}_0$. The mean of the sampling distribution of $\widehat{\beta}_0$ is β_0, and thus $\widehat{\beta}_0$ is an unbiased estimator of β_0, and the standard error of $\widehat{\beta}_0$ is

$$\mathrm{SE}(\widehat{\beta}_0) = \sigma \times \sqrt{\frac{1}{n} + \frac{\bar{x}^2}{\sum(x - \bar{x})^2}}$$

Because σ is unknown, the estimated standard error must be used in practice, and the estimated standard error of $\widehat{\beta}_0$ is

$$\mathrm{se}(\widehat{\beta}_0) = s_e \times \sqrt{\frac{1}{n} + \frac{\bar{x}^2}{\sum(x - \bar{x})^2}}$$

The estimated standard error of $\widehat{\beta}_0$ has $n - 2$ degrees of freedom, the same degrees of freedom as s_e, and is provided in the standard output for a simple linear regression analysis provided by most statistical computing packages.

When the error term in the model is normally distributed with mean 0 and constant standard deviation σ, the sampling distribution of $\widehat{\beta}_0$ follows a normal distribution with mean β_0 and standard error $\mathrm{SE}(\widehat{\beta}_0)$; when the sample size is sufficiently large (i.e., $n \geq 100$), the sampling distribution of $\widehat{\beta}_0$ is approximately normally distributed with mean β_0 and standard error $\mathrm{SE}(\widehat{\beta}_0)$. Furthermore, when the normality assumption is satisfied or the sample is sufficiently large

$$t = \frac{\widehat{\beta}_0 - \beta_0}{\mathrm{se}(\widehat{\beta}_0)}$$

will follow a t distribution with $n - 2$ degrees of freedom. Confidence intervals and hypothesis tests for β_0 will be based on the t distribution. A $(1 - \alpha) \times 100\%$ confidence interval for β_0 when the normality assumption is satisfied or $n > 100$ is

$$\widehat{\beta}_0 \pm t_{\mathrm{crit}} \times \mathrm{se}(\widehat{\beta}_0)$$

where t_{crit} has $n - 2$ degrees of freedom and can be found in Table A.7.

For testing claims about β_0, when the normality assumption is satisfied or $n > 100$, then a hypothesis test about β_0 can also be based on the t distribution. The test statistic for testing claims about β_0 is

$$t = \frac{\widehat{\beta}_0 - \beta_{00}}{\mathrm{se}(\widehat{\beta}_0)}$$

where β_{00} is the null value of β_0. The rejection regions for the upper-, lower-, or two-tail t-test about β_0 are given in Table 8.3, and the value of t_{crit} can be found in Table A.7 for the corresponding significance level α and $n - 2$ degrees of freedom.

Most statistical computing packages report $\widehat{\beta}_0$, $\mathrm{se}(\widehat{\beta}_0)$, and the value of $t_{\mathrm{obs}} = \dfrac{\widehat{\beta}_0}{\mathrm{se}(\widehat{\beta}_0)}$ and its p-value for testing $\beta_0 = 0$ versus $\beta_0 \neq 0$ as part of their standard output in a simple linear regression analysis. Hypothesis tests of β_0 with null values other than 0 (i.e., $\beta_{00} \neq 0$) will generally have to be carried out by hand.

TABLE 8.3 Rejection Regions for the Upper-, Lower-,
and Two-tail t-tests of β_0

Test	H_0	Rejection Region
Upper-tail	$H_0 : \beta_0 \leq \beta_{00}$	Reject H_0 when $t_{obs} > t_{crit}$
Lower-tail	$H_0 : \beta_0 \geq \beta_{00}$	Reject H_0 when $t_{obs} < -t_{crit}$
Two-tail	$H_0 : \beta_0 = \beta_{00}$	Reject H_0 when $|t_{obs}| > t_{crit}$

Example 8.12

The MINITAB output for the simple linear regression analysis of percent body fat modeled as a linear function of chest circumference in Example 8.5 is given in Figure 8.28.

The estimate of β_0 is given both in the regression equation and in the summary table listing the predictors in the model. The row for the predictor labeled `Constant` contains the values of $\widehat{\beta}_0$ under the column head `Coef`, the $se(\widehat{\beta}_0)$ under the column head `SE Coef`, the values of t_{obs}, and the p-value for testing $\beta_0 = 0$ versus $\beta_0 \neq 0$ under the column heads T and P.

Thus, the estimated standard error of $\widehat{\beta}_0$ is 4.520, and since the normality assumption is supported by the normal probability plot given in Figure 8.26, β_0 is significantly different from 0 since $t_{obs} = -11.32$ and its p-value is 0.000. Since it is important to report a confidence interval along with the results of the t-test so that scientific or practical significance of the test results can also be interpreted, a 95% confidence interval for β_0 is

$$-51.172 \pm 1.96 \times 4.52$$

which yields an interval of estimates of β_0 ranging from -60.03 to -42.31.

8.5.2 Inferences about β_1

The slope of the regression model is β_1 that represents the expected change in the mean of the response variable for a one unit increase in the explanatory variable. The least squares estimator the slope of the simple linear regression model is $\widehat{\beta}_1$ that is computed using

$$\widehat{\beta}_1 = \frac{\sum(x - \bar{x})(y - \bar{y})}{\sum(x - \bar{x})^2}$$

```
The regression equation is
PCTBF = - 51.2 + 0.697 Chest


Predictor      Coef  SE Coef        T      P
Constant    -51.172    4.520   -11.32  0.000
Chest       0.69748  0.04467    15.61  0.000


S = 5.96680   R-Sq = 49.4%   R-Sq(adj) = 49.2%


Analysis of Variance


Source           DF       SS      MS       F      P
Regression        1   8678.3  8678.3  243.75  0.000
Residual Error  250   8900.7    35.6
Total           251  17579.0
```

Figure 8.28 The MINITAB output for the simple linear regression analysis of percent body fat modeled as a linear function of chest circumference on the Body Fat data set.

The mean of the sampling distribution of $\widehat{\beta}_1$ is β_1, and thus $\widehat{\beta}_1$ is an unbiased estimator of β_1. The standard error of $\widehat{\beta}_1$ is

$$\mathrm{SE}(\widehat{\beta}_1) = \frac{\sigma}{\sqrt{\sum (x - \bar{x})^2}}$$

Since the value of σ is unknown, the estimated standard error given by

$$\mathrm{se}(\widehat{\beta}_1) = \frac{s_e}{\sqrt{\sum (x - \bar{x})^2}}$$

will be used in practice, and the estimated standard error of $\widehat{\beta}_1$ has $n - 2$ degrees of freedom as do s_e and $\mathrm{se}(\widehat{\beta}_0)$.

When the error term in the model is normally distributed with mean 0 and constant standard deviation σ, the sampling distribution of $\widehat{\beta}_1$ will follow a normal distribution with mean β_1 and standard deviation $\mathrm{SE}(\widehat{\beta}_1)$; when the sample size is sufficiently large (i.e., $n \geq 100$), the sampling distribution of $\widehat{\beta}_1$ is approximately normally distributed with mean β_1 and standard error $\mathrm{SE}(\widehat{\beta}_1)$. Thus, when the normality assumption is satisfied or the sample is sufficiently large,

$$t = \frac{\widehat{\beta}_1 - \beta_1}{\mathrm{se}(\widehat{\beta}_1)}$$

will follow a t distribution with $n - 2$ degrees of freedom, and the confidence intervals and hypothesis tests for β_1 will be based on the t distribution.

When the normality assumption of the simple linear regression model is satisfied or $n > 100$ a $(1 - \alpha) \times 100\%$ confidence interval for β_1 is

$$\widehat{\beta}_1 \pm t_{\mathrm{crit}} \times \mathrm{se}(\widehat{\beta}_1)$$

where t_{crit} has $n - 2$ degrees of freedom and can be found in Table A.7. Since $\beta_1 = 0$ means there is no linear relationship between Y and X, a confidence interval for β_1 that contains the value 0 suggests that the sample data do not support the hypothesized linear relationship between the response and the explanatory variables.

When the normality assumption is satisfied or $n > 100$, a hypothesis test about β_1 can be based on the t distribution, and the test statistic for testing claims about β_1 is

$$t = \frac{\widehat{\beta}_1 - \beta_{10}}{\mathrm{se}(\widehat{\beta}_1)}$$

where β_{10} is the null value of β_1. The rejection regions for the upper-, lower-, or two-tail t-test about β_0 are given in Table 8.3.

In general, the most important test concerning β_1 is the test of $\beta_1 = 0$ versus $\beta_1 \neq 0$ since when $\beta_1 = 0$ there is no linear relationship between Y and X. Thus, the standard output for a simple linear regression analysis provided by most statistical computing packages will include the least squares estimate $\widehat{\beta}_1$, $\mathrm{se}(\widehat{\beta}_1)$, and the values of t_{obs} and its p-value for testing $\beta_1 = 0$ versus $\beta_1 \neq 0$. The value of t_{obs} for testing $\beta_1 = 0$ versus $\beta_1 \neq 0$ is computed using the test statistic

$$t = \frac{\widehat{\beta}_1}{\mathrm{se}(\widehat{\beta}_1)}$$

```
The regression equation is
PCTBF = - 51.2 + 0.697 Chest


Predictor      Coef   SE Coef       T      P
Constant    -51.172     4.520  -11.32  0.000
Chest       0.69748   0.04467   15.61  0.000


S = 5.96680    R-Sq = 49.4%    R-Sq(adj) = 49.2%


Analysis of Variance


Source            DF       SS      MS       F      P
Regression         1   8678.3  8678.3  243.75  0.000
Residual Error   250   8900.7    35.6
Total            251  17579.0
```

Figure 8.29   The MINITAB output for the simple linear regression analysis of percent body fat modeled as a function of chest circumference on the Body Fat data set.

Furthermore, the test of model utility based on the F-ratio in the ANOV table is equivalent to the t-test of $\beta_1 = 0$. In fact, the value the observed F-ratio in the ANOV table is equal of t_{obs}^2 and the p-value for the observed F-ratio is the same as the p-value associated with the value of t_{obs} for testing $\beta_1 = 0$.

Example 8.13
The MINITAB output for the simple linear regression analysis of percent body fat modeled as a linear function of chest circumference in Example 8.5 is given in Figure 8.29.

The least squares estimates of β_0 and β_1 are given both in the regression equation and in the summary table listing the predictors in the model. The row for the predictor labeled Chest contains the values of $\widehat{\beta}_1$ in the column head Coef, the $\text{se}(\widehat{\beta}_1)$ in the column head SE Coef, and the values of t_{obs} and its p-value for testing $\beta_1 = 0$ versus $\beta_1 \neq = 0$ in the columns head T and P.

Thus, the estimated standard error of $\widehat{\beta}_1$ is 0.04467, and since the normality assumption is supported by the normal probability plot given in Figure 8.26, β_1 is significantly different from 0 since $t_{\text{obs}} = 15.61$ and its p-value is 0.000. Also, note that the observed F-ratio is $F_{\text{obs}} = 243.75$ and $t_{\text{obs}}^2 = (15.61)^2 = 243.67$; the small difference between F_{obs} and t_{obs}^2 is due to rounding.

A 95% confidence interval for β_1 is

$$0.69748 \pm 1.96 \times 0.04467$$

which yields an interval of estimates of β_1 ranging from 0.610 to 0.785. Thus, on the basis of the observed data, the expected change in the mean percent body fat for a one unit increase in chest circumference is at least 0.610 percent and possibly as much as 0.785 percent.

Example 8.14
Use the MINITAB output given in Example 8.13 to test $H_0 : \beta_1 \geq 1$ versus $H_A : \beta_1 < 1$ at the $\alpha = 0.01$ level.

Solution   The test statistic for testing $H_0 : \beta_1 \geq 1$ versus $H_A : \beta_1 < 1$ is

$$t = \frac{\widehat{\beta}_1 - 1}{\text{se}(\widehat{\beta}_1)}$$

and the rejection region is

$$\text{Reject } H_0 : \beta \geq 1 \text{ when } t_{\text{obs}} < -1.96$$

The observed value of the t statistic is

$$t_{obs} = \frac{0.69748 - 1}{0.04467} = -6.77$$

Therefore, since $t_{obs} = -6.77 < -1.96$, there is sufficient evidence to reject the null hypothesis $H_0 : \beta_1 \geq 1$ at the $\alpha = 0.01$ level. Using Table A.8, the p-value is approximately 0.000, and therefore, there is strong statistical evidence that β_1 is less than 1. A 95% confidence interval for β_1 is 0.610–0.785. Thus, on the basis of the observed data, the slope β_1 appears to be at least 0.610 and possibly as much as 0.785, but not 1.

8.6 INFERENCES ABOUT THE RESPONSE VARIABLE

The equation of the fitted simple linear regression model is used primarily for estimating the mean value of the response variable for a given value of the explanatory variable and for predicting the value of the response variable for a particular value of the explanatory variable. Thus, the mean value of the response variable Y when the explanatory variable X takes on the value x_0 is

$$\mu_{Y|x_0} = \beta_0 + \beta_1 x_0$$

the estimator of $\mu_{Y|x_0}$ is $\widehat{\mu}_{Y|x_0} = \widehat{\beta}_0 + \widehat{\beta}_1 x_0$. Also, since the value of Y when the explanatory variable X takes on the value x_0 is

$$Y_{x_0} = \beta_0 + \beta_1 x_0 + \epsilon$$

and since ϵ has mean 0, the *predicted* value of Y when $X = x_0$ is $\widehat{y}_{x_0} = \widehat{\beta}_0 + \widehat{\beta}_1 x_0$. Furthermore, because the least squares estimators $\widehat{\beta}_0$ and $\widehat{\beta}_1$ are unbiased estimators of β_0 and β_1, $\widehat{\mu}_{Y|x_0}$ is an unbiased estimator of $\mu_{Y|x_0}$ and $\widehat{y}_{x_0}$ is an unbiased predictor of Y_{x_0}. In fact, $\widehat{\mu}_{Y|x_0}$ is the *best linear unbiased estimator* (BLUE) of $\mu_{Y|x_0}$ and $\widehat{y}_{x_0}$ is the *best linear unbiased predictor* (BLUP) of Y when $X = x_0$.

8.6.1 Inferences About $\mu_{Y|X}$

The sampling distribution of $\widehat{\mu}_{Y|x_0}$ has mean $\mu_{Y|x_0} = \beta_0 + \beta_1 x_0$ and thus $\widehat{\mu}_{Y|x_0}$ is an unbiased estimator of $\mu_{Y|x_0}$. The standard deviation of the sampling distribution of $\widehat{\mu}_{Y|x_0}$ is

$$SE(\widehat{\mu}_{Y|x_0}) = \sigma \times \sqrt{\frac{1}{n} + \frac{(x_0 - \bar{x})^2}{\sum (x - \bar{x})^2}}$$

and the estimated standard error of $\widehat{\mu}_{Y|x_0}$ is

$$se(\widehat{\mu}_{Y|x_0}) = s_e \times \sqrt{\frac{1}{n} + \frac{(x_0 - \bar{x})^2}{\sum (x - \bar{x})^2}}$$

Note that the farther x_0 is from $\bar{x}$, the larger the estimated standard error of $\widehat{\mu}_{Y|x_0}$ will be, and when $x_0 = \bar{x}$

$$se(\widehat{\mu}_{Y|x_0}) = \frac{se}{\sqrt{n}} = se(\bar{y})$$

```
New
Obs    Fit  SE Fit       95% CI              95% PI
 1  11.601   0.612   (10.395, 12.807)   (-0.212, 23.415)
```

Figure 8.30   The MINITAB output for estimating the mean and predicting the value of percent body fat for a chest circumference of 90 cm.

Thus, $\widehat{\mu}_{Y|X}$ is a more accurate estimator of $\mu_{Y|X}$ for values of X near $\bar{x}$ and less accurate for values of X far from $\bar{x}$.

Now, when the error term in the simple linear regression model is normally distributed, the sampling distribution of $\widehat{\mu}_{Y|x_0}$ is normal with mean $\mu_{Y|x_0}$ and standard deviation $SE(\widehat{\mu}_{Y|x_0})$. Also, when $n > 100$ the sampling distribution of $\widehat{\mu}_{Y|x_0}$ is approximately normal with mean $\mu_{Y|x_0}$ and standard deviation $SE(\widehat{\mu}_{Y|x_0})$. Thus, when the error term is normally distributed or $n > 100$,

$$t = \frac{\widehat{\mu}_{Y|x_0} - \mu_{Y|x_0}}{se(\widehat{\mu}_{Y|x_0})}$$

will be distributed as a t distribution with $n - 2$ degrees of freedom, and a $(1 - \alpha) \times 100\%$ confidence interval for $\mu_{Y|x_0}$ is

$$\widehat{\mu}_{Y|x_0} \pm t_{crit} \times se(\widehat{\mu}_{Y|x_0})$$

where t_{crit} has $n - 2$ degrees of freedom and can be found in Table A.7. In general, all of the information needed for computing a confidence interval for $\mu_{Y|X}$ is not given in the standard computer output for a simple linear regression analysis; however, most statistical computing packages will compute a confidence interval for $\mu_{Y|X}$ when asked to.

Example 8.15
MINITAB will compute a confidence interval for $\mu_{Y|X}$ as an additional option in a simple linear regression analysis. The MINITAB output for the confidence interval includes the fitted value $(\widehat{y}_{x_0})$, the estimated standard error of $\widehat{y}_{x_0}$, the confidence interval for $\mu_{Y|x_0}$, and a prediction interval for Y_{x_0}.

For example, the MINITAB output given in Figure 8.30 was included in the simple linear regression analysis of percent body fat and chest circumference with a 95% confidence interval for the mean percent body fat for a chest circumference of 90 cm.

Thus, the fitted value for Chest = 90 is 11.6, the estimated standard error of $\widehat{\mu}_{PCTBF|Chest=90}$ is 0.612, and a 95% confidence interval for the mean percent body fat for a chest circumference of 95 cm based on the simple linear regression model is 10.4%–12.8%.

The MINITAB output given in Figure 8.31 contains the fitted value and a 95% confidence interval for the mean percent body fat for a chest circumference of 125 cm.

Note that because 125 is farther from the mean chest circumference of 100.82 than is 90, the estimated standard error of $\mu_{PCTBF|Chest=125}$ is larger than is the estimated standard error of $\mu_{PCTBF|Chest=90}$, and therefore, the 95% confidence interval for $\mu_{PCTBF|Chest=125}$ is wider than the confidence interval for $\mu_{PCTBF|Chest=90}$.

```
New
Obs    Fit  SE Fit       95% CI              95% PI
 1  36.013   1.144   (33.761, 38.265)   (24.047, 47.978)
```

Figure 8.31   The MINITAB output for estimating the mean and predicting the value of percent body fat for a chest circumference of 125 cm.

In general, values of $\mu_{Y|X}$ should only be estimated for values of X covered by the range of the observed X values for the following two reasons:

1. The variability of $\widehat{\mu}_{Y|X}$ increases as X moves away from $\bar{x}$ and often the resulting estimates of the mean vary too much to provide meaningful estimates.

2. There is no evidence that the linear relationship between Y and X extends beyond the range of the observed X values.

In fact, it is even possible in some cases for extrapolation beyond the range of the observed X values to lead to impossible values of $\mu_{Y|X}$. Therefore, it is never a good idea to use the fitted model to extrapolate beyond the range of the observed X values. A properly designed sampling plan will provide the necessary range of X values so that the means of the response variable can be accurately estimated at a set of prespecified values of X.

8.6.2 Inferences for Predicting Values of Y

In some biomedical studies, one of the goals of fitting a simple linear regression model will be to predict the value of the response variable for a particular value of the explanatory variable, say $X = x_0$. Since the value of Y at $X = x_0$ is

$$Y_{x_0} = \beta_0 + \beta_1 x_0 + \epsilon$$

which can also be expressed as

$$Y_{x_0} = \mu_{Y|x_0} + \epsilon$$

The estimator $\widehat{y} = \widehat{\beta}_0 + \widehat{\beta}_1 x_0$ is used with for estimating the mean of the response variable at x_0 for predicting the value of Y at x_0.

While $\widehat{y}$ is used for estimating both $\mu_{Y|X}$ and Y_X, there is a subtle difference between estimation and prediction. In particular, prediction is used to estimate the value of an unobserved value of a random variable, whereas estimation is used to estimate the unknown value of the mean of a random variable. More importantly, an unobserved value of a random variable is a random unknown quantity, while a parameter is a fixed (i.e., nonrandom) unknown quantity. In general, prediction is the statistical process used for estimating random quantities and estimation is the statistical process used for estimating parameters. The sampling distribution of a predictor is used to judge the accuracy of a predictor, and to distinguish a predictor from estimator, the standard deviation of the sampling distribution of a predictor is called the *prediction error* rather than the standard error.

The prediction error of $\widehat{y}_{x_0}$ is denoted by $\mathrm{PE}(\widehat{y}_{x_0})$ and is

$$\mathrm{PE}(\widehat{y}_{x_0}) = \sigma \times \sqrt{1 + \frac{1}{n} + \frac{(x_0 - \bar{x})^2}{\sum (x - \bar{x})^2}}$$

The estimated prediction error is denoted by $\mathrm{pe}(\widehat{y}_{x_0})$ and

$$\mathrm{pe}(\widehat{y}_{x_0}) = s_e \times \sqrt{1 + \frac{1}{n} + \frac{(x_0 - \bar{x})^2}{\sum (x - \bar{x})^2}}$$

Note that the estimated prediction error can be computed as

$$\mathrm{pe}(\widehat{y}_{x_0}) = \sqrt{s_e^2 + se(\widehat{\mu}_{Y|x_0})^2}$$

```
New
Obs    Fit  SE Fit      95% CI            95% PI
  1  11.601  0.612  (10.395, 12.807)  (-0.212, 23.415)
  2  36.013  1.144  (33.761, 38.265)  (24.047, 47.978)
```

Figure 8.32   The MINITAB output for estimating the mean and predicting the value of percent body fat for a chest circumferences of 90 and 125 cm.

and therefore, the prediction error at $X = x_0$ is always larger than the estimated standard error of estimated mean at $X = x_0$. Even though $\widehat{y}$ is used for both estimating the mean and predicting a value of Y, the reliability of $\widehat{y}$ depends on the application it is being used for, and predictors are always more variable than estimators. Also, the farther x_0 is from $\bar{x}$, the larger the estimated prediction error will be.

When the normality assumption is satisfied or $n > 100$ a $(1 - \alpha) \times 100\%$ *prediction interval* for the value of Y at $X = x_0$ is

$$\widehat{y}_{x_0} \pm t_{\text{crit}} \times \text{pe}(\widehat{y}_{x_0})$$

where t_{crit} has $n - 2$ degrees of freedom and can be found in Table A.7. As is the case with a confidence interval for $\mu_{Y|x_0}$, the information needed for computing a confidence interval for Y_{x_0} is not provided in the standard computer output for a simple linear regression analysis; however, most statistical computing packages will compute prediction intervals for Y values when asked to.

Example 8.16
MINITAB reports both the confidence interval for $\mu_{Y|x_0}$ and a prediction interval for Y_{x_0} when either is requested. For example, the MINITAB output given in Figure 8.32 was generated in the simple linear regression analysis of the model PCTBF $= \beta_0 + \beta_1$Chest $+ \epsilon$ fit to the Body Fat data set. In particular, confidence and prediction intervals are given for Chest $= 90$ cm and Chest $= 125$ cm.

Thus, based on the observed data, the predicted value for percent body fat of an adult males with a chest circumference 90 cm is 11.6% with a 95% prediction interval of 0–23.4%. Because this prediction interval yields a slightly negative lower boundary for percent body fat, which is an impossible value, it should be reported as 0%.

The predicted value for percent body fat of an adult male with a chest circumference 125 cm is 36.0% with a 95% prediction interval of 24.0–48.0%.

Also, note that the prediction intervals are quite a bit wider than the confidence intervals. Also, note that only the estimated standard error of $\widehat{\mu}_{Y|x_0}$ is given in the MINITAB output (i.e., SE Fit) since the value of the estimated prediction error can be computed using

$$\text{pe}(\widehat{y}_{x_0}) = \sqrt{s_{\text{e}}^2 + \text{se}(\widehat{\mu}_{Y|x_0})^2}$$

Thus, since $s_{\text{e}} = 5.96680$

$$\text{pe}(\widehat{y}_{95}) = \sqrt{5.96680^2 + 0.612^2} = 6.00$$

for Chest $= 90$, and when Chest $= 125$ the estimated prediction error is

$$\text{pe}(\widehat{y}_{95}) = \sqrt{5.96680^2 + 1.144^2} = 6.08$$

8.7   SOME FINAL COMMENTS ON SIMPLE LINEAR REGRESSION

Fitting simple linear regression model, or any statistical model for that matter, is usually a dynamic process. Models are fit to the original data, assumptions checked, the residual diagnostics suggest adjustments to the model, and the model is refit and the assumptions rechecked until a good fitting model is found. Only after curing any problem suggested by the residual diagnostics should inferences be drawn from the fitted model about the relationship between the response and the explanatory variables. A simple linear regression analysis should follow the steps outlined below.

SIMPLE LINEAR REGRESSION ANALYSIS

1. Determine the sampling plan that will be used for collecting a random sample on the response and explanatory variables.

2. Collect the data.

3. Investigate the relationship between the response and the explanatory variables using a scatterplot.

4. If the scatterplot suggests a linear relationship between the response and the explanatory variables, fit the simple linear regression model to the observed data.

5. Check the assumptions of the model and identify any problems suggested by the residual diagnostics.

6. Make any adjustments to the model that may cure the problems suggested by the residual diagnostics and refit the model.

7. Repeat steps 5 and 6 until a good fitting model is found.

8. Use the fitted model for making statistical inferences about the relationship between the response and explanatory variable.

It makes no sense to use a poor fitting model to make inferences about the relationship between the response and the explanatory variables or to use a simple linear regression model when the scatterplot suggests the relationship is not linear. Also, while a simple linear regression model can provide important information about the linear relationship between the response and the explanatory variables, confidence intervals and hypothesis tests should not be performed in the presence of nonnormality unless $n > 100$.

It is always important to interpret the results of a hypothesis test and weigh the statistical significance of the test versus the practical significance of the point estimate. For this reason, it is always a good idea to report a confidence interval along with the results of a hypothesis test when testing a claim about the intercept or slope in the simple linear regression model.

Finally, when reporting the results of a simple linear regression analysis, a researcher need not report all of the output provided by a statistical computing package. In particular, the most relevant information in the output from a simple linear regression analysis is whether or not the model has significant utility, the equation of the fitted model provided has significant utility, the standard errors of the coefficients, the value of s_e, the value of R^2, and any specialized inferences made using the model. The equation of any fitted model where the F-ratio suggests that there is no linear relationship between the response and the explanatory variables should not be reported. Also, the residual plot, the normal probability plot, and the ANOV table need not be included in a summary of a simple linear regression analysis; however, it is important to summarize the results of the residual diagnostics. Any adjustments to the original model that are suggested by the residual diagnostics should also be summarized by addressing what the problem was and how it was cured. A scatterplot of fitted line plot of the response versus the explanatory variable should be included in the summary of the simple linear regression analysis. An example of a typical summary report for a simple linear regression analysis is given in Example 8.17.

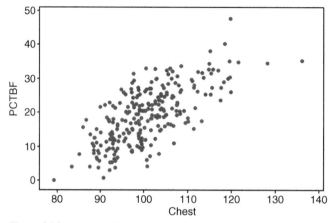

Figure 8.33   A scatterplot of percent body fat versus chest circumference for $n = 252$ adult males.

Example 8.17
The relationship between the percent body fat and the chest circumference was studied for a random sample of $n = 252$ adult males in the Body Fat data set. A scatterplot of percent body fat (PCTBF) versus chest circumference (Chest) is given in Figure 8.33.

Since the scatterplot in Figure 8.33 suggests that there is a linear relationship between percent body fat and chest circumference ($r = 0.703$), the simple linear regression model

$$\text{PCTBF} = \beta_0 + \beta_1 \text{Chest} + \epsilon$$

was fit to the observed data. An analysis of the residuals revealed no problems with the fitted model and a normal probability plot of the residuals supports the normality assumption.

The equation of the fitted model is

$$\widehat{\text{PCTBF}} = -51.2 + 0.675 \text{ Chest}$$

The observed data suggest that there is a significant linear relationship between percent body fat and chest circumference ($F_{\text{obs}} = 243.75$, p-value $= 0.000$). The fitted model is summarized in Table 8.4.

A confidence interval for the mean percent body fat of an adult male with a chest circumference of 95 cm is 10.4–12.8%, and a prediction interval for the percent body fat of an adult male with a chest circumference of 125 cm is 24–48%.

Note that the residual plot and the normal probability plot were presented in the summary of the simple linear regression analysis; however, these plots should be put in an appendix accompanying the summary report. Also, the particular style used in summarizing a simple linear regression analysis is usually determined by the audience the report or article is being written for.

TABLE 8.4   Summary of the Fitted Simple Linear Regression Model for the Model PCTBF= $\beta_0 + \beta_1$Chest + ϵ

Coefficient	Estimate	Standard Error	P-value	95% Confidence Interval
Intercept	−51.2	4.52	0.000	−60.1 to −42.3
Slope	0.697	0.045	0.000	0.587 to 0.763

$s_e = 5.97$ and $R^2 = 49.4\%$.

GLOSSARY

ANOV Table   The sources of variation in a simple linear regression analysis are summarized in an Analysis of Variance or ANOV table.

Autocorrelation   The values of the response variable are said to be autocorrelated when the values of the response variable are not independent.

Best Linear Unbiased Estimator $\widehat{y} = \widehat{\beta}_0 + \widehat{\beta}_1 x$ is the best linear unbiased estimator of $\mu_{Y|x}$.

Best Linear Unbiased Predictor $\widehat{y} = \widehat{\beta}_0 + \widehat{\beta}_1 x$ is the best linear unbiased predictor of Y when $X = x$.

Coefficient of Determination   The coefficient of determination is denoted by R^2 and measures the amount of the total variation in the response variable that is explained by the simple linear regression model. In a simple linear regression model, $R^2 = r^2$ that is also

$$R^2 = \frac{\text{SSReg}}{\text{SSTot}}$$

Data Cloud   The scatter of points in a scatterplot is called a data cloud, and the general shape of the data cloud can be suggestive of a model relating the response and explanatory variables.

Dependent Variable   The response variable is also referred to as the dependent variable.

Fitted Line Plot   A fitted line plot is a scatterplot of the observed data with the least squares regression line drawn through the data cloud.

Homoscedasticity   When the standard deviation of the error term in a simple linear regression model is the same for all values of the explanatory variable, the model is called a homoscedastic model. When the standard deviation varies over the values of the X variable, the model is said to have nonconstant variance.

Independent Variable   An explanatory variable is also referred to as an independent variable or predictor variable.

Least Squares Estimates   The method of least squares produces estimates of the model parameters β_0, β_1, and σ. The resulting estimates of β_0, β_1, and σ produced by using the method of least squares are called the least squares estimates of β_0, β_1, and σ and are denoted by $\widehat{\beta}_0$, $\widehat{\beta}_1$, and s_e, respectively.

Least Squares Method   The method used to determine the equation of the simple linear regression model that best fits the observed data is the least squares method. The least squares method determines the values of β_0 and β_1 that minimize the sum of the squared distance from an observed point to the fitted line. The method of least squares determines the line $\widehat{y} = \widehat{\beta}_0 + \widehat{\beta}_1 x$ that produces the smallest value of

$$\sum_{i=1}^{n}(y - \widehat{y})^2$$

Least Squares Regression Line   The equation of the least squares regression line is $\widehat{y} = \widehat{\beta}_0 + \widehat{\beta}_1 x$.

Line of Means   The line of means is $\mu_{Y|X} = \beta_0 + \beta_1 X$.

Log-Y Model The log-Y model is often used when the simple linear regression model exhibits a nonconstant variance problem and is a model of the form

$$\ln(Y) = \beta_0 + \beta_1 X + \epsilon$$

Measurement Error Modeling When the explanatory variable X is measured with an error, a measurement error modeling approach is used to address this problem.

Pearson's Sample Correlation Coefficient Pearson's sample correlation coefficient r is an estimator of the population correlation coefficient and is computed using

$$r = \frac{1}{n-1} \frac{\sum (x - \bar{x})(y - \bar{y})}{s_x \cdot s_y}$$

where s_x and s_y are the sample standard deviation of the X and Y sample values.

Prediction Error The prediction error is the standard deviation of the sampling distribution of $\widehat{y}$ when used for predicting the value of Y for a particular value of X. The estimated prediction error is denoted by pe and is

$$\text{pe}(\widehat{y}_{x_0}) = s_e \times \sqrt{1 + \frac{1}{n} + \frac{(x_0 - \bar{x})^2}{\sum (x - \bar{x})^2}}$$

Prediction Interval A prediction interval is a confidence interval for a predicted value of the response variable. A $(1 - \alpha) \times 100\%$ prediction interval for the value of Y when $X = x$ and the normality assumption is satisfied is given by

$$\widehat{y}_x \pm t_{\text{crit}} \times \text{pe}(\widehat{y}_{x_0})$$

where t_{crit} is the t-value used for a $(1 - \alpha) \times 100\%$ confidence interval with $n - 2$ degrees of freedom.

Residual Plot A residual plot is a scatterplot of the standardized residuals versus the fitted values or the X values.

Residuals The residuals associated with the fitted model contain information on how well the fitted values $\widehat{y}_1, \widehat{y}_2, \widehat{y}_3, \ldots, \widehat{y}_n$ fit their corresponding observed values $y_1, y_2, y_3, \ldots, y_n$. The ith residual is the difference between y_i and $\widehat{y}_i$ and is denoted by e_i and

$$e_i = y_i - \widehat{y}_i$$

where $\widehat{y}_i = \widehat{\beta}_0 + \widehat{\beta}_i x_i$.

Scatterplot A scatterplot is a graphical, two-dimensional plot of the observed data points $(x_1, y_1), (x_2, y_2), \ldots, (x_n, y_n)$.

Simple Linear Regression Model A simple linear regression model is a model for relating a response variable Y and an explanatory variable X. The form of a simple linear regression model is

$$Y = \beta_0 + \beta_1 X + \epsilon$$

where β_0 is the y-intercept, β_1 is the slope, and ϵ is the error term that explains the disparity between observed points and the linear regression model.

Simple Linear Regression Simple linear regression is a statistical method for building a model that can be used to investigate the strength of the linear relationship between a response variable and an explanatory variable.

Standardized Residuals   The standardized residuals, also called internally studentized residuals, are formed by dividing the residuals by their corresponding standard deviations.

SSE   The sum of squares due to the error term in a simple linear regression model is denoted by SSE and is

$$SSE = \sum e^2$$

SSReg   The sum of squares due to the simple linear regression model is denoted by SSReg and is

$$SSReg = \sum (\hat{y} - \bar{y})^2$$

SSTot   The total variation in the response variable is denoted by SSTot and is

$$SSTot = \sum (y - \bar{y})^2 = SSReg + SSE$$

EXERCISES

8.1   What is the simplest statistical model for relating a response variable to an exploratory variable?

8.2   What are the possible patterns a data cloud can take on in a scatterplot?

8.3   What property does the correlation coefficient measure?

8.4   What is the difference between ρ and Pearson's correlation coefficient r?

8.5   Why is it important to investigate the data cloud in a scatterplot before computing the value of the sample correlation coefficient?

8.6   Use the four scatterplots given in Figure 8.34 having approximate r values of $0.5, 0.8, -0.5$, and -0.8 to answer the following:
(a) Which of the scatterplots suggest positive linear relationships?
(b) Which of the scatterplots suggest negative linear relationships?
(c) In which scatterplot would $r \approx 0.8$? Explain.
(d) In which scatterplot would $r \approx -0.8$? Explain.

8.7   Why is it inappropriate to report the value of r when the data cloud in the scatterplot has a curvilinear data cloud?

8.8   Assuming the data cloud in the scatterplot is linear, summarize the strength of the linear relationship between the two variables according to the guidelines given in Table 8.1 when
(a) $r = 0.42$ (b) $r = 0.93$
(c) $r = 0.23$ (d) $r = -0.89$
(e) $r = -0.57$ (f) $r = -0.08$

8.9   How is a bivariate outlier identified in a scatterplot?

8.10   Why is it possible for the value of r to be approximately 0 when there is a strong relationship between two variables?

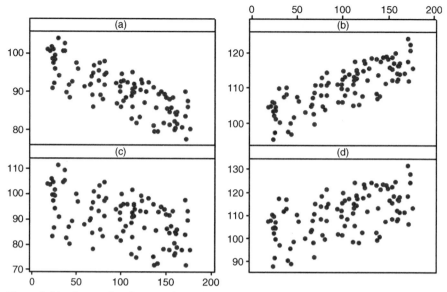

Figure 8.34   Scatterplots for Exercise 8.6.

8.11 In the article "Association of UV index, latitude, and melanoma incidence in nonwhite populations: US surveillance, Epidemiology, and end results (SEER) program, 1992 to 2001" published in the *Archives of Dermatology* (Eide and Weinstock, 2005), the authors report a correlation of $r = -0.85$ between melanoma incidence and the latitude where an individual lives for white men and a correlation of $r = 0.53$ for black men. On the basis of this information does the incidence of melanoma appear to increase or decrease with an increase in latitude for
   (a) white men?
   (b) black men?

8.12 Using the Birth Weight data set
   (a) create a scatterplot of baby's birth weight (BWT) versus mother's weight at the last menstrual period (LWT).
   (b) describe the pattern of the data cloud in the scatterplot created in part (a).
   (c) estimate the correlation between baby's birth weight (BWT) and mother's weight at the last menstrual period (LWT).

8.13 Using the Body Fat data set
   (a) create scatterplots of weight versus height and weight versus chest circumference.
   (b) describe the patterns of the data clouds in the scatterplots created in part (a).
   (c) estimate the correlation between weight and height and weight and chest circumference.
   (d) determine which of the explanatory variables, height or chest circumference, exhibits a stronger linear relationship with an adult male's weight.

8.14 What is the equation of a straight line?

8.15 What is the equation of a simple linear regression model for relating a response variable Y to an explanatory variable X?

8.16   What are the parameters in a simple linear regression model?

8.17   What does the slope in a simple linear regression model measure?

8.18   What does the error term ϵ explain in a simple linear regression model?

8.19   What is the line of means associated with a simple linear regression model?

8.20   What are the assumptions associated with a simple linear regression model?

8.21   What does the term homoscedasticity mean?

8.22   What are the possible problems that can arise when a simple linear regression model
is used when
   (a) the explanatory variable is measured with error?
   (b) there is a nonlinear relationship between the response and the explanatory variable?
   (c) the error term does not have mean 0?
   (d) the standard deviation of the error term is not constant over the range of the
explanatory variable?
   (e) the error term is not approximately normally distributed?

8.23   What is the method of least squares?

8.24   What is the least squares
   (a) estimate of the intercept?
   (b) estimate of the slope?
   (c) estimate of the line of means?

8.25   How is $\widehat{\beta}_0$ different from β_0?

8.26   How is $\widehat{\beta}_1$ different from β_1?

8.27   Compute the values of the least squares estimates of β_0 and β_1 when
   (a) $r = 0.64$, $\bar{x} = 34.5$, $\bar{y} = 122.9$, $s_x = 4.5$, and $s_y = 14.1$.
   (b) $r = -0.73$, $\bar{x} = 52.8$, $\bar{y} = 79.1$, $s_x = 0.53$, and $s_y = 1.14$.

8.28   Using the Body Fat data set, determine the least squares regression line for relating
the response variable weight to
   (a) chest circumference.   **(b)** height.
   (c) abdomen circumference.   **(d)** wrist circumference.

8.29   In the article "Bleeding time and bleeding: an analysis of the relationship of the
bleeding time test with parameters of surgical bleeding" published in the journal
Blood (De Caterina et al., 1994), the authors reported a simple linear regression
model for relating total bleeding (TB) and bleeding time (BT) based on $n = 69$
individuals. The authors reported the least squares line

$$\widehat{TB} = -112.92 + 44.595BT$$

and a correlation coefficient for TB and BT of $r = 0.66$.
   (a) Assuming the scatterplot reveals a linear data cloud, according to the guidelines
on correlations how strong is the linear relationship between total bleeding and
bleeding time?
   (b) What is the value of the least squares estimate of the intercept?
   (c) What is the value of the least squares estimate of the slope?

(d) Estimate the expected change in total bleeding for a one unit increase in bleeding time.

8.30 What is a residual?

8.31 What is a standardized residual?

8.32 How is a standardized residual different from a residual?

8.33 Why is it unlikely for a standardized residual to fall outside of the interval -3 to 3?

8.34 What is a residual plot?

8.35 How is a residual plot used in assessing the validity of the assumptions required of the error term in a simple linear regression model?

8.36 What pattern will be revealed in a residual plot when there
(a) are no apparent problems?
(b) is a violation of the constant variation assumption?
(c) is a violation of the linearity assumption?
(d) is one or more bivariate outliers in the observed data?

8.37 What does it mean when an observed data point has a standardized residual of $e_s = 4.5$?

8.38 What is the procedure that should be used for investigating the influence of an outlier?

8.39 Examine and interpret each of the following residual plots. Be sure to identify any suggested violation of the simple linear regression assumptions and bivariate outliers.

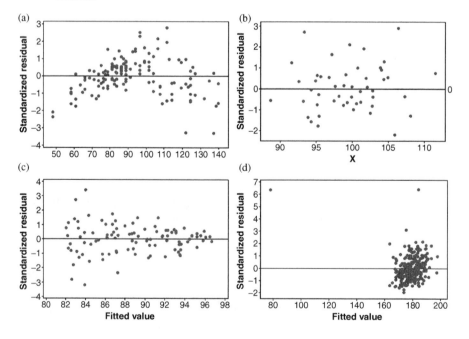

8.40 What is the transformation that might be used to cure a nonconstant variation problem suggested by a residual plot?

8.41   What is the procedure for checking the normality assumption?

8.42   What is the fat pencil test?

8.43   Determine whether each of the following normal probability plots supports the assumption of normality?

(a)   (b)

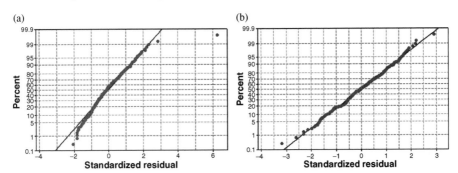

8.44   Using the Body Fat data set with weight as the response variable and chest circumference as the explanatory variable
   (a) fit a simple linear regression model relating weight to chest circumference.
   (b) create a residual for the residuals associated with the fitted model.
   (c) create a normal probability plot for the residuals from the fitted model.
   (d) assess the validity of the simple linear regression model assumptions.
   (e) create a fitted line plot for the simple linear regression model relating weight to chest circumference.

8.45   Using the Body Fat data set with body density as the response variable and abdomen circumference as the explanatory variable
   (a) fit a simple linear regression model relating density to abdomen circumference.
   (b) create a residual for the residuals associated with the fitted model.
   (c) create a normal probability plot for the residuals from the fitted model.
   (d) assess the validity of the simple linear regression model assumptions.
   (e) create a fitted line plot for the simple linear regression model relating density to abdomen circumference.

8.46   What is the least squares estimator of σ?

8.47   How is s_e computed from the information contained in the residuals?

8.48   What are the degrees of freedom associated with s_e.

8.49   What is
   (a) SSTot?   **(b)** SSReg?
   (c) SSE?   **(d)** R^2?

8.50   What does the coefficient of determination measure?

8.51   Determine the value of R^2 when
   (a) SSTot = 1200 and SSReg = 900.
   (b) SSTot = 1200 and SSE = 450.

8.52   Determine the value of R^2 when
   (a) $r = 0.78$.   **(b)** $r = -0.45$.

TABLE 8.5   Partial ANOV Table for Exercise 8.60

Source	df	SS	MS	F
Regression	1			
Error		2450		
Total	118	2760		

8.53   Determine the value of r when
(a) $SSTot = 8100$, $SSReg = 6900$, and $\widehat{\beta}_1 = -6.7$.
(b) $SSTot = 7200$, $SSE = 2900$, and $\widehat{\beta}_1 = 3.1$.

8.54   What is an ANOV table?

8.55   What are the components of an ANOV table?

8.56   What are the null and alternative hypotheses tested by the F-ratio in the ANOV table?

8.57   What are the assumptions of the test based on the F-ratio?

8.58   What does it mean when the F-ratio indicates there is insufficient evidence to reject $H_0 : \beta_1 = 0$?

8.59   What is the data suggesting when the p-value associated with the observed F-ratio is
(a) $p = 0.002$?   (b) $p = 0.125$?

8.60   For the partial ANOV table in Table 8.5, determine the missing entries.

8.61   Use the ANOV table given in Table 8.6 to answer the following:
(a) What is the estimate of σ?
(b) Does the observed F-ratio provide sufficient evidence for rejecting $H_0 : \beta_1 = 0$? Explain.
(c) What is the value of the coefficient of determination?
(d) What is the percentage of the total variation in the observed Y values explained by the simple linear regression model?
(e) If the least squares regression line is $\widehat{y} = 12.8 - 1.21x$, what is the value of the sample correlation coefficient between Y and X?

8.62   What is the formula for the estimated standard error of
(a) $\widehat{\beta}_0$?   (b) $\widehat{\beta}_1$?

8.63   Under what conditions can a t distribution be used for making inferences about either β_0 or β_1?

TABLE 8.6   Partial ANOV Table for Exercise 8.61

Source	df	SS	MS	F	P
Regression	1	14.81	14.81	5.53	0.022
Error	58	155.35	2.68		
Total	59	170.16			

8.64 What is the form of the t statistic for testing
(a) $H_0 : \beta_0 = 0$?
(b) $H_0 : \beta_1 = 0$?
(c) $H_0 : \beta_0 = 10$?
(d) $H_0 : \beta_1 = 2$?

8.65 What is the rejection region for a
(a) upper-tail t-test?
(b) two-tailed t-test?
(c) lower-tail t-test?

8.66 Assuming the normality assumption is valid, what is the formula for computing a $(1 - \alpha) \times 100\%$ confidence interval for

(a) β_0?
(b) β_1?

8.67 Assuming the normality assumption is valid, compute a 95% confidence interval for β_0 when
(a) $\widehat{\beta}_0 = -12.35$, $n = 42$, and se$(\widehat{\beta}_0) = 2.45$.
(b) $\widehat{\beta}_0 = 1587.8$, $n = 150$, and se$(\widehat{\beta}_0) = 158.6$.

8.68 Assuming the normality assumption is valid, compute a 95% confidence interval for β_1 when
(a) $\widehat{\beta}_1 = -3.87$, $n = 32$, and se$(\widehat{\beta}_1) = 0.73$.
(b) $\widehat{\beta}_0 = 73.1$, $n = 62$, and se$(\widehat{\beta}_1) = 23.1$.

8.69 For each part of Exercise 8.68 determine whether or not the confidence interval supports the hypothesis that $\beta_1 \neq 0$.

8.70 Assuming the normality assumption is valid, test $H_0 : \beta_1 = 0$ against $H_A : \beta_1 \neq 0$ at the $\alpha = 0.05$ level when
(a) $\widehat{\beta}_1 = -1.17$, $n = 28$, and se$(\widehat{\beta}_1) = 0.31$.
(b) $\widehat{\beta}_1 = 31.1$, $n = 42$, and se$(\widehat{\beta}_1) = 18.7$.
(c) $\widehat{\beta}_1 = -2.37$, $n = 32$, and se$(\widehat{\beta}_1) = 0.57$.
(d) $\widehat{\beta}_1 = 12.9$, $n = 122$, and se$(\widehat{\beta}_1) = 2.99$.

8.71 Compute the approximate value of the p-value for each of the tests in Exercise 8.70.

8.72 Assuming the normality assumption is valid,
(a) test $H_0 : \beta_0 = 100$ against $H_A : \beta_0 > 100$ at the $\alpha = 0.05$ level when $\widehat{\beta}_0 = 127$, $n = 62$, and se$(\widehat{\beta}_0) = 11.2$.
(b) compute the approximate value of the p-value for the t-test in part (a).
(c) compute 99% confidence interval for β_0.

8.73 Use the MINITAB output given in Figure 8.35 to answer the following:
(a) What are the values of the least squares estimates of β_0 and β_1 and there estimated standard errors?
(b) What is the equation of the least squares regression line?
(c) What is the estimated value of σ?
(d) What is the percentage of the total variation in the observed Y values explained by the simple linear regression model?
(e) Test $H_0 : \beta_1 = 0$ at the $\alpha = 0.05$ level.
(f) Compute a 95% confidence interval for β_1.
(g) Determine the value of r.

```
Regression Analysis: Weight versus Thigh

The regression equation is
Weight = -110+4.86 Thigh


Predictor       Coef  SE Coef       T      P
Constant     -109.96    10.46  -10.51  0.000
Thigh         4.8629   0.1754   27.73  0.000


S = 14.5870    R-Sq = 75.5%    R-Sq(adj) = 75.4%
```
Figure 8.35   MINITAB output for Exercise 8.73.

8.74   Use the MINITAB output given in Figure 8.36 to answer the following:

(a) What are the values of the least squares estimates of β_0 and β_1 and there estimated standard errors?

(b) What is the equation of the least squares regression line?

(c) Determine the estimated value of σ?

(d) Determine the value of the coefficient of determination.

(e) What is the percentage of the total variation in the observed Y values explained by the simple linear regression model?

(f) Test $H_0 : \beta_1 = 0$ at the $\alpha = 0.05$ level.

(g) Compute a 95% confidence interval for β_1.

8.75   In the article "Nonablative facial remodeling: erythema reduction and histologic evidence of new collagen formation using a 300-microsecond 1064-nm Nd:YAG laser" published in the *Archives of Dermatology* (Schmults et al., 2004), the data given in Table 8.7 were reported for a study of the change in collagen fiber diameter and patient's age. Use the data in Table 8.7 to answer the following about the relationship between change in collagen fiber after 3 months of treatment and patient's age:

(a) Draw a scatterplot of diameter change (Y) versus patient's age (X).

(b) Fit a simple linear regression model relating diameter change to patient's age.

(c) Check the validity of the simple linear regression assumptions.

(d) Determine the equation of the least squares regression line.

(e) Determine the value of the coefficient of determination.

(f) Test $H_0 : \beta_1 = 0$ at the $\alpha = 0.05$ level.

```
Predictor       Coef  SE Coef
Constant     -53.813    5.775
Hip         0.73033  0.05766


Analysis of Variance

Source              DF       SS      MS       F      P
Regression           1   6871.2  6871.2  160.43  0.000
Residual Error     250  10707.8    42.8
Total              251  17579.0
```
Figure 8.36   MINITAB output for Exercise 8.74.

**TABLE 8.7   Data on the Change
in Collagen Fiber After 3 Months
of Treatment and Patient's Age**

Patient's Age (X)	Diameter Change (Y)
52	5.8
35	7.2
58	−3.9
31	24.0
44	4.1
67	−10.5
32	14.1
43	9.7
38	15.2

(**g**) Create a fitted line plot for the observed data on diameter change and patient's age.

8.76   Using the Birth Weight data set, fit a simple linear regression model for relating baby's birth weight (Y) to mother's weight at the last menstrual period (X). Then,
(**a**) use the residuals to check the regression assumptions.
(**b**) provided the regression assumptions appear to be satisfied, test whether or not there is a linear relationship between a baby's birth weight and mother's last weight at the last menstrual period.

8.77   Using the Body Fat data set, fit a simple linear regression model for relating body density (Y) to chest circumference (X). Then,
(**a**) use the residuals to check the regression assumptions.
(**b**) provided the regression assumptions appear to be satisfied, test whether or not there is a linear relationship between body density and chest circumference.

8.78   What are the two uses of the least squares regression line?

8.79   What is the estimator of
(**a**) the mean value of Y when $X = x_0$?
(**b**) the value of Y when $X = x_0$?

8.80   Why is it a bad idea to estimate a mean or predict a value of the response variable for a value of the explanatory variable well outside the range of the observed values of the explanatory variable?

8.81   What is the relationship between the estimated standard error of $\mu_{Y|X=x_0}$ and the prediction error for Y when $X = x_0$?

8.82   Why is the prediction error larger than the standard error for a given value of X?

8.83   What happens to the width of a confidence interval for $\mu_{Y|X=x_0}$ as the value of x_0 moves away from $\bar{x}$?

8.84   What happens to the width of a prediction interval for $\mu_{Y|X=x_0}$ as the value of x_0 moves away from $\bar{x}$?

8.85   Why is the prediction interval for the value of Y when $X = x_0$ wider than the confidence interval for $\mu_{Y|X=x_0}$?

```
Predictor      Coef   SE Coef       T      P
Constant     -2.584     5.175   -0.50  0.618
Neck         2.7218    0.1359   20.02  0.000

S = 5.23484    R-Sq = 61.6%    R-Sq(adj) = 61.4%

Analysis of Variance
Source               DF      SS      MS       F      P
Regression            1   10988   10988  400.98  0.000
Residual Error      250    6851      27
Total               251   17839

Predicted Values for New Observations
 X    Fit    SE Fit
35  92.680   0.524
```

Figure 8.37   MINITAB output for fitting a simple linear regression model relating chest circumference to neck circumference.

8.86 The MINITAB output given in Figure 8.37 is based on fitting a simple linear regression model relating chest circumference (Y) to neck circumference (X) using the data in the Body Fat data set. Use the information in figure 8.37 to answer the following:

(a) Compute a 95% confidence interval for the mean chest circumference of an adult male with a neck circumference of 35 cm.

(b) Compute the value of the prediction error for predicting the chest circumference of an adult male with a neck circumference of 35 cm.

(c) Compute a 95% prediction interval for the chest circumference for an adult male with a neck circumference of 35 cm.

8.87 The MINITAB output given in Figure 8.38 is based on fitting a simple linear regression model relating abdomen circumference (Y) to thigh circumference (X) using the data in the Body Fat data set. Use the information in Figure 8.37 to answer the following:

(a) Compute a 95% confidence interval for the mean abdomen circumference for an adult male with a thigh circumference of 55 cm.

(b) Compute a 95% confidence interval for the mean abdomen circumference for an adult male with a thigh circumference of 60 cm.

8.88 Using the data in Figure 8.38 compute

(a) the prediction error for predicting the abdomen circumference for an adult male with a thigh circumference of 55 cm.

(b) a 95% prediction interval for the abdomen circumference for an adult male with an thigh circumference of 55 cm.

(c) the prediction error for predicting the abdomen circumference for an adult male with a thigh circumference of 60 cm.

(d) a 95% prediction interval for the abdomen circumference for an adult male with a thigh circumference of 60 cm.

8.89 Using the Body Fat data set, fit a simple linear regression model for relating weight (Y) to abdomen circumference (X). Then,

(a) use the residuals to check the regression assumptions.

```
Predictor       Coef  SE Coef       T     P
Constant      -0.985    4.974   -0.20  0.843
Thigh        1.57460  0.08341   18.88  0.000


S = 6.93761   R-Sq = 58.8%   R-Sq(adj) = 58.6%


Analysis of Variance
Source              DF      SS     MS       F      P
Regression           1   17152  17152  356.37  0.000
Residual Error     250   12033     48
Total              251   29185


Predicted Values for New Observations
  X    Fit    SE Fit
 55  85.618    0.571
 60  93.491    0.440
```

Figure 8.38   MINITAB output for fitting a simple linear regression model relating abdomen circumference to thigh circumference.

> **(b)** provided the regression assumptions appear to be satisfied, test whether or not there is a linear relationship between weight and abdomen circumference.
>
> **(c)** estimate the mean weight for an adult male having an abdomen circumference of 85 cm.
>
> **(d)** compute a 95% confidence interval for the mean weight for an adult male having an abdomen circumference of 85 cm.
>
> **(e)** predict the weight for an adult male having an abdomen circumference of 85 cm.
>
> **(f)** compute a 95% prediction interval for the mean weight for an adult male having an abdomen circumference of 85 cm.

8.90 Using the Body Fat data set, fit a simple linear regression model for relating chest circumference (Y) to abdomen circumference (X). Then,

> **(a)** use the residuals to check the regression assumptions.
>
> **(b)** provided the regression assumptions appear to be satisfied, test whether or not there is a linear relationship between chest circumference and abdomen circumference.
>
> **(c)** estimate the mean chest circumference for an adult male having an abdomen circumference of 115 cm.
>
> **(d)** compute a 95% confidence interval for the mean chest circumference for an adult male having an abdomen circumference of 115 cm.
>
> **(e)** predict the chest circumference for an adult male having an abdomen circumference of 115 cm.
>
> **(f)** compute a 95% prediction interval for the mean chest circumference for an adult male having an abdomen circumference of 115 cm.

8.91 Using the Body Fat data set, fit a simple linear regression model for relating body density (Y) to abdomen circumference (X). Then,

> **(a)** use the residuals to check the regression assumptions.
>
> **(b)** provided the regression assumptions appear to be satisfied, test whether or not there is a linear relationship between body density and abdomen circumference.

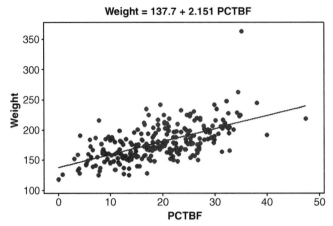

Figure 8.39   Fitted line plot for weight and percent body fat.

(c) estimate the mean body density for an adult male having an abdomen circumference of 100 cm.

(d) compute a 95% confidence interval for the mean body density for an adult male having an abdomen circumference of 100 cm.

(e) predict the body density for an adult male having an abdomen circumference of 100 cm.

(f) compute a 95% prediction interval for the mean body density for an adult male having an abdomen circumference of 100 cm.

8.92   What is the procedure for investigating the influence of a bivariate outlier?

8.93   Under what conditions can a bivariate outlier legitimately be deleted from a data set?

8.94   Figure 8.39 shows a fitted line plot for a simple linear regression model relating weight to percent body fat for adult males based on the Body Fat data set. Note that there is a bivariate outlier at approximately PCTBF $= 35$ and Weight $= 360$. Use the Body Fat data set to answer the following:

(a) Identify the observation that is the bivariate outlier.

(b) Temporarily delete the observation that is the bivariate outlier from the data set.

(c) Refit the simple linear regression model to the reduced data set.

(d) Compare the equations of the least squares regression line based on the complete and the reduced data sets.

(e) Compare the values of s_e and R^2 for the simple linear regression model fit to the complete and the reduced data sets.

(f) Compare the residual plots and normal probability plots for the simple linear regression model fit to the complete and the reduced data sets.

CHAPTER 9

MULTIPLE REGRESSION

IN **THE** previous chapter the simple linear regression model was discussed as a statistical model that could be used for explaining the relationship between a response variable and a single explanatory variable. In this chapter, statistical models for explaining the relationship between a response variable and more than one explanatory variable are discussed. In particular, the statistical models discussed in this chapter are the *multiple regression models*. A multiple regression model for approximating the relationship between a quantitative response variable Y and a set of p quantitative explanatory variables, say $X_1, X_2, X_3, \ldots, X_p$, is a model of the form

$$Y = \beta_0 + \beta_1 X_1 + \beta_2 X_2 + \beta_3 X_3 + \cdots + \beta_p X_p + \epsilon$$

Multiple regression models are often useful in determining the approximate relationship between a response variable and the explanatory variables, and in a well-designed experiment, a multiple regression model can provide strong evidence of a causal relationship between the response variable and the explanatory variables. That is, a multiple regression model cannot prove a cause and effect relationship exists between the response variable and the explanatory variables, however, a good fitting multiple regression model may provide overwhelming evidence supporting the hypothesized causal relationship. In most biomedical research studies it is unlikely for the response variable to be entirely dependent on only a single explanatory variable. Moreover, in a simple linear regression analysis a small coefficient of determination often indicates that the response variable is also dependent on explanatory variables other than the particular explanatory variable that was included in the simple linear regression model.

A *multiple regression analysis* or simply *multiple regression* is a statistical procedure that can be used to build a regression model for predicting the value of a response variable for a particular set of explanatory variables; a simple linear regression model is a multiple regression model that contains only one explanatory variable. Furthermore, a multiple regression is similar to a simple linear regression analysis. An outline of the typical well-planned multiple regression analysis is given below.

THE MULTIPLE REGRESSION PROCEDURE

1. The response variable and the explanatory variables to be considered in the model are identified. It is important at this stage to include any explanatory variable that can be measured and is believed to influence the response variable in the sampling plan.

2. A well-designed sampling plan that will produce sufficient data for building a regression model that can be used for approximating the relationship between the response and the explanatory variables must be developed.

3. The data are observed according to the sampling plan.

4. Scatterplots of the response variable versus each of the explanatory variables should be investigated and correlations for scatterplots with linear data clouds can be computed.

5. The multiple regression model is fit to the observed data using the method of least squares.

6. The model assumptions and residual diagnostics are investigated. Any problems suggested by the residual diagnostics or violations of the model assumptions need to be addressed until a model without any problems is found.

7. A good fitting model can be used to make inferences about the relationship between the response variable and the explanatory variables or for predicting future values of the response variable.

Note that building a multiple regression model is similar to building a simple linear regression model, and thus, building a multiple regression model is an iterative process that generally involves fitting a hypothesized model, checking the assumptions, and examining residual diagnostics until a reasonable model is found. Examples 9.1, 9.2 and 9.3 illustrate studies where multiple regression has been used in biomedical research.

Example 9.1
In the article "Blood mercury levels and neurobehavioral function" published in the *Journal of the American Medical Association* (Weil et al., 2005), the researchers used multiple regression to investigate the relationship between blood mercury level and neurobehavioral test scores, age, race and ethnicity, gender, and educational achievement.

Example 9.2
In the article "Trends in prevalence, awareness, treatment, and control of hypertension in the United States, 1988–2000" published in the *Journal of the American Medical Association* (Hajjar and Kotchen, 2003), the researchers used multiple regression to investigate the relationship between hypertension prevalence and body mass index (BMI), age, race and ethnicity, and gender.

Example 9.3
In the article "Activation of oxidative stress by acute glucose fluctuations compared with sustained chronic hyperglycemia in patients with Type 2 diabetes" published in the *Journal of the American Medical Association* (Monnier et al., 2006), the researchers used multiple regression to investigate the relationship between urinary 8-iso $PGF_{2\alpha}$ excretion and mean glucose concentrations, fasting plasma insulin, and mean amplitude of glycemic excursions.

In each of these studies, the researchers believed that the particular set of explanatory variables was related to the response variable and should produce a better statistical model for explaining the values of the response variable than a simple linear regression model built from any one of these explanatory variables. Also, note that all of the explanatory variables in a multiple regression model must be quantitative variables, however, it is possible to include specialized variables known as *dummy variables* in a regression model to account for the influence of a qualitative variable on the response variable. For example, in Example 9.1, dummy variables were included for the variables gender, race, and educational achievement, and in Example 9.2, dummy variables were included for the variables gender and race. In Example 9.3, all of the explanatory variables are quantitative variables. Dummy variables will be discussed in more detail in Section 9.8.

9.1 INVESTIGATING MULTIVARIATE RELATIONSHIPS

The data set required to fit a multiple regression model consists of a random sample of n multivariate observations where each observation consists of an observed value of the response variable and observed values for each of the explanatory variables that will be used in the model. Thus, when there are p explanatory variables the multivariate data set will consist of n observations of the form $(Y, X_1, X_2, X_3, \ldots, X_p)$. A multivariate data set is usually listed in spreadsheet form with the n rows representing the observed sample values of the variables $Y, X_1, X_2, X_3, \ldots$, and X_p as shown in Table 9.1. The observations on the explanatory variables are double subscripted to identify the explanatory variable and the observation it is associated with. For example, X_{59} represents the value of the ninth observation on the explanatory variable X_5. The response variable only requires a single subscript to identify its observation number. For example, Y_{13} is the value of the response variable measured on the 13th unit in the sample.

Once the data has been collected the first step in a multiple regression analysis is to look at scatterplots of the response variable versus each of the explanatory variables. Throughout this chapter Y will be used to represent the explanatory variable and $X_1, X_2, X_3, \ldots, X_p$ used to represent the explanatory variables believed to influence the response variable. Thus, scatterplots of Y versus X_1, Y versus $X_2, \ldots$, and Y versus X_p should be investigated for linear and nonlinear relationships and outliers. The sample correlation coefficient should also be computed for any scatterplots having linear data clouds.

A scatterplot that reveals a strong linear or strong nonlinear relationship between the response and an explanatory variable should be noted, however, a strong pattern in a scatterplot does not necessarily indicate the explanatory variable will have a strong relationship with the response variable when the other explanatory variables are taken into consideration. In fact, it is not unusual for a scatterplot of the response versus a particular explanatory variable to suggest that there is no obvious relationship between the variables, however, when the multiple regression model is fit, this particular explanatory variable is found to be a significant contributor to the model. Example 9.4 provides an example where Y depends on both the explanatory variables X_1 and X_2, yet the scatterplot of Y versus X_2 suggests there is no linear relationship between Y and X_2.

TABLE 9.1 The Spreadsheet Form of a Multivariate Data Set to be Used in a Multiple Regression Analysis

Observations	Y	X_1	X_2	X_3	$\cdots$	X_p
1	Y_1	X_{11}	X_{21}	X_{31}	$\cdots$	X_{p1}
2	Y_2	X_{12}	X_{22}	X_{32}	$\cdots$	X_{p2}
3	Y_3	X_{13}	X_{23}	X_{33}	$\cdots$	X_{p3}
$\vdots$	$\vdots$	$\vdots$	$\vdots$	$\vdots$	$\cdots$	$\vdots$
n	Y_n	X_{1n}	X_{2n}	X_{3n}	$\cdots$	X_{pn}

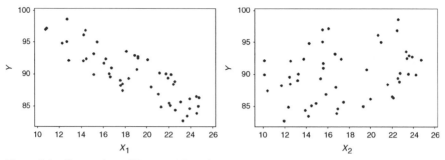

Figure 9.1   Scatterplots of Y versus X_1 and Y versus X_2.

Example 9.4

The scatterplots given in Figure 9.1 are based on explanatory variables X_1 and X_2. The Y values in these scatterplots based on the deterministic relationship

$$Y = 100 - X_1 - 0.5X_2$$

Note that the data cloud in the scatterplot of Y versus X_1 suggests a strong linear relationship ($r = 0.84$), while the data cloud in the scatterplot of Y versus X_2 suggests a weak linear relationship ($r = 0.27$). Thus, if simple linear regression models were fit with both X_1 and X_2 as the explanatory variable, the model using X_1 would explain 71.4% of the total variation in the observed Y values and the model using X_2 would explain only 7.6% of the total variation in the observed Y values. On the other hand, the multiple regression model that includes both X_1 and X_2 as explanatory variables, fits the observed Y values perfectly and explains 100% of the variation in the observed Y values. Figure 9.2, a three-dimensional scatterplot, illustrates the perfect alignment of Y with X_1 and X_2, and hence, the perfect fit.

While scatterplots can be useful in investigating the relationships between the response variable and an explanatory variable, relationships between the response variable and two or more explanatory variables cannot be investigated using a two-dimensional scatterplot. Three-dimensional scatterplots can be used to investigate the response variable and two

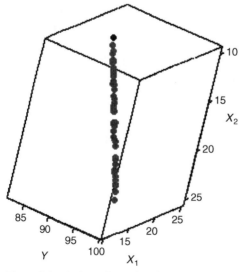

Figure 9.2   A three-dimensional scatterplot of Y versus X_1 and X_2.

explanatory variables, but beyond that there are no graphical methods for representing higher dimensional relationships between the response variable and three or more explanatory variables.

When the data cloud in a scatterplot of the response versus an explanatory variable X suggests a curvilinear relationship, the square of the variable (i.e., X^2) should be considered as an additional explanatory variable to include in a multiple regression model. That is, often adding X^2 to the model will account for the approximate curvilinear relationship between Y and X. For example, if the scatterplot of Y versus X reveals a curvilinear relationship, the model

$$Y = \beta_0 + \beta_1 X + \beta_2 X^2 + \epsilon$$

should be considered as an alternative to the simple linear regression model.

9.2 THE MULTIPLE LINEAR REGRESSION MODEL

A statistical model is said to be a *linear model* for relating a response variable Y to a set of quantitative explanatory variables, say $X_1, X_2, X_3, \ldots, X_p$, when it is a statistical model of the form

$$Y = \beta_0 + \beta_1 X_1 + \beta_2 X_2 + \cdots + \beta_p X_p + \epsilon$$

That is, a linear model is simply the sum of β_0, the products of the explanatory variables and their corresponding βs and an additive random error term. The unknown parameters $\beta_0, \beta_1, \ldots, \beta_p$ are called the *regression coefficients*, β_0 is called the intercept, and $\beta_1, \beta_2, \beta_3, \ldots, \beta_p$ are called the *regression slopes* or simply *slopes*. A multiple regression model is a linear model that defines the equation of a *response surface* rather than a line. Statistical models that are not linear models are called *nonlinear models*.

When the error term has mean 0, an individual regression slope can be interpreted as the expected change in the response variable for a one unit change in the explanatory variable after adjusting for the other explanatory variables in the model. For example, β_3 is the expected change in the response variable when X_3 is increased by one unit and all of the other explanatory variables are held fixed.

Example 9.5
Each of the following statistical models is a linear model.

    a. $Y = \beta_0 + \beta_1 X + \epsilon$
    b. $Y = \beta_0 + \beta_1 X + \beta_2 X^2 + \epsilon$
    c. $Y = \beta_0 + \beta_1 X_1 + \beta_2 X_2 + \beta_3 X_3 + \epsilon$

Note that each of these models is a linear combination of the βs and the explanatory variables and has an additive error term. Moreover, the model in part (b) is a linear model even though it contains the variable X^2. The easiest way to see that the model in part (b) is a linear model is to label X as X_1 and X^2 as X_2. Then, the model in part (b) is $Y = \beta_0 + \beta_1 X_1 + \beta_2 X_2 + \epsilon$ that is clearly a linear model.

Example 9.6
Each of the statistical models listed below is a nonlinear model.

a. $Y = \beta_0 X^{\beta_1} + \epsilon$ is not a linear model because X is raised to the β_1 power.

b. $Y = (\beta_0 + \beta_1 X_1 + \beta_2 X_2)\epsilon$ is not a linear model because the error term is a multiplicative error rather than an additive error.

c. $Y = \beta_0 + (1 - \beta_1 X_1)^{\beta_2(X_2 - \beta_3)} \epsilon$ is not a linear model because β_2, β_3, and X_2 are all in the exponent of the variable X_1. Thus, Y is not a linear combination of the βs and Xs.

Note that the only restriction on the explanatory variables in a linear model is that they are all quantitative variables. Thus, including the square or the square-root of an explanatory variable in a linear model does not change the fact that the model is linear in the βs, and hence, is still a linear model. The components of a multiple regression model are summarized below.

THE BASIC COMPONENTS OF A MULTIPLE REGRESSION MODEL

In the multiple regression model $Y = \beta_0 + \beta_1 X_2 + \beta_2 X_2 + \cdots + \beta_p X_p + \epsilon$

1. there are $p + 1$ unknown parameters, namely, the intercept and p slopes (i.e., $\beta_0, \beta_1, \ldots, \beta_p$).

2. β_0 is the y-intercept.

3. β_i is the expected change in Y for a one unit change in X_i when all of the other explanatory variables are held fixed.

4. ϵ is a random variable that explains the lack of fit of the response surface for approximating the relationship between Y and X.

9.2.1 The Assumptions of a Multiple Regression Model

The standard assumptions placed on a multiple regression model are similar to those of the simple linear regression model. In particular, the explanatory variables are measured without error, the values of the response variable are independent, the mean of the error random variable is 0 (i.e., $\mu_\epsilon = 0$), the standard deviation of the error random variable is exactly the same for each value of the explanatory variable, and the probability distribution of the error random variable is normally distributed with mean zero and standard deviation σ. Nevertheless, there is one additional assumption that must be made when fitting a multiple regression model. In particular, the additional assumption has to do with the explanatory variables, and the assumption is there are no *collinear relationships* between the explanatory variables. A collinear relationship or *collinearity problem* exists among the explanatory variables when one explanatory variable can be explained by a linear combination of the remaining explanatory variables. A collinearity problem among the explanatory variables indicates that there is a high degree of redundancy of some of the information contained in the explanatory variables. The assumptions placed on a multiple regression model

$$Y = \beta_0 + \beta_1 X_1 + \beta_2 X_2 + \cdots + \beta_p X_p + \epsilon$$

are listed below.

THE ASSUMPTIONS FOR A MULTIPLE LINEAR REGRESSION MODEL

The assumptions required for using the multiple regression model

$$Y = \beta_0 + \beta_1 X + \beta_2 X_2 + \cdots + \beta_p X_p + \epsilon$$

are:

A1 The observed values of the explanatory variable X are measured without error.

A2 Each observed value of the response variable Y is independent of the other values of the response variable.

A3 The explanatory variables are not collinear or nearly collinear.

A4 The mean of the error random variable is 0 (i.e., $\mu_\epsilon = 0$).

A5 The standard deviation of the error random variable is exactly the same for each value of the explanatory variable.

A6 The probability distribution of the error random variable is normally distributed with mean zero and standard deviation σ.

The distributional assumptions on ϵ mean that for a given set of values of the explanatory values, say $X_1 = x_1, X_2 = x_2, \ldots, X_p = x_p$, the distribution of Y is normally distributed with mean

$$\mu_{Y|x_1, x_2 \ldots, x_p} = \beta_0 + \beta_1 x_1 + \beta_2 x_2 + \cdots + \beta_p x_p$$

and standard deviation σ. For notational purposes, a given set of values of the explanatory variables $X_1 = x_1, X_2 = x_2, \ldots, X_p = x_p$ will be denoted by $\vec{x}$, and the mean of the response variable given the values in $\vec{x}$ will be denoted by $\mu_{Y|\vec{x}}$.

As was the case with simple linear regression, the use of a multiple regression model when any one of the regression assumptions is violated may produce incorrect or misleading statistical inferences about the relationship between the response and the explanatory variables. In particular,

1. when there is a random error in measuring the value of the explanatory variable, the resulting fitted model may be severely biased.

2. when the values of the response variable are not independent, the estimates of β_0 and β_1 may be biased and any hypothesis tests based on the model may be less reliable than expected.

3. when the explanatory variables are collinear or nearly collinear, there are significant difficulties involved with estimating the regression coefficients and interpreting the resulting estimates.

4. when the random error has mean other than 0, there will be systematic error in the model and the model will be biased.

5. when the standard deviation is not constant over the range of the explanatory variable, this means that the reliability of the model vary from one value of the explanatory variable to another.

6. when the error random variable is not approximately normally distributed, small sample hypothesis tests and confidence intervals may provide unreliable results.

Proper use of a multiple regression model for approximating the relationship between the response variable and a set of explanatory variables requires that a well-planned research project and sampling plan be developed and the sample data are used to assess the validity of the assumptions placed on the error structure of the model. Methods for fitting a multiple regression model and checking the error structure are discussed in detail in Sections 9.3 and 9.4.

9.3 FITTING A MULTIPLE LINEAR REGRESSION MODEL

Fitting a multiple regression model is similar to fitting a simple linear regression model in that the method of least squares is used to actually fit the model. In multiple regression, the least squares procedure is used to determine the response surface that fits the observed data best according to the criterion of minimizing the sum of the squared deviations. That is, for the model

$$Y = \beta_0 + \beta_1 X_1 + \beta_2 X_2 + \cdots + \beta_p X_p + \epsilon$$

least squares procedure determines the equation of the fitted response surface

$$\widehat{y} = \widehat{\beta}_0 + \widehat{\beta}_1 X_1 + \widehat{\beta}_2 X_2 + \ldots + \widehat{\beta}_p X_p$$

that minimizes

$$\text{SSE} = \sum (y - \widehat{y})^2 = \sum (y - \widehat{\beta}_0 - \widehat{\beta}_1 x_1 - \cdots - \widehat{\beta}_p x_p)^2$$

The values of $\widehat{\beta}_0, \widehat{\beta}_1, \widehat{\beta}_2, \ldots, \widehat{\beta}_p$ that minimize SSE are called the *least squares estimates* of the regression coefficients, and the least squares estimates of $\beta_0, \beta_1, \beta_2, \ldots, \beta_p$ are best computed using a statistical computing package.

When the multiple regression model specifies the true relationship between the response variable and the explanatory variable, the least squares estimates $\widehat{\beta}_0, \widehat{\beta}_1, \widehat{\beta}_2, \ldots, \widehat{\beta}_p$ of $\beta_0, \beta_1, \beta_2, \ldots, \beta_p$ are unbiased estimators. However, in most cases the multiple regression model is not the correct model, but is simply a good model that can be used for approximating the relationship between the response and explanatory variables. Moreover, when the multiple regression model does not contain an important explanatory variable that is related to the response variable, the least squares estimators will be biased; the degree of bias will depend on how important the missing variable is. Thus, one of the most critical steps in building a multiple regression model is to have or obtain enough basic information to discern which variables are most likely related to and influence the response variable before the data are collected.

9.4 ASSESSING THE ASSUMPTIONS OF A MULTIPLE LINEAR REGRESSION MODEL

No statistical model should be used for making inferences without first checking the model assumptions and assessing the adequacy of the model's fit. The assumptions of the multiple regression model

$$Y = \beta_0 + \beta_1 X_2 + \beta_2 X_2 + \cdots + \beta_p X_P + \epsilon$$

are

A1 The observed values of the explanatory variable X are measured without error.

A2 Each observed value of the response variable Y is independent of the other values of the response variable.

A3 The explanatory variables are not collinear or nearly collinear.

A4 The mean of the error random variable is 0 (i.e., $E(\epsilon) = 0$).

A5 The standard deviation of the error random variable is exactly the same for each value of the explanatory variable.

A6 The probability distribution of the error random variable is normally distributed with mean zero and standard deviation σ.

Assumptions A1 and A2 should be taken care of in the design stages of the study and by using a well-designed sampling plan. In particular, a researcher must be cognizant of the nature of the variables $X_1, X_2, \ldots, X_p$ and should know whether or not there is a measurement error problem in any one of these explanatory variables. The independence assumption, A2, can easily be satisfied by using a well-designed sampling plan that ensures that independent observations will be observed.

The collinearity assumption, A3, is a much more difficult assumption to anticipate in the planning stages of the research study and needs to be carefully checked before making inferences about the importance of the explanatory variables in the regression model. When there is a collinearity problem in the explanatory variables, the standard error of one or more of the regression slopes will be inflated making the estimation and interpretation of the regression slope difficult and can lead to biased statistical inferences.

The most commonly used collinearity diagnostics are the *variance inflation factors*, and each of the explanatory variables has a variance inflation factor. The variance inflation factor for the ith explanatory variable is denoted by VIF_i and measures the interdependence between X_i and the other explanatory variables. A VIF value of larger than 10 is usually considered to be indicative of a collinearity problem in the explanatory variables. A value of $VIF > 10$ indicates that the relationships among the explanatory variables need to be carefully investigated and a new model without a collinearity problem must be found. Fortunately, most statistical computing packages will provide the VIF values associated with the explanatory variables as part of a multiple regression analysis making it easy to identify a possible collinearity problem. On the other hand, curing a collinearity problem can be a very difficult task.

The simplest type of collinearity that occurs when two of the explanatory variables are causing the problem. Thus, when at least one variance inflation factor greater than 10 occurs when a multiple regression model is fit, the first step in investigating the nature of the collinearity problem is to look at the pairwise correlations among the explanatory variables. Two explanatory variables, say X_1 and X_2, are perfectly collinear when $X_1 = a + bX_2$, and thus, when X_1 and X_2 are highly correlated there will be a potential collinearity problem. Moreover, when X_1 and X_2 are highly correlated there is a redundancy in the information they will provide about the response variable. When the magnitude of the correlation coefficient for X_1 and X_2 is greater than 0.95, the variance inflation factor for both variables will be greater than 10. In this case, deleting either X_1 or X_2 from the model will remove the collinearity problem, and the choice of which variable to remove is left to the researcher.

In many cases, a variance inflation factor greater than 10 is caused by a collinear relationship between more than two explanatory variables. In this case, the information in at least one of the explanatory variables is also contained in some linear combination of the other explanatory variables. This type of collinearity is the most difficult type of collinearity to cure because it is rarely obvious which of the variables are collinear. The following approach is often useful in identifying and curing a collinearity problem.

IDENTIFYING AND CURING A COLLINEARITY PROBLEM

---

1. Compute the correlation coefficients for each pair of explanatory variables and identify any highly correlated pair of explanatory variables. Any two variables with a correlation of magnitude 0.95 or higher will have variance inflation factors greater than 10. Eliminate one of the variables from the model, refit the reduced model, and examine the new VIF values. If all of the new VIF values are less than 10, proceed with the multiple regression analysis on the reduced model; if at least one VIF is greater than 10 in the reduced model, proceed to step 2.

2. Carefully examine the nature of the explanatory variables and try to identify subsets of variables that are closely related and might be causing the collinearity problem. Eliminating some of the variables from a subset of closely related variables often eliminates the collinearity problem, however, the determination of which variables to eliminate from the model is up to the researcher. Variables should be dropped from a model only after carefully considering the scientific importance of each variable. When this approach does not solve the problem, seek the advice and help of a professional statistician for help curing the collinearity problem.

In investigating a collinearity problem, a matrix (i.e., two-dimensional array) of pairwise correlations among the explanatory variables is often helpful in identifying the variables that are causing a collinearity problem. It is also important to look for variables that are naturally related. Example 9.7 illustrates the typical procedure used in analyzing a collinearity problem.

Example 9.7

In the article "Generalized body composition prediction equation for men using simple measurement techniques" published in *Medicine and Science in Sports and Exercise* (Penrose et al., 1985), the Body Fat data set was used to fit a multiple regression model to approximate the relationship between percent body fat (PCTBF) and the explanatory variables listed below.

```
Age (years)
Weight (lbs)
Height (inches)
Neck circumference (cm)
Chest circumference (cm)
Abdomen circumference (cm)
Hip circumference (cm)
Thigh circumference (cm)
Knee circumference (cm)
Ankle circumference (cm)
Biceps (extended) circumference (cm)
Forearm circumference (cm)
Wrist circumference (cm)
```

In particular, the model

$$\text{PCTBF} = \beta_0 + \beta_1 \text{Age} + \beta_2 \text{Weight} + \beta_3 \text{Height} + \beta_4 \text{Neck} + \beta_5 \text{Chest} + \beta_6 \text{Abdomen} + \beta_7 \text{Hip}$$

$$+ \beta_8 \text{Thigh} + \beta_9 \text{Knee} + \beta_{10} \text{Ankle} + \beta_{11} \text{Biceps} + \beta_{12} \text{Forearm} + \beta_{13} \text{Wrist} + \epsilon$$

was fit to the observed data in the Body Fat data set.

TABLE 9.2 Summary of the Regression Coefficients and Variance Inflation Factors for Relating Percent Body Fat (PCTBF) to the Explanatory Variables, Age, Weight, and Several body Measurements

Predictor	Coef	SE Coef	T	P	VIF
Constant	−21.35	22.19	−0.96	0.337	
Age	0.06457	0.03219	2.01	0.046	2.224
Weight	−0.09638	0.06185	−1.56	0.120	44.653
Height	−0.0439	0.1787	−0.25	0.806	2.939
Neck	−0.4755	0.2356	−2.02	0.045	4.432
Chest	−0.0172	0.1032	−0.17	0.868	10.235
Abdomen	0.95500	0.09016	10.59	0.000	12.776
Hip	−0.1886	0.1448	−1.30	0.194	14.542
Thigh	0.2483	0.1462	1.70	0.091	7.959
Knee	0.0139	0.2477	0.06	0.955	4.825
Ankle	0.1779	0.2226	0.80	0.425	1.924
Biceps	0.1823	0.1725	1.06	0.292	3.671
Forearm	0.4557	0.1993	2.29	0.023	2.192
Wrist	−1.6545	0.5332	−3.10	0.002	3.348

The summary of the regression coefficients and variance inflation factors for the fitted model with is given in Table 9.2.

Since the variance inflation factors for the explanatory variables Weight, Chest, Abdomen, and Hip all exceed 10, there is a potential collinearity problem with this particular set of explanatory variables. A matrix of correlations between the explanatory variables is given in Table 9.3. Note that the largest correlation between two of the explanatory variables is 0.941 occurs for the variables Weight and Hip. Thus, since Weight and Hip are highly correlated, it appears that they are also redundant measurements for predicting percent body fat.

The variable Weight will be removed from the model and the model refit to the remaining explanatory variables. In the reduced model the variance inflation factors are still greater than 10 for the variables Abdomen and Hip. The correlation between the variables Abdomen and Hip is

TABLE 9.3 The Matrix of Correlations for the Independent Variables in the Body Fat Data Set

	Age	Weight	Height	Neck	Chest	Abdomen	Hip	Thigh
Weight	−0.013							
Height	−0.245	0.487						
Neck	0.114	0.831	0.321					
Chest	0.176	0.894	0.227	0.785				
Abdomen	0.230	0.888	0.190	0.754	0.916			
Hip	−0.050	0.941	0.372	0.735	0.829	0.874		
Thigh	−0.200	0.869	0.339	0.696	0.730	0.767	0.896	
Knee	0.018	0.853	0.501	0.672	0.719	0.737	0.823	0.799
Ankle	−0.105	0.614	0.393	0.478	0.483	0.453	0.558	0.540
Biceps	−0.041	0.800	0.319	0.731	0.728	0.685	0.739	0.761
Forearm	−0.085	0.630	0.322	0.624	0.580	0.503	0.545	0.567
Wrist	0.214	0.730	0.398	0.745	0.660	0.620	0.630	0.559

	Knee	Ankle	Biceps	Forearm
Ankle	0.612			
Biceps	0.679	0.485		
Forearm	0.556	0.419	0.678	
Wrist	0.665	0.566	0.632	0.586

TABLE 9.4 Summary of the Regression Coefficients and Variance Inflation Factors for Relating Percent Body Fat (PCTBF) to Age and Several Body Measurements

Predictor	Coef	SE Coef	T	P	VIF
Constant	-25.410	8.403	-3.02	0.003	
Age	0.21703	0.03517	6.17	0.000	1.755
Height	-0.1646	0.1053	-1.56	0.119	1.329
Neck	-0.3511	0.2725	-1.29	0.199	3.921
Chest	0.59005	0.07835	7.53	0.000	3.899
Thigh	0.6328	0.1468	4.31	0.000	5.309
Knee	-0.0106	0.2797	-0.04	0.970	4.067
Ankle	-0.0137	0.2674	-0.05	0.959	1.835
Biceps	-0.0337	0.2065	-0.16	0.870	3.480
Forearm	0.2735	0.2423	1.13	0.260	2.142
Wrist	-2.3809	0.6451	-3.69	0.000	3.242

$r = 0.874$. Dropping the variable Hip from the model produces a further reduced model having no variance inflation factors greater than 10, however, there are still two variables with borderline VIF values, namely Abdomen and Chest.

Possible explanations for the collinearity problems among the explanatory variables in the original model include

1. An individual's weight is a function of the body measurement explanatory variables. In fact, 97.7% of the variation in the observed weights is explained by the other body measurements. Thus, the variable Weight appears to be a redundant variable when all of the body measurement variables are included in the model.

2. Chest, Abdomen, and Hip are highly correlated variables since they measure body characteristics in neighboring regions of the body.

A multiple regression model based on excluding the redundant explanatory variables is

$$\text{PCTBF} = \beta_0 + \beta_1 \text{Age} + \beta_2 \text{Height} + \beta_3 \text{Neck} + \beta_4 \text{Chest} + \beta_5 \text{Thigh} + \beta_6 \text{Knee}$$

$$+ \beta_7 \text{Ankle} + \beta_8 \text{Biceps} + \beta_9 \text{Forearm} + \beta_{10} \text{Wrist} + \epsilon$$

The variance inflation factors for this model are listed in Table 9.4, and since none of the explanatory variables in this regression model have variance inflation factors even close to 10, the multiple regression analysis will proceed with this model.

Finally, it is important to note that when a multiple regression model is being built for the sole purpose of predicting values of the response variable, a collinearity problem will have little affect on model's ability to predict. On the other hand, a collinearity problem can lead to inaccurate and unreliable statistical inferences about the regression coefficients in the model.

9.4.1 Residual Diagnostics

The constant variance and normality assumptions placed on the error term in a multiple regression model, assumptions A5 and A6, must be assessed prior to using a fitted multiple regression model. As is the case in a simple linear regression analysis, the validity of the assumption of constant variance and the assumption of normality of the error term are assessed by investigating the behavior of the residuals. The residuals associated with a fitted multiple regression model contain information on how well the fitted values $\hat{y}_1, \hat{y}_2, \hat{y}_3, \ldots, \hat{y}_n$ agree with their corresponding observed values $y_1, y_2, y_3, \ldots, y_n$. In particular, the ith residual is the difference between y_i and $\widehat{y}_i$ and is denoted by e_i. Thus, the ith residual e_i is

$$e_i = y_i - \widehat{y}_i$$

where y_i is the ith observed value of the response variable and $\widehat{y}_i$ is the ith fitted value.

Because each residual has a slightly different standard deviation the standardized residuals, which all have the same standard deviation, will be used in the residual diagnostics. A standardized residual is denoted by e_s and the ith standardized residual by e_{s_i}. Recall from Chapter 8, the standardized residuals all have standard deviation 1, and therefore, it is unlikely for a residual to be outside of the range -3 to 3 when assumptions A5 and A6 are valid. In fact, any observation having a standardized residual with $|e_s| > 3$ should be carefully investigated as a possible outlier since the model is not fitting this observation very well. Furthermore, the standardized residuals can be used to check the constant variance and normality assumptions using graphical diagnostics such as residual plots and normal probability plots.

In a multiple regression analysis, the residual plot of the standardized residuals versus the fitted values can be used to assess the validity of the assumption of constant variance and often used to detect curvilinear relationships not accounted for by the multiple regression model. In particular, systematic patterns in a residual plot are undesirable and suggest a violation of one or more of the assumptions of the multiple regression model. Thus, a "good" fitting model will have a residual plot having (1) no systematic patterns, (2) equal vertical variation across the range of the fitted values (or X values), and (3) all of the standardized residuals falling between -3 and 3. Any patterns in the residual plot are indicative of problems with the fitted model, and the most commonly encountered systematic patterns in a residual plot are the funneling and curvilinear patterns.

A funnel shaped pattern in a residual plot suggests that the variability in the residuals varies over the range of the fitted values, and therefore, is suggesting that the assumption of constant variance may not be valid and there is a potential nonconstant variance problem with the fitted model. Nonconstant variation is often the consequence of having a multiplicative error instead of an additive error and sometimes can be cured by modeling the natural logarithm of Y as a linear function of X with the log Y model, which models the natural logarithm of the response variable with a multiple regression model. The log Y model is

$$\ln(Y) = \beta_0 + \beta_1 X_1 + \beta_2 X_2 + \beta_3 X_3 + \cdots + \beta_p X_p + \epsilon$$

To fit this model, a researcher need only transform the Y values with the natural logarithm function, fit the log Y model, and check the residuals of the fitted log Y model. If the residual plot for this new model still suggests problems with the fitted model, the model should be discarded and another regression model must be tried.

Example 9.8
In the article "Blood mercury levels in US children and women of childbearing age, 1999–2000" published in the *Journal of the American Medical Association* (Schober et al., 2003), the authors were interested in studying the relationship between an individual's blood mercury level (BML) and the explanatory variables age (Age), fish consumption (Fish), and shellfish consumption (Shell). Separate regression models of the form

$$\ln(\text{BML}) = \beta_0 + \beta_1 \text{Age} + \beta_2 \text{Fish} + \beta_3 \text{Shell} + \epsilon$$

were built for each of the study groups consisting of children aged 1–5 years and women aged 16–49 years.

A curvilinear pattern in a residual plot indicates the fitted model does not adequately fit the curved nature of the observed data. When a curvilinear pattern occurs in a residual plot of the standardized residuals versus the fitted values further information about the fitted model can be found by investigating the residual plots formed by plotting the standardized residuals versus each of the explanatory variables. In fact, a curvilinear pattern in a residual plot of the standardized residuals versus the fitted values often suggests that there is at least one explanatory variable that will also have a residual plot with a curvilinear pattern. When the residual plot of the standardized residuals versus the fitted values has a curvilinear pattern, the following approach can often be used to create an alternative regression model that will account for curvilinear relationships between the response variable and some of the explanatory variables.

MODELING CURVILINEAR RELATIONSHIPS

1. For each explanatory variable, examine a residual plot of the standardized residuals versus the explanatory variable.

2. Identify all of the explanatory variables having curvilinear residual plots.

3. For each variable identified as having a curvilinear residual plot, add the square of the explanatory variable (i.e., X^2) to the multiple regression model as a new explanatory variable.

4. Refit the new model and check the residual plots. If no curvilinear pattern appears in the residual plot continue the regression analysis with the new model; however, when there is still a curvilinear pattern in the residual plot further adjustments to the regression model are required.

Note that a residual plot may indicate more than one problem with the fitted model. For example, a residual plot might suggest that the relationship is curvilinear, has nonconstant variance, and/or an outlier. In many regression analyses the original model will not satisfy the error assumptions and will need fine-tuning before the fitted model can be used for making statistical inferences. Example 9.9 illustrates the use of residual plots for fine-tuning a regression model through an iterative process.

Example 9.9

The scatterplot given in Figure 9.3 suggests that a linear relationship between the variables Y and X exists, and therefore, a simple linear regression model will be fit to this set of data. The residual plot for the simple linear regression model

$$Y = \beta_0 + \beta_1 X + \epsilon$$

is given in Figure 9.4 and reveals a fairly strong funnel shape suggesting that there is a nonconstant variance problem with the simple linear regression model.

The response variable was transformed using the natural logarithm and the log Y model $\ln(Y) = \beta_0 + \beta_1 X + \epsilon$ was refit to the observed data. The residual plot for the log Y model is given in Figure 9.5 and now suggests there might be a strong curvilinear relationship between $\ln(Y)$ and X.

In an attempt to explain the curvilinear relationship between $\ln(Y)$ and X, the multiple regression model

$$\ln(Y) = \beta_0 + \beta_1 X + \beta_2 X^2 + \epsilon$$

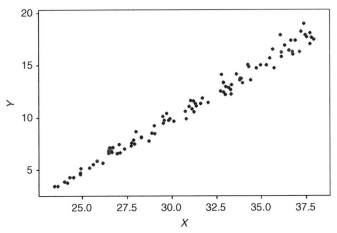

Figure 9.3   A scatterplot of the response variable Y versus the explanatory variable X.

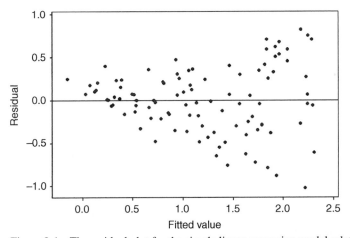

Figure 9.4   The residual plot for the simple linear regression model relating Y to X.

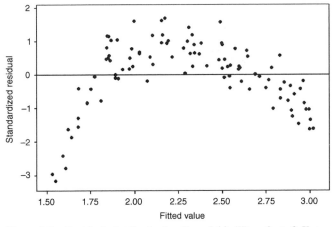

Figure 9.5   Residual plot for the log Y model $\ln(Y) = \beta_0 + \beta_1 X + \epsilon$.

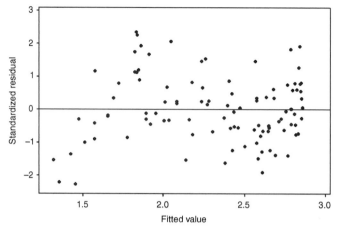

Figure 9.6   Residual plot for the multiple regression model $\ln(Y) = \beta_0 + \beta_1 X + \beta_2 X^2 + \epsilon$.

was fit and the residuals for this model are shown in Figure 9.6. Note that neither of the curvilinear and funneling patterns are present in the residual plot for the model for $\ln(Y)$ that includes the explanatory variables X and X^2. A fitted line plot for the regression model

$$\ln(Y) = \beta_0 + \beta_1 X + \beta_2 X^2 + \epsilon$$

is given in Figure 9.7. Note how well the fitted model agrees with the observed data.

A normal probability plot of the standardized residuals can be used to assess the validity of the normality assumption in a multiple regression model. A valid normality assumption ensures the validity of any confidence intervals, hypothesis tests, or prediction intervals that are part of the planned statistical analysis. The normality assumption can easily be checked by creating a normal probability plot of standardized residuals and using the fat pencil test to assess the validity of this assumption. Thus, a normal probability plot of the standardized residuals supports the assumption of the normality of the error term in the model when the points in the normal plot are roughly linear (i.e., pass the fat pencil test). When the points in the normal probability plot deviate strongly from a straight line there is sufficient evidence to reject the normality assumption.

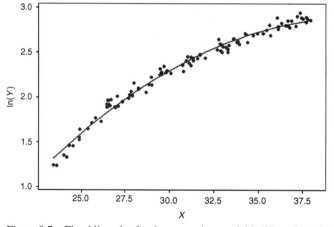

Figure 9.7   Fitted line plot for the regression model $\ln(Y) = \beta_0 + \beta_1 X + \beta_2 X^2 + \epsilon$.

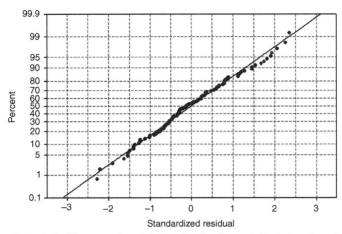

Figure 9.8   The normal probability plot for the model $\ln(Y) = \beta_0 + \beta_1 X + \beta_2 X^2 + \epsilon$ developed in Example 9.9.

Example 9.10

The normal plot of the residuals for the fitted model $\ln(Y) = \beta_0 + \beta_1 X + \beta_2 X^2 + \epsilon$ developed in Example 9.9 is given in Figure 9.8. Clearly, this normal probability plot will pass the fat pencil test, and therefore, the normality assumption of the error term is supported by this normal probability plot.

When the normal probability plot of the standardized residuals does not support the assumption of normality, the estimates of the regression coefficients are unaffected, however, the validity of any confidence intervals or hypothesis tests may be compromised for models based on small samples; for large samples the statistical inferences based on a fitted regression model will not be too sensitive to a violation of the normality assumption. Transformations of the data are often suggested as cures for nonnormality, and taking the natural logarithm of the response variable does sometime cure a nonnormality problem.

Example 9.11

The normal probability plot for the model

$$\text{PCTBF} = \beta_0 + \beta_1 \text{Age} + \beta_2 \text{Height} + \beta_3 \text{Neck} + \beta_4 \text{Chest} + \beta_5 \text{Thigh} + \beta_6 \text{Knee}$$
$$+ \beta_7 \text{Ankle} + \beta_8 \text{Biceps} + \beta_9 \text{Forearm} + \beta_{10} \text{Wrist} + \epsilon$$

fit in Example 9.7 is given in Figure 9.9. Clearly this normal probability plot passes the fat pencil test and supports the assumption of normality.

9.4.2 Detecting Multivariate Outliers and Influential Observations

Detecting multivariate outliers before fitting a multiple regression model is often a very difficult task, since multivariate outliers rarely show up in the scatterplots of the response versus the explanatory variables. Once a multiple regression model has been fit, multivariate outliers can be identified as observations having standardized residuals falling below -3 or above 3. Because the regression coefficients in a multiple regression model can be somewhat sensitive to outliers, it is important to assess the influence any outlier exerts on the fitted model.

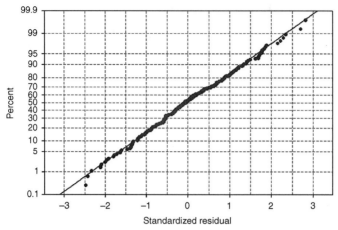

Figure 9.9   The normal plot for the model relating percent body fat to Age and several body measurements in Example 9.7.

When a multivariate outlier is identified the influence of the outlier on the fitted model needs to be investigated. A statistic that is often used to measure the influence that an individual observation has on the fitted model is *Cook's Distance*. Cook's Distance can be computed for each of the n observations and the value of Cook's Distance for the ith observation is denoted by C_i. For the multiple regression model

$$Y = \beta_0 + \beta_1 X_1 + \beta_2 X_2 + \cdots + \beta_p X_p + \epsilon$$

the value of Cook's Distance for the ith observation is

$$C_i = \frac{\sum (\widehat{y} - \widehat{y}_{(i)})^2}{s_e(p + 1)}$$

where $\widehat{y}$ is a fitted value computed using all n observations, $\widehat{y}_{(i)}$ is a fitted value computed using all but the ith observation, and s_e is an estimate of the standard deviation of the random error term ϵ. Cook's Distance can also be interpreted as the cumulative change in the regression coefficients when the ith observation is deleted from the data set, and Cook's Distance can also be expressed as a function of the ith standardized residual. Cook's Distance is typically used for flagging observations that should be further investigated, and fortunately, most statistical computing packages will compute Cook's Distance in a multiple regression analysis.

Any observation that has an unusually large affect on a fitted multiple regression model is called an *influential observation*, and observation having a value of Cook's Distance greater than 1 is identified as a *potentially influential observation*. When an observation has been declared a potentially influential observation, the observation should first be investigated as an impossible value or a mistake in recording the data. Observations that are impossible values should be eliminated from the data set and the model refit on the remaining sample observations. Observations that are clearly due to recording errors should be corrected and the model refit on the corrected data set. When there is no reason justifying the removal of an observation from the data set or its value cannot corrected, the influence of the observation can be investigated by temporarily removing the observation from the data set and refitting the model to the remaining observations. When the estimates of the regression coefficients do not differ much for the model fit on the entire data set and the model fit on the data set without this particular observation, then the observation actually has little influence on the fitted model and does not merit any further consideration. On the other hand, when the estimates of the regression coefficients are significantly different for the models fit on the full and reduced data sets, then the outlier is influencing the fit of the model and more data are needed to resolve this problem.

9.5 ASSESSING THE ADEQUACY OF FIT OF A MULTIPLE REGRESSION MODEL

Once the model assumptions have been validated and any influential observations dealt with the next step in a multiple regression analysis is to assess the adequacy of the fitted multiple regression model. The tools used to assess the fit of a multiple regression model are similar to those used in assessing the fit of a simple linear regression model. In particular, the adequacy of the fit of a regression model can be assessed by computing the values of s_e, R^2, and by testing the utility of the regression model.

9.5.1 Estimating σ

The standard deviation of the random error term ϵ in a multiple regression model is σ and σ is assumed to be the same for every set of values of the explanatory variables. Now, the residuals contain all of the relevant sample information about the error random variable, and thus, the residuals will used for estimating the value of σ. The point estimator of σ is

$$s_e = \sqrt{\frac{e_1^2 + e_2^2 + \cdots + e_n^2}{n - p - 1}} = \sqrt{\frac{\text{SSE}}{n - p - 1}}$$

where $e_1, e_2, e_3, \ldots, e_n$ are the n residuals and SSE is the sum of squared residuals. The degrees of freedom associated with s_e and the sum of squares due to error is $n - p - 1$. That is, since there are $p + 1$ regression coefficients that must be estimated to compute each residual, $p + 1$ degrees of freedom are subtracted from n resulting in a total of $n - p - 1$ degrees of freedom associated with the residual error.

The value of s_e measures how well the observed Y values agree with the fitted Y values, and thus, the smaller the s_e is the better the fitted model is at fitting the observed values of the response variable. The value of s_e is also used in computing the estimated standard error of each of the regression coefficients, and thus, the larger the s_e is the less accurate the estimated regression coefficients will be.

9.5.2 The Coefficient of Determination

Unlike simple linear regression, the correlation coefficients between the response variable and the explanatory variables cannot be used to measure the strength of a multiple regression relationship. A statistic used to measure the strength of a simple linear regression relationship that can also be used for measuring the strength of a multiple regression relationship is the coefficient of determination. In multiple regression the coefficient of determination, R^2, is also referred to as the *multiple correlation coefficient*. The value of R^2 associated with a fitted multiple regression model is

$$R^2 = \text{corr}(Y, \widehat{Y})^2 = \frac{\text{SSReg}}{\text{SSTot}} = 1 - \frac{\text{SSE}}{\text{SSTot}}$$

In both simple linear and multiple regression, the value of R^2 measures the proportion of the total variation in the observed values of the response variable that is explained by the regression model. Thus, the value of R^2 always falls between 0 and 1, and the closer the R^2 is to 1, the better the multiple regression model fits the observed values of the response variable. The magnitude of the correlation between the observed Y values and the fitted values is given by $\sqrt{R^2}$, and thus, when $R^2 > 0.64$ (i.e., $|\text{corr}(Y, \widehat{Y})| > 0.8$) there is a strong linear relationship between observed values of Y and the fitted values. On the other hand, a fitted model having a low value of R^2 is a poor fitting model and most likely does not include the explanatory variables necessary for explaining the response variable.

One problem with using the coefficient of determination as a measure of the strength of a multiple regression relationship is that the value of R^2 can be made as close to 1 as desired by including additional explanatory variables to the model, regardless of their relationship with the response variable. That is, the value of R^2 increases every time an additional variable is added to the model regardless of the variable's importance. In fact, when a data set contains n observations, a multiple regression model with any $n - 1$ explanatory variables produces a model having an R^2 value equal to 1.

A good guideline to use when building a multiple regression model is never to include more explanatory variables than 10% of the sample size (i.e., $p \leq n/10$). Including more explanatory variables than 20% of the sample size will often lead to an artificially high value of R^2 and may overemphasize the importance of the particular explanatory variables used in the model. Furthermore, in a well-designed study where a multiple regression model will be built the sampling plan should be designed so that the number of explanatory variables anticipated in the model is approximately 10% of the sample size. Also, because additional variables are often created from the explanatory variables, such as the square of a variable, and added to the model it is often wise to design the sampling plan so that the number of explanatory variables that are measured is much less 10% of the sample size.

An alternative measure of the adequacy of the fit of a multiple regression model that does measure the importance of the explanatory variables included in a multiple regression model is the *adjusted coefficient of determination* that is denoted by R^2_{adj}. The value of R^2_{adj} is

$$R^2_{\text{adj}} = 1 - (1 - R^2)\frac{n - 1}{n - p - 1} = 1 - \frac{\text{MSE}}{\text{MSTot}}$$

where p is the number of explanatory variables in the multiple regression model, MSE is the mean squared error, and $\text{MSTot} = \text{SSTot}/(n - 1)$ is the mean squared total variation. The value of R^2_{adj} is always less than the value of R^2, and unlike R^2 the value of R^2_{adj} can be negative.

One advantage of using R^2_{adj} instead of R^2 is that R^2_{adj} penalizes a model for including explanatory variables that do not improve the performance of the fitted model. That is, when the sum of squares due to error (SSE) is not significantly reduced by including a particular explanatory variable the value of R^2_{adj} will be smaller for the model with this variable than it is for the model that does not include this explanatory variable. In fact, the larger the value of R^2_{adj} is the smaller the value of s_e will be, however, the same is not true for R^2. Furthermore, R^2_{adj} is a statistic that can be used for comparing the adequacy of fit of two different regression models; R^2 values are not designed for and should not be used for comparing the adequacy of fit of two or more regression models and is particularly useful for comparing nested models.

Most statistical computing packages report both R^2_{adj} and R^2 as part of their standard multiple regression analysis output. Since R^2_{adj} increases or decreases with the addition of a new explanatory variable to the model it is always better to report the value of R^2_{adj}, rather than R^2, as the measure of adequacy of fit of a model. Also, a large discrepancy between the values of R^2_{adj} and R^2 indicates that there are explanatory variables in the model that are not necessary, and in this case, these variables should be identified and deleted from the model.

9.5.3 Multiple Regression Analysis of Variance

The analysis of variance (ANOV) table for summarizing the sources of variation in a multiple regression analysis is similar to the analysis of variance table for a simple linear regression analysis. The ANOV table for a multiple regression analysis is a summary table that lists the degrees of freedom, sums of squares, and mean squares for the decomposition of total variation into a source of variation due to the regression model and a source of variation due to residual error.

The total variation in the observed values of the response variable (SSTot) is decomposed into sum of squares due to regression (SSReg) and sum of squares due to error (SSE) according to

---

MULTIPLE REGRESSION SUM OF SQUARES

$$SSReg = \sum (\hat{y} - \bar{y})^2$$

$$SSE = \sum (y - \hat{y})^2$$

$$SSTot = \sum (y - \bar{y})^2 = SSReg + SSE$$

Note that for a multiple regression model with p explanatory variables there are $n - p - 1$ degrees of freedom associated with SSE and $n - 1$ degrees of freedom with SSTot. Therefore, because the degrees of freedom associates with the regression and error sources of variation add to the total degrees of freedom there are $p = (n - 1) - (n - p - 1)$ degrees of freedom associated with the regression source of variation (i.e., SSReg). The decomposition of the total variation in a multiple regression analysis is usually summarized in an analysis of variance table, and most statistical computing packages report an ANOV table of the form given in Table 9.5 in their multiple regression analysis output.

The most important information given in an analysis of variance table are the values of MSE and the p-value associated with the observed F-ratio. In particular, $s_e^2 = MSE$ and is unbiased estimator of σ^2, and the observed F-ratio and its p-value are used to test the significance of the regression model. It is also important to note that the values of s_e, R^2,

TABLE 9.5 The ANOV Table for a Multiple Regression Analysis

Source	df	SS	MS	F	P
Regression	p	SSReg	$MSReg = \dfrac{SSReg}{p}$	$F_{obs} = \dfrac{MSReg}{MSE}$	p
Error	$n - p - 1$	SSE	$MSE = \dfrac{SSE}{n - p - 1}$		
Total	$n - 1$	SSTot			

and R^2_{adj} can be easily computed from the information in an ANOV table since

$$s_e = \sqrt{\text{MSE}}$$

$$R^2 = \frac{\text{SSReg}}{\text{SSTot}}$$

$$R^2_{\text{adj}} = 1 - \frac{\text{MSE}}{\text{MSTot}}$$

When the assumptions of a multiple regression model are satisfied, an F-test can be used to test whether or not the multiple regression model is more useful than a model containing no explanatory variables for explaining the observed values of the response variable. In particular, the null and alternative hypotheses being tested in a multiple regression F-test are

$$H_0 : \text{ All of the regression slopes are 0}$$

$$H_A : \text{ At least one of the regression slopes is not 0}$$

For example, with the multiple regression model

$$Y = \beta_0 + \beta_1 X_1 + \beta_2 X_2 + \beta_3 X_3 + \cdots + \beta_p X_p + \epsilon$$

an equivalent form of the null hypothesis is $H_0 : \beta_1 = \beta_2 = \beta_3 = \cdots = \beta_p = 0$. When H_0 is true and $\beta_1 = \beta_2 = \beta_3 = \cdots = \beta_p = 0$, the regression model reduces to the *null model* $Y = \beta_0 + \epsilon$. Thus, the F-test is actually testing the joint significance of all of the explanatory variables in the model. When the p-value associated with the observed F-ratio is significant (i.e., smaller than α), the multiple regression model is significantly better than the null model. On the other hand, when the p-value for the observed F-ratio is not significant (i.e., larger than α) the multiple regression model is no better than the null model for explaining the values of the response variable. Therefore, when the observed F-ratio has a small p-value, the multiple regression will have some utility for explaining the response variable, however, a small p-value does not suggest the model is a good fitting model.

Careful selection of the explanatory variables in the planning stages of a research study usually leads to a significant F-ratio. It is important to note that the F-test is a test of the null hypothesis that all of the regression slopes are 0, and a significant F-ratio does not suggest that all of the regression slopes are non-zero. Furthermore, a significant F-ratio does not imply that the multiple regression model is a good model; a good multiple regression model will also explain a large proportion of the variation in the response variable and will be based on meaningful explanatory variables. And finally, it is important to note that the F-test can be sensitive to violations of the model assumptions unless the sample size is sufficiently large.

Example 9.12

The multiple regression model fit in Example 9.7 that had no collinearity problems was

$$\text{PCTBF} = \beta_0 + \beta_1 \text{Age} + \beta_2 \text{Height} + \beta_3 \text{Neck} + \beta_4 \text{Chest} + \beta_5 \text{Abdomen}$$

$$+ \beta_6 \text{Thigh} + \beta_7 \text{Knee} + \beta_8 \text{Ankle} + \beta_9 \text{Biceps} + \beta_{10} \text{Forearm}$$

$$+ \beta_{11} \text{Wrist} + \epsilon$$

The residual plot of the standardized residuals versus the fitted values for this model are given in Figure 9.10. Since all of the assumptions appear to be satisfied for this model, the regression analysis will proceed.

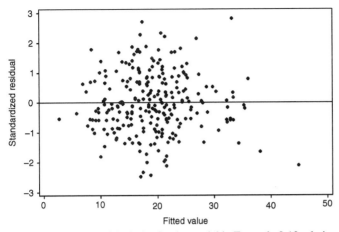

Figure 9.10 The residual plot for the model in Example 9.12 relating percent body fat to age and several body measurements with no collinearity problems.

The equation of the fitted model is

```
PCTBF = -25.4+0.217 Age - 0.165 Height - 0.351 Neck + 0.590 Chest
      + 0.633 Thigh - 0.011 Knee - 0.014 Ankle - 0.034 Biceps
      + 0.273 Forearm - 2.38 Wrist
```

The MINITAB summary of the regression coefficients is given in Table 9.6 and the analysis of variance table is given in Table 9.7.

Based on the output in ANOV table, the F-ratio is significant ($p = 0.000$), which means that this regression model is significantly better than the null model that contains no explanatory variables. Furthermore, since $R^2_{adj} = 59.9\%$ and $R^2 = 61.5$, this model is explaining about 60% of the total variation in the observed values of percent body fat.

Note that in Example 9.12 the value of R^2_{adj} is 59.9% and the value of R^2 is 61.5%, which suggests there might be one or more explanatory variables in the fitted model that are not actually needed in the model. Thus, when the regression assumptions are satisfied

TABLE 9.6 **The MINITAB Summary of Regression Coefficients for the Multiple Regression Model Fit in Example 9.12**

Predictor	Coef	SE Coef	T	P	VIF
Constant	-25.410	8.403	-3.02	0.003	
Age	0.21703	0.03517	6.17	0.000	1.755
Height	-0.1646	0.1053	-1.56	0.119	1.329
Neck	-0.3511	0.2725	-1.29	0.199	3.921
Chest	0.59005	0.07835	7.53	0.000	3.899
Thigh	0.6328	0.1468	4.31	0.000	5.309
Knee	-0.0106	0.2797	-0.04	0.970	4.067
Ankle	-0.0137	0.2674	-0.05	0.959	1.835
Biceps	-0.0337	0.2065	-0.16	0.870	3.480
Forearm	0.2735	0.2423	1.13	0.260	2.142
Wrist	-2.3809	0.6451	-3.69	0.000	3.242

S = 5.29946   R-Sq = 61.5%   R-Sq(adj) = 59.9%

TABLE 9.7 **The Analysis of Variance table for the Multiple Regression Model Fit in Example 9.12**

Analysis of Variance

Source	DF	SS	MS	F	P
Regression	10	10810.7	1081.1	38.49	0.000
Residual Error	241	6768.3	28.1		
Total	251	17579.0			

the multiple regression model is significant, the next step is to investigate the importance of the explanatory variables in the model and remove the explanatory variables that do not appear to be needed in the model.

9.6 STATISTICAL INFERENCES-BASED MULTIPLE REGRESSION MODEL

Once a multiple regression model has been fit, the assumptions checked and validated, and the model is found to be significant, the regression model can be used for making inferences about the relationship between the response variable and the explanatory variables, the likely values of the regression coefficients, the mean value of the response variable for a given set of values of the explanatory variables, and for predicting future values of the response variable.

9.6.1 Inferences about the Regression Coefficients

The regression coefficients in a multiple regression model are the intercept β_0 and the regression slopes $\beta_1, \beta_2, \ldots, \beta_p$. Because the error term in a multiple regression model has mean 0, the ith regression slope represents the expected change in the response variable when the ith explanatory variable is increased by 1 unit while all of the other explanatory variables are held fixed. Thus, when it is possible to increase the value of the ith explanatory variable by 1 unit without changing the values of the other explanatory variables, β_i measures the effect the explanatory variable X_i has on the response variable.

Recall that the regression coefficients $\beta_0, \beta_1, \beta_2, \ldots, \beta_p$ are estimated by the least squares estimators $\widehat{\beta}_0, \widehat{\beta}_1, \widehat{\beta}_2, \ldots, \widehat{\beta}_p$. The sampling distribution $\widehat{\beta}_i$ has mean β_i and standard deviation SE($\widehat{\beta}_i$). The estimated standard error of $\widehat{\beta}_i$, SE($\widehat{\beta}_i$), must be estimated in practice since σ is unknown; the estimated standard error of $\widehat{\beta}_i$ is denoted by se($\widehat{\beta}_i$). Because of computational considerations a statistical computing package should always be used to find the values of the least squares estimates and their estimated standard errors.

When the error term in a multiple regression model is normally distributed or the sample size is sufficiently large, the sampling distribution of

$$t = \frac{\widehat{\beta}_i - \beta_i}{\text{se}(\widehat{\beta}_i)}$$

will follow a t distribution with $n - p - 1$ degrees of freedom. Thus, when the normality assumption is satisfied the t distribution can be used for testing claims and computing confidence intervals for the regression coefficients. The test statistic for testing a claim about the ith regression coefficient with the null value β_{i0} is

$$t = \frac{\widehat{\beta}_i - \beta_{i0}}{\text{se}(\widehat{\beta}_i)}$$

which has $n - p - 1$ degrees of freedom. A $(1 - \alpha) \times 100\%$ confidence interval for the ith regression coefficient is

$$\widehat{\beta}_i \pm t_{\text{crit}} \times \text{se}(\widehat{\beta}_i)$$

where t_{crit} has $n - p - 1$ degrees of freedom and is found in Table A.7.

Since the ith explanatory variable drops out of the multiple regression model when the ith regression slope is 0 (i.e., $\beta_i X_i = 0$), testing the importance of ith explanatory variable in the multiple regression model simply amounts to testing $H_0 : \beta_i = 0$ versus $H_A : \beta_i \neq 0$. The test statistic for testing $H_0 : \beta_i = 0$ versus $H_A : \beta_i \neq 0$ is

$$t = \frac{\widehat{\beta}_i}{\text{se}(\widehat{\beta}_i)}$$

which also has $n - p - 1$ degrees of freedom.

The standard multiple regression output provided by a statistical computing package includes the least squares estimates, the estimated standard errors, t_{obs} for testing $\beta_i = 0$ and its p-value, and may or may not include the VIF values for each explanatory variable along with the values of s_e, R^2, R^2_{adj}, and the ANOV table. On the other hand, a confidence interval for any of the regression coefficients will generally need to be computed by hand.

Example 9.13

The MINITAB summary of the regression coefficients for the multiple regression model fit in Example 9.7 is given in Table 9.8. In particular, MINITAB reports the estimated regression coefficient and its standard error, t_{obs}, for testing the coefficient is equal to 0 with its p-value, and the variance inflation factor for each explanatory variable. Use the information in Table 9.8 to

a. test the importance of the explanatory variable Knee in the regression model.

b. compute a 95% confidence interval for the regression slope associated with the explanatory variable Age.

TABLE 9.8 The MINITAB Summary of Regression Coefficients for the Multiple Regression Model Fit in Example 9.7

Predictor	Coef	SE Coef	T	P	VIF
Constant	-25.410	8.403	-3.02	0.003	
Age	0.21703	0.03517	6.17	0.000	1.755
Height	-0.1646	0.1053	-1.56	0.119	1.329
Neck	-0.3511	0.2725	-1.29	0.199	3.921
Chest	0.59005	0.07835	7.53	0.000	3.899
Thigh	0.6328	0.1468	4.31	0.000	5.309
Knee	-0.0106	0.2797	-0.04	0.970	4.067
Ankle	-0.0137	0.2674	-0.05	0.959	1.835
Biceps	-0.0337	0.2065	-0.16	0.870	3.480
Forearm	0.2735	0.2423	1.13	0.260	2.142
Wrist	-2.3809	0.6451	-3.69	0.000	3.242

S = 5.29946   R-Sq = 61.5%   R-Sq(adj) = 59.9%

Solutions   Since the normality assumption is satisfied (see Example 9.11), using the information in Table 9.8

    a. the p-value for testing the importance, the explanatory variable Knee in the regression model is $p = 0.970$. Thus, the regression slope for Knee is not significantly different from 0 and therefore Knee does not appear to be an important explanatory variable and could be dropped from the model.

    b. a 95% confidence interval for the regression slope associated with Age has $252 - 10 - 1 = 241$ degrees of freedom since $n = 252$ and $p = 10$. The resulting 95% confidence interval is $0.22 \pm 1.96 \times 0.035$ that yields an interval of 0.15–0.29. Thus, based on the observed data, the expected difference in percent body fat for two individuals whose age differs by 1 year, but whose other body measurements are the same, differ by at least 0.15% and possibly as much as 0.29%.

After fitting a regression model it is often tempting to remove all of the explanatory variables whose regression coefficients are not significantly different from 0 from the model and refit a reduced regression model without these variables, however, this is not an appropriate statistical method of fine-tuning a regression model since the t-tests for the regression coefficients are not independent of one another. A method for testing the importance of more than one variable at a time will be discussed in Section 9.7.

9.6.2 Inferences about the Response Variable

Because the error term in a multiple regression model has mean 0, the mean of the response variable Y for a given set of values of the explanatory variable, say $\vec{x} = (x_1, x_2, x_3, \ldots, x_p)$, is

$$\mu_{Y|\vec{x}} = \beta_0 + \beta_1 x_1 + \beta_2 x_2 + \beta_3 x_3 + \cdots + \beta_p x_p$$

The least squares estimate of $\mu_{Y|\vec{x}}$ is

$$\widehat{\mu}_{Y|\vec{x}} = \widehat{\beta}_0 + \widehat{\beta}_1 x_1 + \widehat{\beta}_2 x_2 + \widehat{\beta}_3 x_3 + \cdots + \widehat{\beta}_p x_p$$

and when the normality assumption is satisfied or n is sufficiently large, a $(1 - \alpha) \times 100\%$ confidence interval for $\mu_{Y|\vec{x}}$ is

$$\widehat{\mu}_{Y|\vec{x}} \pm t_{\text{crit}} \times \text{se}(\widehat{\mu}_{Y|\vec{x}})$$

where t_{crit} has $n - p - 1$ degrees of freedom and can be found in Table A.7 and $\text{se}(\widehat{\mu}_{Y|\vec{x}})$ is the estimated standard error of $\widehat{\mu}_{Y|\vec{x}}$. Most statistical computing packages will compute a confidence interval for the mean value of the response variable given the values in $\vec{x}$ when asked to.

As is the case in simple linear regression, the predicted value of the response variable for a given set of values of explanatory variable is the same as the estimate of the mean of the response variable for $\vec{x}$. The predicted value of Y for a particular set of values of the explanatory variable $\vec{x}$ is

$$\widehat{y}_{\vec{x}} = \widehat{\beta}_0 + \widehat{\beta}_1 x_1 + \widehat{\beta}_2 x_2 + \widehat{\beta}_3 x_3 + \cdots + \widehat{\beta}_p x_p$$

Thus, the predicted value of Y and the estimate of the mean value of Y for the set of explanatory variables $\vec{x}$ are both calculated using

$$\widehat{\beta}_0 + \widehat{\beta}_1 x_1 + \widehat{\beta}_2 x_2 + \widehat{\beta}_3 x_3 + \cdots + \widehat{\beta}_p x_p$$

However, because a Y value includes the error term and the mean does not, the prediction error, denoted by $\text{pe}(\widehat{y}_{\vec{x}})$, must account for this extra source of variation. The prediction

Predicted Values for New Observations

```
New
Obs     Fit  SE Fit        95% CI            95% PI
 1   11.743   1.800   (8.199, 15.288)   (0.719, 22.768)
```

Figure 9.11   The MINITAB summary of the predicted values for Example 9.14.

error for the set of explanatory variables $\vec{x}$ is

$$\text{pe}(\widehat{y}_{\vec{x}}) = \sqrt{s_e^2 + \text{se}(\widehat{\mu}_{Y|\vec{x}})^2}$$

When normal assumption is satisfied a $(1 - \alpha) \times 100\%$ prediction interval for the value of Y for a particular set of explanatory variables $\vec{x}$ is

$$\widehat{y}_{\vec{x}} \pm t_{\text{crit}} \times \text{pe}(\widehat{y}_{\vec{x}})$$

where t_{crit} has $n - p - 1$ degrees of freedom and can be found in Table A.7. Again, since the formulas for the standard error of $\widehat{\mu}_{Y|\vec{x}}$ and the prediction error of $\widehat{y}$ are computationally difficult, a statistical computing package should be used for computing confidence intervals for a mean and prediction intervals for the response variable given the values in $\vec{x}$.

Example 9.14
MINITAB was used to produce a 95% confidence interval for the mean percent body fat based on the model fit in Example 9.7 for an individual with

Age	Height	Neck	Chest	Thigh	Knee	Ankle	Biceps	Forearm	Wrist
35.0	70.0	30.0	90.0	56.0	38.0	23.0	30.0	28.0	18.0

The MINITAB output given in Figure 9.11 includes the fitted value, the estimated standard error of the fitted value, a confidence interval for the mean, and a prediction interval.

Thus, an interval of estimates of the mean percent body fat for this set of values of the explanatory variables Age, Height, Neck Chest, Thigh, Knee, Ankle, Biceps, Forearm, and Wrist is 8.2–15.3%, and a 95% prediction interval for the percent body fat of an individual for this same set of values of Age, Height, Neck Chest, Thigh, Knee, Ankle, Biceps, Forearm, and Wrist is 0.7–22.8%.

Note that the prediction interval for an individual value percent body fat in Example 9.14 is much wider than the confidence interval for the mean percent body fat. The reason why a prediction interval is larger than a confidence interval for mean is that the estimated prediction error is always larger than the estimated standard error. That is,

$$\text{pe}(\widehat{y}_{\vec{x}}) = \sqrt{s_e^2 + \text{se}(\widehat{\mu}_{Y|\vec{x}})^2} \geq \text{se}(\widehat{\mu}_{Y|\vec{x}})$$

While MINITAB does not report the value of the estimated prediction error it can easily be computed using the MINITAB output from Examples 9.13 and 9.14. In particular, from Example 9.13 the value of s_e is 5.3 and from Example 9.14 the value of $\text{se}(\widehat{\mu}_{Y|\vec{x}})$ is 1.8, and therefore, the estimated prediction error in Example 9.14 is

$$\text{pe} = \sqrt{5.3^2 + 1.8^2} = 5.6$$

Thus, the predicted value of an individual's percent body fat is about three times as variable as the estimate of the mean percent body fat for these particular values of the explanatory variables.

9.7 COMPARING MULTIPLE REGRESSION MODELS

In many biomedical studies the effects or influence of a particular set of explanatory variables on the response variable is one of the primary research questions that is being investigated and one of the main reasons multiple regression is used for modeling the approximate relationship between the response and explanatory variables. That is, when the slope of an explanatory variable is actually 0 the variable drops completely out of the model. Thus, when all of the regression slopes for a particular subset of the explanatory variables are not significantly different from 0, the utility of these variables for explaining the values of the response variable is in doubt. Furthermore, in many studies the researcher will have a good idea of the explanatory variables that are important for explaining the response variable, but at the same time may be interested in exploring the relationship between some additional explanatory variables whose relationship to the response has not been previously studied. In this case, a researcher will often want to test the importance of these additional variables.

The regression model containing all of the explanatory variables is called the *full model*. Suppose the full model contains p explanatory variables of which the first k variables listed in the model are believed or known to be the important variables and the variables $X_{k+1}, \ldots, X_p$ are the variables whose importance is being tested. Then, a convenient way to write the full model is

$$Y = \beta_0 + \underbrace{\beta_1 X_1 + \cdots + \beta_k X_k}_{\text{important variables}} + \underbrace{\beta_{k+1} X_{k+1} + \beta_{k+2} X_{k+2} + \cdots + \beta_p X_p}_{\text{variables being tested}} + \epsilon$$

The model including only the important explanatory variables $X_1, X_2, \ldots, X_k$ is called the *reduced model*, and thus the reduced model is

$$Y = \beta_0 + \beta_1 X_1 + \cdots + \beta_k X_k + \epsilon$$

which is nested in the full model. In fact, the reduced model is simply the full model when $\beta_{k+1} = \beta_{k+2} = \cdots = \beta_p = 0$. Furthermore, since the reduced model is nested in the full model, testing $H_0 : \beta_{k+1} = \beta_{k+2} = \cdots = \beta_p = 0$ is equivalent to testing the importance of the explanatory variables $X_{k+1}, X_{k+2}, \ldots, X_p$.

When no problems are indicated by the residual diagnostics, there are no collinearity problems, and the normality assumption is satisfied an *extra sum of squares F-test* can be used to test

$$H_0 : \beta_{k+1} = \beta_{k+2} = \cdots = \beta_p = 0$$

versus the alternative hypothesis

$$H_A : \text{At least one of } \beta_{k+1}, \beta_{k+2}, \ldots, \beta_p \text{ is not } 0$$

Moreover, the extra sum of squares F-test compares how well the full and reduced models fit the observed data.

Let SSE_p be the sum of squares due to error and MSE_p is the mean square error for the full model and let SSE_k be the sum of squares for the reduced model. Then, the extra sum of squares F-test statistic for testing $H_0 : \beta_{k+1} = \beta_{k+2} = \cdots = \beta_p = 0$ is

$$F = \frac{(SSE_k - SSE_p)/(p - k)}{MSE_p}$$

which follows an F distribution with $p - k$ and $n - p - 1$ degrees of freedom. Note that an F distribution is referenced by two sets of degrees of freedom where the first set of degrees of freedom associated with the numerator of the F-ratio and the second set of degrees of freedom are associated with the denominator of the F-ratio.

The p-value for an extra sum of squares F-test will require a statistical computing package and is generally not part of a standard multiple regression analysis. For this reason, a rejection region will be used for the extra sum of squares F-test. The rejection region for the extra sum of squares F-test is

$$\text{Reject } H_0 \text{ when } F_{obs} > F_{crit, \alpha}$$

where $F_{crit, \alpha}$ has $p - k$ and $n - p - 1$ degrees of freedom and can be found in Table A.11. Note that the degrees of freedom of the numerator is simply the number of explanatory variables being considered for removal from the full model, and the denominator degrees of freedom are the degrees of freedom of the SSE in the full model.

The procedure for testing comparing $H_0 : \beta_{k+1} = \beta_{k+2} = \cdots = \beta_p = 0$ versus the alternative hypothesis H_A : At least one of $\beta_{k+1}, \beta_{k+2}, \ldots, \beta_p$ is not 0 with an extra sum of squares F-test is outlined below.

THE EXTRA SUM OF SQUARES F-TEST

1. Fit the full model.

2. Check the assumptions and perform a residual analysis on the fitted full model.

3. Cure any problems suggested by the residual analysis and refit the a new version of the full model if needed.

4. Fit the reduced model.

5. Determine the rejection region for the F-test used for comparing these two models.

6. Compute the observed value of the extra sum of squares F statistic for comparing these two models.

7. Reject or fail to reject H_0 according to whether or not F_{obs} is in the rejection region.

Provided that the multiple regression assumptions are satisfied for the full model, there is no need to check either the residual diagnostics or the normality assumption for the reduced model. Example 9.15 illustrates the use of the extras sum of squares F-test for comparing a full model with a reduced model.

Example 9.15

In modeling the percent body fat of an adult male, the multiple regression model with explanatory variables Age, Height, Neck, Chest, Thigh, Knee, Ankle, Biceps, Forearm, and Wrist was fit in Example 9.7. Because a large percentage of an individual's body fat is often found in the torso region, a researcher might want to test the importance of the body measurements taken on the extremities for modeling percent body fat. In particular, the importance of the variables Knee, Ankle, Biceps, Forearm, and Wrist might be tested since these are not areas of the body that typically contain a large amount of fat. Thus, an extra sum of squares F-test will be used to test the importance of the variables Knee, Ankle, Biceps, Forearm, and Wrist.

TABLE 9.9 **The ANOV Table for the Reduced Regression Model Resulting when Knee, Ankle, Biceps, Forearm, and Wrist are Removed from the Full Model**

```
Analysis of Variance

Source                   DF        SS       MS       F       P
Regression                5   10358.4   2071.7   70.58   0.000
Residual Error          246    7220.6     29.4
Total                   251   17579.0
```

From Example 9.7, the values of SSE and MSE for the full model are 6768.3 and 28.1, respectively. The ANOV table for the reduced model is given in Table 9.9.

The full model has 10 explanatory variables (i.e., $p = 10$) and the reduced model has 5 explanatory variable in it. Thus, the rejection region for an $\alpha = 0.01$ level extra sum of squares F-test of the reduced model versus the full model has $10 - 5 = 5$ and $252 - 10 - 1 = 241$ degrees of freedom, and therefore, the rejection region for this extra sum of squares F-test is

$$\text{Reject } H_0 \text{ when } F_{\text{obs}} > 4.10$$

The observed value of the extra sum of squares F-test statistic is

$$F_{\text{obs}} = \frac{(7220.6 - 6768.3)/10 - 5}{28.1} = 3.22$$

Therefore, because $3.22 < 4.10$, there is insufficient evidence to reject H_0 at the $\alpha = 0.01$ level. Thus, there is no statistical evidence that the full model is any better than the reduced model for explaining an adult male's percent body fat. In fact, R^2_{adj} for the full model is 59.9% and R^2_{adj} for the reduced model is 58.1%. Thus, the value of R^2_{adj} is roughly the same with or without the variables Knee, Ankle, Biceps, Forearm, and Wrist in the model.

The fitted equation of the reduced model is

```
PCTBF = - 33.2 + 0.174 Age - 0.279 Height - 0.713 Neck
        + 0.574 Chest + 0.562 Thigh
```

and the estimated standard errors of the regression coefficients are given in Table 9.10.

The extra sum of squares F-test is a test of the simultaneous importance of the explanatory variables being tested since it is a test of $\beta_{k+1} = \beta_{k+2} = \cdots = \beta_p$ are all equal to 0. Thus, when the extra sum of squares F-test is significant, it supports keeping the variables being tested in the model, it is incorrect to assume that each and every variable tested has a regression coefficient that is significantly different from 0. The alternative hypothesis in an extra sum of squares F-test simply specifies that at least one of the regression slopes is different from 0 and does not provide any further information about the model. Thus, the importance of an individual variable, say X_i, should be investigated with a t-test of $\beta_i = 0$.

TABLE 9.10 **The Estimated Regression Coefficients for the Reduced Model**

```
Predictor        Coef    SE Coef        T       P
Constant      -33.236      7.907    -4.20   0.000
Age           0.17432    0.03266     5.34   0.000
Height       -0.27917    0.09961    -2.80   0.005
Neck          -0.7129     0.2474    -2.88   0.004
Chest         0.57388    0.07710     7.44   0.000
Thigh          0.5617     0.1156     4.86   0.000
```

9.8   MULTIPLE REGRESSION MODELS WITH CATEGORICAL VARIABLES

In many biomedical research studies the researcher will need to account for differences in the response variable that are due to one or more categorical variables. For example, variables such as gender, ethnicity, and smoking status are often believed to be important explanatory variables for explaining some of the variation in a response variable. However, since categorical variables do not take on quantitative values their categorical values cannot be used in a regression model. By creating a special set of variables that take on the values 0 and 1, the information provided by a categorical variable included in a multiple regression model.

The specialized variables that are created to account for the different values of a categorical variable are called *dummy variables* or *indicator variables*. In particular, a dummy variable is a dichotomous variable that takes on the value 1 when a particular condition is satisfied and 0 when the condition is not satisfied. For example, a dummy variable that can be used for the categorical variable Gender is

$$G = \begin{cases} 1 & \text{if the individual is male} \\ 0 & \text{if the individual is female} \end{cases}$$

and an equally valid gender dummy variable is

$$G^\dagger = \begin{cases} 1 & \text{if the individual is female} \\ 0 & \text{if the individual is male} \end{cases}$$

Note that it would not make any difference which form of the gender dummy variable is used in a regression model since the fitted values and the significance of the gender dummy variable will be the same whether G or $G^\dagger$ is used. Also, a dummy variable uses the values 1 and 0 only to designate whether or not the particular condition is satisfied. It is fairly common to use a dummy variable where the dummy variable is 1 when the condition is present, and when the condition is absent the dummy variable is 0.

When a categorical variable has more than two categories, say k categories, a set of $k - 1$ dummy variables must be created to account for the k different values of the variable. When a categorical variable takes the $c_1, c_2, \ldots, c_k$, the dummy variables that will account for these k are $Z_1, Z_2, \ldots, Z_{k-1}$, where $Z_i = 1$ when the value of categorical variable has value c_i and 0 otherwise; the value c_k is accounted for when all the dummy variables have the value 0. For example, suppose the categorical variable Obesity takes on the values "not obese", "obese", and "extremely obese". Then, the dummy variables Z_1 and Z_2 defined below can be used to account for all three values of the variable Obesity.

$$Z_1 = \begin{cases} 1 & \text{if an individual is not obese} \\ 0 & \text{otherwise} \end{cases}$$

and

$$Z_2 = \begin{cases} 1 & \text{if an individual is obese} \\ 0 & \text{otherwise} \end{cases}$$

Note that when $Z_1 = Z_2 = 0$, the value of the categorical variable is identified as "extremely obese" since the individual is neither obese nor not obese.

Example 9.16

Create dummy variables for each of the following categorical variables.

   a. The variable C that represents the stage of cancer of a cancer patient. The variable C takes on the values I, II, III, and IV.

   b. The variable B that represents the blood type of an individual. The variable B takes on the A, B, AB, and O.

   c. The variable T that represents whether or not an individual received a treatment. The variable T takes on the values yes and no.

   d. The variable L that represents the dose level of an experimental drug that is applied to an individual in an experiment. The variable L takes on the values low, medium, and high.

Solutions

   a. The following three dummy variables will be needed to account for the categorical variable C since C takes on the four values I, II, III, and IV.

$$Z_1 = 1 \text{ if the patient's cancer stage is I and 0 otherwise.}$$

$$Z_2 = 1 \text{ if the patient's cancer stage is II and 0 otherwise.}$$

$$Z_3 = 1 \text{ if the patient's cancer stage is III and 0 otherwise.}$$

   b. The following three dummy variables will be needed to account for the variable B since B takes on the four values A, B, AB, and O.

$$Z_1 = 1 \text{ if A if the individual's blood is type A and 0 otherwise.}$$

$$Z_2 = 1 \text{ if B if the individual's blood is type B and 0 otherwise.}$$

$$Z_3 = 1 \text{ if AB if the individual's blood is type AB and 0 otherwise.}$$

   c. The following dummy variable will account for T since T takes on the two values yes and no.

$$Z = 1 \text{ if the patient was treated and 0 otherwise.}$$

   d. The following two dummy variables will be needed to account for the variable L since L takes on the three values low, medium, and high.

$$Z_1 = 1 \text{ if the individual received a low dose of the drug and 0 otherwise.}$$

$$Z_2 = 1 \text{ if the individual received a medium dose of the drug and 0 otherwise.}$$

Coding the data for the dummy variables in a data set can be done at either the data entry stage or after the data has been imported into a statistical computing package for analysis; most statistical computing packages have routines for converting the data for a categorical variable into the appropriate set of dummy variables for use in a multiple regression model. For example, when the gender of an individual is recorded in the data set and the coding for the gender dummy variable assigns the value 1 to females and 0 to males, the observed data might look like

Gender	Z
Female	1
Male	0
Female	1
Female	1
Male	0
$\vdots$	$\vdots$

Example 9.17

Suppose the explanatory variable Race is collected in a random sample, and an individual's race is classified as "Caucasian", "African-American", "Asian", or "Other". The coded data for the observed data might look like

Race	Z_1	Z_2	Z_3
Asian	0	1	0
Asian	0	1	0
African-American	0	0	1
Caucasian	1	0	0
African-American	0	0	1
African-American	0	0	1
Other	0	0	0
$\vdots$	$\vdots$	$\vdots$	

Note that Z_1 is the indicator for "Caucasian", Z_2 is the indicator for "Asian", Z_3 is the indicator for "African-American", and $Z_1 = Z_2 = Z_3 = 0$ indicates an individual's race was classified as "Other".

9.8.1 Regression Models with Dummy Variables

Dummy variables are often used in regression models to account for categorical variables that identify specific subpopulations that are of particular interest in a research study. In fact, using dummy variables to account for subpopulations in a multiple regression model is one of the most efficient ways to use the information contained in the sample for comparing two or more distinct subpopulations. For example, suppose the gender of an individual defines the two subpopulations that are being studied and compared in a research project. One approach to modeling the response variable for both subpopulations would be to take a stratified random sample of males and females and build regression models for the response variable separately from the strata samples. A more efficient approach to modeling the response variable is to use the combined samples for males and females to build a regression model that includes a dummy variable for the gender of an individual. The use of dummy variables in a multiple regression model will increase the information available for estimating the regression coefficients providing more accurate estimates and more powerful tests of the regression coefficient, also.

The simplest form of a dummy variable regression model is the *no-interaction model* that contains all of the quantitative explanatory variables and the dummy variables associated with the categorical variable of interest. The no-interaction model is a regression model with a different y-intercept for each of the values of the categorical variable. For example, with a single dummy variable Z, which accounts for the values of a dichotomous categorical variable, and a single quantitative explanatory variable X, the no-interaction model is

$$Y = \beta_0 + \beta_1 Z + \beta_2 X + \epsilon$$

When $Z = 1$, the regression model is

$$Y = \beta_0 + \beta_1 + \beta_2 X + \epsilon$$

and when $Z = 0$, the model is

$$Y = \beta_0 + \beta_2 X + \epsilon$$

Note that in both cases the regression slope for the explanatory variable X is β_2, however, when $Z = 1$ the y-intercept is $\beta_0 + \beta_1$ and when $Z = 0$ the y-intercept is β_0.

The second form of a dummy variable regression model is the *interaction model* that contains all of the quantitative explanatory variables, the dummy variables associated with a categorical variable, and the products of the quantitative explanatory variables and dummy variables. The product of an explanatory variable and a dummy variable is called an *interaction term*. In the interaction model, both the y-intercept and the regression slopes for each of the quantitative explanatory variables will depend on the values of the dummy variables. For example, with a single dummy variable Z, which accounts for the values of a dichotomous categorical variable, and a single quantitative explanatory variable X, the interaction model is

$$Y = \beta_0 + \beta_1 Z + \beta_2 X + \beta_3 ZX + \epsilon$$

where ZX is the interaction term for the variables Z and X. When $Z = 1$, the regression model is

$$Y = \beta_0 + \beta_1 + \beta_2 X + \beta_3 X + \epsilon$$
$$= (\beta_0 + \beta_1) + (\beta_2 + \beta_3)X + \epsilon$$

and when $Z = 0$, the model is

$$Y = \beta_0 + \beta_2 X + \epsilon$$

Note the regression slope for the explanatory variable X is $\beta_2 + \beta_3$ and the y-intercept is $\beta_0 + \beta_1$ when $Z = 1$, and when $Z = 0$, the y-intercept is β_0 and the slope for X is β_2. Figures 9.12 and 9.13 illustrate the difference between the no-interaction and interaction model when there is one dummy variable and one quantitative explanatory variable in the regression model.

Example 9.18
Suppose X_1 and X_2 are quantitative explanatory variables and Z_1 and Z_2 are dummy variables. Determine

    a. the equation of the no-interaction model.
    b. the y-intercept when $Z_1 = 1$ and $Z_2 = 1$.
    c. the equation of the interaction model.
    d. the y-intercept and regression slopes for X_1 and X_2 when $Z_1 = 0$ and $Z_2 = 1$.

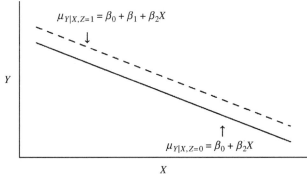

Figure 9.12 The no-interaction dummy variable regression model with one explanatory variable and one dummy variable.

Solutions

a. The equation of the no-interaction model is

$$Y = \beta_0 + \beta_1 Z_1 + \beta_2 Z_2 + \beta_3 X_1 + \beta_4 X_2 + \epsilon$$

b. The y-intercept when $Z_1 = 1$ and $Z_2 = 1$ is $\beta_0 + \beta_1 + \beta_2$.

c. The equation of the interaction model is

$$Y = \beta_0 + \beta_1 Z_1 + \beta_2 Z_2 + \beta_3 X_1 + \beta_4 X_2 + \beta_5 Z_1 X_1$$

$$+ \beta_6 Z_1 X_2 + \beta_7 Z_2 X_1 + \beta_8 Z_2 X_2 + \epsilon$$

d. The y-intercept and regression slopes for X_1 and X_2 when $Z_1 = 0$ and $Z_2 = 1$ are $\beta_0 + \beta_2$, $\beta_3 + \beta_7$, and $\beta_4 + \beta_8$, respectively.

Note that the interaction model in Example 9.18 has nine regression coefficients. In general, when there are p quantitative explanatory variables and d dummy variables in the interaction model, the regression model will have $(p + 1)(d + 1)$ regression coefficients. For example, when there are $p = 8$ explanatory variables and $d = 3$ dummy variable, the interaction model will have $(8 + 1)(3 + 1) = 36$ regression coefficients. Furthermore, because the number of regression coefficients in the interaction model can be quite large and the number of variables in a model should never exceed 10% of the sample size, the use of an interaction model must be anticipated by a researcher in determining the sample size to be used in the research study.

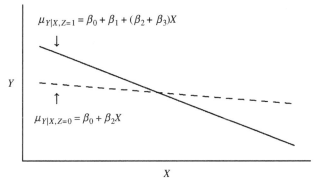

Figure 9.13 The interaction dummy variable regression model with one explanatory variable and one dummy variable.

9.8.2 Testing the Importance of Categorical Variables

Once a dummy variable regression model has been fit and the model assumptions checked and verified, the extra sum of squares F-test can be used to test the relationship between the response variable and the categorical variables by testing the appropriate hypotheses concerning the dummy variables. In particular, an extra sum of squares F-test can be used to test the importance of the categorical variable or for comparing the interaction model with the no-interaction model.

Provided the normality assumption is satisfied or a large sample is being used, the overall importance of the categorical variable associated with the dummy variables can be tested with an extra sum of squares F-test. Since, the general model building strategy is to start with a full model and reduce the model from there, the full interaction model should be considered the full model when dummy variables are being included in the model. The reduced model for testing whether or not the categorical variable is important in explaining the response variable is the model that includes only the quantitative explanatory variables. For example, when there are three quantitative explanatory variables, say X_1, X_2, and X_3, and a single dummy variable Z, the full model will be

$$Y = \beta_0 + \beta_1 X_1 + \beta_2 X_2 + \beta_3 X_2 + \beta_4 Z + \beta_5 Z X_1 + \beta_6 Z X_2 + \beta_7 Z X_3 + \epsilon$$

and the reduced model is

$$Y = \beta_0 + \beta_1 X_1 + \beta_2 X_2 + \beta_3 X_3 + \epsilon$$

When the extra sum of squares F-test for comparing the interaction model with the model having no dummy variables is significant, then the dummy variables are important to the fit of the model and the categorical variable has some utility for explaining the response variable. On the other hand, when the F-test is not significant, there is no statistical evidence supporting the use of the categorical variable in the model.

Example 9.19

Suppose a multiple regression model based on two quantitative explanatory variables and a single dummy variable was fit. Use the ANOV table for the dummy variable regression model

$$Y = \beta_0 + \beta_1 X_1 + \beta_2 X_2 + \beta_3 Z + \beta_4 Z X_1 + \beta_5 Z X_2 + \epsilon$$

given in Table 9.11, and the ANOV table for the reduced model

$$Y = \beta_0 + \beta_1 X_1 + \beta_2 X_2 + \epsilon$$

which is given in Table 9.12 to answer the following:

a. Compute the values of R^2 and R^2_{adj} for the interaction model.

b. Compute the values of R^2 and R^2_{adj} for the reduced model.

c. Test the importance of the categorical variable associated with the dummy variable Z at the $\alpha = 0.05$ level.

TABLE 9.11 The ANOV Table for the Interaction Model

Source	df	SS	MS	F	P
Regression	5	2150	430	27.17	0.000
Error	109	1725	15.83		
Total	114	3875			

TABLE 9.12   The ANOV Table for the Reduced Model

Source	df	SS	MS	F	P
Regression	2	1550	775	37.26	0.000
Error	112	2325	20.8		
Total	114	3875			

Solutions   Using the information in the ANOV in Tables 9.11 and 9.12

a. the values of R^2 and R^2_{adj} for the interaction model are $R^2 = \frac{2150}{3875} = 0.55$ and $R^2_{\text{adj}} = 1 - \frac{15.83}{33.99} = 0.53$.

b. the values of R^2 and R^2_{adj} for the reduced model are $R^2 = \frac{1550}{3875} = 0.40$ and $R^2_{\text{adj}} = 1 - \frac{20.8}{33.99} = 0.39$.

c. the rejection region for testing $H_0 : \beta_3 = \beta_4 = \beta_5 = 0$ at the $\alpha = 0.05$ level is based on 3 and 109 degrees of freedom and is

$$\text{Reject } H_0 \text{ when } F_{\text{obs}} > 2.68$$

Note that 100 degrees of freedom are used for $F_{\text{crit},0.05}$ since the F-values for 109 degrees of freedom are not listed in Table A.11.

The observed value of the extra sum of squares F statistic for testing of the importance of the categorical variable associated with the dummy variable Z is

$$F_{\text{obs}} = \frac{(2325 - 1725)/3}{15.83} = 12.63$$

Thus, since $12.63 > 2.68$ there is sufficient evidence to reject H_0, which means that the interaction model is a better model than the reduced model. Hence, the categorical variable associated with the dummy variable Z appears to be useful in explaining the response variable Y.

The general approach to take when comparing dummy variable regression models is outlined below.

COMPARING DUMMY VARIABLE MODELS

---

1. Test the overall importance of categorical variable in the model by comparing the interaction model with the reduced model that only includes the quantitative explanatory variable.

   (a) When the extra sum of squares F-test for comparing these two models is not significant, the reduced model, based on only the quantitative explanatory variables, is a better model than the interaction model.

   (b) When the extra sum of squares F-test is significant, the dummy variable terms should not be dropped from the model. In this case, the interaction model should be compared to the no-interaction model as outlined in step 2.

2. When the extra sum of squares F-test in step 1 is significant, the interaction model and the no-interaction model should be compared.

   (a) When the extra sum of squares F-test for comparing these two models is not significant, the interaction terms can be dropped from the model and the no-interaction model is a better model than the interaction model.

   (b) When the extra sum of squares F-test is significant, the interactions are important to the model and the interaction model is a better fitting model than the no-interaction model.

TABLE 9.13 The ANOV Table for the Interaction Model

```
Analysis of Variance
```

Source	DF	SS	MS	F	P
Regression	9	10940.8	1215.6	44.4	0.000
Residual Error	242	6638.2	27.4		
Total	251	17579.0			

TABLE 9.14 The ANOV Table for the No-Interaction Model

```
Analysis of Variance
```

Source	DF	SS	MS	F	P
Regression	5	9987.8	1997.6	64.65	0.000
Residual Error	246	7591.1	30.9		
Total	251	17579.0			

Note that the first comparison made when investigating the importance of a categorical variable is whether or not the variable is important at all, and the second comparison investigates how the categorical variable affects the response variable.

Example 9.20

Suppose that a regression model for approximating an individual's percent body fat is going to be built for both adult males and adult females using the explanatory variables height (Height), neck circumference (Neck), chest circumference (Chest), thigh circumference (Thigh), and gender (G) where

$$G = \begin{cases} 0 & \text{if the individual is male} \\ 1 & \text{if the individual is female} \end{cases}$$

The analysis of variance tables for the interaction model, the no-interaction model, and the model based on only the quantitative variables Height, Neck, Chest, and Thigh are given in Tables 9.13, 9.14, and 9.15, respectively.

Assuming the residual diagnostics suggest no problems with the interaction model and the normality assumption is satisfied, use the dummy variable analysis outlined above to determine the most appropriate model for approximating the percent body fat for adult males and females. Use $\alpha = 0.05$ for the significance level in all of the model comparison tests.

Solutions First compare the interaction model with the model based on only the quantitative explanatory variables. The extra sum of squares F-test for comparing these two models is based on the information in Tables 9.13 and 9.15, and the rejection region for this test is based on 5 and 241 degrees of freedom and is

$$\text{Reject } H_0 \text{ when } F_{\text{obs}} > 2.71$$

TABLE 9.15 The ANOV Table for the Model with only the Quantitative Explanatory Variables Height, Neck, Chest, and Thigh

```
Analysis of Variance
```

Source	DF	SS	MS	F	P
Regression	4	9522.4	2380.6	72.99	0.000
Residual Error	247	8056.6	32.6		
Total	251	17579.0			

Note that 200 degrees of freedom are used for $F_{\text{crit},0.05}$ since the F-values for 241 degrees of freedom are not listed in Table A.11.

The observed value of the extra sum of squares F statistic for testing of the importance of the categorical variable associated with the dummy variable G is

$$F_{\text{obs}} = \frac{(8056.6 - 6638.2)/5}{27.4} = 10.35$$

Since $10.35 > 2.71$, the F statistic is significant and it appears that the interaction model is a significantly better model than the model based on only the variables Height, Neck, Chest, and Thigh. Thus, the gender of an individual does appear to be useful in explaining percent body fat based on the observed data.

Since the interaction model is significantly better than the model without the dummy variable G, the next step in the analysis is to compare the interaction and no-interaction models. The information in Tables 9.13 and 9.14 will be used in the extra sum of squares F-test for comparing these two models, and the rejection region for this test is

$$\text{Reject } H_0 \text{ when } F_{\text{obs}} > 2.87$$

using 4 and 200 degrees of freedom for $F_{\text{crit},0.05}$.

The observed value of the extra sum of squares F statistic for testing of the importance of the interaction terms is

$$F_{\text{obs}} = \frac{(7591.1 - 6638.2)/4}{27.4} = 8.69$$

Since $8.69 > 2.87$, the F statistic is significant and it appears that the interaction model is a significantly better model than the no-interaction model. Therefore, based on the observed data the best fitting regression model is

$$Y = \beta_0 + \beta_1 G + \beta_2 \text{Height} + \beta_3 \text{Neck} + \beta_4 \text{Chest} + \beta_5 \text{Thigh}$$

$$+ \beta_6 G \cdot \text{Height} + \beta_7 G \cdot \text{Neck} + \beta_8 G \cdot \text{Chest} + \beta_9 G \cdot \text{Thigh} + \epsilon$$

9.9 VARIABLE SELECTION TECHNIQUES

In exploratory research studies involving a large number of explanatory variables one of the primary goals of the statistical analysis is to screen the explanatory variables to identify the explanatory variables that have the most utility for explaining the response variable. When a researcher does not have enough information on the importance of the explanatory variables before collecting to determine a set of models to be compared, a *variable selection procedure* can be used to investigate the importance of the explanatory variables. In particular, a variable selection procedure is an algorithmic procedure that is used for investigating the importance of the explanatory variables available for inclusion in the full multiple regression model. While there are many different variable selection procedures that could be used, only the *Maximum R^2_{adj}* and *Bayes Information Criterion* (BIC) will be discussed in this section.

A variable selection procedure should only be used as a screening device for investigating the relationship between the response variable and the explanatory variables and should never be used blindly for determining the model in a regression analysis. That is, because a variable selection procedure is based on the information in the observed data, it will tend to overemphasize the importance of some of the explanatory variables in the model best fitting the selection criterion. A fitted model that contains explanatory variables whose true regression slopes are 0 is said to be an *overfit model*, and a fitted model that excludes explanatory variables whose regression slopes are not 0 is said to be an *underfit model*. In an overfit model the precision of the estimates of the regression coefficients is reduced, and in an underfit model the estimates of the regression coefficients are biased. Thus, because a regression model is built from a sample rather than a census, fitted models should always be subjected to scientific scrutiny to make sure the fitted model is scientifically reasonable. In some research studies there are theoretical reasons for keeping certain explanatory variables in a regression model, regardless of what the observed data suggests.

A variable selection procedure should be used to identify the models containing the fewest explanatory variables that do a good job of modeling the response variable according to the selection criterion. Generally, a variable selection procedure will identify several competing models that will need to be further investigated when choosing a final model. The basic steps that should be followed when using any of the variable selection methods are outlined below.

THE GENERAL VARIABLE SELECTION PROCEDURE

1. Develop a "good" fitting full model containing all of the predictors of interest. The full model should have no residual problems, all influential points must have been dealt with, and there should not be any collinearity problems among the explanatory variables.

2. Apply the variable selection procedure.

3. Identify the best models according to the variable selection criterion, and choose a small number of models to consider as candidates for the final model.

4. Select the final model. The selection of the final should be based on scientific knowledge rather than purely based on the variable selection procedure.

The choice of the final model must be made using sound statistical and scientific reasoning. The final model should contain only the important explanatory variables and explanatory variables that are scientifically plausible. Since there will often be several good candidates for the final model, the final model should be selected on scientific terms rather than statistical terms. That is, the selection procedure criterion should never be used as the sole mechanism for determining the final model. Also, since there are many different variable selection methods that can be used and each method may lead to a different model, a researcher should only use a single variable selection procedure for screening the importance of the explanatory variables.

9.9.1 Model Selection Using Maximum R^2_{adj}

Because a good model should explain a large proportion of the observed variation in the response variable, one approach to the variable selection problem is to chose the model or models that explain the largest proportion of the variation in the Y's. However, because the proportion of the total variation explained by a model is measured by R^2 and the value of R^2 always increases when explanatory variables are added to the model, the largest value of R^2 always occurs with the full model. Thus, a variable selection procedure based upon comparing the values of R^2 is not appropriate. On the other hand, the value decreases when unimportant explanatory variables are included in a model. Therefore, a variable selection procedure that compares models on the basis of R^2_{adj} is preferable to one that uses R^2.

The *Maximum R^2_{adj} variable selection procedure* is one of the simplest variable selection procedures and typically one of the variable selection procedures available in a statistical computing package. The Maximum R^2_{adj} variable selection procedure compares the values of R^2_{adj} for all possible models based on a particular set of explanatory variables and is outlined below.

THE MAXIMUM R_{adj}^2 VARIABLE SELECTION PROCEDURE

Step 0 Fit the full model, check the model assumptions, and cure any problems suggested by the residual diagnostics, before proceeding to step 1.

Step 1 Fit all possible regression models based on the p explanatory variables in the full model and compute the value of R_{adj}^2 for each model.

Step 2 Determine the models having the largest values of R_{adj}^2. These models are the candidates for the final model.

Step 3 Select the final model based upon the value of R_{adj}^2, the number of variables in the model, and scientific reasoning.

The final model based on the Maximum R_{adj}^2 procedure should have a large value of R_{adj}^2, be based on a few explanatory variables, and make sense scientifically. The models having the largest values of R_{adj}^2 will also have the smallest values of MSE since

$$R_{adj}^2 = 1 - \frac{\text{MSE}}{\text{MSTot}}$$

and MSTot is same for all of models being compared. Furthermore, when using the Maximum R_{adj}^2 procedure, a researcher must determine the minimum level of R_{adj}^2 that is acceptable for a model and the difference between two values of R_{adj}^2 that has practical significance. For example, based on past experience a researcher might decide that a reasonable model will have a value of R_{adj}^2 of at least 0.60 (i.e., 60%), and any two values of R_{adj}^2 that differ by more than 0.02 (i.e., 2%) are practically different.

Because fitting all possible models can be computationally impossible, statistical computing packages often address the computational complexity of the problem by fitting only the best b models when there are $k = 1, 2, 3, \ldots$, and p explanatory variables in the model. For example, with 20 explanatory variables there are 1,048,576 possible models that need to be compared. By fitting only the best $b = 5$ models for models containing $k = 1, 2, 3, \ldots$, or 20 explanatory variables less than 100 models will need to be fit and compared.

Example 9.21
The MINITAB output given in Table 9.16 resulted from using the Maximum R_{adj}^2 variable selection procedure on the $n = 252$ observations on adult male percent body fat (PCTBF) and the explanatory variables Age, Height, Chest, Neck, Thigh, Knee, Ankle, Biceps, Forearm, and Wrist contained in the Body Fat data set. Note that MINITAB only reported the best two models for each possible number of explanatory variables in a model.

Based on the information in Table 9.16, the best model is the seven variable model with the explanatory variables Age, Height, Chest, Neck, Thigh, Forearm, and Wrist ($R_{adj}^2 = 60.8$). Also, the best fitting models are based on 6, 5, and 4 explanatory variables. In particular, the best four models according to the maximum R_{adj}^2 criterion are the models based on the explanatory variables

1. Age, Height, Chest, Neck, Thigh, Forearm, and Wrist ($R_{adj}^2 = 60.8$).
2. Age, Height, Chest, Neck, Thigh, and Wrist ($R_{adj}^2 = 60.7$).
3. Age, Height, Chest, Neck, and Thigh ($R_{adj}^2 = 60.6$).
4. Age, Chest, Neck, and Thigh ($R_{adj}^2 = 59.9$).

Note that each of the best models contain the variables Age, Chest, Neck, and Thigh and the difference between the R_{adj}^2 values for the best five models differ by less than 2%. Thus, without

TABLE 9.16 The MINITAB Output for the Maximum R^2_{adj} Variable Selection Procedure for the Response Variable PCTBF and Explanatory Variables Age, Height, Chest, Neck, Thigh, Knee, Ankle, Biceps, Forearm, and Wrist

Vars	R-Sq	R-Sq (adj)	S	Age	Height	Neck	Chest	Thigh	Knee	Ankle	Biceps	Forearm	Wrist
1	49.4	49.2	5.9668				X						
1	31.3	31.0	6.9495					X					
2	53.0	52.6	5.7626		X		X						
2	52.3	51.9	5.8053	X			X						
3	55.5	55.0	5.6161	X			X						X
3	55.3	54.7	5.6300	X			X	X					
4	60.6	59.9	5.2968	X			X	X					X
4	58.2	57.5	5.4537	X	X		X	X					
5	61.4	60.6	5.2525	X	X		X	X					X
5	60.9	60.1	5.2882	X		X	X	X					X
6	61.6	60.7	5.2460	X	X	X	X	X					X
6	61.5	60.6	5.2531	X	X		X	X				X	X
7	61.9	60.8	5.2413	X	X	X	X	X				X	X
7	61.7	60.6	5.2526	X	X	X	X	X	X				X
8	61.9	60.7	5.2486	X	X	X	X	X	X			X	X
8	61.9	60.6	5.2517	X	X	X	X	X			X	X	X
9	61.9	60.5	5.2591	X	X	X	X	X	X		X	X	X
9	61.9	60.5	5.2594	X	X	X	X	X	X	X		X	X
10	61.9	60.3	5.2700	X	X	X	X	X	X	X	X	X	X

considering any scientific or theoretical reasons for having a particular explanatory variable in the model, the best model having a large R^2_{adj} value and the fewest explanatory variables is

$$\text{PCTBF} = \beta_0 + \beta_1 \text{Age} + \beta_2 \text{Chest} + \beta_3 \text{Neck} + \beta_4 \text{Thigh} + \epsilon$$

9.9.2 Model Selection using BIC

The *Bayes Information Criterion* is a variable selection procedure that was developed to control for the overfitting of a model when a variable selection procedure is used. The formula for computing the value of BIC for a particular model is

$$\text{BIC} = n \ln\left(\frac{\text{SSE}}{n}\right) + (k+1)\ln(n)$$

where n is the sample size, k is the number of explanatory variables in the model, and SSE is the sum of squares due to error for the model. The value of BIC is increases when either the sum of squares error or the number of variables in the model is increased, and thus, the smaller the value of BIC, the better the model is fitting the observed data according to the BIC criterion. Thus, when comparing two models, the model with the smaller BIC fits observed data better, has fewer explanatory variables, or both. Similar to R^2_{adj} the BIC statistic also penalizes models for including uninformative explanatory variables. The BIC variable selection procedure is outlined below.

THE BIC VARIABLE SELECTION PROCEDURE

Step 0 Fit the full model, check the model assumptions, and cure any problems suggested by the residual diagnostics, before proceeding to step 1.

Step 1 Fit all possible regression models based on the p explanatory variables in the full model and compute the value of BIC for each model.

Step 2 Determine the models having the smallest values of BIC. These models are the candidates for the final model.

Step 3 Select the final model based upon the value of BIC, the number of variables in the model, and scientific reasoning.

Again, the final model should be selected according the BIC variable selection criterion and scientific reasons. Also, when selecting the final model, values of BIC that differ by less than 2 are not generally considered statistically different. Thus, when comparing two models that have BIC values differing by less than 2, chose the model that contains fewer explanatory variables as the better candidate for the final model. Unfortunately, not all statistical computing packages have routines using BIC as the variable selection procedure, however, the BIC value of a particular model is easily computed from the values of n and s_e for the model being considered. In particular, for a model having k explanatory variables, the value of BIC for the model is

$$\text{BIC} = n \ln \left(\frac{(n - k - 1)}{n} s_e^2 \right) + (k + 1) \ln(n)$$

Example 9.22

The Bayes Information Criterion values and the MINITAB output for the Maximum R_{adj}^2 variable selection procedure for fitting models to percent body fat (PCTBF) based on the explanatory variables Age, Height, Chest, Neck, Thigh, Knee, Ankle, Biceps, Forearm, and Wrist in the Body Fat data set are given in Table 9.17.

Based on the BIC values in Table 9.17, the best two models are

$$\text{PCTBF} = \beta_0 + \beta_1 \text{Age} + \beta_2 \text{Chest} + \beta_3 \text{Neck} + \beta_4 \text{Thigh} + \epsilon$$

which has a BIC value of 861.8 and

$$\text{PCTBF} = \beta_0 + \beta_1 \text{Age} + \beta_2 \text{Chest} + \beta_3 \text{Neck} + \beta_4 \text{Thigh} + \beta_5 \text{Height} + \epsilon$$

which has a BIC value of 862.1. All of the other models considered have BIC values that are larger than 862.1 by at least 2, and therefore, are not competitors for the final model.

Thus, without considering scientific or theoretical reasons for having a particular explanatory variable in the model, the best model having a large BIC value and the fewest explanatory variables is the model

$$\text{PCTBF} = \beta_0 + \beta_1 \text{Age} + \beta_2 \text{Chest} + \beta_3 \text{Neck} + \beta_4 \text{Thigh} + \epsilon$$

9.10 SOME FINAL COMMENTS ON MULTIPLE REGRESSION

Fitting multiple regression model is a dynamic process. A multiple regression model is fit to the original data, the model assumptions are checked, the residual diagnostics are examined, adjustments may or may not be made to the model, and models are refit and the assumptions rechecked until a good fitting model is found. Only after curing any problems suggested by the residual or collinearity diagnostics should inferences be drawn from the fitted model

TABLE 9.17 The BIC Values and the Output for the Maximum R^2_{adj} Variable Selection Procedure for the Response Variable PCTBF and Explanatory Variables Age, Height, Chest, Neck, Thigh, Knee, Ankle, Biceps, Forearm, and Wrist

Vars	R-Sq	R-Sq (adj)	BIC	S	Age	Height	Neck	Chest	Thigh	Knee	Ankle	Biceps	Forearm	Wrist
1	49.4	49.2	908.3	5.9668				X						
1	31.3	31.0	985.1	6.9495					X					
2	53.0	52.6	895.3	5.7626			X	X						
2	52.3	51.9	899.0	5.8053	X			X						
3	55.5	55.0	886.8	5.6161	X			X						X
3	55.3	54.7	888.0	5.6300	X			X	X					
4	60.6	59.9	861.8	5.2968	X			X	X					X
4	58.2	57.5	876.5	5.4537	X	X		X	X					
5	61.4	60.6	862.1	5.2525	X	X		X	X					X
5	60.9	60.1	865.5	5.2882	X		X	X	X					X
6	61.6	60.7	865.9	5.2460	X	X	X	X	X					X
6	61.5	60.6	866.6	5.2531	X	X		X	X				X	X
7	61.9	60.8	870.0	5.2413	X	X	X	X	X				X	X
7	61.7	60.6	871.1	5.2526	X	X	X	X	X	X				X
8	61.9	60.7	875.2	5.2486	X	X	X	X	X	X			X	X
8	61.9	60.6	875.5	5.2517	X	X	X	X	X			X	X	X
9	61.9	60.5	880.7	5.2591	X	X	X	X	X	X		X	X	X
9	61.9	60.5	880.7	5.2594	X	X	X	X	X	X	X		X	X
10	61.9	60.3	886.2	5.2700	X	X	X	X	X	X	X	X	X	X

about the relationship between the response and the explanatory variables. The steps for a typical multiple regression analysis are outlined below.

THE MULTIPLE REGRESSION PROCEDURE

1. Determine the sampling plan that will be used for collecting a random sample on the response and explanatory variables.

2. Collect the data.

3. Investigate the relationship between the response and explanatory variables using scatterplots.

4. Fit the full model.

5. Check the assumptions of the model and identify any problems suggested by the residual and collinearity diagnostics.

6. Make any adjustments to the model that may cure the problems suggested by the residual and collinearity diagnostics and refit the model.

7. Repeat steps 5 and 6 until a good fitting model is found.

8. Use the fitted model for making statistical inferences about the relationship between the response and explanatory variable.

Before testing any hypotheses about the model, making inferences about the response variable, or using a variable selection procedure it is critical to develop a full model that satisfies the multiple regression assumptions. A poor fitting model should never be used for make inferences about the relationship between the response and the explanatory variables, and confidence intervals and hypothesis tests should not be performed in the presence of nonnormality unless $n > 100$. Also, the number of variables used in a multiple regression model should not exceed 10% of the sample size (i.e., $p < n/10$).

When the relationship between the response variable and a large number of explanatory variables is being investigated a variable selection procedure is commonly used to screen the explanatory variables, however, no variable selection procedure should be used blindly for determining the final regression model. In general, the model that best satisfies the variable selection criterion will not be superior to any of the competing models which also fare well under the selection criterion. The scientific merit of all of the models competing to be the final model must be evaluated in selecting the final model. Again, it is important to keep the following George Box statements in mind, "Essentially, all models are wrong, but some are useful" and "Remember that all models are wrong; the practical question is how wrong do they have to be to not be useful" (Box et al., 1987). Thus, the ultimate goal of a multiple regression analysis is to determine a parsimonious model that fits the observed data well and makes scientific sense.

Finally, when reporting the results of a multiple regression analysis a researcher need only provide the most relevant information from the multiple regression output. In particular, a researcher should report the equation of the fitted model provided it has significant utility, the standard errors of the coefficients, the value of s_e, the value of R^2, and any specialized inferences made using the model. On the other hand, the residual plots, the normal probability plot, and the ANOV table need not be included in summarizing the multiple regression analysis; however, it is important to summarize the results of the residual diagnostics when they suggest adjustments to the original model were needed.

GLOSSARY

Adjusted Coefficient of Determination The adjusted coefficient of determination measures is denoted by R^2_{adj} and is

$$R^2_{adj} = 1 - (1 - R^2)\frac{n - 1}{n - p - 1} = 1 - \frac{\text{MSE}}{\text{MSTot}}$$

where p is the number of explanatory variables in the multiple regression model, $\text{MSE} = \frac{\text{SSE}}{n-p-1}$ is the mean squared error, and $\text{MSTot} = \frac{\text{SSTot}}{n-1}$ is the mean squared total variation.

Bayes Information Criterion The Bayes Information Criterion is associated with a model is

$$\text{BIC} = n \ln\left(\frac{\text{SSE}}{n}\right) + (k + 1)\ln(n)$$

where n is the sample size and k is the number of explanatory variables in the model.

BIC Variable Selection Procedure The BIC variable selection procedure is based on comparing the values of BIC for all possible models based on a particular set of explanatory variables.

Collinear Relationship A collinear relationship or collinearity problem exists among the explanatory variables when one explanatory variable can be explained by a linear combination of the remaining explanatory variables.

Cook's Distance The value of Cook's Distance for the ith observation is denoted by C_i, and for the multiple regression model

$$Y = \beta_0 + \beta_1 X_1 + \beta_2 X_2 + \cdots + \beta_p X_p + \epsilon$$

Cook's Distance is

$$C_i = \frac{\sum (\widehat{y} - \widehat{y}_{(i)})^2}{s_e(p+1)}$$

where $\widehat{y}$ is a fitted value computed using all n observations, $\widehat{y}_{(i)}$ is a fitted value computed using all but the ith observation, and s_e is an estimate of the standard deviation of the random error term ϵ.

Dummy Variable Regression Model A regression model that includes one or more dummy variables is called a dummy variable regression model.

Dummy Variable A dummy variable that is also called an indicator variable is created to account for the different values of a categorical variable and is a dichotomous variable that takes on the value 1 when a particular condition is satisfied and 0 when the condition is not satisfied.

Extra sum of Squares F-test The extra sum of squares F-test is a test that is used for testing a reduced model versus the full model.

Full Model The regression model containing all of the explanatory variables is called the full model.

Influential Observation Any observation that has an unusually large affect on a fitted multiple regression model is called an influential observation.

Interaction Model The interaction model is a dummy variable regression model that contains all of the quantitative explanatory variables, the dummy variables associated with the categorical variable, and the products of the quantitative explanatory variables and dummy variables.

Interaction Term An explanatory variable that is formed from the product of an explanatory variable and a dummy variable is called an interaction term.

Linear Model A statistical model is said to be a linear model for relating a response variable Y to a particular set of quantitative explanatory variables, say $X_1, X_2, X_3, \ldots, X_p$ when it is a statistical model of the form

$$Y = \beta_0 + \beta_1 X_1 + \beta_2 X_2 + \cdots + \beta_p X_p + \epsilon$$

Statistical models that are not linear models are called nonlinear models.

Maximum R^2_{adj} Variable Selection Procedure The Maximum R^2_{adj} variable selection procedure is based on comparing the values of R^2_{adj} for all possible models based on a particular set of explanatory variables.

Multiple Correlation Coefficient The multiple correlation coefficient measures the proportion of the total variation in the observed values of the response variable that is explained by a regression model and is denoted by R^2. The value of R^2 is

$$R^2 = \text{corr}(Y, \widehat{Y})^2 = \frac{\text{SSR}}{\text{SSTot}} = 1 - \frac{\text{SSE}}{\text{SSTot}}$$

Multiple Regression Model A multiple regression model for approximating the relationship between a quantitative response variable Y and a set of p quantitative explanatory variables $X_1, X_2, X_3, \ldots, X_p$ is a model of the form

$$Y = \beta_0 + \beta_1 X_1 + \beta_2 X_2 + \beta_3 X_3 + \cdots + \beta_p X_p + \epsilon$$

where the explanatory variables $X_1, X_2, X_3, \ldots, X_p$ are quantitative variables.

No-interaction Model The no-interaction model is a dummy variable regression model that contains all of the quantitative explanatory variables and the dummy variables associated with the categorical variable of interest.

Null Model The regression model that includes no explanatory variables is called the null model. The equation for the null model is $Y = \beta_0 + \epsilon$.

Overfit Model A fitted model that contains explanatory variables whose true regression slopes are 0 is said to be an overfit model.

Reduced Model Any multiple regression model that excludes one or more of the explanatory variables included in the full model is called a reduced model.

Regression Coefficients The unknown parameters $\beta_0, \beta_1, \ldots, \beta_p$ are called the regression coefficients, β_0 is the y-intercept, and $\beta_1, \beta_2, \beta_3, \ldots, \beta_p$ are the regression slopes.

Response Surface A multiple regression model based on two or more explanatory variables defines the equation of a response surface.

Variable Selection Procedure A variable selection procedure is an algorithmic procedure that is used for investigating the importance of the explanatory variables available for the full model.

Variance Inflation Factor The variance inflation factor associated with the ith explanatory variable measures the interdependence between X_i and the other explanatory variables. The variance inflation factor for the explanatory variable X_i is denoted by VIF_i.

Underfit Model A fitted model that excludes explanatory variables whose true regression slopes are not 0 is said to be an underfit model.

EXERCISES

9.1 What is a multivariate data set?

9.2 What is a graphical approach that can be used to investigate the possible pairwise relationships between a response variable Y and a set of explanatory variables $X_1, X_2, \ldots, X_p$?

9.3 What is the general form of a multiple regression model for relating a response variable Y to a set of explanatory variables $X_1, X_2, \ldots, X_p$?

9.4 What is the form of the simplest multiple regression model that might be used to explain a curvilinear relationship between a response variable Y and an explanatory variable X?

9.5 What are the
(a) parameters in a multiple regression model?
(b) regression coefficients in a multiple regression model?
(c) regression slopes in a multiple regression model?

9.6 For the multiple regression model $Y = \beta_0 + \beta_1 X_1 + \beta_2 X_2 + \epsilon$ what is the expected change in Y when

(a) X_1 is increased by one unit and X_2 is held fixed?

(b) X_2 is increased by one unit and X_1 is held fixed?

(c) X_1 and X_2 are both increased by one unit?

9.7 Determine whether or not each of the following statistical models is a linear model.

(a) $Y = \beta_1 X_1 + \beta_2 X_2 + \epsilon$.

(b) $Y = \beta_0(\beta_1 X_1 + \beta_2 X_2) + \epsilon$.

(c) $Y = \beta_0 + \beta_1 X_1 + \beta_2 X_2 + \beta_3 X_1 X_2 + \epsilon$.

(d) $Y = \beta_0 + \beta_1 X_1^{\beta_2} + \epsilon$.

(e) $Y = (\beta_0 + \beta_1 X_1 + \beta_2 X_2)^2 + \epsilon$.

9.8 What are the assumptions required of a multiple regression model?

9.9 How do the assumptions required of a multiple regression model and a simple linear regression model differ?

9.10 What does it mean when there is a collinear relationship in a set of explanatory variables?

9.11 Assuming that the error term ϵ has mean 0 in the regression model

$$Y = \beta_0 + \beta_1 X_1 + \beta_2 X_2 + \beta_3 X_3 + \epsilon$$

(a) what is the mean of Y when $X_1 = 3$, $X_2 = 10$, and $X_3 = 2$?

(b) what is the mean of Y when $X_1 = 0$, $X_2 = 5$, and $X_3 = 10$?

9.12 What is the least squares procedure for fitting a multiple regression model?

9.13 Are the least squares estimates of the regression coefficients in a multiple regression model always unbiased estimators?

9.14 Why is it important to investigate the pairwise correlations between the explanatory variables?

9.15 If all of the pairwise correlations between the explanatory variables are between -0.5 and 0.7, is it still possible for there to be a collinearity problem with the explanatory variables? Explain.

9.16 What is a procedure that can be used to check for collinearity problems in the explanatory variables?

9.17 How can the VIF values be used to check for collinearity problems in the explanatory variables?

9.18 Suppose when the multiple regression model

$$Y = \beta_0 + \beta_1 X_1 + \beta_2 X_2 + \beta_3 X_3 + \beta_4 X_4 + \epsilon$$

was fit the pairwise correlations between the explanatory variables $X_1, X_2, X_3,$ and X_4 given in Table 9.18 were also computed. Based on the correlations in

TABLE 9.18 Sample Correlations Between the Explanatory Variables X_1, X_2, X_3, and X_4

	Correlations			
	X_1	X_2	X_3	X_4
X_1	0.077			
X_2	−0.368	−0.794		
X_3	−0.043	0.967	−0.691	
X_4	0.388	0.832	−0.913	0.679

TABLE 9.19 MINITAB Output for Exercise 9.19

```
Predictor      Coef  SE Coef      T      P      VIF
Constant     188.70    22.75   8.30  0.000
X1        -0.01211  0.02206  -0.55  0.585    1.560
X2         0.38058  0.07867   4.84  0.000  130.053
X3        -1.2528    0.2367  -5.29  0.000   71.959
X4        -1.8553    0.2058  -9.01  0.000   18.199
```

Table 9.18 do any of the explanatory variables appear to be nearly collinear? Explain.

9.19 Suppose the multiple regression model

$$Y = \beta_0 + \beta_1 X_1 + \beta_2 X_2 + \beta_3 X_3 + \beta_4 X_4 + \epsilon$$

was fit. Based on the MINITAB output in Table 9.19, is there evidence of a collinearity problem with the explanatory variables? Explain.

9.20 What is a

(a) residual?   (b) standardized residual?

9.21 How can the residuals be used to check the assumptions required of a multiple regression model?

9.22 What is a large standardized residual?

9.23 What does it mean when observation has a standardized residual $e_s = -8.19$?

9.24 What is a residual plot and how is a residual plot used?

9.25 What
(a) does a "good" residual plot look like?
(b) patterns should be looked for in a residual plot?
(c) is the purpose of plotting the residuals versus each explanatory variable?

9.26 Determine whether or not each of the following residual plots suggests there is a particular violation of the regression assumptions, and when there is an apparent violation be sure to identify the assumption being violated.

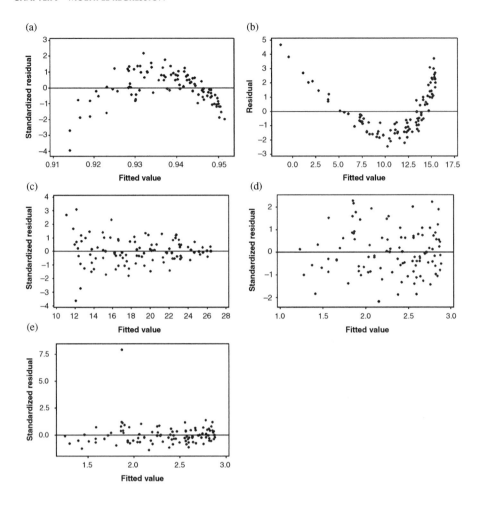

9.27 When a residual plot of the standardized residuals versus the fitted values reveals a funnel-shaped pattern what is the

(a) problem being suggested by the residual plot?

(b) transformation that might be used to cure the problem suggested by the residual plot?

9.28 When a residual plot of the standardized residuals versus a particular explanatory variable reveals a curvilinear pattern what is the

(a) problem being suggested by the residual plot?

(b) variable or might be added to the model to cure the problem suggested by the residual plot?

9.29 In the article "Sensitivity to reward and body mass index: evidence for a nonlinear relationship" published in *Appetite* (Davis and Fox, 2008), the authors reported the fitted multiple regression model $\widehat{SR} = 6.72 + 1.77 \times \text{Sex} - 5.19 \times B - 8.47 \times B^2$, where SR is a measure of sensitivity to reward, Sex is a dummy variable that is 1 for a male and 0 for a female, and B is the standardized value of BMI.

(a) If the author's model is the best fitting model, what would the residual plot for the model $SR = \beta_0 + \beta_1 \text{Sex} + \beta_2 B + \epsilon$ be expected to look like?

(b) Determine the fitted value for a male with a $B = 0.25$

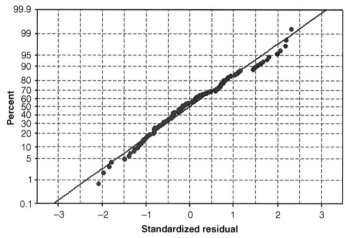

Figure 9.14   Normal probability plot for the model $Y = \beta_0 + \beta_1 X_1 + \beta_2 X_2 + \epsilon$.

     (c) Determine the residual for an observation with Sex $= 1$, $B = 0.25$, and SR $= 7.3$.

9.30   How can the normality assumption be checked after fitting a multiple regression model?

9.31   What statistical inferences is the normality assumption required for?

9.32   Does the normal probability plot given in Figure 9.14, which resulted from fitting the model $Y = \beta_0 + \beta_1 X_1 + \beta_2 X_2 + \epsilon$, support the normality assumption? Explain.

9.33   What is a statistic that can be used to identify influential observations?

9.34   What is the cutoff value that is used with Cook's Distance to identify an influential observation.

9.35   What is the procedure that should be used to investigate the influence of an observation that has been identified as an influential observation?

9.36   Why is it inappropriate to simply eliminate all influential observations from a data set and refit the multiple regression model to the reduced data set?

9.37   The residual plot in Figure 9.15 reveals a multivariate outlier with a value of Cook's Distance of 1.087. Table 9.20 contains summaries of the fitted model for the complete data set and Table 9.21 contains summary information for the model fit without this observation. Use the information in Tables 9.20 and 9.21 to answer the following:

    (a) How much influence does this observation exert over the estimates of the slope and intercept? Explain.

    (b) How much influence does this observation exert over the values of s_e and R^2? Explain.

    (c) How much influence does this observation exert over the estimated standard errors of the slope and intercept estimates? Explain.

    (d) How much influence does this observation exert over the predicted value of Y when $X = 10$? Explain.

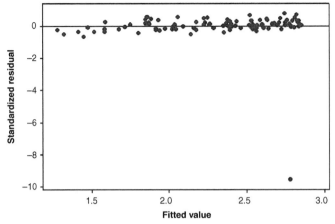

Figure 9.15   Residual plot for Exercise 9.37.

TABLE 9.20   Summary Statistics for the Full Data Set

Predictor	Coef	SE Coef	T	P
Constant	-0.7003	0.1281	-5.47	0.000
X	0.1824	0.0077	23.61	0.000

S = 0.178064   R-Sq = 85.0%   R-Sq(adj) = 84.9%

9.38   Use the Body Fat data set to answer the following:
  (a) Regress Weight on Age, Height, Neck, Chest, Abdomen, Hip, Thigh, Knee, Ankle, Biceps, Forearm, Wrist.
  (b) Check the assumptions associated with this model. Be sure to plot the standardized residuals versus each of the explanatory variables, check for collinearity, and check the normality assumption.
  (c) Identify any influential observations.

9.39   Use the Body Fat data set to answer the following:
  (a) Regress Density on Age, Height, Neck, Chest, Abdomen, Hip, Thigh, Knee, Ankle, Biceps, Forearm, Wrist.
  (b) Check the assumptions associated with this model. Be sure to plot the standardized residuals versus each of the explanatory variables, check for collinearity, and check the normality assumption.
  (c) Identify any influential observations.

9.40   How are the residuals used in estimating σ?

9.41   How many degrees of freedom does s_e have?

9.42   What is the coefficient of determination and how is it computed?

TABLE 9.21   Summary Statistics for the Data Set Without the Influential Observation

Predictor	Coef	SE Coef	T	P
Constant	-0.82447	0.03454	-23.87	0.000
X	0.19106	0.00209	91.52	0.000

S = 0.0477717 R-Sq = 98.9% R-Sq(adj) = 98.8%

9.43   What does the coefficient of determination measure?

9.44   What is the adjusted coefficient of determination and how is it computed?

9.45   Why is R^2_{adj} preferred over R^2 as a measure of the adequacy of fit of a multiple regression model?

9.46   Explain why the number of explanatory variables in a multiple regression model should not exceed 10% of the number of observations used to fit the model.

9.47   Compute the value of R^2_{adj} for the model $Y = \beta_0 + \beta_1 X_1 + \beta_2 X_+ \cdots + \beta_p X_p + \epsilon$ in each of the following scenarios.
(a) $R^2 = 0.81, n = 56, p = 5$.
(b) $R^2 = 0.68, n = 88, p = 6$.
(c) MSE $= 50$, SSTot $= 13560$, $n = 61$, and $p = 5$.
(d) MSE $= 1.15$, SSTot $= 560$, $n = 211$, and $p = 10$.

9.48   The partial ANOV table given in Table 9.22 resulted from fitting the multiple regression model $Y = \beta_0 + \beta_1 X_1 + \beta_2 X_2 + \beta_3 X_3 + \beta_4 X_4 + \epsilon$. Use the information in Table 9.22 to answer the following:
(a) Fill in the missing entries in the ANOV table.
(b) What is the estimate of σ?
(c) Compute the value of R^2 and R^2_{adj}.

9.49   Suppose SSE $= 522.1$, SSTot $= 1037.8$, $n = 231$, and there are $p = 12$ explanatory variables in the model.
(a) Construct the ANOV table.
(b) Estimate σ.
(c) Compute the value of R^2_{adj}.

9.50   What are the null and alternative hypotheses in the F-test summarized in the ANOV table?

9.51   What is the rejection region for the F-test used to test all of the regression slopes are equal to 0?

9.52   Why does a variable drop out of a multiple regression model when its slope is equal to 0?

9.53   Test the hypothesis that all of the regression slopes are 0 using the information in

(a) Exercise 9.48.   (b) Exercise 9.49.

9.54   What does it mean when $100 \times R^2\%$ is more than $100 \times R^2_{adj}\%$ by at least 5%?

TABLE 9.22   Partial ANOV Table for Exercise 9.48

Source	df	SS	MS	F
Regression				
Error		6050		
Total	124	7682		

TABLE 9.23 MINITAB Output Resulting from Fitting the Regression Model for Y with Explanatory Variables X_1, X_2, and X_3

Predictor	Coef	SE Coef	T	P
Constant	58.88	10.78	5.46	0.000
X1	0.0633	0.01015	6.24	0.000
X2	-0.1215	0.03167	-3.84	0.000
X3	0.0144	0.00432	3.32	0.002

S = 3.78525   R-Sq = 67.6%   R-Sq(adj) = 65.5%

Analysis of Variance

Source	DF	SS	MS	F	P
Regression	3	1376.31	458.77	32.02	0.000
Residual Error	46	659.09	14.33		
Total	49	2035.40			

9.55 What is the sampling distribution of $\dfrac{\widehat{\beta}_i - \beta_i}{se(\widehat{\beta}_i)}$ when

(a) the normality assumption is valid?

(b) n is large?

9.56 What is the form of

(a) a $100 \times (1 - \alpha)\%$ confidence interval for a regression coefficient.

(b) the test statistic for testing a regression coefficient is equal to 0?

(c) the test statistic for testing all of the regression slopes are equal to 0?

9.57 The MINITAB output given in Table 9.23 resulted from fitting the multiple regression model relating Y to the explanatory variables X_1, X_2, and X_3. Assuming that the assumptions of the model are valid, use the information in Table 9.23 to answer the following:

(a) Test $H_0 : \beta_1 = \beta_2 = \beta_3 = 0$ at the $\alpha = 0.01$ level.

(b) Estimate the expected change in Y for a one unit increase in X_3 when X_1 and X_2 are held fixed.

(c) Test $H_0 : \beta_3 = 0$ at the $\alpha = 0.05$ level.

(d) Compute a 95% confidence interval for β_3.

9.58 The MINITAB output given in Table 9.24 resulted from fitting the multiple regression model relating Y to the explanatory variables N, D, S, U, and R. Assuming that the assumptions of the model are valid, use the information in Table 9.24 to answer the following:

(a) Do the VIF statistics suggest there are any possible collinearity problems? Explain.

(b) Test $H_0 : \beta_N = \beta_D = \beta_S = \beta_U = \beta_R = 0$ at the $\alpha = 0.01$ level.

(c) Estimate the expected change in Y for a one unit increase in R when all of the other explanatory variables are held fixed.

(d) Test $H_0 : \beta_S = 0$ at the $\alpha = 0.05$ level.

(e) Compute a 95% confidence interval for β_R.

(f) Which explanatory variable should be dropped from the model first?

9.59 In the article "Passive cigarette smoke exposure of Infants" published in the *Archives of Pedriatric and Adolescent Medicine* (Ownby et al., 2000), the authors reported

TABLE 9.24   MINITAB Output Resulting from Fitting the Regression Model for Y with Explanatory Variables N, D, S, U, and R

```
Predictor          Coef        SE Coef       T       P      VIF
Constant         7.2313        0.1258    57.46   0.000
N            0.00000268   0.00000192     1.40   0.163    2.340
D            0.00000288   0.00000170     1.69   0.092    2.983
S            0.00000017   0.00000153     0.11   0.911    4.184
U            0.00000198   0.00000131     1.51   0.134    1.782
R            0.00005135   0.00000921     5.57   0.000    2.333

S = 1.48314     R-Sq = 51.9%     R-Sq(adj) = 50.6%


Analysis of Variance

Source              DF      SS       MS       F      P
Regression           5   413.656   82.731   37.61  0.000
Residual Error     174   382.750    2.200
Total              179   796.405
```

the estimated regression coefficients and standard errors given in Table 9.25 for a regression model relating the logarithm of an infant's cotinine–creatinine ratio for $n = 97$ infants. Use the information in Table 9.25 to answer the following:

(a) Compute the value of the t statistic for each of the regression coefficients.

(b) Approximate the p-value associate with each of the t statistics in part (a).

(c) Does it appear that the sex of a child is important in predicting the logarithm of an infant's cotinine–creatinine ratio? Explain.

9.60 What are the two uses of the least squares response surface $\hat{y}$ in a multiple regression analysis?

9.61 What is the relationship between the prediction error and the standard error of $\hat{\mu}_{Y|\vec{X}=\vec{x}}$?

9.62 Suppose that the model $Y = \beta_0 + \beta_1 X_1 + \beta_2 X_2 + \beta_3 X_3 + \epsilon$ was fit to $n = 43$ observations yielding the $\hat{y} = -12.2 + 1.2X_1 - 0.8X_2 + 5.6X_3$.

(a) Estimate the mean value of Y when $X_1 = 2$, $X_2 = 5$, and $X_3 = 4$.

(b) If the estimated standard error of the estimate in part (a) is se $= 1.3$, compute a 95% confidence interval for the mean of Y when $X_1 = 2$, $X_2 = 5$, and $X_3 = 4$.

TABLE 9.25   Regression Coefficients for Predicting the Logarithm of an Infant's Cotinine–Creatinine Ratio

Variable	Coefficient	SE
Intercept	1.64	0.25
Mother's smoking frequency	2.69	0.51
Father's smoking frequency	2.36	0.40
Mother 3 father interaction	−1.25	0.74
Smoking frequency of persons visited away from home	1.15	0.39
Smoking frequency of other people in home	1.64	0.59
Smoking frequency of persons providing child care away from home	2.76	0.80
Child's sexë 3 child care away from home interaction	−1.93	1.07
Child's sex	−0.24	0.26

TABLE 9.26 ANOV Table for Regressing Y on the All Nine Explanatory Variables

Source	DF	SS	MS	F	P
Regression	9	16.1233	1.7915	13.34	0.000
Residual Error	50	6.7165	0.1343		
Total	59	22.8398			

(c) Predict the value of Y when $X_1 = 2$, $X_2 = 5$, and $X_3 = 4$.

(d) If the $s_e = 0.65$, compute a 95% prediction interval for the value of Y when $X_1 = 2$, $X_2 = 5$, and $X_3 = 4$.

9.63 In the article "Sensitivity to reward and body mass index: evidence for a nonlinear relationship" published in *Appetite* (Davis and Fox, 2008), the authors reported the fitted multiple regression model

$$\widehat{SR} = 6.72 + 1.77\text{Sex} - 5.19B - 8.47B^2$$

where SR is a measure of sensitivity to reward, Sex is a dummy variable that is 1 for a male and 0 for a female, B is the standardized value of BMI, and $n = 366$ observations.

(a) Estimate the mean value of SR for a male with a value of $B = 0.2$.

(b) If the estimated standard error of the estimate in part (a) is $\text{se}(\widehat{SR}) = 0.7$, compute a 95% confidence interval for the mean value of SR for a male with a value of $B = 0.2$.

(c) Predict the value of SR for a male with a value of $B = 0.2$.

(d) If the $s_e = 2.5$, compute a 95% prediction interval for the value of SR for a male with a value of $B = 0.2$.

9.64 What is the procedure for testing the importance of two or more variables in a multiple regression model?

9.65 For the regression model $Y = \beta_0 + \beta_1 X_1 + \cdots + \beta_{k+1} X_{k+1} + \cdots + \beta_p X_p + \epsilon$, what is the test statistic for testing $H_0 : \beta_{k+1} = \beta_{k+2} = \cdots = \beta_p = 0$?

9.66 The ANOV table given in Table 9.26 resulted from fitting the multiple regression model $Y = \beta_0 + \beta_1 X_1 + \cdots + \beta_9 X_9 + \epsilon$, and the ANOV table in Table 9.27 resulted from fitting the reduced model that excluded the explanatory variables X_6, X_7, X_8, and X_9. Use the information in Tables 9.26 and 9.27 to test the importance of the explanatory variables X_6, X_7, X_8, and X_9 (i.e., $H_0 : \beta_6 = \beta_7 = \beta_8 = \beta_9 = 0$).

9.67 The ANOV table given in Table 9.28 resulted from fitting the multiple regression model $Y = \beta_0 + \beta_1 X_1 + \cdots + \beta_9 X_9 + \epsilon$, and the ANOV table in Table 9.29 resulted from fitting the reduced model that excluded the explanatory variables X_7, X_8,

TABLE 9.27 ANOV Table for Regressing Y on only X_1, X_2, X_3, X_4, and X_5

Source	DF	SS	MS	F	P
Regression	5	15.4331	3.0866	22.50	0.000
Residual Error	54	7.4067	0.1372		
Total	59	22.8398			

TABLE 9.28   **ANOV Table for Regressing Y on the All Nine Explanatory Variables**

Source	DF	SS	MS	F	P
Regression	9	25867.0	2874.1	64.47	0.000
Residual Error	70	2984.9	42.6		
Total	79	28851.9			

and X_9. Use the information in Tables 9.28 and 9.29 to test the importance of the explanatory variables X_7, X_8, and X_9 (i.e., $H_0 : \beta_7 = \beta_8 = \beta_9 = 0$).

9.68   Using the Body Fat data set
(a) regress Density on the explanatory variables Age, Height, Neck, Chest, Knee, Ankle, Biceps, and Forearm.
(b) regress Density on the explanatory variables Age, Height, Neck, and Chest.
(c) determine the importance of the explanatory variables Knee, Ankle, Biceps, and Forearm for predicting Density.

9.69   Using the Body Fat data set
(a) regress Density on the explanatory variables Age, Height, Neck, Chest, Hip, Biceps, and Forearm.
(b) regress Density on the explanatory variables Age, Height, Neck, Chest, and Hip.
(c) determine the importance of the explanatory variables Biceps and Forearm for predicting Density.

9.70   What is a dummy variable?

9.71   How many dummy variables are needed to account for a categorical variable with
(a) four different categories?
(b) five different categories?
(c) three different categories?

9.72   In the Birth Weight data set the variable Race is a categorical variable that takes on the values 1, 2 and 3. If Race = 1 is used to represent a white mother, Race = 2 represents a black mother, and Race = 3 represents a mother of any other ethnicity, create two dummy variables that could be used in a multiple regression model to account for the race of a baby's mother.

9.73   For a dummy variable multiple regression model based on one dummy variable and three explanatory variables write down the equation of the
(a) no-interaction model.
(b) interaction model.

TABLE 9.29   **ANOV Table for Regressing Y on Only X_1, X_2, X_3, X_4, X_5, and X_6**

Source	DF	SS	MS	F	P
Regression	6	25843.8	4307.3	104.55	0.000
Residual Error	73	3008.1	41.2		
Total	79	28851.9			

9.74 For a dummy variable multiple regression model based on the dummy variables Z_1 and Z_2 and a single quantitative explanatory variable X

(a) write down the equation of the interaction model.

(b) determine the slope of the regression line when $Z_1 = Z_2 = 1$ for the interaction model.

(c) determine the slope of the regression line when $Z_1 = Z_2 = 0$ for the interaction model.

(d) determine the slope of the regression line when $Z_1 = 1$ and $Z_2 = 0$ for the interaction model.

9.75 Suppose a dummy variable multiple regression model is fit with a single dummy variable Z and a single explanatory variable X. If the resulting fitted model is

$$\widehat{y} = 10.2 - 2.1Z + 4.5X + 1.1XZ$$

(a) determine the equation of the fitted regression line for $Z = 0$.

(b) determine the equation of the fitted regression line for $Z = 1$.

(c) determine the difference between the predicted values of Y when $X = 4$ for $Z = 0$ and $Z = 1$.

9.76 Using the interaction model as the full model, determine which models will need to be fit when testing whether or not

(a) the dummy variable is needed in the regression model.

(b) the interaction model is a better fitting model than the no-interaction model?

9.77 In the article "Age as a prognostic factor for complications of major head and neck surgery" published in the *Archives of Otolaryngology – Head & Neck Surgery* (Boruk et al., 2005), the authors reported the results given in Table 9.30 for a regression model to predict the hospital length of stay that included a dummy variable for the sex of an individual (Sex) and a dummy variable indicating whether or not an individual was younger than 70 or older (Age). Use the information in Table 9.30 to answer the following:

(a) Does the sex of an individual appear to be an important variable for predicting the hospital length of stay? Explain.

(b) Does it appear that knowing whether or not an individual is younger than 70 is useful in predicting the hospital length of stay? Explain.

(c) Can the simultaneous importance of the dummy variables Sex and Age be tested? Explain.

TABLE 9.30 Regression Coefficients for Modeling Hospital Length of Stay

Variable	Coefficient (SE)	t	p
Sex	0.729 (1.132)	0.644	0.52
CCI score	0.883 (0.356)	2.482	0.01
TUGA in min	0.017 (0.003)	5.689	< 0.001
ASA class	1.308 (1.119)	1.168	0.24
Age < 70 years versus older	−0.960 (1.405)	−0.683	0.50
Constant	−4.322 (2.467)	−1.752	0.08

TABLE 9.31   Regression Coefficients for a Multiple Regression Model of the Number of Hours Per Week Spent Seeing Patients

Variable	Estimate (SE)	t-Value	P-Value
Intercept	33.81 (8.49)	3.98	< 0.01
Sex	-2.17 (2.56)	-0.85	0.40
Age	-0.14 (0.25)	-0.57	0.57
Marital status	-0.03 (2.34)	-0.01	0.99
Parental status	4.99 (3.46)	1.44	0.15
Interaction of sex and parental status	-7.63 (4.14)	-1.84	0.07

(d) Based on the information in Table 9.30 which variables appear to be important for predicting the hospital length of stay?

9.78   In the article "Gender and Parenting significantly affect work hours of recent dermatology program graduates" published in the *Archives of Dermatology* (Jacobson et al., 2004), the authors reported the results given in Table 9.31 for a regression model to predict the number of hours per week spent seeing patients for recent dermatology program graduates. The multiple regression model reported by the authors included dummy variables for the sex of an individual, marital status, parental status, and the interaction between sex and parental status. Use the information in Table 9.31 to answer the following:

(a) Does the marital status of a recently graduated dermatologist appear to be an important variable for predicting the number of hours per week spent seeing patients? Explain.

(b) Does the parental status of a recently graduated dermatologist appear to be an important variable for predicting the number of hours per week spent seeing patients? Explain.

(c) Does the sex of a recently graduated dermatologist appear to be an important variable for predicting the number of hours per week spent seeing patients? Explain.

(d) How could the simultaneous importance of the dummy variables for the sex, marital status, parental status, and interaction between sex and parental status be tested?

9.79   In the article "Sensitivity to reward and body mass index: evidence for a nonlinear relationship" published in *Appetite* (Davis and Fox, 2008), the authors reported the ANOV table given in Table 9.32 for the multiple regression model

$$SR = \beta_0 + \beta_1 \text{Sex} + \beta_2 B + \beta_3 B^2 + \beta_4 \text{SEX} \cdot B + \beta_5 \text{Sex} \cdot B^2 + \epsilon$$

TABLE 9.32   ANOV Table for Model $SR = \beta_0 + \beta_1$ Sex $+ \beta_2 B + \beta_3 B^2 + \beta_4 \text{SEX} \cdot B + \beta_5 \text{Sex} \cdot B^2 + \epsilon$

Source	df	SS	MS
Regression	5	429.8	85.96
Error	360	4021.9	11.2
Total	365	4451.7	

TABLE 9.33   ANOV Table for the Model SR $= \beta_0 + \beta_1$ Sex $+ \beta_2 B + \beta_3 B^2 + \epsilon$

Source	df	SS	MS
Regression	3	403.3	85.96
Error	362	4048.4	11.3
Total	365	4451.7	

where SR is a measure of sensitivity to reward, Sex is a dummy variable that is 1 for a male and 0 for a female, and B is the standardized value of BMI. Suppose the ANOV table given in Table 9.33 resulted from fitting the model

$$SR = \beta_0 + \beta_1 \text{Sex} + \beta_2 B + \beta_3 B^2 + \epsilon$$

Use the information in Tables 9.32 and 9.33 to answer the following:

(a) Test $H_0 : \beta_4 = \beta_5 = 0$.

(b) Using the model suggested by the test in part (a), predict the value of SR when Sex $= 1$ and $B = 0.3$.

9.80 What are the two statistics that the variable selection procedures are based on?

9.81 What is an

(a) overfit model?   (b) undefit model?

9.82 Why must a good fitting full model be found before applying a variable selection procedure?

9.83 Why is it inappropriate to simply apply a variable selection procedure and accept the model that best satisfies the selection criterion as the final model?

9.84 After applying a variable selection procedure for screening the explanatory variables, what is the procedure used for selecting the final model?

9.85 What are the two formulas that can be used for computing BIC?

9.86 Use the variable selection summary output given in Table 9.34 for 10 screening explanatory variables on a data set having $n = 70$ observations to answer the following:

(a) Which of the 10 explanatory variables has the highest correlation with the response variable? Explain.

(b) If any two models with R^2_{adj} values differing by less than 0.02 (2%) are not practically different, which model having the fewest variables is the best model?

(c) Compute the value of BIC for each of the models listed in Table 9.34.

(d) If any two models with BIC values differing by less than 2 are not practically different, which model having the fewest variables is the best model?

9.87 In the article " Glucose metabolism and coronary heart disease in patients with normal glucose tolerance" published in the *Journal of the American Medical Association*, (Sasso et al., 2004) used a stepwise regression procedure to model the response variable Duke Myocardial Jeopardy Score as a function of 11 available explanatory variables based on a sample of $n = 234$ observations. The authors began

TABLE 9.34   Variable Selection Output for Exercise 9.34

Variables in the Model	R^2	R^2_{adj}	s_e
X_5	41.8	40.8	48.035
X_3	25.8	24.5	54.233
$X_3, X_5 5$	56.4	54.8	41.969
X_5, X_9	54.2	52.6	42.988
X_3, X_5, X_9	63.7	61.7	38.646
X_4, X_5, X_9	59.4	57.2	40.832
X_3, X_4, X_5, X_9	66.3	63.8	37.572
X_3, X_5, X_9, X_{10}	65.3	62.7	38.115
X_2, X_4, X_5, X_6, X_9	68.2	65.2	36.803
$X_3, X_4, X_5, X_9, X_{10}$	67.7	64.7	37.108
$X_2, X_4, X_5, X_6, X_9, X_{10}$	70.2	66.7	36.010
$X_2, X_3, X_4, X_5, X_9, X_{10}$	69.8	66.4	36.209
$X_2, X_3, X_4, X_5, X_6, X_9, X_{10}$	71.2	67.2	35.731
$X_2, X_3, X_4, X_5, X_7, X_9, X_{10}$	70.6	66.6	36.064
$X_2, X_3, X_4, X_5, X_6, X_7, X_9, X_{10}$	71.9	67.4	35.661
$X_2, X_3, X_4, X_5, X_6, X_8, X_9, X_{10}$	71.2	66.6	36.070
$X_1, X_2, X_3, X_4, X_5, X_6, X_7, X_9, X_{10}$	71.9	66.8	35.970
$X_2, X_3, X_4, X_5, X_6, X_7, X_8, X_9, X_{10}$	71.9	66.7	36.022
All 10	71.9	66.1	36.343

with an empty model and at each successive step of their model building approach a new variable was added to the model. Use the summary statistics given in Table 9.35 to answer the following:

(a) Determine the value of R^2_{adj} for each of the 11 models that were fit.

(b) Which model has the highest R^2_{adj} value?

(c) If there is no scientific reason to include any particular explanatory variable in the final model, is there any to use a model with more than eight variables? Explain.

(d) The authors claimed that all 11 explanatory variables are important for explaining the Duke Myocardial Jeopardy Score. If any two models with R^2_{adj} values differing by less than 0.02 (2%) are not practically different, which model is the best model?

9.88   Use the information given in Table 9.35 and SSTot $= 1208$ to answer the following:

TABLE 9.35   Summary of a Stepwise Approach to Building a Regression Model for the Response Variable Duke Myocardial Jeopardy Score

No. of Variables	R^2	No. of Variables	R^2
1	0.364	7	0.679
2	0.521	8	0.685
3	0.620	9	0.687
4	0.641	10	0.688
5	0.661	11	0.688
6	0.672		

(a) Determine the value of SSE for each of the 11 models that were fit.

(b) Determine the BIC value for each of the 11 models that were fit.

(c) Which model has the highest BIC value?

(d) If there is no scientific reason to include any particular explanatory variable in the final model is there any reason to use a model with more than eight variables? Explain.

(e) If any two models with BIC values differing by less than 2 are not practically different, which model having the fewest variables is the best model?

9.89 Use the Body Fat data set with Density as the response variable and Age, Height, Neck, Chest, Abdomen, Knee, Ankle, Biceps, and Forearm as the explanatory variables to answer the following:

(a) Fit the full model and check the regression assumptions.

(b) Apply the maximum R_{adj}^2 variable selection procedure and determine the three best fitting models.

(c) Based on the three best fitting models does it appear that age is an important variable for predicting body density? Explain.

(d) Based on the three best fitting models does it appear that forearm circumference is an important variable for predicting body density? Explain.

(e) If any two models with R_{adj}^2 values differing by less than 0.02 (2%) are not practically different, which model having the fewest variables should be considered the best model?

9.90 Use the Body Fat data set with Weight as the response variable and Age, Height, Neck, Chest, Abdomen, Knee, Ankle, Biceps, and Forearm as the explanatory variables to answer the following:

(a) Fit the full model and check the regression assumptions.

(b) Apply the maximum R_{adj}^2 variable selection procedure and determine the three best fitting models.

(c) Based on the three best fitting models does it appear that age is an important variable for predicting Weight? Explain.

(d) Based on the three best fitting models does it appear that biceps circumference is an important variable for predicting Weight? Explain.

(e) If any two models with R_{adj}^2 values differing by less than 0.02 (2%) are not practically different, which model having the fewest variables is the best model?

9.91 Use the Body Fat data set with Density as the response variable and Age, Height, Neck, Chest, Abdomen, Thigh, Ankle, Biceps, and Forearm as the explanatory variables to answer the following:

(a) Fit the full model and check the regression assumptions.

(b) Apply the BIC variable selection procedure and determine the three best fitting models.

(c) Based on the three best fitting models does it appear that age is an important variable for predicting body density? Explain.

(d) Based on the three best fitting models does it appear that biceps circumference is an important variable for predicting body density? Explain.

(e) If any two models with BIC values differing by less than 2 are not practically different, which model having the fewest variables is the best model?

9.92 Use the Body Fat data set with Weight as the response variable and Age, Height, Neck, Chest, Abdomen, Thigh, Ankle, Biceps, and Forearm as the explanatory variables to answer the following:

(a) Fit the full model and check the regression assumptions.

(b) Apply the BIC variable selection procedure and determine the three best fitting models.

(c) Based on the three best fitting models does it appear that the explanatory variable Age is an important variable for predicting Weight? Explain.

(d) Based on the three best fitting models does it appear that the explanatory variable Ankle is an important variable for predicting Weight? Explain.

(e) If any two models with BIC values differing by less than 2 are not practically different, which model having the fewest variables is the best model?

LOGISTIC REGRESSION

IN CHAPTERS 8 AND 9, linear regression models were discussed for building statistical models that could be used to explain how a quantitative response variable is related to a set of explanatory variables. In this chapter, statistical models for a dichotomous qualitative response variable will be discussed. In particular, the statistical models that will be discussed in Chapter 10 are *logistic regression models* or *binary regression models*. Moreover, analogous to linear regression, a logistic regression model can be a simple linear logistic regression model or a multiple logistic regression model. The use of logistic regression has only recently been made possible with the widespread availability of microcomputers and statistical computing packages, and as a result, logistic regression models are now commonly used in biomedical research for modeling a dichotomous response variable as a function of a set of explanatory variables.

Example 10.1
Logistic regression models could be used to model the response variable when investigating

  a. the survival of an individual after receiving a particular treatment.
  b. the presence of a disease based on the presence or absence of a particular gene.
  c. the presence of severe side effects after receiving a particular treatment.
  d. whether an individual's blood pressure can be lowered by a new drug.
  e. the presence of coronary heart disease is related to the age of an individual.

As is the case with linear regression models, one of the primary uses of logistic regression is to build a statistical model that can be used to understand how a dichotomous response variable varies over a set of explanatory variables. The main difference between a logistic regression model and a linear regression model is that a logistic regression model models the probabilities associated with the response variable rather than modeling the actual values of the response variable. While there are some important differences between the statistical analysis of a logistic regression model and a linear regression model, there are many similarities used in building, assessing, and using the fitted model in logistic and linear regression.

Because the response variable in a logistic regression model is a dichotomous variable it is convenient to code the response variable as a *binary variable* that takes on the value 1 when a particular characteristic is present and 0 when the characteristic is absent. For example, a researcher studying cancer may be interested in whether or not a patient's cancer has gone into remission after treatment. In this case, the response variable could be coded as 1 when a patient's cancer is in remission and 0 when it is not. Throughout Chapter 10 the response variable will be treated as a binary variable with

$$Y = \begin{cases} 1 & \text{when the characteristic is present} \\ 0 & \text{when the characteristic is absent} \end{cases}$$

10.1   ODDS AND ODDS RATIOS

A logistic regression model for a binary response variable is a model based on the *odds* that the response variable has the characteristic of interest (i.e., $Y = 1$). The odds that the response variable has the characteristic (i.e., $Y = 1$) is the ratio of the probability that the characteristic is present and the probability that the characteristic is absent. In particular,

$$\text{odds}(Y = 1) = \frac{P(Y = 1)}{P(Y = 0)}$$

The odds that $Y = 1$ ranges between 0 and ∞ and can be interpreted as the likelihood of the event $Y = 1$ relative to the event $Y = 0$. When the odds that $Y = 1$ is larger than 1, the event $Y = 1$ is more likely to occur than the event $Y = 0$, and when the odds is less than 1 the event $Y = 1$ is likely to occur than is $Y = 0$. Thus, the larger the odds of $Y = 1$ the more likely the event $Y = 1$ to occur.

Example 10.2
Suppose the probability that $Y = 1$ is 0.75. Then, the probability that $Y = 0$ is 0.25 and the odds that $Y = 1$ is

$$\text{odds}(Y = 1) = \frac{P(Y = 1)}{P(Y = 0)} = \frac{0.75}{0.25} = 3$$

In this case, $Y = 1$ is three times as likely to occur as $Y = 0$.

In most biomedical research studies, the goal is to investigate how the response variable Y depends on a particular set of explanatory variables. When a binary response variable is expected to depend on the values of the explanatory variable, the most relevant odds are the odds that $Y = 1$ conditioned on a particular set of values of the explanatory variable. That is, the odds that are generally studied in a biomedical research study are

$$\text{odds}(Y = 1 | X = x) = \frac{P(Y = 1 | X = x)}{P(Y = 0 | X = x)}$$

Note that when there are two or more explanatory variables being used to explain Y, X will be a vector of values of the explanatory variables.

Example 10.3

In a study on health problems associated with smoking, a researcher might be interested in the relationship between the response variable

$$Y = \begin{cases} 1 & \text{Individual has lung cancer} \\ 0 & \text{Individual does not have lung cancer} \end{cases}$$

and the explanatory variable

$$\text{Smokes} = \begin{cases} 1 & \text{Individual smokes 1 or more packs of cigarettes per day} \\ 0 & \text{Individual does not smoke 1 or more packs of cigarettes per day} \end{cases}$$

In this case, there are two odds that could be computed, namely, the odds that $Y = 1|\text{Smokes} = 0$ and the odds that $Y = 1|\text{Smokes} = 1$, and a comparison of these two odds will provide important information on whether or not the explanatory variable Smokes is associated with the incidence of lung cancer.

Comparing the odds that $Y = 1$ for several different values of an explanatory variable can be used to determine how the odds that $Y = 1$ varies over a set of values of an explanatory variable. In particular, when the odds that $Y = 1$ are the same for all of the values of explanatory variable X, the variables Y and X will be independent. On the other hand, when the odds that $Y = 1$ vary over the different values of an explanatory variable X, the response variable and explanatory variable will be associated (i.e., dependent). The comparison of the odds that $Y = 1$ for two different values on an explanatory variable is usually based on the ratio of the odds and is called the *odds ratio*. In particular, the odds ratio for two values of an explanatory variable, $X = x_1$ and $X_2 = x_2$ is

$$\text{odds ratio} = \text{OR} = \frac{\text{odds}(Y = 1|X = x_1)}{\text{odds}(Y = 1|X = x_2)}$$

Note that the odds ratio is a measure of the relative likelihood that $Y = 1$ for $X = x_1$ and $X = X_2$, and the odds ratio takes on values between 0 and ∞. Furthermore, when the odds ratio is

- equal to 1, the likelihood that $Y = 1$ is the same for these two values of X.
- less than 1, the likelihood that $Y = 1$ is smaller when $X = x_1$ than it is when $X = x_2$.
- greater than 1, the likelihood that $Y = 1$ is larger when $X = x_1$ than it is when $X = x_2$.

Note that the odds ratio measures only the relative likelihood that $Y = 1$, and not the likelihood that $Y = 1$ for either of the two values x_1 and x_2. For example, if the odds ratio for comparing the odds when $X = x_1$ and when $X = x_2$ is $\text{OR} = 4$, then this means that event $Y = 1$ is four times as likely to occur when $X = x_1$ than it is when $X = x_2$; however, in no way does $\text{OR} = 4$ measure the likelihood that $Y = 1$ since the odds ratio can be 4 when $P(Y = 1|X = x_1) = 0.6$ and $P(Y = 1|X_2 = x_2) = 0.15$ or when $P(Y = 1|X = x_1) = 0.16$ and $P(Y = 1|X_2 = x_2) = 0.04$.

Example 10.4

Use the probabilities given in Table 10.1 to answer the following:

    a. Compute odds that $Y = 1$ when $X = 0$.
    b. Compute odds that $Y = 1$ when $X = 1$.
    c. Compute odds ratio when $X = 0$ and $X = 1$.

TABLE 10.1   2 × 2 Table of Probabilities for the Variables *Y* and *X*

X	*Y*	
	0	1
0	0.10	0.90
1	0.40	0.60

Solutions Using the probabilities in Table 10.1,

a. the odds that $Y = 1$ when $X = 0$ is odds$(Y = 1|X = 0) = \frac{0.90}{0.10} = 9$. Thus, the event that $Y = 1$ is nine times as likely as the event $Y = 0$ when $X = 0$.

b. the odds that $Y = 1$ when $X = 0$ is odds$(Y = 1|X = 1) = \frac{0.60}{0.40} = 1.5$. Thus, the event that $Y = 1$ is 1.5 times as likely as the event $Y = 0$ when $X = 1$.

c. the odds ratio when $X = 0$ and $X = 1$ is OR $= \frac{9}{1.5} = 6$. Thus, the event $Y = 1$ is six times as likely to occur when $X = 0$ than it is when $X = 1$.

Example 10.5

In the article "Deep vein thrombosis in stroke: the use of plasma D-dimer level as a screening test in the rehabilitation setting" published in *Stroke* (Harvey et al., 1996), the authors reported the results of a study on 105 patients having deep vein thrombosis (DVT) identified by a venous duplex ultrasound (VDU). The results of the study are summarized in Table 10.2.

Based on the information in Table 10.2, the estimated odds ratio for comparing the odds that the VDU test is positive for the two D-dimer cutoff values is

$$\widehat{OR} = \frac{0.12 \times 0.69}{0.18 \times 0.01} = 46$$

and therefore, it appears that a positive VDU test for deep vein thrombosis using a D-dimer cutoff of >1591 is 46 times as likely as a positive VDU test for deep vein thrombosis using a D-dimer cutoff of ≤ 1591.

Finally, the relative risk and the odds ratio are both measures of the association between a response variable and an explanatory variable, and the odds ratio is approximately equal to the relative risk when the probabilities associated with $Y = 1$ are small. One advantage of using the odds ratio in biomedical research is that the odds ratio can be used in prospective, case control, and retrospective studies while the relative risk is appropriate only in prospective studies. Moreover, because logistic regression models are directly related to the odds and odds ratio, the odds ratio is a commonly reported statistic in biomedical research studies involving a binary response variable.

TABLE 10.2   Results of a Study on 105 Patients Having Deep vein Thrombosis

D-dimer Cutoff	Positive VDU	Negative VDU
D-dimer >1591 ng/mL	0.12	0.18
D-dimer ≤ 1591 ng/mL	0.01	0.69

10.2   THE LOGISTIC REGRESSION MODEL

When the response variable Y is a binary variable, the important parameters associated with the distribution of Y are $p = P(Y = 1)$ and $1 - p = P(Y = 0)$. Two reasons why a linear regression model is not appropriate for modeling a binary response variable Y or $p = P(Y = 1)$ as a function of a set of explanatory variables are

1. a good model for Y would return only predicted values of 1 and 0 that is unlikely and nearly impossible for a linear regression model to do.

2. a good model for $P(Y = 1)$ would return only estimated probability values between 0 and 1 that is unlikely and nearly impossible for a linear regression model to do.

Logistic regression is one of the most common statistical approaches used for modeling the probabilities associated with a binary response variable. The *logistic regression model* for modeling $P(Y = 1)$ as a function of a set of explanatory variables, say $X_1, X_2, \ldots, X_p$, is given by

$$P(Y = 1 | X_1, X_2, \ldots, X_p) = \frac{e^{\beta_0 + \beta_1 X_1 + \beta_2 X_2 + \beta_3 X_3 + \cdots + \beta_p X_p}}{1 + e^{\beta_0 + \beta_1 X_1 + \beta_2 X_2 + \beta_3 X_3 + \cdots + \beta_p X_p}}$$

However, a simpler form of the model can be expressed in terms of the *logit* of the probability that $Y = 1$. The *logit transformation* of $p = P(Y = 1)$ is

$$\text{logit}(p) = \ln\left(\frac{p}{1 - p}\right)$$

and the inverse of the logit function is called the *logistic function*. That is, when $\text{logit}(p) = \lambda$ it follows from the logistic function that $p = \frac{e^\lambda}{1 + e^\lambda}$.

When the logit transformation is used for modeling p than the odds that $Y = 1$ in a logistic regression model are

$$\text{odds}(Y = 1 | X_1, X_2, \ldots, X_p) = e^{\beta_0 + \beta_1 X_1 + \beta_2 X_2 + \beta_3 X_3 + \cdots + \beta_p X_p}$$

and therefore, the logarithm of the odds (i.e., the logit of p) is

$$\text{logit}[\, p(Y = 1 | X_1, X_2, \ldots, X_p)\,] = \ln[\text{odds}(Y = 1 | X_1, X_2, \ldots, X_p)]$$

$$= \beta_0 + \beta_1 X_1 + \beta_2 X_2 + \beta_3 X_3 + \cdots + \beta_p X_p$$

Thus, the logit of p is linear in the explanatory variables $X_1, X_2, \ldots, X_p$. Furthermore, the values of the *logit* function can range from $-\infty$ to ∞, which leaves the βs free to range over $-\infty$ and ∞ and the corresponding values of p free to range from 0 to 1.

In general, a logistic regression model is stated in terms of the logit of the probability that $Y = 1$ because it produces a simpler form than does the logistic model for the probability that $Y = 1$. Thus, the logistic regression model based on the explanatory variables $X_1, X_2, \ldots, X_p$ is

$$\text{logit}[\, p(\vec{X})\,] = \beta_0 + \beta_1 X + \beta_2 X_2 + \cdots + \beta_p X_p$$

where $\vec{X} = (X_1, X_2, \ldots, X_p)$. The *logistic regression coefficients* are $\beta_0, \beta_1, \beta_2, \ldots, \beta_p$, where β_0 is called the intercept and $\beta_1, \beta_2, \ldots, \beta_p$ are called the *logistic regression slopes*. Also, because a logistic regression model is a model for a probability rather than a value of the response variable, there is no error term in a logistic regression model. That is,

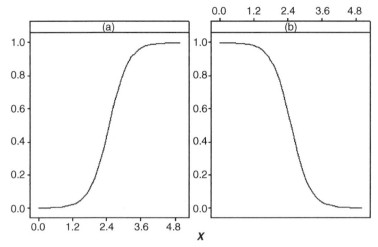

Figure 10.1   Logistic curves for $\beta_1 > 0$ (a) and $\beta_1 < 0$ (b).

probabilities, unlike a response variable, are not random variables and do not require a random error term.

The simplest form of a logistic regression model is the *simple linear logistic regression model* that has a single explanatory variable X. A simple linear logistic regression model is

$$\text{logit}[\,(p(X)\,] = \beta_0 + \beta_1 X$$

Note that in a simple linear logistic regression model the logit is modeled with a straight line. The logit line slopes upward when $\beta_1 > 0$ that also means the probability that $Y = 1$ increases as the variable X increases, and the logit line slopes downward for $\beta_1 < 0$ meaning that the probability that $Y = 1$ decreases as the variable X increases. Examples of logistic curves associated with logit lines having positive and negative slopes are shown in Figure 10.1.

In a linear regression model, the ith regression slope measures the expected change in the response variable for a one unit change in the explanatory variable X_i when all of the other explanatory variables are held fixed. In a logistic regression model, the ith logistic regression slope measures the change in the logit of $P(Y = 1)$ for a one unit change in the explanatory variable X_i when all of the other explanatory variables are held fixed. Furthermore, in a logistic regression model, e^{β_i} corresponds to the odds ratio for comparing $X_i = x + 1$ and $X_i = x$ since the difference of two logits corresponds to the logarithm of a ratio. In general, the odds ratio for comparing $X_i = s$ and $X_i = t$ when all of the other explanatory variables are held fixed is

$$\text{OR} = e^{\beta_i(s-t)}$$

Example 10.6
The logistic model $\text{logit}[\,p(\text{Age})\,] = \beta_0 + \beta_1 \times \text{Age}$ might be used for modeling the probability of the presence $(Y = 1)$ or absence $(Y = 0)$ of coronary heart disease as a function of the explanatory variable Age. The odds ratio that coronary heart disease is present for Age $= 55$ and Age $= 56$ is e^{β_1}, and the odds ratio that coronary heart disease is present for Age $= 55$ and Age $= 56$ is $e^{\beta(60-55)} = e^{5\beta_1}$.

Like linear regression models, logistic regression models can include dummy variables, interaction terms, and transformed explanatory variables such as X^2. In fact, the

TABLE 10.3 Odds Ratios For the Variables Age, Hypertension, and Stenosis ICA for the Incidence of Leukoaraiosis

Variable	Leukoaraiosis Odds Ratio
Age	1.06
Hypertension	2.33
Stenosis ICA	2.23

dummy variable interaction model is a commonly used as logistic regression model in many biomedical research studies; the interaction logistic regression model based on a single dummy variable and p explanatory variables includes all of the explanatory variables, the dummy variable, and the interaction terms formed by multiplying the dummy variable times each of the explanatory variable. For example, the dummy variable interaction model for a single dummy variable Z and two explanatory variables X_1 and X_2 is

$$\text{logit}[\,p(X_1, X_2, Z)\,] = \beta_0 + \beta_1 X_1 + \beta_2 X_2 + \beta_3 Z + \beta_4 X_1 Z + \beta_5 X_2 Z$$

The no interaction dummy variable logistic regression model includes only the dummy variable and the explanatory variables and is often compared with the interaction model when investigating the importance of a dummy variable.

Example 10.7
In the article "What is the significance of leukoaraiosis in patients with acute ischemic stroke?" published in the *Archives of Neurology* (Wiszniewska et al., 2000), the authors reported the odds ratios given in Table 10.3 for a fitted logistic regression model for the probability of leukoaraiosis in stroke patients. Based on the variables listed in Table 10.3, the logistic regression model was

$$\text{logit}(p) = \beta_0 + \beta_1 \text{Age} + \beta_2 \text{Hypertension} + \beta_3 \text{Stenosis ICA}$$

where hypertension and stenosis ICA are dummy variables.

Since the odds ratio for the explanatory variable X_i in a logistic regression model is e^{β_i}, based on the odds ratios given in Table 10.3, the estimated logistic regression slopes are $\ln(1.06) = 0.058$ for the variable Age, $\ln(2.33) = 0.846$ for Hypertension, and $\ln(2.23) = 0.802$ for Stenosis ICA. Note that the estimated intercept cannot be determined from the information in Table 10.3.

It is fairly common practice in biomedical articles for the authors to report the estimated odds ratio $e^{\widehat{\beta_i}}$ rather than the estimated logistic regression coefficient $\widehat{\beta_i}$ when summarizing a fitted logistic regression model.

10.2.1 Assumptions of the Logistic Regression Model

As is the case with any statistical model, there are several assumptions associated with a logistic regression model. The assumptions required of the logistic regression model are listed below.

ASSUMPTIONS OF A LOGISTIC REGRESSION MODEL

The assumptions associated with the logistic regression model

$$\text{logit}[\,p(\vec{X})\,] = \beta_0 + \beta_1 X_1 + \beta_2 X_2 + \cdots + \beta_p X_p$$

are

A1 The observations $Y_1, Y_2, \ldots Y_n$ are independent of one another.

A2 The explanatory variables are measured without error.

A3 There are no collinear relationships among the explanatory variables.

A4 The variation in the response variable follows the binomial variance function $\text{Var}(Y|\vec{X}) = p(\vec{X})(1 - p(\vec{X}))$.

A5 The sample size is sufficient for using large sample testing procedures.

Note that independence assumption, the assumption that the explanatory variables are measured without error, and the assumption that there are no collinear relationships between the explanatory variables, assumptions A1, A2, and A3 are also assumptions of a linear regression model. On the other hand, assumptions A4 and A5 are not assumptions associated with a linear regression model. In particular, assumption A4 states that the variability in the response variable will vary for different values of $\vec{X}$, whereas in a linear regression model the variance of the response variable is assumed to be the same for each value of $\vec{X}$.

When any of the assumptions required of a logistic regression model is violated, the validity of any inferences made from the fitted logistic regression model will be questionable. In particular when assumption the Y values are not independent, the estimated standard errors and the p-values associated with any hypothesis tests will be unreliable. A logistic regression model built on explanatory variables measured with error often leads to inaccurate and misleading statistical inferences. When there are collinear relationships between the explanatory variables, the estimated logistic regression coefficients, the estimated standard errors, and the p-values associated with any hypothesis test will be unreliable. When the variance of the response variable is larger than is predicted by the binomial variance function, the estimated logistic regression coefficients are unaffected, but the estimated standard errors of the logistic regression coefficients are underestimated, and the p-values associated with a hypothesis test may be unreliable. When the variance is larger than expected with binomial, the model is said to have *extrabinomial variation* or has an *overdispersion* problem. Finally, the large sample properties of the estimators of the logistic regression coefficients, such as large sample confidence intervals and hypothesis tests, will be reliable only when a sufficiently large sample is used.

Note that assumption A4 is an assumption about the variability of the response variable that is given by

$$\text{Var}(Y|\vec{X}) = p(\vec{X})(1 - p(\vec{X}))$$

and hence, in logistic regression the variance of the response variable varies with the values of the explanatory variables. When an extrabinomial variation is present, there is an overdispersion problem and the variance of the response variable is

$$\text{Var}(Y|\vec{X}) = \sigma^2 p(\vec{X})(1 - p(\vec{X}))$$

where $\sigma^2 > 1$; σ^2 is called the *dispersion parameter*. Extrabinomial variation often occurs when the observations on the response variable are not independent (i.e., assumption A1 is not valid) or when the model is incorrectly specified.

Because the violation of any of the assumptions required of a logistic regression model will affect the reliability of the inferences made from the fitted model, each of the five logistic regression assumptions must be checked, and an assumptions that is violated must be dealt with before using the fitted model to make inferences about the relationship between the response variable and the explanatory variables. Methods for checking the assumptions of a logistic regression model will be discussed in Section 10.4.

10.3   FITTING A LOGISTIC REGRESSION MODEL

The sample data for fitting the logistic regression model

$$\text{logit}[\, p(\vec{X})\,] = \beta_0 + \beta_1 X_1 + \beta_2 X_2 + \cdots + \beta_p X_P$$

consists of a sample of n independent multivariate observations on a binary response variable Y and the p explanatory variables. That is, the observed sample consists of n independent multivariate observations of the form $(Y, X_1, X_2, \ldots, X_p) = (Y, \vec{X})$. Note that the data structure for fitting a logistic regression model is similar to the data structure used in fitting a multiple linear regression model. The only difference between the two data structure is that the response variable in logistic regression is a binary variable and in a multiple linear regression model the response variable is a quantitative variable.

Unfortunately, the method of least squares cannot be used to fit a logistic regression model primarily because there is no additive error term in a logistic regression model. The method that is used to determine the estimates of the logistic regression coefficients and fit a logistic regression model is the method of *maximum likelihood estimation*. The maximum likelihood procedure is to choose the values of the logistic regression coefficients that maximize the *likelihood function*. The likelihood function for a logistic regression model is the product of the probabilities of the observed values of the response variable that is

$$L = \prod p_i^{y_i} (1 - p_i)^{1-y_i}$$

where $\prod$ is mathematical shorthand for product, $p_i = P(Y = 1 | \vec{X} = \vec{x}_i)$, and $\vec{x}_i$ is the vector of values of the explanatory variables for Y_i. In terms of the logistic regression coefficients, the likelihood function is

$$L = \prod \left(\frac{e^{\beta_0 + \beta_1 x_1 + \beta_2 x_2 + \cdots + \beta_p x_p}}{1 + e^{\beta_0 + \beta_1 x_1 + \beta_2 x_2 + \cdots + \beta_p x_p}} \right)^{y_i} \left(\frac{1}{1 + e^{\beta_0 + \beta_1 x_1 + \beta_2 x_2 + \cdots + \beta_p x_p}} \right)^{1-y_i}$$

The estimates of the logistic regression coefficients that maximize the likelihood function are called the *maximum likelihood estimates* or *MLEs* of the logistic regression coefficients. The maximum likelihood estimates of the logistic regression coefficients are denoted by $\widehat{\beta}_0, \widehat{\beta}_1, \widehat{\beta}_2, \ldots, \widehat{\beta}_p$ that are $\beta_0, \beta_1, \beta_2, \ldots, \beta_p$ that best agree with the observed data. Unfortunately, there are no closed form solutions (i.e., formulas) that can be used to compute the maximum likelihood estimates of the logistic regression coefficients, and hence, they must be found using a statistical computing package that will also provide information on the estimated standard errors, measures of the adequacy of the model's fit, and diagnostics for checking the assumptions.

When the sample size is sufficiently large and the model has been correctly specified, the maximum likelihood estimates are nearly unbiased, their standard errors can be easily computed, and their sampling distributions will be approximately normally distributed. Finally, the least squares estimates of the regression coefficients in a linear regression model are maximum likelihood estimates as well as least squares estimates when the normality assumption is valid. As always, no inferences should be made with a fitted statistical model until the model's fit and the assumptions of the model have been assessed.

Once a good fitting model has been found odds, ratios and probabilities can be estimated and inferences about the relationship between the response variable and the explanatory variables can be made. In particular, the maximum likelihood estimate of the odds ratio associated with a one unit change in the explanatory variable X_i when all of the other explanatory variables are held fixed is

$$\widehat{OR} = e^{\widehat{\beta_i}}$$

The maximum likelihood estimate of the probability that $Y = 1$ when $\vec{X} = (x_1, x_2, \ldots, x_p)$ is

$$\widehat{p}(x_1, x_2, \ldots, x_p) = \frac{e^{\widehat{\beta_0}+\widehat{\beta_1}x_1+\widehat{\beta_2}x_2+\cdots+\widehat{\beta_p}x_p}}{1 + e^{\widehat{\beta_0}+\widehat{\beta_1}x_1+\widehat{\beta_2}x_2+\cdots+\widehat{\beta_p}x_p}}$$

Example 10.8

The Coronary Heart Disease data set contains information on the presence or absence of coronary heart disease (CHD) and the age (Age) of $n = 100$ individuals. The response variable CHD is coded as

$$CHD = \begin{cases} 1 & \text{when coronary heart disease is present} \\ 0 & \text{when coronary heart disease is absent} \end{cases}$$

The results of the maximum likelihood procedure for fitting for the logistic regression model

$$\text{logit}[\, p(\text{Age})\,] = \beta_0 + \beta_1 \text{Age}$$

are summarized in Table 10.4.

Assuming the logistic regression assumptions are satisfied and the model's fit is acceptable, the summary statistics in Table 10.4 provide information that can be used to compute the equation of the fitted model, estimating the odds ratios, and for estimating the probability that $CHD = 1$ as a function of the explanatory variable Age. In particular,

1. the equation of the fitted logistic regression model is

$$\text{logit}[\, p(\text{Age})\,] = -5.310 + 0.111\text{age}$$

2. the odds ratio for comparing the odds of the presence of coronary heart disease for two ages separated by 1 year is

$$\widehat{OR} = e^{0.111} = 1.117$$

and the odds ratio for comparing the odds of the presence of coronary heart disease for two ages separated by 5 years is

$$\widehat{OR} = e^{5 \times 0.111} = 1.742$$

TABLE 10.4   The Results of the Maximum Likelihood Fit for the Logistic Regression Model logit[p(Age)] = $\beta_0 + \beta_1$Age

```
          Logistic Regression Table
```

Predictor	Coef	SE Coef
Constant	−5.30945	1.13365
AGE	0.110921	0.0240598

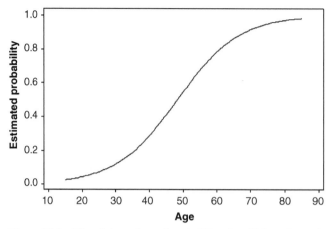

Figure 10.2   Plot of the estimated probability that CHD $= 1$ as a function of Age.

3. the estimate of the probability that coronary heart disease is present (i.e., CHD $= 1$) for an individual with Age $= 55$ is

$$\widehat{p}(55) = \frac{e^{-5.31+0.11\times55}}{1 + e^{-5.31+0.11\times55}} = 0.69$$

4. the graph of the estimated probability that coronary heart disease is present (i.e., CHD $= 1$) as a function of the age of an individual is given in Figure 10.2.

Note that the graph of the estimated probability that coronary heart disease is present (i.e., CHD $= 1$) as a function of the age shows that the presence of coronary heart disease is increasing with the age of an individual.

10.4   ASSESSING THE FIT OF A LOGISTIC REGRESSION MODEL

Before proceeding to make any inference with a fitted logistic regression model, the adequacy of the fitted model must be assessed. In particular, the validity of the logistic regression assumptions must be checked, the adequacy of the model's fit assessed, and the model's utility tested. In assessing the adequacy of the fit of a logistic regression model, the first step is to check the assumptions of the model, and when the assumptions appear to be valid then the fit of the model to the observed data is tested with a *goodness of fit test*. The residual diagnostics are investigated only for models that fit reasonably well since a poorly fitting model should never be used for making inferences about the relationship between the response and the explanatory variables.

10.4.1   Checking the Assumptions of a Logistic Regression Model

Recall that the five assumptions of a logistic regression model are independence of observations (A1), the explanatory variables are measured without error (A2), there are no collinear relationships between the explanatory variables (A3), there is no extrabinomial variation in the response variable (A4), and the sample size is sufficient for using the large sample properties of the maximum likelihood estimates and the likelihood function (A5).

The assumptions of the independence of observations and sufficient sample size should be accounted for in the design of the sampling plan used to collect the sample data used to fit the model. In fact, when the observations are not independent or the sample size is not sufficient for using the large sample properties of the maximum likelihood estimates, any statistical inference made from the fitted model will be highly unreliable. To ensure that the large sample properties of likelihood estimation are appropriate, the sample size should be relatively large and the number of variables in the fitted model should be less than 10% of the sample size (i.e., $p \leq \frac{n}{10}$).

The assumption that there is no measurement error in the explanatory variables is an important assumption that requires the researcher to have a clear understanding of the explanatory variables. In particular, the researcher should design the study so that only explanatory variables that can be measured without error are used in a logistic regression model. When the explanatory variable is known or even suspected of being measured with an error, a *measurement error modeling* approach should be used for building a logistic regression model. For more information on the effects and cures of measurement error problems in a logistic regression model see *Measurement Error in Nonlinear Models* (Carroll et al., 2006).

As is the case in linear regression, collinear relationships among the explanatory variables cause the estimated logistic regression coefficients, the estimated standard errors, and the *p*-values associated with a hypothesis test are to be unreliable and can lead to inaccurate and misleading inferences. Unfortunately, at the current time, most statistical computing packages do not include any collinearity diagnostics as part of their logistic regression fitting procedures. Since a collinearity problem is a problem that is based on the relationships between the observed values of the explanatory variables and does not involve the response variable, the variance inflation factors (VIF), which are widely available for fitting linear regression models, can be used to detect a collinearity problem in the explanatory variables as outlined below.

DETECTING COLLINEARITIES IN LOGISTIC REGRESSION

An approach that can be used for detecting collinearity problems in the explanatory variables $X_1, X_2, \ldots, X_p$ is to

1. first compute the pairwise correlations between the explanatory variables. Any two explanatory variables having a correlation of $|r| \geq 0.95$ are nearly collinear and should not be used together in the logistic regression model.

2. fit the linear regression model $Y = \beta_0 + \beta_1 x_1 + \beta_2 x_2 + \cdots + \beta_p x_p + \epsilon$, where Y is the binary response variable. If there are any *VIF* values that are greater than 10 for this regression model, then there is a collinearity problem with the explanatory variables that must be fixed before fitting the corresponding logistic regression model.

Note that the procedure outlined above is exactly the same procedure that was used when fitting a multiple linear regression model. Furthermore, the approaches used to eliminate collinearity problems in a multiple linear regression model can also be used to eliminate collinearity problems in a logistic regression model. In general, curing a collinearity problem is a difficult task and is best approached by carefully analyzing the relationships between the explanatory variables and by only fitting logistic regression models based on scientifically relevant subsets of the explanatory variables with no collinearity problems.

The assumption that the variation follows the binomial variance model is an important assumption that must be checked and dealt with in building a logistic regression model. Extrabinomial variability can seriously reduce the reliability of the maximum likelihood estimates of the logistic regression coefficients and any statistical inference based on the maximum likelihood estimates. The detection of an extrabinomial variation problem and methods for curing extrabinomial variation are beyond the scope of this text. For more information on detecting and curing extrabinomial variation, see *The Statistical Sleuth* (Ramsey, 2002).

10.4.2 Testing for the Goodness of Fit of a Logistic Regression Model

Once the assumptions have been checked and any violation of the assumptions have been dealt with appropriately, the next step in a logistic regression analysis is to assess the agreement between the fitted model and the observed data. Tests used to assess the agreement between the fitted model and the observed data are called *goodness-of-fit tests* and are used to test the following null and alternative hypotheses:

H_0: The response variable follows binomial distributions with probabilities specified by the logistic regression model.

H_A: The response variable does not follow binomial distributions with probabilities specified by the logistic regression model.

When the sample is sufficiently large and the number of variables in the model is not too large (i.e., $p < \frac{n}{10}$), a test statistic that can be used to test the goodness of fit for a logistic regression model is the *Hosmer–Lemeshow test statistic*. The Hosmer–Lemeshow test statistic is based on partitioning the observations into 10 groups according to their estimated probabilities and comparing the estimated probabilities with the observed proportions in each group. The goodness-of-fit test is carried out by simply comparing the p-value for the Hosmer–Lemeshow test statistic with a prespecified significance level α. That is, for an α level goodness-of-fit test, reject H_0 when the p-value associated with the Hosmer–Lemeshow test statistic is less than α; fail to reject H_0 when the p-value associated with the Hosmer–Lemeshow test statistic is greater than or equal to α. Fortunately, the Hosmer-Lemeshow test statistic and its p-value are generally included as part of the logistic regression output in most of the commonly used statistical computing packages.

When the Hosmer–Lemeshow p-value is less than α, conclude that there is a significant lack of agreement between the fitted logistic regression model and the observed data; when the p-value is greater than α, conclude that there is an adequate agreement (i.e., no significant lack of fit) between the fitted model and the observed data to proceed with the analysis of the logistic model. A model that exhibits significant lack of fit (i.e., p-value greater than α) should not be used for making inferences about the relationship between the response variable and the explanatory variables. Also, a p-value greater than α suggests that there is no significant lack of fit; however, this neither does mean that the model is the correct model nor does it necessarily mean that it fits the data all that well. Failing to reject the null hypothesis in a Hosmer–Lemeshow goodness-of-fit test simply means that the logistic regression analysis of the model that was fit should continue. Examples of the use of the Hosmer–Lemeshow goodness-of-fit test and its p-value are given in Examples 10.8 and 10.9

Example 10.9
For the logistic model

$$\text{logit}[\, p(\text{Age})\,] = \beta_0 + \beta_1 \text{Age}$$

TABLE 10.5 The Hosmer–Lemeshow Goodness of Fit Statistic and Its p-Value for the Model logit[p(Age)] $= \beta_0 + \beta_1$Age

```
Goodness-of-Fit Tests
Method                 Chi-Square    DF        P
Hosmer-Lemeshow           0.8900      8    0.999
```

that was fit to the Coronary Heart Disease data set in Example 10.8, the value of the Hosmer–Lemeshow goodness-of-fit test statistic and its p-value, computed by the statistical computing package MINITAB, are given in Table 10.5.

On the basis of the Hosmer–Lemeshow test statistic and its p-value of 0.999, there is no significant evidence of lack of fit in this model, and thus, it is reasonable to proceed with further analysis of this model.

Example 10.10

Using the Birth Weight data set to explore the relationship between low birth weight (LOW) and the explanatory variables mother's age (AGE), mother's weight at last menstrual period (LWT), and mother's smoking status during pregnancy (Smoke), the logistic regression model

$$\text{logit}(p) = \beta_0 + \beta_1\,\text{Age} + \beta_2\,\text{LWT} + \beta_3\,\text{Smoke}$$

was fit. Table 10.6 contains the maximum likelihood estimates of the logistic regression coefficients and Table 10.7 contains a summary of the Hosmer–Lemeshow goodness-of-fit test.

On the basis of the Hosmer–Lemeshow test statistic and its p-value of 0.550, there is no significant evidence of lack of fit in this model, and thus, it is reasonable to proceed with further analysis of this model.

10.4.3 Model Diagnostics

After developing a model that passes the goodness-of-fit test, the next step is to examine the residuals and residual-based diagnostics to identify any point that the model is not fitting well. Recall that the residuals of a fitted regression model contain the relevant information on how well the model is fitting the observed data. Similarly, the residuals of a fitted logistic regression model can also be used to assess the fit of a logistic regression model. The residuals associated with a logistic regression model are based on comparing the value of the response variable with the estimated probability of the response based on the fitted model.

A residual that is often used in assessing the fit of a logistic regression model is the *Pearson residual* that will be denoted by r. In particular, the Pearson residuals are computed for each of the distinct values of the explanatory variables and the value of r is

$$r = \frac{t - m\widehat{p}(\vec{x})}{\sqrt{m\widehat{p}(\vec{x})(1 - \widehat{p}(\vec{x}))}}$$

TABLE 10.6 Results of the Maximum Likelihood Fit for the Logistic Regression Model logit(p) $= \beta_0 + \beta_1$Age $+ \beta_2$LWT $+ \beta_3$Smoke

Predictor	Coef	SE Coef
Constant	1.36823	1.01426
AGE	−0.03900	0.03273
LWT	−0.01214	0.00614
SMOKE	0.67076	0.32588

TABLE 10.7   The Hosmer–Lemeshow Goodness-of-Fit Statistic and Its
p-Value for the Model $\text{logit}(p) = \beta_0 + \beta_1\text{Age} + \beta_2\text{LWT} + \beta_3\text{Smoke}$

```
Goodness-of-Fit Tests
Method                    Chi-Square        DF            P
Hosmer-Lemeshow               6.876          8        0.550
```

where t is the sum of the Y values for the set of explanatory variables $\vec{x}$, $\hat{p}(\vec{x})$ is the estimated probability of Y for $\vec{x}$, and m is the number of observations having the explanatory condition $\vec{x}$. It is important to note that unlike the residuals in a regression analysis, the Pearson residuals are not computed for every observation of the response variable in the data set. That is, they are only computed for the values of the response variable having a distinct set of explanatory conditions $\vec{x}$. For example, for the logistic regression model fit to the binary variable CHD in Example 10.8, the residuals are computed for each value of the variable Age. Example 10.11 illustrates how the Pearson residuals are computed for two different ages for the model fit in Example 10.8.

Example 10.11
In Example 10.8, a logistic regression model was fit to the response variable CHD with the explanatory variable Age. The first observation in the Coronary Heart Disease data set is CHD = 0 and Age = 20, and this the only observation for which AGE = 20. Thus, Age = 20 is a distinct explanatory condition.

In order to compute the Pearson residual for the explanatory condition Age = 20, an estimate of the probability that CHD = 1 must be computed first. The estimate of the probability that CHD = 1 when Age = 20 is

$$\hat{p}(20) = \frac{e^{-5.31+0.11\times20}}{1+e^{-5.31+0.11\times20}} = 0.043$$

Since the number of observations with Age = 20 is $m = 1$ and this observation has CHD = 0, the sum of the CHD values for Age = 20 is $t = 0$. Thus, the Pearson residual for the explanatory condition Age = 20 is

$$r = \frac{0 - 1 \times 0.043}{\sqrt{1 \times 0.043(1 - 0.043)}} = -0.21$$

Note that there are six observations with Age = 30 of which five are CHD = 0 and 1 is CHD = 1. Thus, for the explanatory condition Age = 30, the values of t and m are $t = 1$ and $m = 6$. The estimate of the probability that CHD = 1 when Age = 30 is

$$\hat{p}(30) = \frac{e^{-5.31+0.11\times30}}{1+e^{-5.31+0.11\times30}} = 0.12$$

and thus, the Pearson residual for Age = 30 is

$$r = \frac{0 - 6 \times 0.12}{\sqrt{6 \times 0.12(1 - 0.12)}} = 0.35$$

To judge whether or not a Pearson residual is large they will be standardized so that they all have common standard deviation 1. A standardized Pearson residual is denoted by r_s and is available in most of the commonly used statistical computing packages, and the standardized residuals can be used to identify points that the model is not fitting well. In particular, any standardized Pearson residual with $|r_s| \gg 3$ should be considered a large standardized residual and the observation associated with this residual investigated. Useful residual plots in a linear regression analysis are the plots of the standardized residuals versus the fitted values and versus each of the explanatory variables; however, because of the nature of the response variable (i.e., $Y = 0$ or $Y = 1$) in a logistic regression analysis, these plots are often hard to interpret and are not generally used. One type of residual plot that can be useful in identifying observations having large standardized Pearson residuals is a plot of the standardized residuals versus the observation indexes.

Example 10.12
A plot of the standardized residuals versus the observation indexes is given in Figure 10.3 for the model logit[$p(\text{Age})$] $= \beta_0 + \beta_1 \text{Age}$ for the binary response variable CHD in the Coronary Heart Disease data set.

Note that all of the standardized Pearson residuals fall between -3 and 3, and therefore, there is no evidence of any unusual observations based on the analysis of the standardized Pearson residuals. However, there is one residual that stands out from the others. In particular, the residual for the experimental condition Age $= 25$ has a standardized residual of $r_s = 2.37$ that is not unusually large but does stand out from the others. The reason why this standardized residual is large is that the estimated probability of CHD $= 1$ when Age $= 25$ is 0.07, and thus the model is saying that it is unlikely for CHD $= 1$ when Age $= 25$; however, one of the two observations in the data set for which Age $= 25$ did have evidence of coronary heart disease (i.e., CHD $= 1$). Thus, the model does not fit the observations on Age $= 25$ as well as it fits the observations on the other values of the variable Age.

Two residual diagnostics that can be used to detect outliers and observations that may have a large influence on the fitted logistic regression model are the $\Delta \chi^2$ statistic and the $\Delta \beta$ statistics. Both the $\Delta \chi^2$ and $\Delta \beta$ statistics are based on the standardized Pearson residuals, and when used together, can be powerful tools for identifying observations that might be strongly influencing the fit of the logistic regression model. Moreover, both $\Delta \chi^2$ and $\Delta \beta$ are available options in a logistic regression analysis in most of the commonly used statistical computing packages.

The $\Delta \chi^2$ statistic measures the change in the Pearson χ^2 statistic when all of the observations with the jth explanatory conditions are deleted. Pearson's χ^2 statistic is the sum of the squared Pearson residuals that can also be used for testing the goodness of fit of a logistic regression model. Explanatory conditions that have a large $\Delta \chi^2$ value identify explanatory conditions where the model is not fitting very well. In general, $\Delta \chi^2$ values tend

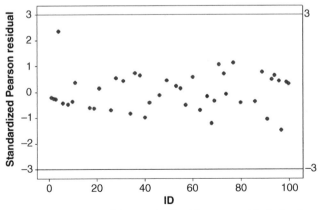

Figure 10.3 A plot of the standardized Pearson residuals for the model fit in Example 10.7 to the binary response variable CHD.

to be large when the estimated probability is between 0.0 and 0.1 and there are observed values of the response variable equal to 1. The values of $\Delta\chi^2$ may also be large when the estimated probability is between 0.9 and 1.0, and there are observed values of the response variable equal to 0. When the value of $\Delta\chi^2$ is large, the Pearson residual is generally also relatively large. That is, when $\widehat{p}$ is close to 0, the event $Y = 1$ should be very unlikely, and hence, the model may not fit well when there are too many observed values where $Y = 1$; similarly, when $\widehat{p}$ is close to 1, the event $Y = 0$ should be very unlikely, and hence, the model may not fit well when there are too many observed values where $Y = 0$.

Plots of the $\Delta\chi^2$ values that should be investigated include plots of the $\Delta\chi^2$ values versus the fitted probabilities and $\Delta\chi^2$ versus the observation index. The analysis of a $\Delta\chi^2$ plot is performed by looking for extremely large values of $\Delta\chi^2$ in a plot. The best approach in analyzing a $\Delta\chi^2$ plot is to look for observations with $\Delta\chi^2$ values much larger than the rest of the $\Delta\chi^2$ values. Experimental conditions where the fitted model does not appear to be fitting well should be carefully investigated.

Example 10.13
A plot of the $\Delta\chi^2$ values versus the observation index is given in Figure 10.4 for the model

$$\text{logit}(p) = \beta_0 + \beta_1 \text{Age}$$

fit in Example 10.8.

Note that there is one set of explanatory conditions that has a $\Delta\chi^2$ value that stands out from the rest. In particular, $\Delta\chi^2 = 5.6$ value for Age = 25 that also had a large standardized Pearson residual. As seen in Example 10.12, there is one observation with Age = 25 and CHD = 1 that the model does not fit well. The influence of this point should be further investigated.

Another diagnostic tool used to assess a model's fit is the $\Delta\beta$ statistic that is analogous to Cook's distance. The $\Delta\beta$ statistic measures the change in the estimated logistic regression coefficients when all of the observations with a particular explanatory condition are deleted from the analysis. In general, the standardized values of $\Delta\beta$ are used to detect potentially influential explanatory conditions. The value of $\Delta\beta$ tends to be large when the estimated probability is between 0.1 and 0.3 and there are observed values of the response variable equal to 1. The value of $\Delta\beta$ may also be large when the estimated probability is between 0.7 and 0.9, and there are observed values of the response variable equal to 0.

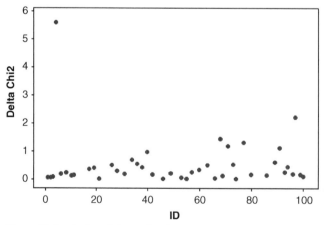

Figure 10.4   A plot of the $\Delta\chi^2$ values versus the observation index for the model $\text{logit}[\,p(\text{Age})\,] = \beta_0 + \beta_1 \text{Age}$.

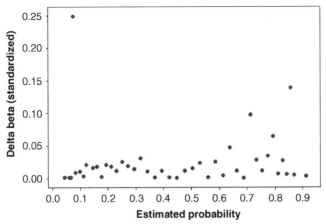

Figure 10.5   A plot of the $\Delta\beta$ values versus the estimated probability that CHD $= 1$ for the model logit[p(Age)] $= \beta_0 + \beta_1$Age.

Two plots that can be used to investigate the $\Delta\beta$ values are plots of $\Delta\beta$ versus the fitted probabilities and $\Delta\beta$ versus the observation index. Look for observations with $\Delta\beta$ values much larger than the rest of the $\Delta\beta$ values. Experimental conditions where $\Delta\beta$ is large suggest there is a large enough change in the estimated logistic regression coefficients that observations for these experimental conditions should be carefully investigated.

Example 10.14
A plot of the $\Delta\beta$ values versus the estimated probabilities is given in Figure 10.5 for the model

$$\text{logit}(p) = \beta_0 + \beta_1\text{Age}$$

fit in Example 10.8 using the Coronary Heart Disease data set.

Note that there is one set of explanatory conditions that has a $\Delta\beta$ value that stands out from the rest. In particular, $\Delta\beta = 0.25$ value for Age $= 25$ that also had a large standardized Pearson residual and a large $\Delta\chi^2$ value. As seen in Example 10.12, there is one observation with Age $= 25$ and CHD $= 1$ that the model does not fit well. The influence of this point should be further investigated.

To investigate the influence of the observations with explanatory conditions Age $= 25$, the model was refit without the observations for Age $= 25$. The resulting fitted logistic regression model without the observations with Age $= 25$ has an intercept $\widehat{\beta}_0 = -5.90$ and slope $\widehat{\beta}_1 = 0.123$; the slope and intercept for the full data set are -5.31 and 0.11. The estimated probability curves based on the fitted model with and without the observations with Age $= 25$ are given in Figure 10.6.

Since the slope, intercept, and more importantly the estimated probabilities do not differ much when the model is fit with or without the observations on Age $= 25$, the influence of these observations appears to be minor. Hence, the model fit to the full data set will be used for making statistical inferences.

Example 10.15
In Example 10.10, the logistic regression model

$$\text{logit}(p) = \beta_0 + \beta_1\text{AGE} + \beta_2\text{LWT} + \beta_3\text{SMOKE}$$

was fit using the Birth Weight data set. The p-value for the Hosmer–Lemeshow goodness-of-fit test was 0.550 suggesting there is no significant evidence of lack of fit in this model.

A plot of the standardized Pearson residuals versus observation index is given in Figure 10.7, and Figure 10.8 contains the model diagnostic plots of the $\Delta\chi^2$ and $\Delta\beta$ values versus the observation index.

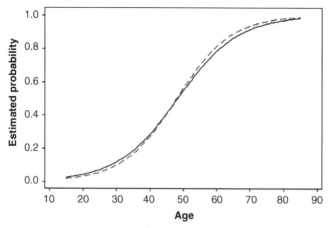

Figure 10.6 Plots of the estimated probability that CHD $= 1$ with the full data set represented by the solid line and without the observations for Age $= 25$ represented by the dashed line.

Note that all of the standardized residuals are between -3 and 3; however, there are one value of $\Delta \chi^2 > 6$ and two values of $\Delta \beta$ standing out from the rest of the observations. The influence of the two sets of explanatory conditions with large $\Delta \beta$ values, which includes the explanatory conditions for the largest value of $\Delta \chi^2$, can be investigated by deleting all of the points with these explanatory conditions and then refitting the model to the reduced data set.

The model fit to the reduced data set should be examined for large changes in the values of the logistic regression coefficients and the estimated probabilities. When the differences between the values of the logistic regression coefficients and the estimated probabilities are large for the full and reduced data sets, these two points are highly influential and must be further investigated.

Finally, because the model diagnostics used in a logistic regression analysis are interpreted visually, declaring a point an outlier or an influential point must be made subjectively. Assessing a multicollinearity or an extrabinomial variation problem in a logistic regression model is made somewhat subjectively. For these reasons, the fitting of a logistic regression model should be carried out only by an experienced and well-trained statistician.

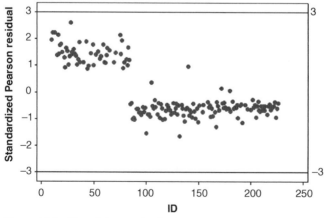

Figure 10.7 Plot of the standardized Pearson residuals against observation index for the model fit in Example 10.10 using the Birth Weight data set.

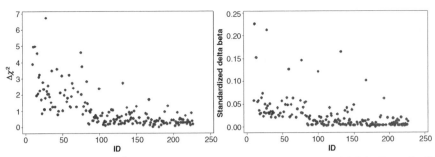

Figure 10.8   Plots of $\Delta \chi^2$ and $\Delta \beta$ against observation index for the model fit in Example 10.10 using the Birth Weight data set.

10.5   STATISTICAL INFERENCES BASED ON A LOGISTIC REGRESSION MODEL

After fitting and assessing the fit of a logistic regression model, provided none of the assumptions is violated and the model is fitting the observed data adequately, the fitted model can be used for making statistical inferences about the relationship between the response variable and the explanatory variables. In particular, inferences can be made about the importance of a single explanatory variable through the use of confidence intervals and hypothesis tests. Nested models can also be compared and used to test the importance of two or more explanatory variables included in the larger model, simultaneously.

10.5.1   Inferences about the Logistic Regression Coefficients

One of the advantages of using maximum likelihood estimation to fit a logistic regression model is that the large sample distribution of an estimate of a logistic regression coefficient (i.e., $\widehat{\beta}_i$) is known to be approximately normally distributed with mean β_i and standard deviation approximately $\text{se}(\widehat{\beta}_i)$ when the model is correctly specified. Thus, for sufficiently large samples, the sampling distribution of

$$Z = \frac{\widehat{\beta}_i - \beta_i}{\text{se}(\widehat{\beta}_i)}$$

will be approximately distributed as a standard normal, and the Z statistic can be used in hypothesis tests and confidence intervals for making statistical inferences about a logistic regression coefficient.

When the sample is sufficiently large an upper, lower, or two-tailed test about the ith regression coefficient β_i can be carried out using the Z statistic. In particular, when the null value of β_i is β_{i0} the Z test statistic is

$$Z = \frac{\widehat{\beta}_i - \beta_{i0}}{\text{se}(\widehat{\beta}_i)}$$

Since the explanatory variable X_i contributes nothing to a logistic regression model when $\beta_i = 0$, the most common hypothesis tested about a logistic regression slope is $H_0 : \beta_i = 0$.

The test statistic for testing $H_0 : \beta_i = 0$ is

$$Z = \frac{\widehat{\beta}_i}{\text{se}(\widehat{\beta}_i)}$$

A statistical computing package will typically report the maximum likelihood estimates of the logistic regression coefficients, their estimated standard errors, the value of the Z statistic for testing $H_0 : \beta_i = 0$ for each coefficient, and the p-values associated with the observed Z-values. Thus, testing the importance of the explanatory variable X_i in a logistic regression model simply amounts to examining the p-value associated with the Z test of $H_0 : \beta_i = 0$. When the p-value is less than the prespecified value of α, $H_0 : \beta_i = 0$ is rejected and the variable appears to be important variable in the logistic regression model; when the p-value is larger than the prespecified value of α there is no evidence that the variable is an important variable in the logistic regression model.

Example 10.16

The MINITAB output for the logistic regression model fit in Example 10.8 using the Coronary Heart Disease data set for relating the binary response variable CHD to the explanatory variable Age is given in Table 10.8.

Note that the MINITAB output includes the estimates of the logistic regression coefficients, their estimated standard errors, and the value of the Z statistic and its p-value for testing $H_0 : \beta_i = 0$. Since the p-value for testing the slope of the explanatory variable Age is $p = 0.000$, according to the observed data it appears that there is a significant relationship between the response variable CHD and the explanatory variable Age.

Note that the standard MINITAB output given in Table 10.8 also contains information on the odds ratio for the variable Age including a 95% confidence interval for the odds ratio. In this case, a 95% confidence interval for the odds ratio associated with a one unit increase in Age is 1.07–1.11.

The estimated odds ratio associated with the explanatory variable X_i is $\widehat{\text{OR}} = e^{\widehat{\beta}_i}$. The odds ratio is an important parameter in biomedical research that is used to measure the strength of the relationship between a response variable and an explanatory variable. Measures of the strength of the relationship between a response variable and an explanatory variable are often referred to as measures of the *effect size*. When the odds ratio is significantly different from 1, the effect size is said to be significant. A confidence interval for the odds ratio is based on the confidence interval for the logistic regression slope β_i.

Now, the formula for computing a large sample $(1 - \alpha) \times 100\%$ confidence interval for a logistic regression coefficient β_i is

$$\widehat{\beta}_i \pm z_{\text{crit}} \times \text{se}(\widehat{\beta}_i)$$

where the value of z_{crit} can be found in Table A.4. A $(1 - \alpha) \times 100\%$ confidence interval for the odds ratio associated with the explanatory variable X_i is computed by exponentiating the lower and upper end points of the confidence interval for β_i. That is, a $(1 - \alpha) \times 100\%$

TABLE 10.8   MINITAB Output for the Logistic Regression Model Fit in Example 10.8

Logistic Regression Table

Predictor	Coef	SE Coef	Z	P	Odds Ratio	95% CI Lower	Upper
Constant	−5.30945	1.13365	−4.68	0.000			
AGE	0.11092	0.02406	4.61	0.000	1.12	1.07	1.17

TABLE 10.9   MINITAB Output for the Logistic Regression Model Fit in Example 10.10

```
Logistic Regression Table

                                               Odds      95% CI
Predictor      Coef   SE Coef      Z       P   Ratio   Lower   Upper
Constant    2.06239   1.09516    1.88   0.060
AGE        -0.04478   0.03391   -1.32   0.187   0.96    0.89    1.02
LWT        -0.01701   0.00686   -2.48   0.013   0.98    0.97    1.00
SMOKE       0.65480   0.33297    1.97   0.049   1.92    1.00    3.70
```

confidence interval for the odds ratio associated with a one unit increase in the explanatory variable X_i when all of the other explanatory variables are held fixed is

$$e^{\widehat{\beta}_i - z_{\text{crit}} \times \text{se}(\widehat{\beta}_i)} \quad \text{to} \quad e^{\widehat{\beta}_i + z_{\text{crit}} \times \text{se}(\widehat{\beta}_i)}$$

Example 10.17
The MINITAB output for the logistic regression model fit in Example 10.10 using the Birth Weight data set for relating the binary response variable LOW to the explanatory variables AGE, LWT, and SMOKE is given in Table 10.9.

Based on the information in Table 10.9, the slope for the explanatory variable AGE is not significantly different from 0 ($p = 0.187$), but the slopes associated with the explanatory variables LWT ($p = 0.013$) and SMOKE ($p = 0.049$) are significantly different from 0 when $\alpha = 0.05$.

The estimated odds ratio for the dummy variable SMOKE is 1.92 with a confidence interval of 1.00–3.70. Thus, according to this logistic regression model, it appears that the odds of a low birth weight baby for a mother who smoked during pregnancy is possibly as much as 3.7 times the odds of having a low birth weight baby for a mother who did not smoke during pregnancy.

10.5.2 Comparing Models

When building a logistic regression model for a response variable based on a set of explanatory variables, it is often important to compare several different models. In a logistic regression analysis model, comparisons are based on the *log-likelihood statistic* that is the logarithm of the likelihood function evaluated at the parameter estimates or the *deviance* of the model that is $-2 \times$ log-likelihood. In general, the deviances of two models are used to compare two nested models using a drop-in-deviance test that is analogous to the extra sums of squares F statistic used to compare nested models in a linear regression analysis. The drop-in-deviance tests the simultaneous importance of a set of explanatory variables in a logistic regression model. For example, a drop-in-deviance test can be used to assess the importance of a categorical variable in a logistic regression model by testing the interaction model against the no-interaction model.

The drop-in-deviance test can be used to compare the fit of two models only when one of the models is nested in the other. A model is said to be nested in another when all of the variables in the reduced model are also included in the larger model. That is, the two models that can be tested with a drop-in-deviance test are

$$\text{Full model: } \text{logit}(p) = \beta_0 + \beta_1 X_1 + \cdots + \beta_k X_k + \cdots + \beta_p X_p$$

$$\text{Reduced model: } \text{logit}(p) = \beta_0 + \beta_1 X_1 + \cdots + \beta_k X_k$$

Note that there are p explanatory variables in the full model and k explanatory variables in the reduced model. In terms of the logistic regression slopes, the drop-in-deviance test for comparing the full and reduced model is a test of the null hypothesis

$$H_0 : \beta_{k+1} = \beta_{k+2} = \cdots = \beta_p = 0$$

The drop-in-deviance test statistic for comparing the full and reduced models is

drop-in-deviance = deviance (full model) − deviance (reduced model)

For sufficiently large samples, the drop-in-deviance statistic is approximately distributed as a χ^2 distribution with $p - k$ degrees of freedom. When the drop in deviance test statistic is large relative to the χ^2 distribution, then the p-value will be small and the drop-in-deviance statistic provides evidence against H_0. The four steps that must be carried out to test $H_0 : \beta_{k+1} = \beta_{k+2} = \cdots = \beta_p = 0$ (i.e., model I versus model II) are outlined below.

DROP-IN-DEVIANCE TEST

---

1. Fit the full model and assess the adequacy of fit. Do not proceed with the drop-in-deviance test until the full model adequately fits the observed data.

2. Fit the reduced model.

3. Compute the value of the drop-in-deviance test statistic, which has $p - k$ degrees of freedom.

4. Compute the p-value for this observed value of the drop-in-deviance test statistic the χ^2 distribution with $p - k$ degrees of freedom. Reject

$$H_0 : \beta_{k+1} = \beta_{k+2} = \cdots = \beta_p = 0$$

when the p-value is less than the prespecified value of α.

The drop-in-deviance test is often used to test all of the logistic regression slopes are equal to 0 (i.e., $H_0 : \beta_1 = \beta_2 = \cdots = \beta_p = 0$) that is known as the *model utility test*. The model utility test is a test of the full model that was fit against a model containing none of the explanatory variables at all. Thus, the model utility test in logistic regression is analogous to the model utility F-test in a linear regression analysis. The test statistic for the model utility test is based on the drop-in-deviance test statistic and is usually denoted by G. Large values of G will have small p-values, and H_0 is rejected for p-values smaller than the prespecified value of α. A significant model utility test suggests that at least one of the logistic regression slopes is significantly different from 0; however, it does not imply that the fitted model is a good fitting model. On the other hand, a nonsignificant model utility test suggests that the fitted model is no better than the empty model that contains none of the explanatory variables that were included in the fitted model, and in this case, the fitted model has no apparent utility for explaining the response variable.

Example 10.18

The MINITAB output for the model

$$\text{logit}(p) = \beta_0 + \beta_1 \text{AGE} + \beta_2 \text{LWT} + \beta_3 \text{SMOKE}$$

fit to the response variable LOW on the Birth Weight data set is given in Figure 10.9.

The MINITAB output contains the log-likelihood statistic and the results of the model utility test. For this model, the log-likelihood is -107.332 that means the deviance for this model is $-2 \times (-107.332) = 214.664$. Also, for the test of the model's utility is significant since the p-value associated with G is $p = 0.002$, and hence, $H_0 : \beta_1 = \beta_2 = \beta_3 = 0$ should be rejected. Thus, the logistic regression model with the explanatory variables AGE, LWT, and SMOKE fits better than a model with no explanatory variables at all.

Predictor	Coef	SE Coef	Z	P	Odds Ratio	95% CI Lower	Upper
Constant	2.06239	1.09516	1.88	0.060			
AGE	-0.04478	0.03391	-1.32	0.187	0.96	0.89	1.02
LWT	-0.01701	0.00686	-2.48	0.013	0.98	0.97	1.00
SMOKE	0.65480	0.33297	1.97	0.049	1.92	1.00	3.70

```
Log-Likelihood = -107.332
Test that all slopes are zero: G = 15.303, DF = 3, P-Value = 0.002
```

Figure 10.9   The MINITAB output for the model $logit(p) = \beta_0 + \beta_1 AGE + \beta_2 LWT + \beta_3 SMOKE$ fit to the Birth Weight data set.

Note a significant model utility test does not mean the model is the best model or even a good model; it simply means that the fitted model is a significantly better fitting model than is the model having no explanatory variables in it. For example, it is possible, and even common, to have a significant model utility test and a significant Hosmer–Lemeshow goodness-of-fit test. In this case, the fitted model has a significant lack of fit and does not fit the observed data very well even though it fits better than an empty model. Regardless of the model significance test, the model is a poorly fitting model and should not be used in making statistical inferences about the relationship between the response variable and the explanatory variables.

Example 10.19 illustrates how the importance of a dummy variable can be tested using a drop-in-deviance test.

Example 10.19
The Prostate Cancer Study data set contains data from a study carried out at the Ohio State University Comprehensive Cancer Center on prostate cancer patients. One of the goals of the study was to determine whether a set of variables measured during an initial exam can be used to determine whether or not a cancerous tumor has penetrated the prostatic capsule. The response variable in this study is

$$Capsule = \begin{cases} 1 & \text{if the tumor has penetrated the prostatic capsule} \\ 0 & \text{if the tumor has not penetrated the prostatic capsule} \end{cases}$$

Three explanatory variables that were measured at the initial exam that might be useful in predicting whether or not a cancerous tumor has penetrated the prostatic capsule are age (AGE), race (RACE), and prostatic specific antigen level (PSA). The dummy variable Race is coded as 1 when the subject is black and 0 when the subject is white.

The first model to be considered is the interaction model that is

$$logit(p) = \beta_0 + \beta_1 AGE + \beta_2 PSA + \beta_3 RACE$$
$$+ \beta_4 Race \times AGE + \beta_5 RACE \times PSA$$

The MINITAB output for the interaction model is given in Figure 10.10.

Note that the p-value for the Hosmer–Lemeshow goodness-of-fit test is $p = 0.183$, and therefore, there is no evidence of significant lack of fit with the interaction model.

Table 10.10 contains the values of the log-likelihood statistic for the interaction model and the no-interaction model. Using the information in Table 10.10 and a drop-in-deviance test to compare the fit of the interaction model with the no-interaction model, the drop-in-deviance test

```
Predictor          Coef    SE Coef     Z      P
Constant       -0.30044    1.14814  -0.26  0.794
AGE             0.00237    0.01741   0.14  0.892
PSA            -0.01687    0.00673  -2.51  0.012
RACE            7.92729    4.31765   1.84  0.066
RACE*AGE       -0.12936    0.06652  -1.94  0.052
RACE*PSA        0.02396    0.01808   1.33  0.185


Log-Likelihood = -247.598
Test that all slopes are zero: G = 11.391, DF = 5, P-Value = 0.044


Goodness-of-Fit Tests
Method             Chi-Square    DF      P
Hosmer-Lemeshow       11.336      8  0.183
```

Figure 10.10 MINITAB output for the interaction model.

statistic is

$$\text{drop-in-deviance} = 501.200 - 495.196 = 6.004$$

which has $5 - 3 = 2$ degrees of freedom. The p-value associated with a drop-in-deviance of 6.004 with 2 degrees of freedom is $p = 0.0497$ that is barely significant at the $\alpha = 0.05$ level. Thus, it appears that the interaction model fits slightly better than the no-interaction model, and race does have some value as a predictor of prostatic capsule penetration.

10.6 VARIABLE SELECTION

When building a logistic regression model from a large number of explanatory variables one of the primary goals of the statistical analysis will be to screen the explanatory variables and identify the explanatory variables that are most useful for explaining or predicting the response variable. In this case, a variable selection procedure can be used to investigate the importance of the explanatory variables, however, a variable selection procedure should only be used as a screening device and should never be used blindly as the method of determining the final model for relating the response variable to the explanatory variables. Furthermore, any model produced by a variable selection procedure should be subjected to scientific scrutiny to make sure the model is scientifically sound.

The goal of a variable selection procedure in a logistic regression analysis is to find a small set of models containing the fewest number of explanatory variables which do a good job of modeling the probability that the response variable $Y = 1$. The basic steps that should be followed when using a variable selection method for building a logistic regression model are outlined below.

TABLE 10.10 The Log-Likelihood and Deviance Statistics for the Interaction Model and the No-Interaction Model

Model	Number of Variables in the Model	Log-Likelihood	Deviance
Interaction	5	−247.598	495.196
No-interaction	3	−250.600	501.200
Without Race	2	−252.896	505.792

1. Develop a "good" fitting full model containing all of the predictors of interest. The full model should have no violations of the model assumptions, all influential points must have been dealt with, and there should be no collinearity problems among the explanatory variables.

2. Apply the variable selection procedure.

3. Identify the best models according to the variable selection criterion.

4. Choose a small number of models to consider as candidates for the final model.

5. Select and report the final model. The selection should be based on the outcome of the variable selection procedure and scientific reasoning.

A commonly used variable selection procedure in fitting logistic regression models is based on the *Bayes Information Criterion* (BIC). An advantage of using the BIC variable selection procedure is that it can be used with any statistical model that is fit using maximum likelihood estimation. The BIC procedure also tends to control against overfitting the true model. The formula for computing the BIC value associated with a logistic regression model is

$$\text{BIC} = \text{deviance} + (k + 1) \times \ln(n)$$

where k is the number of explanatory variables in the model and n is the sample size.

The BIC variable selection procedure is to select the models with lowest BIC values as competitors for the final model. Of course, the choice of the final model must be based on scientific reasons rather than purely statistical reasons. The steps that must be carried out when using the BIC variable selection procedure in a logistic regression analysis are outlined below.

THE BIC VARIABLE SELECTION PROCEDURE FOR LOGISTIC REGRESSION

Step 0 Fit the full model, check the model assumptions, and cure any problem suggested by the model diagnostics, before proceeding to step 1.

Step 1 Fit all possible logistic regression models based on the p explanatory variables in the full model and compute the value of BIC for each model.

Step 2 Determine the models having the smallest values of BIC. These models are the candidates for the final model.

Step 3 Select the final model based upon the value of BIC, the number of variables in the model, and scientific reasoning.

Note that the BIC variable selection procedure outlined above is exactly the same procedure that was used in Chapter 9 for a multiple regression model.

The final model should be selected according to the BIC criterion and scientific reasons. Also, when selecting the final model, values of BIC that differ by less than 2 are not generally considered statistically different. Thus, when comparing two models that have BIC values differing by less than 2, choose the model that contains fewer explanatory variables as the better candidate for the final model. Unfortunately, not all statistical computing packages have routines using BIC as the variable selection procedure; however, the BIC value of a particular model is easily computed from the values of n and the log-likelihood for any model being considered. In particular, for a model having k explanatory variables, the value

TABLE 10.11 The VIF Values for the Explanatory Variables Age, Height, Chest, and Abdomen

Predictor	Coef	SE Coef	T	P	VIF
Constant	-0.0264	0.6210	-0.04	0.966	
Age	0.0027	0.0018	1.53	0.126	1.165
Height	-0.0298	0.0086	-3.47	0.001	1.157
Chest	-0.0056	0.0062	-0.90	0.368	6.332
Abdomen	0.0305	0.0049	6.25	0.000	6.395

of BIC is

$$\text{BIC} = n \ln(-2\log\text{-likelihood}) + (k+1)\ln(n)$$

$$= n \times \text{deviance} + (k+1)\ln(n)$$

Example 10.20

Suppose that a logistic regression model is to be built for the binary response variable

$$\text{BF} = \begin{cases} 1 & \text{if percent body fat is} \leq 25 \\ 0 & \text{if percent body fat is} > 25 \end{cases}$$

as a function of the explanatory variables Age, Height, Chest, and Abdomen using the Body Fat data set ($n = 252$) and the BIC variable selection procedure.

The first step is to check for collinearity among the explanatory variables by fitting the linear regression model

$$\text{BF} = \beta_0 + \beta_1 \text{Age} + \beta_2 \text{Height} + \beta_3 \text{ Chest} + \beta_4 \text{ Abdomen}$$

and by inspecting the VIF values for these explanatory variables. The results of fitting the linear regression model are shown in Table 10.11. Note that all of the VIF values are less than 10, and thus, there is no evidence of a collinearity problem with the explanatory variables Age, Height, Chest, and Abdomen.

The second step in the BIC variable selection procedure is to fit and assess the logistic regression model

$$\text{logit}(p) = \beta_0 + \beta_1 \text{Age} + \beta_2 \text{Height} + \beta_3 \text{Chest} + \beta_4 \text{Abdomen}$$

The p-value for the Hosmer–Lemeshow goodness of fit test is $p = 0.903$ and the model diagnostics $\Delta\chi^2$ and $\Delta\beta$ do not indicate that there are any outliers or influential points that need to be dealt with. Thus, the BIC variable selection procedure will proceed, and the BIC values for the top models are given in Table 10.12.

Now, based on the BIC values in Table 10.12, the best model according to the BIC criterion is the model with the explanatory variables Abdomen and Height since it has the lowest value of BIC and no other model has a BIC value within 2 of this model.

The MINITAB output for this model is given in Figure 10.11. Output for best model. Note that the p-value for Hosmer–Lemeshow goodness-of-fit test for the model $\text{logit}(p) = \beta_0 + \beta_1 \text{Height} +$

TABLE 10.12 Best Two Models for $k = 1,2,3,4$ Explanatory Variables

Number of Variables in the Model	Variables in Model	Deviance	BIC
1	Chest	205.136	216.195
1	Abdomen	163.494	174.553
2	Abdomen, Age	155.898	172.486
2	Abdomen, Height	142.386	158.974
3	Abdomen, Height, Age	139.994	162.174
3	Abdomen, Height, Chest	139.210	161.328
4	Abdomen, Height, Chest, Age	136.986	164.633

```
                                       Odds      95% CI
Predictor       Coef    SE Coef     Z     P  Ratio  Lower  Upper
Constant    -0.410896   5.97869  -0.07  0.945
Abdomen      0.304446   0.04258   7.15  0.000  1.36   1.25   1.47
Height      -0.424259   0.10349  -4.10  0.000  0.65   0.53   0.80


Log-Likelihood = -71.193
Test that all slopes are zero: G = 147.434, DF = 2, P-Value = 0.000


Goodness-of-Fit Tests
Method              Chi-Square    DF      P
Hosmer-Lemeshow         5.826      8   0.667
```

Figure 10.11   The MINITAB output for the logistic regression model
$\text{logit}(p) = \beta_0 + \beta_1 \text{Height} + \beta_2 \text{Abdomen}$.

β_2Abdomen is $p = 0.667$ that suggests this model fits the observed data adequately well. Also, both of the explanatory variables are significant in this model.

The final step in the BIC variable selection procedure would be to examine this model and to assess the model on scientific grounds.

10.7   SOME FINAL COMMENTS ON LOGISTIC REGRESSION

Fitting a logistic regression model is a dynamic process with a model fit to the original data, assumptions checked, the model diagnostics often suggest adjustments to the model, and new models are fit until a good fitting model is found. Only after curing problems suggested by the residual or collinearity diagnostics should inferences be drawn from the fitted model about the relationship between the response and the explanatory variables.

Before testing any hypothesis about the model, making inferences about the response variable, or using a variable selection procedure, it is critical to develop a full model that satisfies the logistic regression assumptions. A poor fitting model should never be used for making inferences about the relationship between the response and the explanatory variables, and confidence intervals and hypothesis tests should not be performed unless the assumptions of the model are valid and the model adequately fits the observed data. The steps that should be carried out in a typical logistic regression analysis are outlined below.

THE LOGISTIC REGRESSION PROCEDURE

---

1. Determine the sampling plan that will be used for collecting a random sample on the response and explanatory variables.

2. Collect the data.

3. Investigate the possibility of collinear relationships between the explanatory variables using multiple regression, scatterplots, and correlations. Cure any collinearity problems before proceeding.

4. Fit the full model and test the goodness of fit of the model.

5. Check the assumptions of the model and identify any problems suggested by the model diagnostics.

6. Make any adjustments to the model that are needed and refit the model.

7. Repeat steps 4, 5, and 6 until a good fitting model is found.

8. Use the fitted model for making statistical inferences about the relationship between the binary response and explanatory variables.

When the BIC variable selection procedure is used to investigate the relationship between the response variable and a large number of explanatory variables, the model that best satisfies the variable selection criterion will not be superior to any of the competing models that also fare well under the selection criterion. The scientific merit of all of the models competing to be the final model must be evaluated in selecting the final model. Thus, the goal of a logistic regression analysis is to determine a parsimonious model that fits the observed data well and makes scientific sense.

Finally, when reporting the results of a logistic regression analysis, a researcher should only provide the most relevant information from the logistic regression output. In particular, a researcher should report the equation of the fitted model provided it does not have significant lack of fit, the standard errors of the coefficients, the estimated odds ratios, and any specialized inferences made using the model. Diagnostic plots need not be included in summarizing a logistic regression analysis.

GLOSSARY

Bayes Information Criterion The Bayes Information Criterion for a logistic regression model is

$$\text{BIC} = \text{deviance} + (k + 1) \times \ln(n)$$

Binary Variable A binary variable is a dichotomous variable that takes on the values 0 and 1.

Deviance The deviance of a fitted model is $-2 \times$ log-likelihood.

Drop-in-deviance Test A drop-in-deviance test is used to compare two logistic regression models when one model is nested in the other. The drop-in-deviance test statistic for comparing a reduced model that is nested in the full model is

$$\text{drop-in-deviance} = \text{deviance (full model)} - \text{deviance (reduced model)}$$

Extrabinomial Variation There is an extrabinomial variation when the variance of the response variable is

$$\text{Var}(Y|\vec{X}) = \sigma^2 p(\vec{X})(1 - p(\vec{X}))$$

and $\sigma^2 > 1$; σ^2 is called the dispersion parameter.

Goodness-of-Fit Test A goodness-of-fit test is used to assess the fit of a model to the observed data.

Likelihood Function The likelihood function for a logistic regression model is the product of the probabilities of the observed values of the response variable that is

$$L = \prod p_i^{y_i}(1 - p_i)^{1-y_i}$$

where $\prod$ is mathematical shorthand for product, $p_i = P(Y = 1|\vec{X} = \vec{x}_i)$, and $\vec{x}_i$ is the vector of values of the explanatory variables for Y_i. In terms of the logistic regression coefficients, the likelihood function is

$$L = \prod \left(\frac{e^{\beta_0 + \beta_1 x_1 + \beta_2 x_2 + \cdots + \beta_p x_p}}{1 + e^{\beta_0 + \beta_1 x_1 + \beta_2 x_2 + \cdots + \beta_p x_p}} \right)^{y_i} \left(\frac{1}{1 + e^{\beta_0 + \beta_1 x_1 + \beta_2 x_2 + \cdots + \beta_p x_p}} \right)^{1-y_i}$$

Log-likelihood Statistic The log-likelihood statistic for a fitted model is the logarithm of the likelihood function evaluated at the parameter estimates.

Logistic Function The inverse of the logit function is the logistic function. When $\text{logit}(p) = \lambda$ applying the logistic function to the $\text{logit}(p)$ produces $p = \frac{e^{\lambda}}{1+e^{\lambda}}$.

Logistic Regression Model The logistic regression model for modeling the probabilities of a binary response variable as a function of a set of explanatory variables, say $X_1, X_2, \ldots, X_p$, is given by

$$P(Y = 1|\vec{X}) = p(\vec{X}) = \frac{e^{\beta_0 + \beta_1 X_1 + \beta_2 X_2 + \beta_3 X_3 + \cdots + \beta_p X_p}}{1 + e^{\beta_0 + \beta_1 X_1 + \beta_2 X_2 + \beta_3 X_3 + \cdots + \beta_p X_p}}$$

The logistic regression model is usually stated in terms of the *logit* of $p(\vec{X})$ and is written as

$$\text{logit}[\, p(\vec{X}) \,] = \beta_0 + \beta_1 X_1 + \beta_2 X_2 + \beta_3 X_3 + \cdots + \beta_p X_p$$

Logit Transformation The logit transformation of a probability p is

$$\text{logit}(p) = \ln\left(\frac{p}{1-p}\right)$$

Maximum Likelihood Procedure The maximum likelihood procedure is used to determine the estimates of the logistic regression coefficients and fit a logistic regression model. The estimates of the logistic regression coefficients that maximize the likelihood function are called the maximum likelihood estimates of the logistic regression coefficients.

Model Utility Test The model utility test is a test of the null hypothesis that all of the logistic regression slopes are 0.

Odds Ratio The odds ratio for two values of an explanatory variable, $X = x_1$ and X_2, is defined to be

$$\text{odds ratio} = \text{OR} = \frac{\text{odds}(Y = 1|X = x_1)}{\text{odds}(Y = 1|X = x_2)}$$

and is a measure of the relative likelihood that $Y = 1$ for $X = x_1$ and $X = X_2$.

Odds The odds that the response variable has the characteristic of interest (i.e., $Y = 1$) is the ratio of the probability that $Y = 1$ and the probability that $Y = 0$. That is,

$$\text{odds}(Y = 1) = \frac{P(Y = 1)}{P(Y = 0)}$$

Pearson Residuals A Pearson residual is

$$r = \frac{t - m\widehat{p}(\vec{x})}{\sqrt{m\widehat{p}(\vec{x})(1 - \widehat{p}(\vec{x}))}}$$

where t is the sum of the Y values for the set of explanatory conditions $\vec{x}$, $\widehat{p}(\vec{x})$ is the estimated probability of Y for $\vec{x}$, and m is the number of observations having the explanatory condition $\vec{x}$. A standardized Pearson residual is formed by dividing a Pearson residual by its standard deviation.

$\Delta\beta$ Statistic The $\Delta\beta$ statistic measures the change in the estimated logistic regression coefficients when all of the observations with a particular explanatory condition are deleted from the analysis.

$\Delta\chi^2$ Statistic The $\Delta\chi^2$ statistic measures the change in the Pearson χ^2 statistic when all of the observations with the jth explanatory conditions are deleted.

EXERCISES

10.1 What is the difference between a dichotomous and a binary variable?

10.2 What is the difference between the type of response variable that is modeled with a linear regression model and a logistic regression model?

10.3 In a study of obesity, a researcher is interested in factors that influence the probability that an individual has a body mass index (BMI) of 30 or more. Create a binary response variable that could be used in modeling the probability that an individual has a BMI of 30 or more.

10.4 For a binary response variable Y, how are the odds that $Y = 1$ computed?

10.5 For a binary response variable Y, what
(a) does it mean when the odds that $Y = 1$ is 5?
(b) is the probability that $Y = 1$ when the odds that $Y = 1$ is 5?

10.6 For a binary variable Y compute the odds that $Y = 1$ when

(a) $P(Y = 1) = 0.5$ (b) $P(Y = 1) = 0.8$
(c) $P(Y = 1) = 0.1$ (d) $P(Y = 1) = 0.9$
(e) $P(Y = 0) = 0.2$ (f) $P(Y = 0) = 0.66$

10.7 For a binary variable Y and a dichotomous explanatory variable X, how is the odds ratio computed.

10.8 What does it mean when the odds ratio is
(a) less than 1.
(b) equal to 1.
(c) more than 1.

10.9 Use the information in Table 10.13 to compute the odds ratio for $X = 0$ and $X = 1$.

10.10 Using the information in Table 10.14 compute the odds ratio.

10.11 In the article "Identification of patients at low risk for recurrent venous thromboembolism by measuring thrombin generation" published in the *Journal of the American Medical Association* (Hron et al., 2006), the authors reported the data given in Table 10.15 on the recurrence of venous thromboembolism (VTE) and peak thrombin level. Use this data to answer the following:
(a) Assuming that the $n = 914$ observations resulted from a simple random sample estimate, the probability of recurrence when the peak thrombin level is at least 400.

TABLE 10.13 Table of Probabilities for Exercise 10.9

X	Y	
	1	0
1	0.25	0.75
0	0.10	0.90

TABLE 10.14   Table of Probabilities for Exercise 10.10

X	Y	
	1	0
1	0.45	0.15
0	0.10	0.30

TABLE 10.15   Data on the Recurrence of Venous Thromboembolism (VTE) and Peak Thrombin Level

Peak Thrombin Level	VTE Recurrence	
	Yes	No
≥ 400	61	244
< 400	39	570

(b) Assuming that the $n = 914$ observations resulted from a simple random sample estimate, the probability of recurrence when the peak thrombin level is less than 400.

(c) Estimate the odds ratio for comparing the odds of recurrence for these two peak thrombin levels.

10.12 In the article "Improving the health of African-american men: experiences for the Targeting Cancer in Blacks (TCiB) Project" published in *The Journal of Men's Health & Gender* (Fort, 2007), the author reported the data given in Table 10.16 summarizing the responses of $n = 937$ African-American men who were asked to respond to the statement "What people eat or drink doesn't affect whether they will get cancer."

(a) Estimate the odds that a low income African-American male will agree with this statement.

(b) Estimate the odds that a high income African-American male will agree with this statement.

(c) Estimate the odds ratio for comparing the odds of agreement with the statement for these two income levels.

TABLE 10.16   Summary of the Responses of $n = 937$ African-American Men Who Were Asked to Respond to the Statement "What People Eat or Drink Doesn't Affect Whether They Will Get Cancer"

Income Level	Opinion	
	Agree	Disagree
Low	30%	70%
High	16%	84%

TABLE 10.17   Data on the Relationship Between the Presence of the Antigen TA-90 and the Results of a Lymphadenectomy Operation

TA-90 Antigen	Lynphadenectomy	
	Positive	Negative
Present	0.149	0.376
Absent	0.030	0.446

10.13 In the article "Tumor-associated antigen TA-90 immune complex assay predicts subclinical metastasis and survival for patients with early stage melanoma" published in the journal *Cancer* (Kelley et al., 1998), the authors reported the data given in Table 10.17 for a study investigating the relationship between the presence of the antigen TA-90 and the results of a lymphadenectomy operation. Use the information in Table 10.16 to compute the odds ratio of having a positive nodes in a lymphadenectomy operation for the presence and absence of the TA-90 antigen.

10.14 Using the Birth Weight data set
(a) create a 2×2 contingency table that summarizes the percentage of babies weight classification (LOW) by mother's smoking status (SMOKE).
(b) estimate the odds ratio for LOW=1 for comparing smoking status.

10.15 What is the logit transformation for a probability p?

10.16 Compute the value of logit(p) when

(a) $p = 0.25$ (b) $p = 0.90$

10.17 Write down the form of the logistic regression model in terms of logit(p)
(a) for the model based on a single explanatory variable X.
(b) for the model based on the explanatory variables X_1, X_2, X_3.
(c) for the interaction model based on a single dummy variable Z and a single explanatory variable X.
(d) for the interaction model based on two dummy variables, Z_1 and Z_2, and a single explanatory variable X.

10.18 In a logistic regression model what is the form of
(a) logit[$P(Y = 1 | \vec{X})$].
(b) $P(Y = 1 | \vec{X})$.

10.19 If the logit[$p(X)$] $= 2 - 1.1X$, what
(a) is the probability that $Y = 1$ when $X = 2$?
(b) is the probability that $Y = 1$ when $X = 5$?
(c) happens to the probability that $Y = 1$ as the value of X increases?
(d) is the odds ratio for the probability that $Y = 1$ when $X = 2$ and $X = 5$?

10.20 What are the assumptions of a logistic regression model.

10.21 What are the steps that must be carried out before using a fitted logistic regression model for making statistical inferences?

10.22 What does it mean when the explanatory variables are collinear?

TABLE 10.18   The Estimated Odds Ratios from a Logistic Regression Model for the Incidence of Leukoaraiosis

Variable	Odds Ratio	P-Value
Age	1.06	<0.001
Hypertension	2.33	<0.001
Stenosis ICA	2.23	0.003

10.23   How can the explanatory variables be checked for collinearity?

10.24   What does it mean when there is extrabinomial variation in the response variable?

10.25   What method is used for fitting a logistic regression model?

10.26   What is the likelihood function for a logistic regression model?

10.27   What is the relationship between the maximum likelihood estimates of the logistic regression coefficients and the likelihood function?

10.28   In the article "Risk factors for the development of pedal edema in patients using pramipexole" published in *Archives of Neurology* (Kleiner-Fisman and Fisman, 2007), the authors reported the results of a logistic regression analysis and an estimated odds ratio of $\widehat{OR} = 3.12$ for the binary explanatory variable history of diabetes mellitus. Based on the value of estimated odds ratio, what is the estimate of the slope for the variable history of diabetes mellitus in the fitted logistic regression model?

10.29   In the article "What is the significance of leukoaraiosis in patients with acute ischemic stroke?" published in the *Archives of Neurology* (Wiszniewska et al., 2000), the authors reported the estimates of the odds ratios from a logistic regression model for modeling the probability of the incidence of leukoaraiosis given in Table 10.18. Use the information in Table 10.18 to answer the following:
   (a) Determine the estimate of the logistic regression coefficient for the variable Age.
   (b) Determine the estimate of the logistic regression coefficient for the variable Hypertension.
   (c) Estimate the odds ratio for a difference in age of 1 year when hypertension and stenosis ICA are held fixed.
   (d) Estimate the odds ratio for a difference in age of 5 years when hypertension and stenosis ICA are held fixed.

10.30   Use the MINITAB output for the logistic regression model

$$\text{logit}(p) = \beta_0 + \beta_1 X$$

given in Figure 10.12 to answer the following:
   (a) Write down the equation of the fitted logistic regression model.
   (b) Test the goodness of fit for this model.
   (c) Determine the maximum likelihood estimate of the odds ratio associated with the explanatory variable X.
   (d) Estimate the probability that $Y = 1$ when $X = 5$.
   (e) Plot the estimated probability that $Y = 1$ as a function of X.

```
Logistic Regression Table

Predictor       Coef    SE Coef      Z      P
Constant    -0.767781   0.130326  -5.89  0.000
X           -0.074958   0.024681  -3.04  0.002


Log-Likelihood = -320.945
Test that all slopes are zero: G = 11.839, DF = 1, P-Value = 0.001


Goodness-of-Fit Tests
Method           Chi-Square  DF     P
Hosmer-Lemeshow     4.2476    5  0.514
```

Figure 10.12 MINITAB output for Exercise 10.30.

10.31 Use the MINITAB output for the logistic regression model

$$\text{logit}(p) = \beta_0 + \beta_1 X + \beta_2 X_2$$

given in Figure 10.13 to answer the following:

(a) Write down the equation of the fitted logistic regression model.

(b) Test the goodness of fit for this model.

(c) Determine the maximum likelihood estimate of the odds ratio associated with the explanatory variable X_2.

(d) Estimate the probability that $Y = 1$ when $X_1 = 35$ and $X_2 = 5$.

10.32 What is the formula for computing a Pearson residual?

10.33 Why are the standardized Pearson residuals generally used instead of the Pearson residuals?

10.34 Use the plot of the standardized Pearson residuals versus the observation index given in Figure 10.14 to answer the following:

(a) Does this residual plot suggest there are explanatory conditions for which the model is not fitting well?

(b) How should the influence of the explanatory condition for which there is an unusually large standardized Pearson residual be investigated further?

10.35 What are the two model diagnostics that can be used to detect outliers and influential explanatory conditions?

```
Logistic Regression Table

Predictor       Coef    SE Coef      Z      P
Constant    -1.76192   0.517697  -3.40  0.001
X1          -0.08629   0.026048  -3.31  0.001
X2           0.03192   0.015980   2.00  0.046


Log-Likelihood = -318.951
Test that all slopes are zero: G = 15.827, DF = 2, P-Value = 0.000


Goodness-of-Fit Tests
Method           Chi-Square  DF     P
Hosmer-Lemeshow    15.281    8  0.054
```

Figure 10.13 MINITAB output for Exercise 10.31.

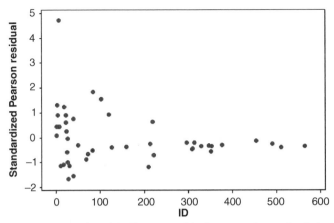

Figure 10.14   Plot of the Pearson residuals versus observation index.

10.36 What is the general rule for identifying points to be investigated using the $\Delta\chi^2$ and $\Delta\beta$ model diagnostics?

10.37 Using the Birth Weight data set with the response variable LOW, fit the model

$$\text{logit}(p) = \beta_0 + \beta_1 \text{AGE} + \beta_2 \text{ LWT} + \beta_3 \text{ SMOKE}$$

and then
(a) test the goodness of fit for this model.
(b) create and interpret a plot of the standardized residuals versus the observation index.
(c) create and interpret a plot of $\Delta\chi^2$ versus the observation index.
(d) create and interpret a plot of $\Delta\beta$ versus the observation index.

10.38 For the logistic regression model $\text{logit}(p) = \beta_0 + \beta_1 X_1 + \beta_2 X_2 + \cdots + \beta_p X_p$, what is the formula for computing a $(1 - \alpha) \times 100\%$ confidence interval for
(a) the logistic regression coefficient associated with the explanatory variable X_1?
(b) an odds ratio associated a one unit increase in the explanatory variable X_1 when all of the other explanatory variables are held fixed?

10.39 For the logistic regression model $\text{logit}(p) = \beta_0 + \beta_1 X_1 + \beta_2 X_2 + \cdots + \beta_p X_p$ and a sufficiently large sample, compute a 95% confidence interval for the odds ratio associated with the explanatory variable X_1 when maximum likelihood estimation produces
(a) $\widehat{\beta}_1 = 0.58$ and $\text{se}(\widehat{\beta}_1) = 0.21$.
(b) $\widehat{\beta}_1 = -1.83$ and $\text{se}(\widehat{\beta}_1) = 0.41$.

10.40 For each of the scenarios in Exercise 10.39 test $H_0 : \beta_1 = 0$ and compute the p-value associated with the test.

10.41 The MINITAB output given in Figure 10.15 resulted from fitting a logistic regression model to the binary response variable vital status (STA) and the explanatory variables age (AGE), systolic blood pressure (SYS), and heart rate (HRA) on the Intensive Care Unit data set. Use the information in Figure 10.15 to answer the following:
(a) Test the goodness of fit of this model.

```
Predictor         Coef    SE Coef       Z     P
Constant      -1.06127    1.22819   -0.86  0.388
AGE            0.02837    0.01078    2.63  0.009
SYS           -0.01676    0.00587   -2.85  0.004
HRA            0.00093    0.00670    0.14  0.890


Log-Likelihood = -91.618
Test that all slopes are zero: G = 16.925, DF = 3, P-Value = 0.001


Goodness-of-Fit Tests

Method            Chi-Square    DF     P
Hosmer-Lemeshow       8.630      8  0.374
```
Figure 10.15   MINITAB output for the logistic regression model with response variable STA and the explanatory variables AGE, SYS, and HRA.

(b) Test the utility of this model.

(c) Are there any explanatory variables that could be dropped from the model? Explain.

(d) Compute a 95% confidence interval for the odds ratio associated with the explanatory variable AGE.

10.42 The MINITAB output given in Figure 10.16 resulted from fitting a logistic regression model to the binary response variable prostatic capsule tumor penetration (CAPSULE) and the explanatory variables age (AGE) and prostatic specific antigen (PSA) on the Prostate Cancer Study data set. Use the information in Figure 10.16 to answer the following:

(a) Test the goodness of fit of this model.

(b) Test the utility of this model.

(c) Does the age of a male appear to influence the probability of prostatic capsule tumor penetration? Explain.

(d) Compute a 95% confidence interval for the odds ratio associated with a one unit increase in the explanatory variable PSA when the value of AGE is held constant.

10.43 In the article "Hypoglycemia in patients with type 2 diabetes mellitus" published in the *Archives of Internal Medicine* (Miller et al., 2001), the authors reported the odds

```
Predictor          Coef    SE Coef       Z     P
Constant      0.0913247    1.06955    0.09  0.932
AGE          -0.0041247   0.0162116  -0.25  0.799
PSA          -0.0136647   0.0061460  -2.22  0.026


Log-Likelihood = -252.896
Test that all slopes are zero: G = 5.464, DF = 2, P-Value = 0.065

Goodness-of-Fit Tests
Method            Chi-Square    DF     P
Hosmer-Lemeshow       7.258      8  0.509
```
Figure 10.16   MINITAB output for the logistic regression model with response STA and the explanatory variables AGE, SYS, and HRA.

TABLE 10.19   Odds Ratios for a Logistic Regression Model for Predicting the Occurrence of Hypoglycemia

Variable	Odds Ratio	P-value
Constant	1.42	$\cdots$
Age	0.98	0.03
Male Sex	0.81	0.25
Race: White	1.15	0.78
Race: Hispanic	0.68	0.65
Race: Other	1.34	0.65
Diabetes duration	0.99	0.31
HbA_{1c}	0.87	0.006
Sulfibylurea therapy	1.54	0.08
Insulin therapy	3.44	<0.001
Baseline hypoglycemia	2.65	<0.001
Medicinal therapy	1.00	>0.99

ratios for a logistic regression model for predicting the occurrence of hypoglycemia given in Table 10.19. Use Table 10.19 to answer the following:

(a) Does the sex of an individual appear to be an important explanatory variable for predicting the occurrence of hypoglycemia?

(b) Does the race of an individual appear to be an important explanatory variable for predicting the occurrence of hypoglycemia?

(c) Based on the information in Table 10.19 which explanatory variables do not appear to be important for predicting the occurrence of hypoglycemia?

10.44 Using Prostate Cancer Study data set, fit a logistic regression model with capsule penetration (CAPSULE) as the response variable with explanatory variables age (AGE), prostatic specific antigen (PSA), and tumor volume (VOL). For the resulting fitted model

(a) test the goodness of fit of this model.

(b) create and examine plots of the standardized Pearson residuals, $\Delta\chi^2$, and $\Delta\beta$ versus the observation index. Are there any observations that need to be investigated further?

(c) test the utility of the fitted model.

(d) compute the deviance of this model.

(e) are there any explanatory variables that should be dropped from the model?

10.45 How is the deviance of a model computed?

10.46 What is the form of the drop-in-deviance test statistic for comparing the models

$$\text{logit}(p) = \beta_0 + \beta_1 X_1 + \beta_2 X_2 + \beta_3 X_3 + \beta_4 X_4$$

and

$$\text{logit}(p) = \beta_0 + \beta_1 X_1$$

10.47 How many degrees of freedom would the drop-in-deviance have in Exercise 10.46?

```
Predictor          Coef    SE Coef      Z      P   Ratio  Lower  Upper
Constant       -1.06127    1.22819  -0.86  0.388
AGE             0.02837    0.01078   2.63  0.009   1.03   1.01   1.05
SYS            -0.01676    0.00587  -2.85  0.004   0.98   0.97   0.99
HRA             0.00093    0.00670   0.14  0.890   1.00   0.99   1.01


Log-Likelihood = -91.618


Predictor          Coef    SE Coef      Z      P   Ratio  Lower  Upper
Constant       -3.05851   0.696109  -4.39  0.000
AGE             0.02754   0.010565   2.61  0.009   1.03   1.01   1.05


Log-Likelihood = -96.153
```

Figure 10.17   MINITAB output for Exercise 10.47.

10.48   The MINITAB output given in Figure 10.17 summarizes the fit of the logistic regression models

$$\text{logit}(p) = \beta_0 + \beta_1 \text{AGE} + \beta_2 \text{SYS} + \beta_3 \text{HRA}$$

and

$$\text{logit}(p) = \beta_0 + \beta_1 \text{AGE}$$

Use the information in Figure 10.17 to test $H_0 : \beta_2 = \beta_3 = 0$.

10.49   The MINITAB output given in Figure 10.18 summarizes the fit of the logistic regression models

$$\text{logit}(p) = \beta_0 + \beta_1 \text{NDRUGTX} + \beta_2 \text{RACE} + \beta_3 \text{RACE*NDRUGTX} + \beta_4 \text{TREAT}$$

and

$$\text{logit}(p) = \beta_0 + \beta_1 \text{NDRUGTX} + \beta_4 \text{TREAT}$$

Use the information in Figure 10.17 to test $H_0 : \beta_2 = \beta_3 = 0$.

```
                                                    Odds      95% CI
Predictor          Coef    SE Coef      Z      P   Ratio  Lower  Upper
Constant       -0.991883  0.191483  -5.18  0.000
NDRUGTX        -0.098734  0.031738  -3.11  0.002   0.91   0.85   0.96
RACE            0.046381  0.282811   0.16  0.870   1.05   0.60   1.82
RACE*NDRUGTX    0.092851  0.052578   1.77  0.077   1.10   0.99   1.22
TREAT           0.397955  0.196333   2.03  0.043   1.49   1.01   2.19


Log-Likelihood = -315.508
Logistic Regression Table
                                                    Odds      95% CI
Predictor          Coef    SE Coef      Z      P   Ratio  Lower  Upper
Constant       -0.999072  0.169077  -5.91  0.000
NDRUGTX        -0.073922  0.024470  -3.02  0.003   0.93   0.89   0.97
TREAT           0.434794  0.194780   2.23  0.026   1.54   1.05   2.26


Log-Likelihood = -318.430
```

Figure 10.18   The MINITAB output for Exercise 10.49.

10.50   Use the Intensive Care Unit data set to answer the following:

   (a) Fit the logistic regression interaction model with vital status (STA) as the response variable with age (AGE) and CPR prior to admission (CPR) as the explanatory variables.

   (b) Test the goodness of fit of the model in part(a).

   (c) Fit the no-interaction model.

   (d) Compare the fit of the interaction model against the no-interaction model using a drop-in-deviance test.

   (e) Which model appears to be a better model for explaining the response variable? Explain.

10.51   Use the Intensive Care Unit data set to answer the following:

   (a) Fit the logistic regression interaction model with vital status (STA) as the response variable with age (AGE), CPR prior to admission (CPR), systolic blood pressure at admission (SYS), and heart rate at admission (HRA) as the explanatory variables.

   (b) Test the goodness of fit of the model in part(a).

   (c) Fit the logistic regression model with vital status (STA) as the response variable with age (AGE) and CPR prior to admission (CPR) as the explanatory variables.

   (d) Compare the fit of the model in part(a) against the model fit in part(c) using a drop-in-deviance test.

   (e) Which model appears to be a better model for explaining the response variable? Explain.

10.52   Use the Intensive Care Unit data set to answer the following:

   (a) Fit the logistic regression interaction model with vital status (STA) as the response variable with age (AGE), CPR prior to admission (CPR), systolic blood pressure at admission (SYS), and heart rate at admission (HRA) as the explanatory variables.

   (b) Test the goodness of fit of the model in part(a).

   (c) Fit the logistic regression model with vital status (STA) as the response variable with age (AGE) and CPR prior to admission (CPR) as the explanatory variables.

   (d) Compare the fit of the model in part(a) against the model fit in part(c) using a drop-in-deviance test.

   (e) Which model appears to be a better model for explaining the response variable? Explain.

10.53   Use the Birth Weight data set to answer the following:

   (a) Fit the logistic regression interaction model with birth weight classification (LOW) as the response variable with mother's smoking status (SMOKE) and mother's race (RACE) as the explanatory variables.

   (b) Test the goodness of fit of the model in part(a).

   (c) Fit the logistic regression model with birth weight classification (LOW) as the response variable with explanatory variable mother's smoking status (SMOKE).

   (d) Compare the fit of the model in part(a) against the model fit in part(c) using a drop-in-deviance test.

   (e) Which model appears to be a better model for explaining the response variable? Explain.

TABLE 10.20 Explanatory Variables and the Log-Likelihood Statistic for the Best Two Logistic Regression Models

k	Variables in the Model	Log-Likelihood
1	X_7	-215.67
1	X_5	-241.12
2	X_7, X_3	-203.78
2	X_7, X_1	-205.63
3	X_7, X_3, X_1	-190.22
3	X_7, X_1, X_2	-199.81
4	X_7, X_3, X_1, X_5	-191.18
4	X_7, X_3, X_2, X_5	-193.65
5	X_7, X_3, X_1, X_4, X_5	-187.07
5	X_7, X_2, X_3, X_4, X_5	-186.33
6	$X_7, X_1, X_2, X_3, X_4, X_5$	-182.88
6	$X_7, X_1, X_2, X_3, X_4, X_6$	-182.87
7	$X_7, X_1, X_2, X_3, X_3, X_4, X_5, X_6$	-182.13

10.54 What is the formula for computing the BIC value associated with a logistic regression model?

10.55 Suppose the BIC statistic value for a logistic regression model with five explanatory variables is $BIC_5 = 234.56$ and the BIC statistic value for a logistic regression model with only three of the five explanatory variables is $BIC_3 = 235.19$, which model would be best according to the Bayes Information Criterion?

10.56 Table 10.20 contains summary information on the fit of the best two logistic regression models based on a sample of $n = 313$ observations for models including $k = 1, 2, \ldots, 7$ explanatory variables. Use the information in Table 10.20 to answer the following:

(a) Compute the deviance associated with each of the models summarized in Table 10.20.

(b) Compute the value of BIC for each model listed in Table 10.20.

(c) If there are no scientific reasons for including any particular explanatory variable in the final model, which model is best according to the BIC variable selection procedure?

(d) If there are scientific reasons why the explanatory variable X_4 should be included in the final model, which model is best according to the BIC variable selection procedure?

CHAPTER 11

DESIGN OF EXPERIMENTS

THE GOAL of any research project or study is to obtain relevant information about the target population and the research questions concerning the target population. When two or more populations are being studied and the researcher controls the assignment of the units of the study to the different groups being studied, the study is called an *experiment*, and experiments performed on humans to assess the efficacy of a treatment or medical procedure are called *clinical trials*. In Chapter 3, the principles and sampling methods that can be used to obtain a representative sample from the target population were discussed, and in this chapter, the principles and techniques that are used in designing an experiment for comparing two or more populations are discussed.

Experiments are performed for several reasons including (1) for comparing how different treatments affect a response variable, (2) for screening the importance of the explanatory variables that are believed to affect the response variable, and (3) for building a statistical model such as a linear or logistic regression model that relates the response variable to a set of explanatory variables. Regardless of the reason for performing an experiment, the goal of an experiment is to obtain data that are representative of the populations being studied for making statistical inferences about the differences between the populations.

11.1 EXPERIMENTS VERSUS OBSERVATIONAL STUDIES

Recall from Chapter 1, the two types of statistical studies are experiments that are studies where the researcher controls the assignment of the units to the treatment groups and observational studies that are studies where the units come to the researcher already assigned to the treatment groups. For example, in a retrospective study of the risk factors associated with the incidence of lung cancer the subjects in the study will already belong to the groups formed according to the risk factors that are being compared, and hence, this retrospective study would be an observational study. On the other hand, a prospective study where the researcher assigned the subjects to a particular diet and then followed their weight loss over a period of time would be an experiment.

Applied Biostatistics for the Health Sciences. By Richard J. Rossi
Copyright © 2010 by John Wiley & Sons, Inc.

Example 11.1

Consider each of the following proposed research projects and determine whether an experiment or an observational study must be used.

  a. A medical researcher is going to study the risk factors associated with coronary heart disease in a case–control study.

  b. A medical researcher is going to study the efficacy of the Atkins, South Beach, and Mediterranean diets for producing weight loss in a prospective study.

  c. A medical researcher is going to study the effective lifetime of human blood stored at several different temperatures.

  d. A medical researcher is going to study the relationship between cholesterol levels and coronary heart disease in a retrospective case–control study.

  e. A medical researcher is going to study the relationship between the use of echinacea and the duration of a common cold in a retrospective study.

  f. A medical researcher is going to study the relationship between the use of echinacea and the duration of a common cold in a prospective study.

Solutions

  a. Because case–control studies are retrospective studies and the subjects come predetermined as cases or controls, this study would have to be performed as an observational study.

  b. Since the researcher could assign the subjects to the diets, this study could be performed as an experiment.

  c. Since the researcher could assign the blood samples to the different temperatures, this study could be performed as an experiment.

  d. Because case–control studies are retrospective studies and the subjects come predetermined as cases or controls, this study would have to be performed as an observational study.

  e. Because case–control studies are retrospective studies, this study would have to be performed as an observational study.

  f. Since the researcher could assign the subjects an echinacea group and nonechinacea group, this study could be performed as an experiment.

Because a researcher assigns the units to the groups in an experiment, the researcher has more control over any factors that may influence the response variable. The factors that are not controlled for in an experiment or observational study are called *extraneous*, *confounding*, or *lurking* variables and may be the cause of misleading statistical inferences. In a well-designed experiment, a researcher can minimize the effects of any extraneous factors that may be present in the units, however, in an observational study the researcher has little control over any extraneous factors. When the effects of the explanatory variables are mixed with the effects of uncontrolled extraneous factors, the effects of the explanatory variables are said to be *confounded* with the effects of extraneous variables. That is, when an explanatory variable is confounded with an extraneous variable, the effects of the explanatory variable on the response variable cannot be distinguished or separated from the effects of the extraneous variable. Confounding factors are often present in observational studies and may also be present in poorly designed experiments. Confounding factors can usually be controlled for through the careful planning and execution of a well-designed experiment.

Example 11.2

It has been hypothesized that one reason why people living in the Mediterranean region have a long life expectancy and age well is that their diet mainly consists of vegetables, legumes, fruits, nuts, whole grains, fish, moderate alcohol use, a high ratio of unsaturated fats to saturated fats, and lean meat.

Suppose random samples of people living in the Mediterranean region and people living in the United States yield a significant difference in mean longevity. It would be hard to attribute the difference in longevity to diet alone since there are many other differences between people living in the Mediterranean and the United States. For example, two sources of confounding factors might be lifestyle and genetic variables that may also account for the observed difference in longevity. Therefore, in this study the explanatory variable diet would most likely be confounded with several extraneous variables.

Because a well-designed experiment controls for the possibility of extraneous factors, experiments may be able to establish strong evidence that changing the value of one explanatory variable, while no other changes take place in the experimental conditions, causes a change in the response variable. A *causal relationship* between a response variable and the explanatory variables is a relationship where changing the experimental conditions causes changes in the value of the response variable. Furthermore, in a well-designed experiment, any significant differences observed in the response variable for two different experimental conditions will most likely be due to the difference in the values of the explanatory variables and not chance error. However, in a poorly designed experiment or an observational study there is often confounding between extraneous factors and the explanatory variables, and therefore, causal relationships are much harder to establish with poorly designed experiments or observational studies.

Example 11.3
A large prospective study might be used to investigate whether or not there is causal relationship between coronary heart disease and diet in a well-designed experiment. If the experiment is designed properly, extraneous factors due to lifestyle and genetic factors could be controlled for. In this case, any significant differences in longevity would most likely be due to diet and not some other factor. In fact, a well-designed experiment was conducted to compare the rate of coronary events for individuals who have had a previous heart attack for individuals on the Mediterranean diet and individuals receiving no dietary advice from the researchers in the Lyon Diet Heart Study. The results of this experiment were reported in the article "Mediterranean alpha-linolenic acid-rich diet in secondary prevention of coronary heart disease" published in *Lancet* (de Lorgeril et al., 1994). The conclusion drawn by the authors from this experiment was that the Mediterranean diet appears to have some utility in the prevention of coronary heart disease.

In some research studies, it would be unethical, impractical, or extremely costly to use an experiment. For example, in an epidemiological study, it would be highly unethical to infect a group of people with a disease in order to test the efficacy of a potential cure for the disease. In fact, the medical profession is held to the World Medical Association Declaration of Helsinki and its amendments that outline the ethical principles for research involving human subjects. For this reason, retrospective and case–control studies, which are observational studies, are frequently used in epidemiological and medical studies. Furthermore, when it is impossible or impractical to use an experiment, a well-planned observational study can often be used to obtain relevant information as long as special care is taken to control for extraneous factors.

EXPERIMENTS VERSUS OBSERVATION STUDIES

Whenever possible a well-designed experiment should be used instead of an observational study for the following reasons.

1. Extraneous factors can be controlled for in an experiment.

2. When the units have been randomly assigned to the treatment groups, any significant differences in the response variable for units assigned to different groups is most likely be due to the treatments and not an extraneous variable.

3. The results of a well-designed experiment are generally free from bias and repeatable.

4. Experiments can be useful in establishing causal relationships.

11.2 THE BASIC PRINCIPLES OF EXPERIMENTAL DESIGN

In a comparative experiment two or more explanatory conditions are imposed on a group of units so that the effects of the explanatory conditions on the response variable may be compared. The *experimental design* in a comparative experiment is a plan detailing how the experiment will be carried out. In particular, the experimental design should includes a clear statement of the research goals, identify the response variable being studied, the explanatory variables believed to influence the response variable, the extraneous variables that must be controlled, a description of the units that will be used in the experiment, a detailed plan outlining how the units will be assigned to the experimental conditions, a plan for collecting the data, and a detailed plan for the statistical analysis of the observed data.

11.2.1 Terminology

Before discussing the aspects of a well-designed experiment, the basic concepts and terminology used in designing experiments and observational studies will be introduced.

Experimental Unit   An *experimental unit* is the smallest unit in the population to which a set of experimental conditions can be applied so that two different units may receive different experimental conditions.

Response Variable   The *response variable* is the outcome variable in an experiment. The response variable is sometimes referred to as a dependent variable.

Explanatory Variable   An *explanatory variable* is a variable that is believed to cause or be related to changes in the response variable. The explanatory variables in an experiment are often called *factors* and the values that a factor takes on in an experiment are called the *levels* of the factor.

Treatment   A *treatment* is any experimental condition that is applied to the experimental units. A *treatment group* is the collection of experimental units assigned to a particular treatment. Special types of treatments include a *placebo treatment* that is an inert treatment and a *control treatment* that is a baseline treatment that all the other treatments will be compared against.

Experimental design   The *experimental design* is the plan used to allocate the experimental units to the different treatments being compared in the experiment.

Block   A *block* of experimental units is a subgroup of the experimental units that are homogeneous. That is, the experimental units in the blocks are more alike within the block than they are when compared to the experimental units in the other blocks.

Blinded Experiment   An experiment is called a *blinded experiment* when measures are taken to prevent the experimental units and researchers who apply the treatments to the experimental units from knowing which treatment has been applied. Blinded experiments are generally used when the experimental units are human and are used to eliminate possible sources of bias from the experiment. A blinded experiment is called a *single-blind* experiment when only the subjects are blinded, and an experiment is called a *double-blind* experiment when both the subjects and the researchers are blinded.

Randomization   *Randomization* is a probability based method of allocating the experimental units to the different experimental conditions.

Replicated Experiment   An experiment is said to be *replicated* when two or more experimental units receive the same treatment. An experiment is said to be *balanced* when each treatment receives the same number of replicates. Experiments that are not balanced are said to be *unbalanced*.

Experimental Error   *Experimental error* is a measure of the variation that exists among the measurements made on the experimental units that have been treated alike. Experimental error comes from the inherent variability in the experimental units and the variability induced by performing the experiment.

Example 11.4

To study whether vitamin C is effective in preventing the common cold, a random sample of 200 volunteers is taken. The 200 subjects are divided into two groups of size 100. Each group is given a year's supply of 1000 mg pills and instructed to take a pill each night before going to bed for a period of 1 year. The pills assigned to one group of subjects contain 1000 mg of vitamin C, while the pills assigned to the other group contain 1000 mg of an inert substance, and the subjects in neither group knows which type of pill they have been given. At the end of the 1-year period the subjects are asked how many colds they had contracted during the year.

   a. What are the experimental units in this experiment?
   b. What is the response variable in this experiment?
   c. What are the treatments in this experiment?
   d. Is this a blinded experiment?

Solutions

   a. The experimental units in this experiment are the 200 volunteers. Because the experimental units are human, this is a clinical trial.
   b. The response variable in this experiment is the number of colds contracted during the 1-year period.
   c. The treatments in this experiment are 1000 mg of vitamin C and a placebo treatment of 1000 mg of an inert substance.
   d. This experiment is being conducted as a single-blind experiment since the subjects in each group do not know which treatment they have been assigned to.

11.2.2 Designing an Experiment

In a well-designed experiment there should be at least two groups being compared, the pool of experimental units should be representative of the target population, the experimental units should be as similar as possible before they are assigned to the treatment groups, the experiment should be designed so that it will have implications in real-life settings, and the experiment should be designed to control for extraneous factors. Furthermore, a well-designed experiment will be free from systematic error, attain a prespecified degree of accuracy, and have a range of validity that will provide relevant information about the research questions of interest.

   The three principles that form the foundation of a well-designed experiment are *control, randomization,* and *reduction of error*. A *controlled experiment* is an experiment where the researcher controls for the effects of extraneous variables and a *randomized controlled experiment* is a controlled experiment where the experimental units are randomly assigned to the treatments. An experiment is said to be controlled because the researcher controls how the experimental units are assigned to groups and also determines which treatment each group will receive. The experimental error is a measure of the variation that exists among the observations on the experimental units that have been treated alike, and a well-designed experiment will be designed to minimize the experimental error.

To make fair and unbiased comparisons between the values of the response variable in two treatment groups, it is imperative that the experimental units in the different treatment groups be as similar as possible before the treatments are applied. In an ideal experimental, the experimental units in a comparative experiment would be perfectly identical before the treatments were applied, so that it would be clear that any significant differences showing up in the values of the response variable for two different treatments are due to the treatments and not an extraneous factor. Because it is generally impossible to use identical experimental units in an experiment, randomization and control are the two methods that are used to make the units assigned to each treatment group as similar as possible and for controlling confounding factors.

Randomly assigning the experimental units to the treatments is done to ensure that the experimental units in the treatment groups are as alike as possible before the treatments are applied. That is, by randomly assigning the experimental units to the treatments it will be unlikely for the experimental units to align in an unfavorable pattern due to an extraneous factor. The advantages of using an experiment where the experimental units are randomly assigned to the treatment groups are listed below.

ADVANTAGES OF RANDOMIZATION

---

1. Randomly assigning the experimental units to the treatments prevents systematic error from entering the experiment by treating all of the experimental units the same way before the treatments are applied.

2. Randomly assigning the experimental units to the treatments produces a predictable pattern of results over the different possible randomizations.

3. Randomly assigning the experimental units to the prevents makes it possible to assess the reliability of any treatment comparisons made in the experiment.

4. Using a larger number of experimental units in an experiment where the units are randomly assigned to the treatment groups decreases the variability of the estimates and increases the likelihood that the units in the treatment groups are alike apart from the treatments.

5. Any significant differences in the values of the response variable for two treatments will most likely be due to the treatments, and not extraneous factors, when the experimental units are randomly assigned to the treatment groups.

Thus, the most important reason for randomly assigning the units to the treatment groups is to have a fair and unbiased assignment of the experimental units to each group so that any significant differences in the values of the response variable will most likely be due to the treatments and not some other factor.

While randomization produces treatment groups that are as similar as possible before the treatments are applied, it does not minimize the experimental error in a comparative experiment. The experimental error in an experiment is due to the inherent variability in the experimental units and the variation that is induced by performing the experiment. Furthermore, the desired precision of the experiment can only be attained when the experimental error is minimized. Two ways of minimizing the experimental error are (1) to use the most efficient experimental design and (2) by replicating the treatments. In particular, the optimal experimental design for a research study will depend primarily on the nature of the experimental units and the extraneous factors that need to be controlled.

A treatment is replicated when two or more experimental units are assigned to the treatment. Replicating the treatments provides important information that is used in estimating the experimental error, increases the reliability of any comparisons made between two treatment means, and broadens the base of inference by bringing a wider variety of units into the experiment. When the treatments are not replicated there will be no way to estimate the experimental error, and hence, no statistical comparisons of the treatments will be possible. The factors that affect the number of replicates used in an experiment include the cost of an experimental unit, the number of experimental units available, the physical and logistical conditions in which the experiment will be performed, and the level of reliability expected in the experiment. However, it is important to note that increasing the number of replicates in an experiment will only increase the reliability of an experiment when the units are representative of the target population and are assigned using a randomization scheme.

In many experiments where the response variable is a quantitative variable, the goal of the experiment is to compare the means of the treatment groups in order to determine which treatment is the most beneficial. Since the estimated standard error of the sample mean $\bar{y}$ is

$$se(\bar{y}) = \frac{s}{\sqrt{n}}$$

the accuracy of a treatment sample mean is related to the number of replicates assigned to the treatment by the Square Root Law. Thus, four times as many replicates will be needed to halve the estimated standard error or bound on the error of estimation associated with $\bar{y}$.

11.3 EXPERIMENTAL DESIGNS

An experimental design is simply the plan used to allocate the experimental units to the treatment groups. A good experimental design will control for unwanted sources of variability and control for extraneous factors. The sources of variation in an experiment are (1) the variability due to the different experimental conditions (i.e., treatments) of interest, (2) the variability due to the measurement process, and (3) the inherent variability in the experimental units. The variability due to different treatments is used in determining whether the treatment effects are significantly different from one another. The variability due to the measurement process and the variability in the experimental units is the experimental error variability that should be minimized in order to ensure that any differences in the treatment effects will be detected. A well-designed experiment provides estimates of each of these sources of variability and at the same time controls the experimental error variability.

There are many different experimental designs that can be used to control for extraneous factors and the different sources of experimental variability. The experimental design that is appropriate for a particular experiment will depend on the nature of the experimental units, the extraneous factors to control, the physical and logistical constraints required to perform the experiment, and the treatment structure.

The first step in determining the appropriate design for an experiment is to examine the experimental units. Since one of the goals of an experimental design is to assign the experimental units so that the treatment groups are as similar as possible before the treatments are applied, it is critical to examine the experimental units and determine whether the units are homogeneous, heterogeneous, or align in blocks of units.

When the experimental units are a homogeneous or heterogeneous collection of units, randomly assigning the units to the treatment groups will usually control for any extraneous factors within the units. Because homogeneous experimental units have less inherent variability than heterogeneous units, experiments based on a homogeneous experimental units will have a smaller experimental error than experiments based on a collection of heterogeneous experimental units. However, if the experimental units are too homogeneous they may not be representative of the population being studied, and therefore, the uniformity of the experimental units must be balanced with the range of units in the target population. An experimental design that can be used with homogeneous or heterogeneous experimental units is the *Completely Randomized Design* (CRD) that is discussed in Section 11.3.1.

When the experimental units can be sorted into groups of homogeneous units called *blocks*, then there is an extraneous factor present in the experimental units causing them to align in blocks that must be controlled for. A pre-existing characteristic of the experimental units or the experimental process that is not assigned by the researcher is called a *blocking factor*, and the values of a blocking factor are used to sort the units into blocks of units that are alike. Note that blocking factors are extraneous factors that are being controlled for, and there may be more than one blocking factor present in an experiment.

In biomedical research with human experimental units, blocks of units are often formed according to blocking factors which are associated with physical characteristics of humans such as age, sex, race, risk levels, and prior history. For example, a matched pairs experiment is an experiment used to compare two treatments where the pool of experimental units is carefully examined and pairs of experimental units that are alike are formed to control for extraneous factors. Each pair of units constitutes a block of units, and within each pair experimental units one of the units receives one treatment and the other unit receives the other treatment.

Blocks of experimental units sometimes exist because of the physical process used in the experiment. Examples of some blocking factors that can arise in the experimental process are given in Example 11.5.

Example 11.5
In each of the following scenarios the experimental units can be sorted into blocks according to a blocking factor.

    a. The experimental units in the experiment come from different lots. Here the blocking factor is lot.

    b. The experiment is large enough that it must be run over several different time periods due to physical or logistical constraints. Here the blocking factor is time period.

    c. The experiment is performed at different locations (i.e., clinics, laboratories, or hospitals). Here the blocking factor is location.

    d. The experiment uses different machines to analyze the results. Here the blocking factor is machine.

Physical and logistical constraints often require that an experiment to be run in sets of trials or at different locations to attain the necessary number of replicates of each treatment required to produce the desired level of reliability in the experiment.

Example 11.6
Suppose that a study on the effects of three different treatments and rapid eye movement (REM) is to be carried out at a clinic having only three specialized sleeping beds. To achieve replication in the experiment, the experiment will be carried out by assigning each treatment to a different sleeping bed, running this trial of the experiment, and then repeating this process until the desired number of replicates is obtained. In this case, the time period of a trial is an extraneous factor whose effects could be confounded with the treatment effects that must be controlled. The trials in this experiment are the blocks and each block will consist of three units, and the replicates of each treatment in this experiment come from repeating the experiment over several different time periods.

The presence of a blocking factor or blocks of experimental units requires an experimental design that takes into account the systematic variation due to the block and must control for it. Furthermore, in a well-designed experiment, the block variation is extracted from the experimental error increasing the reliability and validity of the point estimates, confidence intervals, and hypothesis tests. Any minor differences in the experimental units within a block will be controlled for by randomly assigning the units within the block to the treatments. An experimental design that can be used when the experimental units align in blocks or units is the *Randomized Block Design* (RBD), which is discussed in Section 11.3.2.

11.3.1 The Completely Randomized Design

One of the simplest experimental designs is the completely randomized design. A completely randomized design is the least restrictive design since any number of treatments may be studied and the number of replicates on each treatment may be different in a completely randomized design. The completely randomized design is an appropriate experimental design when the experimental units are either homogeneous or heterogeneous on the whole and the experimental process controls for any extraneous factors. On the other hand, a completely randomized design is not an appropriate experimental design when the experimental units align in blocks. A completely randomized design relies on randomization to control for any differences in the experimental units. In particular, by randomly assigning the experimental units to the treatment groups, the effects of any extraneous factors tend to average out over the treatment groups making the groups as similar as possible before the treatments are applied to the units.

A completely randomized design is simply a plan for allocating the n experimental units to the treatment groups. In an experiment designed as an unbalanced completely randomized design, the experiment will have t treatments, n experimental units available for the experiment, and the number of replicates of the ith treatment is n_i, where $\sum n_i = n$. In an experiment designed as a balanced completely randomized design, the experiment will have t treatments that are each replicated r times, and thus the experiment requires $n = r \times t$ experimental units. Also, that the number of replicates required in a completely randomized design to achieve a prespecified level of accuracy will be smaller when the experimental units are homogeneous rather than heterogeneous. Also, when the experimental units are heterogeneous more units will be required to average out effects of the extraneous variables causing the units to be heterogeneous.

Two methods of randomly allocating the experimental units to the treatments in a completely randomized design are outlined below.

CRD RANDOMIZATION METHOD I

---

1. Label the experimental units from 1 to n.

2. Draw a simple random sample of n_1 labels from the n labels. The labels drawn correspond to the labels of the units that will be allocated to treatment 1.

3. Draw a simple random sample of n_2 labels from the remaining $n - n_1$ labels. The labels drawn correspond to the labels of the units that will be allocated to treatment 2.

4. Draw a simple random sample of n_3 labels from the remaining $n - n_1 - n_2$ labels. The labels drawn correspond to the labels of the units that will be allocated to treatment 3.

5. Repeat this process until there are only n_t labels left that correspond to the labels of the units that will be allocated to treatment t.

CRD RANDOMIZATION METHOD II

1. Label the experimental units from 1 to n.

2. Create a random ordering of the n experimental units.

3. The first n_1 labels in the random ordering correspond to the labels of the units that will be allocated to treatment 1.

4. The next n_2 labels in the random ordering correspond to the labels of the units that will be allocated to treatment 2.

5. The first n_3 labels in the random ordering correspond to the labels of the units that will be allocated to treatment 3.

6. Repeat this process until there are only n_t labels left that correspond to the labels of the units that will be allocated to treatment t.

Both randomization methods are appropriate for allocating the experimental units to the treatment groups in a completely randomized design, and the choice of the particular randomization plan a researcher chooses to use should be based on convenience and the statistical computing package that will be used for analyzing the observed experimental data; some statistical computing packages even have built in randomization routines for the most commonly used experimental designs.

Example 11.7
Suppose that a completely randomized design is going to be used in an experiment with $t = 4$ treatments and $n = 24$ experimental that will be replicated according to $n_1 = 5, n_2 = 6, n_3 = 5, n_4 = 8$. Using randomization method I the units would be labeled 1–24. Then,

1. 5 labels would be randomly selected from the 24 labels to represent the units allocated to treatment 1.

2. 6 labels would be randomly selected from the remaining 19 labels to represent the units allocated to treatment 2.

3. 5 labels would be randomly selected from the 13 labels to represent the units allocated to treatment 3.

4. the remaining 8 labels would be randomly selected from the 24 labels to represent the units allocated to treatment 4.

Using method II a random ordering of the 24 labels would be created. Then,

1. the first 5 labels would represent the units allocated to treatment 1.

2. labels ordered 6 through 11 would to represent the units allocated to treatment 2.

3. labels 12 through 16 would represent the units allocated to treatment 3.

4. the last 8 labels would represent the units allocated to treatment 4.

A completely randomized design is a design that can be used to study any number of treatments, with any number of replicates, has a simple, straightforward, and easily interpreted statistical analysis, is least affected by missing data, and is the design that provides the most information per experimental unit about the experimental error. The only disadvantage of using a completely randomized design occurs when the units are not fairly homogeneous. In this case, comparative precision may be lost and another design might be a more appropriate design. Also, when a large number of treatments are being compared a completely randomized design experiment can become hard to manage and extraneous factors will be more likely to enter the experiment.

Finally, in designing an experiment that controls for both internal and external factors, it is often useful to summarize the degrees of freedom that are allocated to each source of

TABLE 11.1   Degrees of Freedom Table for a Completely Randomized Design

Source of Variation	Degrees of Freedom
Treatments	$t - 1$
Error	$n - t$
Total	$n - 1$

variation in a *degrees of freedom table*. A degrees of freedom table summarizes each source of variation and its associated degrees of freedom in a fashion similar to that used in an ANOV table. In fact, when the response variable is a quantitative variable and means are being compared, once the data from the experiment are observed the degrees of freedom table will be converted into an ANOV table summarizing the breakdown or the total variation in the response variable. The ANOV tables for designed experiments are discussed in Chapter 12.

The degrees of freedom table for a completely randomized design with t treatments and n experimental units is given in Table 11.1.

Note that the allocation of the degrees of freedom in a completely randomized design only depends on the number of treatments being compared and the number of experimental units being used in the experiment, and the allocation does not depend on in any way on the number of replicates used for the treatments. Furthermore, the reliability of a designed experiment depends on the degrees of freedom for error. When the number of experimental units is small, the degrees of freedom allocated to the experimental error will also be small compromising the accuracy and power of any comparisons made between the treatments. A good rule of thumb is to use enough experimental units so that there will be at least 12 degrees of freedom for the experimental error, however, it is always best to determine the number of experimental units that will be needed to achieve a prespecified level of accuracy and reliability in the design stage of the experiment.

Example 11.8

For a completely randomized design experiment that has 5 treatments and uses 36 experimental units, the degrees of freedom table is given in Table 11.2.

Example 11.9

For a balanced completely randomized design experiment that has six treatments that will each be replicated 10 times, determine

a. the number of experimental units that are required in this experiment.

b. the degrees of freedom table for this experiment.

TABLE 11.2   Degrees of Freedom Table for a Completely Randomized Design with 5 Treatments and 36 Experimental Units

Source of Variation	Degrees of Freedom
Treatments	$5 - 1 = 4$
Error	$36 - 5 = 31$
Total	$36 - 1 = 35$

TABLE 11.3 Degrees of Freedom Table for a Balanced Completely Randomized Design with six Treatments each Replicated 10 times

Source of Variation	Degrees of Freedom
Treatments	5
Error	54
Total	59

Solutions For a balanced completely randomized design experiment that has six treatments that will each be replicated 10 times

a. the number of experimental units required in this experiment is $6 \times 10 = 60$.

b. the degrees of freedom table for this experiment is given in Table 11.3.

Once the experimental data are observed, the degrees of freedom table will be converted into its corresponding analysis of variance table. The statistical analysis of experimental data resulting from a completely randomized design experiment and the sample size requirements for a completely randomized design are discussed in Chapter 12.

11.3.2 The Randomized Block Design

When the experimental units can be sorted into blocks of units according to a single blocking factor, a randomized block design should be used to assign the experimental units to the treatments to control for the effects of the blocking factor. Moreover, when the variability between the blocks is larger than the variability within the blocks, a randomized block design will reduce the experimental error and increase the reliability of any comparisons of the treatments. In this case, a randomized block design is more efficient than a completely randomized design.

In a randomized block design with t treatments and r blocks each block must consist of t experimental units so that each treatment will be replicated once in each of the r blocks. By assigning each treatment to one experimental unit within each block, the block affects will be equally distributed over the units in each treatment group making the treatment groups as similar as possible before the treatments are applied. A randomized block design is a balanced design where each treatment is replicated r times and the number of experimental units required in the experiment is $n = t \times r$.

The randomization plan used to allocate the experimental units to the treatments in a randomized block design must satisfy the requirement that each treatment is assigned to one and only one experimental unit within each block. In essence, each block is a completely randomized design with only one replicate of each treatment. The algorithm for randomly assigning the experimental units to the treatments in a randomized block design is outlined below.

RBD RANDOMIZATION

---

1. Sort the experimental units into the r blocks of t experimental units according to the blocking factor.

2. Within each block of units, randomly assign each treatment to one experimental unit.

TABLE 11.4 Degrees of Freedom Table for a Randomized Block Design

Source of Variation	Degrees of Freedom
Blocks	$r - 1$
Treatments	$t - 1$
Error	$(r - 1)(t - 1)$
Total	$rt - 1$

The advantages of using a randomized block design to control for a blocking factor are that blocking can increase the reliability of the experiment, there is no restriction on the number of blocks (i.e., replicates) used in a randomized block design nor is there any restriction on the number of treatments that can be studied, and the statistical analysis of the data resulting from a randomized block design experiment is relatively simple, straightforward, and easy to interpret. The only real disadvantage of using a randomized block design occurs when the blocks of experimental units are nearly similar. In this case, a completely randomized design would provide more degrees of freedom for estimating the experimental error, and hence, be a more efficient design and produce more accurate treatment comparisons than does the randomized block design.

The sources of variation and their associated degrees of freedom for a randomized block design with t treatments and r blocks are summarized in the degrees of freedom table given in Table 11.4.

In a randomized block design a good rule of thumb is to use enough experimental units so that there will be at least 12 degrees of freedom for the experimental error, however, it is always best to determine the number of experimental units that will be needed to achieve a prespecified level of accuracy and reliability in the design stage of the experiment.

Example 11.10

The degrees of freedom table for a randomized block design with $t = 6$ treatments and $r = 4$ blocks is given in Table 11.5.

Example 11.11

For a randomized block design experiment that has five treatments that will each be replicated 15 times, determine

  a. the number of experimental units that are required in this experiment.

  b. the number of blocks in this experiment.

  c. the number of experimental units in each block.

  d. the degrees of freedom table for this experiment.

TABLE 11.5 Degrees of Freedom Table for a Randomized Block Design with $t = 6$ Treatments and $r = 4$ Blocks

Source of Variation	Degrees of Freedom
Blocks	$4 - 1 = 3$
Treatments	$6 - 1 = 5$
Error	$(4 - 1)(6 - 1) = 15$
Total	$24 - 1 = 23$

TABLE 11.6 Degrees of Freedom Table for a Randomized Block Design with 5 Treatments and 15 Blocks

Source of Variation	Degrees of Freedom
Blocks	14
Treatments	4
Error	56
Total	74

TABLE 11.7 Degrees of Freedom Table for a Matched Pairs Design

Source of Variation	Degrees of Freedom
Blocks	$r - 1$
Treatments	1
Error	$r - 1$
Total	$2r - 1$

Solutions For a randomized block design experiment that has five treatments that will each be replicated 15 times

a. the number of experimental units required in this experiment is $5 \times 15 = 75$.

b. the number of blocks in this experiment is the number of replicates of each treatment, and hence, $r = 15$.

c. the number of experimental units in each block is the number of treatments being compared in the experiment, and hence, is 5.

d. the degrees of freedom table for this experiment is given in Table 11.6.

A matched pairs design is a special case of a randomized block design where there are only two treatments and the experimental units are matched in similar pairs according to a particular matching criterion. The experiment is carried out by randomly assigning each member of the pair one of the two treatments. The degrees of freedom table for a matched-pairs design is given in Table 11.7.

The statistical analysis of the experimental data resulting from a randomized block design experiment and the sample size requirements for a randomized block design are discussed in Chapter 12.

11.4 FACTORIAL EXPERIMENTS

In many research experiments there will be two or more factors that are being studied. When the treatments are formed from the combinations of the factor levels, the experiment is called a *factorial experiment* and the treatments are said to have a *factorial treatment structure*. For example, a triple HIV cocktail treatment consists of taking two nucleoside analogue drugs and a protease inhibitor, and the treatments in an experiment designed to find the optimal cocktail treatment would be formed by taking combinations of the dosage

TABLE 11.8   The Six Different Possible Antibiotic Treatments

Treatment	Dose	Form
1	Low	Liquid
2	Low	Capsule
3	Medium	Liquid
4	Medium	Capsule
5	High	Liquid
6	High	Capsule

levels of each of these drugs. In this example, each drug is a factor and the different dosages of a drug are the factor levels.

Example 11.12
Suppose that in a study of the efficacy of a particular antibiotic, the antibiotic treatments being compared in the study are based on the dosage and the form in which the antibiotic is administered. In particular, suppose that the three dosages being studied are a low, medium, and high dose and the two forms in which the drug can be administered are liquid that is injected and capsular that is taken orally. In this experiment the factors are Dose with levels low, medium, and high and Form that has levels liquid and capsule, and thus, there are six treatments that result from crossing the factors Dose and Form in a factorial experiment. The six treatments are listed in Table 11.8.

The factors in a factorial experiment can be quantitative or qualitative factors and each factor must have at least 2 levels. An experiment where the treatment combinations are formed from the levels of two factors is called a *two-factor experiment*, an experiment where the treatment combinations are formed from the levels of three factors is called a *three-factor experiment*, and in general, an experiment where the treatment combinations are formed from the levels of k factors is called a *k-factor experiment*.

In a two-factor experiment with factors A and B, when factor A has a levels and factor B has b levels, the number of treatments in the experiment is $a \times b$, and hence, the experiment is referred to as $a \times b$ *factorial experiment*. Similarly, a three-factor experiment with factors A, B, and C has $a \times b \times c$ treatments and is referred to as $a \times b \times c$ *factorial experiment* when factor A has a levels, factor B has b levels, and factor C has c levels.

Example 11.13
A factorial experiment where

- **a.** factor A has 3 levels and factor B has 2 levels is a 3×2 factorial experiment. In this experiment there are six treatments that are being studied.

- **b.** factor A has 5 levels and factor B has 3 levels is a 5×3 factorial experiment. In this experiment there are 15 treatments that are being studied.

- **c.** factor A has 2 levels, factor B has 2 levels, and factor C has 2 levels is a $2 \times 2 \times 2$ three-factor factorial experiment. In this experiment there are eight treatments that are being studied.

- **d.** factor A has 2 levels, factor B has 3 levels, and factor C has 3 levels is a $2 \times 3 \times 3$ three-factor factorial experiment. In this experiment there are 18 treatments that are being studied.

Example 11.14
Suppose in determining the optimal treatment combination for a triple HIV cocktail a factorial treatment experiment will be performed with a low and a high dose of each of the three drugs N1, N2, and P. The eight treatments in this experiment that are formed by taking combinations of the 2 levels of each drug are listed in Table 11.9.

TABLE 11.9 The Eight Treatments in the Triple HIV Factorial Experiment

Treatment	N1	N2	P
1	Low	Low	Low
2	Low	Low	High
3	Low	High	Low
4	Low	High	High
5	High	Low	Low
6	High	Low	High
7	High	High	Low
8	High	High	High

With a large number of factors being studied, the number of treatments and experimental units needed in an experiment grows large rather quickly. For this reason, in exploratory research factorial experiments in which each of the k factors has only 2 levels are fairly common and are referred to as 2^k *factorial experiments*. For example, the factorial experiment described in Example 11.14 is a 2^3 factorial experiment. Adding more levels to each factor can greatly increase the cost of the experiment and is often responsible for a reduction in the number of replicates used with each treatment. For example, a five-factor experiment with run as a 2^5 factorial experiment with three replicates requires 96 experimental units, however, when all of factors have 3 levels, the number of experimental units needed for the experiment is 729.

The reasons for using a factorial experiment over studying the factors one at a time are (1) the factors impact on the response variable can be investigated simultaneously providing for a greater degree of validity of the results, (2) the impact of the different levels of the factor on the response variable can be investigated, (3) the interactions among the factors can be investigated, and (4) factorial experiments make more efficient use of the experimental units available for experimentation. Also, factorial experiments are generally run as balanced experiments, and therefore, it will be assumed throughout Section 11.4 that all of the factorial experiments are balanced.

11.4.1 Two-Factor Experiments

In a $a \times b$ two-factor experiment with factors A and B, the goals of the experiment are to determine the impacts of the factors A and B on the response variable. In particular, a factorial experiment is designed for investigating the interaction between the two factors. When the two factors interact their effects on the response variable depend on each other and cannot be separated. On the other hand, when the two factors do not interact it is possible to investigate the importance of each of the two factors separately, and in some cases, it is possible to determine whether or not one factor is more important than the other. Thus, a factorial design is specifically designed for comparing an interaction model with a no-interaction model, and when the factors do not interact, a two-factor experiment can be used to investigate the importance of each factor in the no-interaction model.

The degrees of freedom for the treatment structure in a factorial experiment can be subdivided into sources of variation due to the *main effects* of each of the factors A and B and the *interaction* between the factors. In a two-factor experiment, a factor main effect is the effect of the factor on the response variable when averaged over the levels of the other factor, and the AB interaction is present when the difference in the response variable among

TABLE 11.10 Subdivision of the Treatment Degrees of Freedom Table for a Two-Factor Experiment

Source of Variation	Degrees of Freedom
Treatments	$ab - 1$
A	$a - 1$
B	$b - 1$
AB	$(a - 1)(b - 1)$

the levels of one factor depends on the particular level of the other factor. Thus, when the factors A and B interact the effect of one factor cannot be separated from the other and the main effects are not meaningful.

The subdivision of the treatment degrees of freedom for a $a \times b$ two-factor experiment is given the degrees of freedom table shown in Table 11.10. Note that the treatment degrees of freedom is the sum of the degrees of freedom for the factor A main effects, the factor B main effects, and the AB interactions. Also, when a separate line for the treatment source of variation is included in a degree of freedom table, the sources in subdivision of the treatment degrees of freedom are usually offset to make it clear that the treatment degrees of freedom have been subdivided. On the other hand, it is not necessary to offset the main effect and interaction sources of variation when a separate line for the treatment source of variation is not included in the table. The main effects and interaction sources of variation will be discussed in more detail in Section 11.5.

The corresponding degree of freedom tables for a two-factor completely randomized design and a two-factor randomized block design formed by replacing the treatment source of variation with the subdivision of the treatment degrees of freedom due to factors A and B in Table 11.10. Thus, the degree of freedom tables for a two-factor completely randomized design and a two-factor randomized block design are given in Tables 11.11 and 11.12, respectively.

Example 11.15

Suppose the effects of temperature and light intensity on the shelf life of fresh blood plasma are to be studied in a two-factor experiment with three different temperatures and two different light intensities. To carry out the experiment, 48 bags of blood plasma will be randomly assigned to a temperature and light intensity so that each treatment is replicated eight times. The degrees of freedom table for this 3×2 completely randomized design experiment is given in Table 11.13.

Example 11.16

Suppose the effects of temperature and light intensity on the shelf life of fresh blood plasma are to be studied in a two-factor experiment with three different temperatures and two different light intensities.

TABLE 11.11 Degrees of Freedom Table for a Two-Factor Completely Randomized Design

Source of Variation	Degrees of Freedom
A	$a - 1$
B	$b - 1$
AB	$(a - 1)(b - 1)$
Error	$ab(r - 1)$
Total	$abr - 1$

TABLE 11.12 Degrees of Freedom Table for a Two-Factor Randomized Block Design

Source of Variation	Degrees of Freedom
Blocks	$r - 1$
A	$a - 1$
B	$b - 1$
AB	$(a - 1)(b - 1)$
Error	$(r - 1)(ab - 1)$
Total	$abr - 1$

TABLE 11.13 Degrees of Freedom Table for the 3 × 2 Two-Factor Blood Plasma Shelf Life Experiment

Source of Variation	Degrees of Freedom
Temp	2
Light	1
Temp*Light	2
Error	42
Total	47

To carry out the experiment, 48 bags of blood plasma will be randomly assigned to a temperature and light intensity so that each treatment is replicated eight times, however, due to logistical constraints the experiment can only be performed on six bags of blood at one time. Thus, the experiment will be run as a randomized block design with eight blocks. The degrees of freedom table for this 3×2 randomized block design experiment is given in Table 11.14.

11.4.2 Three-Factor Experiments

In a three-factor experiment with factors A, B, and C the goals of the experiment are to determine the impacts of the three factors on the response variable and whether or not the factors interact. Unlike the two-factor experiment where there is only one possible type of interaction, with three factors there are four possible types of interaction. In particular, the interactions possible in a three-factor experiment are the AB interaction, the AC interaction, the BC interaction, and the ABC interaction. The AB, AC, and BC interactions are called *two-way interactions* because they involve only two factors at a time, and the ABC interaction is called a *three-way interactions* because it involves all three factors.

TABLE 11.14 Degrees of Freedom Table for the 3 × 2 Two-Factor Blood Plasma Shelf Life Experiment

Source of Variation	Degrees of Freedom
Blocks	7
Temp	2
Light	1
Temp*Light	2
Error	35
Total	47

TABLE 11.15   Subdivision of the Treatment Degrees of Freedom Table for a Three-Factor Experiment

Source of Variation	Degrees of Freedom
Treatments	$abc - 1$
A	$a - 1$
B	$b - 1$
C	$c - 1$
AB	$(a - 1)(b - 1)$
AC	$(a - 1)(c - 1)$
BC	$(b - 1)(c - 1)$
ABC	$(a - 1)(b - 1)(c - 1)$

The degrees of freedom for the treatment structure in a three-factor experiment can be subdivided into sources of variation due to the effects of the factors A, B, and C and the interactions. In a three-factor experiment a factor main effect is the effect of the factor on the response variable when averaged over all of the levels of the other factors, a two-way interaction is present when the difference in the response variable among the levels of one factor depends on the particular level of the other factor, and a three-way interaction is present when difference in the response variable among the levels of one factor depends on the particular levels of the other two factors. As in a two-factor experiment, when any of the factors interact the effects of one factor cannot be separated from the others and the main effects of these factors will not be meaningful.

The subdivision of the $abc - 1$ treatment degrees of freedom for a $a \times b \times c$ three-factor experiment is shown in Table 11.15.

Similar to a two-factor experiment, in a three-factor experiment the subdivision of the treatment degrees of freedom should be included in the degrees of freedom table for the completely randomized design and the randomized block design. In general, the line for the treatment degrees of freedom is dropped from the table and replaced with the subdivided treatment degrees of freedom as listed in Table 11.15.

Example 11.17

In Example 11.14 an experiment for determining the optimal treatment combination for a triple HIV cocktail was described as a factorial treatment experiment with a low and a high dose of each of the three drugs N1, N2, and P. The degrees of freedom table for running this 2^3 factorial experiment as a completely randomized design with five replicates of each treatment is given in Table 11.16.

TABLE 11.16   The Degrees of Freedom Table for the Triple Cocktail Experiment Run as a Completely Randomized Design

Source of Variation	Degrees of Freedom
N1	1
N2	1
P	1
N1*N2	1
N1*P	1
N2*P	1
N1*N2*P	1
Error	32
Total	39

TABLE 11.17 The Degrees of Freedom Table for the Triple Cocktail Experiment Run as a Completely Randomized Design

Source of Variation	Degrees of Freedom
Blocks	4
N1	1
N2	1
P	2
N1*N2	1
N1*P	2
N2*P	2
N1*N2*P	2
Error	44
Total	59

Example 11.18

Suppose that the experiment for determining the optimal treatment combination for a triple HIV cocktail is to be performed as a randomized block factorial treatment experiment with a low and a high dose of each of the drugs N1, N2, and low, medium, and high doses of the drug P. This experiment has $2 \times 2 \times 3 = 12$ treatments that are being studied, and the degrees of freedom table for a randomized block $2 \times 2 \times 3$ factorial experiment with five replicates (i.e., blocks) of each treatment is given in Table 11.17.

11.5 MODELS FOR DESIGNED EXPERIMENTS

Linear models are often used to model the quantitative observations on a response variable that result from a designed experiment. In particular, a statistical model for a designed experiment is similar to a regression model, linear or logistic, and accounts for all aspects of the design including treatments, factors, blocks, and experimental error. In particular, the statistical model for a designed experiment reflects all of the sources of variation listed in the degree of freedom table. When the response variable is a quantitative variable, the statistical model for a designed experiment modeling the response variable Y is a linear model, and when the response variable is a binary variable then the statistical model for a designed experiment is a logistic regression model for the probability that $Y = 1$.

Throughout this section only the models for a quantitative response variable will be discussed. The two main differences between the linear model for a quantitative response and a logistic regression model for a binary response variable are (1) a linear model is a model of Y while a logistic regression model is a model for the logit of $P(Y = 1)$ and (2) a linear model has an additive error term and there is no error term in a logistic regression model. In either case, the parameters of the model will be the same in the model associated with a designed experiment.

11.5.1 The Model for a Completely Randomized Design

The linear model used to model a quantitative response variable in a completely randomized design experiment with t treatments is given below.

THE LINEAR MODEL FOR A COMPLETELY RANDOMIZED DESIGN

The linear model for a completely randomized design is

$$Y_{ij} = \mu + \tau_i + \epsilon_{ij}$$

where

$Y_{ij} =$ the response of jth experimental unit receiving the ith treatment

$\mu =$ the overall mean of the untreated experimental units

$\tau_i =$ the ith treatment effect

$\epsilon_{ij} =$ the experimental error for the jth unit receiving the ith treatment

---

In general, the subscripts are usually dropped from the Y, τ, and ϵ terms in the model and the model for a completely randomized design is written as $Y = \mu + \tau + \epsilon$. Note that this linear model states that each observation on the response variable is the sum of an overall mean, a treatment effect for the treatment applied to the experimental unit, and experimental error that accounts for inherent variability in experimental units and the experimental process.

The assumptions on error term (i.e., ϵ) in the model are that the errors are independent random variables with mean 0 and the same standard deviation. When hypothesis tests and confidence intervals will be performed in the statistical analysis of a completely randomized design experiment the error term must also be normally distributed. Note that these are the same assumptions placed on the error term in a linear regression model.

Now, since $\mu_\epsilon = 0$, the mean of the response variable for the units receiving the ith treatment is $\mu + \tau_i$, and therefore, the difference between the means of the response variable for two units receiving different treatments

$$(\mu + \tau_i) - (\mu + \tau_j) = \tau_i - \tau_j$$

Thus, any comparisons of the treatment means can be rewritten in terms of the treatment effects (i.e., the τs). In fact, one of the important hypotheses that is tested in a designed experiment is

$$H_0 : \text{The treatment means are all equal}$$

which can be restated in terms of the treatment effects as

$$H_0 : \text{The treatment effects are all equal}$$

The analysis of the experimental data resulting from a completely randomized design experiment generally includes model fitting, assumption checking, and confidence intervals and hypothesis tests on the treatment effects. A detailed discussion of the analysis of a completely randomized design experiment with a quantitative explanatory variable is given in Chapter 12.

Example 11.19

The model for a binary response variable in a completely randomized design is

$$\text{logit}(p) = \mu + \tau$$

where τ represents the treatment effects and μ is the overall mean. Note that there is no error term in a logistic regression model. Also, if there are t treatments, the logistic regression model for a completely randomized design defines t probabilities associated with $Y = 1$ of the form

$$p(Y = 1 | \text{treatment } i) = \frac{e^{\mu + \tau_i}}{1 + e^{\mu + \tau_i}}$$

11.5.2 The Model for a Randomized Block Design

The linear model used to model a quantitative response variable in a randomized block design experiment with t treatments and b blocks is

---

THE LINEAR MODEL FOR A RANDOMIZED BLOCK DESIGN

The linear model for a randomized block design is

$$Y_{ij} = \mu + \rho_j + \tau_i + \epsilon_{ij}$$

where

Y_{ij} = the response of the unit in the jth block receiving the ith treatment

μ = the overall mean of the untreated experimental units

ρ_j = the jth block effect

τ_i = the ith treatment effect

ϵ_{ij} = the experimental error for the unit in the jth block with the ith treatment

---

Dropping the subscripts, the model for a randomized block design can be written as $Y = \mu + \rho + \tau + \epsilon$. Thus, in a randomized block design the observation on response variable is the sum of an overall mean, a block effect, a treatment effect, and experimental error. The assumptions on error term (i.e., ϵ) in the model for a randomized block design are the same as they were for the model in a completely randomized design. That is, the error terms are assumed to be independent random variables with mean 0 and the same standard deviation, and when hypothesis tests and confidence intervals will be performed in the statistical analysis, the error term must also be normally distributed.

Additional assumptions must also be placed on the block effects in the model for a randomized block design since the block effects are generally considered random sources of variation. In particular, the two assumptions placed on the blocks are (1) blocks and treatments do not interact and (2) the block effects are normally distributed with mean 0 and standard deviation σ_B.

Now, since the error term and the block terms have mean 0, the mean of the response variable for an experimental unit receiving the ith treatment is $\mu + \tau_i$ and the difference between the means of two experimental units receiving different treatments is

$$(\mu + \tau_i) - (\mu + \tau_j) = \tau_i - \tau_j$$

as it was in the completely randomized design model. Hence, any comparisons of the treatment means in a randomized block design experiment can be rewritten in terms of the treatment effects τ, and the null hypothesis

$$H_0 : \text{The treatment means are all equal}$$

can also be restated in terms of the treatment effects as

$$H_0 : \text{The treatment effects are all equal}$$

A detailed discussion of the analysis of a randomized block design experiment with a quantitative explanatory variable is given in Chapter 12.

Example 11.20

The model for a binary response variable in a randomized block design is

$$\text{logit}(p) = \mu + \rho + \tau$$

where ρ represents the block effects, τ represents the treatment effects, and μ is the overall mean. Again, there is no error term in a logistic regression model.

11.5.3 Models for Experimental Designs with a Factorial Treatment Structure

When the treatments in a designed experiment have a factorial treatment structure, additional terms can be added to the model that more fully explain the sources of variation in the experiment. In particular, terms will be added to the model to account for the main effects of each factor and interactions effects.

In a two-factor experiment with factors A and B where the ith treatment is comprised of the jth level of factor A and the kth level of factor B, the ith treatment effect is described below.

THE LINEAR MODEL FOR A TWO-FACTOR TREATMENT STRUCTURE

The linear model for a two-factor factorial treatment structure is

$$\tau_i = \gamma_j + \beta_k + \gamma\beta_{jk}$$

where

$\gamma_j = $ the main effect of factor A at level j

$\beta_k = $ the main effect of factor B at level k

$\gamma\beta_{jk} = $ the interaction effect of factor A at level j and factor B at level k

---

Again, it is standard practice to drop the subscripts and write the treatment effect τ as $\gamma + \beta + \gamma\beta$ in a model for a factorial experiment. Thus, the model for a completely randomized design two-factor experiment is

$$Y = \mu + \gamma + \beta + \gamma\beta + \epsilon$$

and the model for two-factor randomized block design experiment is

$$Y = \mu + \rho + \gamma + \beta + \gamma\beta + \epsilon$$

Furthermore, the difference between two treatment means, $\tau_r - \tau_s$, in either the completely randomized or randomized block model is

$$(\gamma_j - \gamma_l) + (\beta_k - \beta_m) + (\gamma\beta_{jk} - \gamma\beta_{lm})$$

where the rth treatment is formed from level j of factor A and level k of factor B and sth treatment is formed from level l of factor A and level m of factor B. Note that the difference between two treatment means is now based on the difference between the main effects and the interaction effects in the model. Furthermore, the difference between two treatment means will only be the difference between the main effects when the factors do not interact. Thus, an important hypothesis that is tested in a two-factor experiment is

$$H_0 : \text{Factors } A \text{ and } B \text{ do not interact}$$

which can be restated in terms of the interaction effects as

$$H_0 : \text{all of the } \gamma\beta \text{ terms are equal to } 0.$$

When the test of the interaction is significant there is evidence that the factors A and B interact, and therefore, the factor main effects are not meaningful and should not be tested.

On the other hand, when there is no significant evidence that factors A and B interact it will be important to test the factor A and factor B main effects. That is, when the factors do not interact the difference of the treatment means is simple the sum of the differences of the factor A and B main effects. In particular, when the factors do not interact the difference of the treatment means is

$$(\gamma_i - \gamma_l) + (\beta_j - \beta_m)$$

where the first treatment is formed from the ith level of factor A and the jth level of factor B and the second treatment is formed from the lth level of factor A and the mth level of factor B. Tests of interaction and main effects in a factorial experiment will be discussed in detail in Chapter 12.

The model for the factorial treatment structure in a three-factor experiment with factors A, B, and C is described below.

THE LINEAR MODEL FOR A THREE-FACTOR TREATMENT STRUCTURE

The linear model for a three-factor factorial treatment structure is

$$\tau_i = \gamma_j + \beta_k + \delta_l + \gamma\beta_{jk} + \gamma\delta_{jl} + \beta\delta_{kl} + \gamma\beta\delta_{jkl}$$

where

$\gamma_j =$ the main effect of factor A at level j

$\beta_k =$ the main effect of factor B at level k

$\delta_l =$ the main effect of factor C at level l

$\gamma\beta_{jk} =$ the two-way interaction effects of factors A and B at levels j and k

$\gamma\delta_{jl} =$ the two-way interaction effects of factors A and C at levels j and l j and l

$\beta\delta_{kl} =$ the two-way interaction effects of factors B and C at levels k and l k and l

$\gamma\beta\delta_{jkl} =$ three-way interaction effects of factors A, B, and C at levels j, k, l j, k, l

---

Again the subscripts are usually dropped and the three-factor model for the treatment effects can be written as

$$\tau = \gamma + \beta + \delta + \gamma\beta + \gamma\delta + \beta\delta + \gamma\beta\delta$$

Thus, the model for a completely randomized design three-factor experiment is

$$Y = \mu + \gamma + \beta + \delta + \gamma\beta + \gamma\delta + \beta\delta + \gamma\beta\delta + \epsilon$$

and the model for three-factor randomized block design experiment is

$$Y = \mu + \rho + \gamma + \beta + \delta + \gamma\beta + \gamma\delta + \beta\delta + \gamma\beta\delta + \epsilon$$

Furthermore, the difference between two treatment means, $\tau_r - \tau_s$, under each of these models is the difference between the main effects and all of the two and three-way interaction effects for the factors in the model. The difference between two treatment means will only be a function of the main effects when there are no two-way or three-way interactions in the model, and hence, the importance of the main effects of the factors A, B, and C can only be tested when the data suggests there is no evidence of any two-way or three-way interactions. The testing procedure for a three-factor model will be discussed in Chapter 12.

11.6 SOME FINAL COMMENTS OF DESIGNED EXPERIMENTS

The main reason that a well-designed experiment is more reliable than an observational study is that in an experiment the researcher can control for extraneous factors. In designing an experiment that will provide sufficient data for investigating the research questions the researcher must first select a set experimental units that is representative of the target population. When the pool of experimental units is not representative of the target population the experiment may produce misleading inferences about the target population. Furthermore, the nature of the experimental units will also influence the experimental design that will be used and the accuracy of the experiment.

In choosing the appropriate experimental design the researcher must also decide on the treatments that will be studied and whether or not there are any extraneous factors that must be controlled for. The goal of an experimental design is to allocate the experimental units to the treatment groups so that they are as similar as possible before the treatments are applied. When the experimental units in each of the treatment groups are similar, any difference in the response variable for two experimental units assigned different treatments is most likely due to treatments and not an extraneous factor. Thus, the researcher must examine the experimental units and determine whether they are homogeneous, heterogeneous, or align in blocks of units. When the experimental units are homogeneous or heterogeneous randomization may be used to control for any extraneous factors in a completely randomized design, and when the units align in blocks a restricted randomization should be used such as a randomized block design. The examination of the experimental units and the choice of an appropriate design are important steps in minimizing the experimental error.

The reliability of an experiment depends on the number of replicates used in the experiment, and therefore, an important step in designing the experiment is to prespecify the level of reliability. Once the desired level of reliability of an experiment has been set, the number of replicates that are required to attain this level of reliability can be determined. The cost of performing an experiment is clearly a limiting factor on the number of experimental units that can be used, but on the other hand, performing an experiment with an insufficient number of experimental units would also be a waste of money. Methods for determining the necessary number of experimental units for a prespecified level of reliability in a completely randomized or a randomized block design are discussed in Chapter 12.

Finally, while only the completely randomized and the randomized block experimental designs were discussed in this chapter, there are many other experimental designs that exist. A good source of information on a wide variety of experimental designs that can be used to control for extraneous factors is the experimental design book *Design and Analysis of Experiments* (Petersen, 1985).

GLOSSARY

Blinded Experiment   An experiment is called a blinded experiment when measures are taken to prevent the experimental units and researchers who apply the treatments to the experimental units from knowing which treatment has been applied. A blinded experiment is called a single-blind experiment when only the subjects are blinded, and an experiment is called a double-blind experiment when both the subjects and the researchers are blinded.

Block A block of experimental units is a subgroup of the experimental units that are homogeneous.

Blocking Factor A pre-existing characteristic of the experimental units or the experimental process that is not assigned by the researcher is called a blocking factor.

Completely Randomized Design A completely randomized design is an experimental design where the experimental units are randomly assigned to the treatment groups without restriction.

Confounding When the effects of an explanatory variable on the response variable cannot be distinguished or separated from the effects of an extraneous variable, the variables are said to be confounded.

Control Treatment A control treatment is a baseline treatment that all the other treatments will be compared against.

Controlled Experiment A controlled experiment is an experiment where the researcher controls for the effects of extraneous variables, and a randomized controlled experiment is a controlled experiment where the experimental units are randomly assigned to the treatments.

Experiment An experiment is any study where the researcher assigns the units of the study to the treatment groups. Experiments performed on humans to assess the efficacy of a treatment or treatments are called clinical trials.

Experimental design The experimental design is the plan used to allocate the experimental units to the different treatments being compared in the experiment.

Experimental Error Experimental error is a measure of the variation that exists among the measurements made on the experimental units that have been treated alike.

Experimental Unit An experimental unit is the smallest unit in the population to which a set of experimental conditions can be applied so that two different units may receive different experimental conditions.

Extraneous Variable Factors that are not controlled for in an experiment or observational study are called extraneous, confounding, or lurking variables.

Factorial Experiment An experiment where the treatments are formed from the combinations of the factor levels the experiment is called a factorial experiment.

Factorial Treatment Structure Treatments that are formed from the combinations of the factor levels are said to have a factorial treatment structure.

Interaction Effects An interaction is present when the difference in the response variable among the levels of one factor depends on the particular levels of another factor or other factors.

Main Effects A factor main effect is the effect of the factor on the response variable when averaged over all of the levels of the other factors.

Observational Study An observational study is any study where the units come to the researcher already assigned to the treatment groups.

Placebo A placebo treatment is an inert treatment.

Randomization Randomization is a probability based method of allocating the experimental units to the different treatments.

Randomized Block Design A randomized block design is an experimental design where the experimental units are sorted into blocks and each treatment is randomly assigned to one and only one experimental unit within each block.

Replicated Experiment   An experiment is said to be replicated when two or more experimental units receive the same treatment. An experiment is said to be balanced when each treatment receives the same number of replicates, and experiments that are not balanced are said to be unbalanced.

Three-way Interaction   A three-way interaction is an interaction between three factors in factorial experiment.

Treatment   A treatment is any experimental condition that is applied to the experimental units. A treatment group is the collection of experimental units assigned to a particular treatment.

Two-way Interaction   A two-way interaction is an interaction between two factors in factorial experiment.

EXERCISES

11.1   What is an experiment?

11.2   What is an observational study?

11.3   What distinguishes an experiment from an observational study?

11.4   What is

    (a) an extraneous variable?   **(b)** confounding variable?

11.5   What does it mean when the effects of two variables are said to be confounded?

11.6   Determine whether each of the following studies is an experiment or an observational study.

    (a) A medical researcher is going to study the relationship between cell phone use and Alzheimer's disease.

    (b) A medical researcher is going to study the relationship between recovery time after heart bypass surgery and age.

    (c) A fertility clinic is going to study the optimal temperature in which to store frozen sperm.

    (d) A medical researcher at a pharmaceutical lab has developed a new synthetic antibiotic and needs to determine the appropriate dosage of this antibiotic.

11.7   Why is a well-designed experiment preferred over an observational study?

11.8   Why is a retrospective study always an observational study?

11.9   Can an experiment always be used in a prospective study? Explain.

11.10   A medical researcher wants to study the long-term effects of the regular smoking of marijuana. In a retrospective study a random sample of 200 adults is selected and surveyed on their use of marijuana and their health. Determine whether this study is an observational study or an experiment. If this study is an observational study explain why it was not performed as an experiment.

11.11   A medical researcher wants to investigate the relationship between increased dietary intake of fiber and cholesterol level. The three treatments being studied are a control treatment where a subject maintains their current diet and two increased fiber treatments where a subject increases their dietary intake of fiber by either 10% or 25%. A simple random sample of size 300 is selected from a list of 500 volunteers to make up the pool of experimental units. Each subject will have their cholesterol level measured prior to the start of the experiment to serve as a baseline comparison and then again after a 3-month treatment period, and the change in cholesterol level after the 3-month treatment period will be studied. The 300 subjects are randomly assigned to the three groups and the subjects are given detailed instructions on how they are to alter their dietary regimen.

(a) Is this study an experiment or an observational study?

(b) What are the treatments in this study?

(c) What are the experimental units in this study?

(d) What is the response variable in this study?

11.12 A medical researcher wants to investigate the relationship between the duration of the common cold and the use of echinacea and vitamin C. The three treatments being studied are echinacea, 1000 mg of vitamin C, and a control treatment where a subject receives a placebo. A simple random sample of size 90 is selected from a list of volunteers to make up the pool of experimental units. Each subject will record the length of the duration of any colds they have in a one-year period. The 90 subjects are randomly assigned to the three groups and the subjects are given identical capsules containing their respective treatments in a fashion so that a subject will not know which treatment they have received.

(a) Is this study an experiment or an observational study?

(b) What are the treatments in this study?

(c) What are the experimental units in this study?

(d) What is the response variable in this study?

(e) Is this a blinded experiment?

11.13 A physical therapist is interested in comparing three different physical therapy regimens for patients recovering from knee replacement surgery. The three treatment to be studied are weight training, aquatic exercise, and walking. Each treatment group will consist of eight subjects who have recently had knee surgery. Each subject will be measured and given a condition score before starting their rehabilitation program and then measured again at the end of the program. The change in an individual's condition score will be analyzed.

(a) Is this study an experiment or an observational study?

(b) What are the treatments in this study?

(c) What are the experimental units in this study?

(d) What is the response variable in this study?

(e) Is this a blinded experiment?

11.14 What is

(a) an experimental unit?

(b) a treatment?

(c) a block?

(d) a blinded experiment?

(e) a placebo?

(f) a replicate?

(g) a balanced experiment?

(h) an experimental error?

(i) a randomized controlled experiment?

(j) an experimental design?

11.15 What is the purpose of replicating the treatments in an experiment?

11.16 What are the factors that limit the number of experimental units and replicates of each treatment that can be used in an experiment?

11.17 What is the purpose of randomly assigning the experimental units to the treatment groups?

11.18 What are the two sources of experimental error?

11.19 What is a blocking factor?

11.20 What is the purpose of sorting the experimental units into blocks of units that are alike?

11.21 Under what conditions is it appropriate to consider using a

(a) completely randomized design?   (b) randomized block design?

11.22 Determine the random allocation of the experimental units to the treatments in a completely randomized design with

(a) $t = 4$ treatments, $n = 25$ experimental units, and treatment replications $n_1 = 6, n_2 = 5, n_3 = 5, n_4 = 9$.

(b) $t = 3$ treatments, $n = 25$ experimental units, and treatment replications $n_1 = 8, n_2 = 9, n_3 = 5, n_4 = 8$.

(c) $t = 3$ treatments, $n = 27$ experimental units, and balanced treatment replication.

(d) $t = 4$ treatments, $n = 32$ experimental units, and balanced treatment replication.

11.23 Determine the degrees of freedom table associated with each of the completely randomized designs in Exercise 11.22.

11.24 Determine the degrees of freedom table for a completely randomized design with

(a) $t = 4$ treatments and $n = 36$ experimental units.

(b) $t = 5$ treatments and $n = 50$ experimental units.

(c) $t = 3$ treatments and $n = 30$ experimental units.

(d) $t = 10$ treatments and $n = 40$ experimental units.

11.25 A balanced completely randomized design is going to be used to study four treatments. Determine

(a) the number of replicates needed so that there will be at least 20 degrees associated with experimental error.

(b) the degrees of freedom table for this experiment using the number of replicates from part (a).

11.26 A balanced completely randomized design is going to be used to study six treatments. Determine

(a) the number of replicates needed so that there will be at least 32 degrees associated with experimental error.

(b) the degrees of freedom table for this experiment using the number of replicates from part (a).

11.27 For a randomized block design with five treatments and six blocks, determine

(a) the number of experimental units needed to perform this experiment.

    (b) the number of experimental units in each block.

    (c) the number of replicates of each treatment.

11.28 For a randomized block design with 6 treatments and 12 blocks, determine
    (a) the number of experimental units needed to perform this experiment.
    (b) the number of experimental units in each block.
    (c) the number of replicates of each treatment.

11.29 Determine the randomization for a randomized block design with
    (a) $t = 4$ treatments and $r = 6$ blocks.
    (b) $t = 3$ treatments and $r = 5$ blocks.
    (c) $t = 3$ treatments and $r = 7$ blocks.
    (d) $t = 5$ treatments and $r = 4$ blocks.

11.30 Determine the degrees of freedom table associated with each of the randomized block designs in Exercise 11.29.

11.31 Determine the degrees of freedom table for a randomized block design with
    (a) $t = 4$ treatments and $r = 6$ blocks.
    (b) $t = 6$ treatments and $r = 4$ blocks.
    (c) $t = 7$ treatments and $r = 8$ blocks.
    (d) $t = 10$ treatments and $r = 10$ blocks.

11.32 An experiment is going to be performed to compare five treatments, however, only six experimental units may be studied at any one time. Determine
    (a) the number of blocks needed so that there will be at least 25 degrees associated with experimental error.
    (b) the degrees of freedom table for this experiment using the number of blocks from part (a).

11.33 An experiment is going to be performed to compare 8 treatments, however, only 12 experimental units may be studied at any one time. Determine
    (a) the number of blocks needed so that there will be at least 40 degrees associated with experimental error.
    (b) the degrees of freedom table for this experiment using the number of blocks from part (a).

11.34 What are the advantages of a completely randomized design?

11.35 What is the advantage of using a randomized block design over a completely randomized design when the units align in blocks?

11.36 What is the disadvantage of using a randomized block design over a completely randomized design when the units do not align in blocks?

11.37 What is the experimental design that is used in a matched pairs study?

11.38 Determine the degrees of freedom table for a matched pairs experiment when there are

    (a) 10 pairs.   **(b)** 25 pairs.

11.39 Suppose a researcher is going to study the effects of alcohol on motor function skills. Twenty subjects of different motor function skills are available for the experiment, and each subject will be tested before receiving any alcohol and after their blood alcohol level (BAC) reaches a level 0.08%.

(a) What is the blocking factor in this experiment?

(b) How many blocks are there in this experiment?

(c) What are the treatments in this experiment?

11.40 What is a

(a) factorial experiment?

(b) factorial treatment structure?

(c) two-factor experiment?

(d) two-factor treatment structure?

11.41 Determine the treatments in a two-factor experiment when

(a) factor A has levels low, medium, and high and factor B has levels low and high.

(b) factor A has levels 10%, 15%, and 20% and factor B has levels water, alcohol, glycerine.

11.42 Determine the treatments in a three-factor experiment when

(a) factor A has levels low and high, factor B has levels wet and dry, and factor C has levels 10% and 20%.

(b) factor A has levels low, medium, and high, factor B has levels light and dark, and factor C has levels 10% and 20%.

11.43 Determine the number of treatments in a

(a) 4×2 factorial experiment.

(b) 3×4 factorial experiment.

(c) $4 \times 2 \times 2$ factorial experiment.

(d) $2 \times 2 \times 5$ factorial experiment.

(e) 2^4 factorial experiment.

(f) 2^5 factorial experiment.

11.44 In a 2^4 factorial experiment how many

(a) factors are being studied?

(b) levels does each factor have?

(c) treatments are being studied?

11.45 Determine the degrees of freedom table for a completely randomized design experiment run as a

(a) 4×3 factorial experiment with $r = 6$ replicates of each treatment.

(b) 3×3 factorial experiment with $r = 5$ replicates of each treatment.

(c) 2×5 factorial experiment with $r = 10$ replicates of each treatment.

11.46 A completely randomized design is going to be used to study the treatments in a 4×2 factorial experiment. Determine

(a) the number of replicates needed so that there will be at least 26 degrees associated with experimental error.

(b) the degrees of freedom table for this experiment using the number of replicates from part (a).

11.47 A completely randomized design is going to be used to study the treatments in a 5×2 factorial experiment. Determine

(a) the number of replicates needed so that there will be at least 35 degrees associated with experimental error.

(b) the degrees of freedom table for this experiment using the number of replicates from part (a).

11.48 Determine the degrees of freedom table for a randomized block design experiment run as a

(a) 2×3 factorial experiment with $r = 4$ blocks.

(b) 4×4 factorial experiment with $r = 5$ blocks.

(c) 3×6 factorial experiment with $r = 12$ blocks.

11.49 A randomized block design is going to be used to study the treatments in a 2×3 factorial experiment. Determine

(a) the number of blocks needed so that there will be at least 35 degrees associated with experimental error.

(b) the degrees of freedom table for this experiment using the number of blocks from part (a).

11.50 A randomized block design is going to be used to study the treatments in a 3×3 factorial experiment. Determine

(a) the number of blocks needed so that there will be at least 35 degrees associated with experimental error.

(b) the degrees of freedom table for this experiment using the number of blocks from part (a).

11.51 If the response variable is a quantitative variable, what are the assumptions made on the error term in the model for a

(a) completely randomized design?

(b) randomized block design?

11.52 If the response variable is a quantitative variable, what are the assumptions made on the block term in the model for a randomized block design?

11.53 Determine the degrees of freedom table for a completely randomized design experiment run as a

(a) $4 \times 3 \times 2$ factorial experiment with $r = 5$ replicates of each treatment.

(b) $3 \times 3 \times 2$ factorial experiment with $r = 6$ replicates of each treatment.

(c) $2 \times 2 \times 5$ factorial experiment with $r = 8$ replicates of each treatment.

11.54 A completely randomized design is going to be used to study the treatments in a $4 \times 2 \times 3$ factorial experiment. Determine

(a) the number of replicates needed so that there will be at least 25 degrees associated with experimental error.

(b) the degrees of freedom table for this experiment using the number of replicates from part (a).

11.55 A completely randomized design is going to be used to study the treatments in a 2^3 factorial experiment. Determine

(a) the number of replicates needed so that there will be at least 30 degrees associated with experimental error.

(b) the degrees of freedom table for this experiment using the number of replicates from part (a).

11.56 Determine the degrees of freedom table for a randomized block design experiment run as a

(a) $2 \times 3 \times 3$ factorial experiment with $r = 5$ blocks.

(b) $2 \times 4 \times 4$ factorial experiment with $r = 8$ blocks.

(c) $3 \times 2 \times 2$ factorial experiment with $r = 10$ blocks.

11.57 A randomized block design is going to be used to study the treatments in a $2 \times 3 \times 2$ factorial experiment. Determine
  (a) the number of blocks needed so that there will be at least 25 degrees associated with experimental error.
  (b) the degrees of freedom table for this experiment using the number of blocks from part (a).

11.58 A randomized block design is going to be used to study the treatments in a 2^3 factorial experiment. Determine
  (a) the number of blocks needed so that there will be at least 30 degrees associated with experimental error.
  (b) the degrees of freedom table for this experiment using the number of blocks from part (a).

11.59 What is a main effect?

11.60 What is an interaction effect?

11.61 If the response variable is a quantitative variable, determine the model for
  (a) a completely randomized design.
  (b) a randomized block design.
  (c) a completely randomized design in a two-factor factorial experiment.
  (d) a randomized block design in a two-factor factorial experiment.
  (e) a completely randomized design in a three-factor factorial experiment.
  (f) a randomized block design in a three-factor factorial experiment.

11.62 If the response variable is a quantitative variable, what is the difference between two treatment means in a two-factor experiment when
  (a) the factors interact?
  (b) the factors do not interact?

11.63 If the response variable is a quantitative variable, what is the difference between two treatment means in a three-factor experiment when
  (a) all of the interactions are present?
  (b) only the two-way interactions are present?
  (c) none of the factors interact?

11.64 If the response variable is a quantitative variable, determine the model for a four-factor factorial experiment run as a
  (a) a completely randomized design.
  (b) a randomized block design.

11.65 If the response variable is a binary variable, determine the model for
  (a) a completely randomized design.
  (b) a randomized block design.
  (c) a completely randomized design in a two-factor factorial experiment.
  (d) a randomized block design in a two-factor factorial experiment.
  (e) a completely randomized design in a three-factor factorial experiment.
  (f) a randomized block design in a three-factor factorial experiment.

CHAPTER 12

ANALYSIS OF VARIANCE

 IN **CHAPTER** 11, the design of experiments was discussed and in this chapter the analysis of data resulting from a designed experiment or a well-designed observational study will be discussed. In particular, the statistical method used to analyze data from a designed experiment that will be discussed is *analysis of variance* that is also referred to as ANOV. Analysis of variance can be used when the response variable is a quantitative variable and the objective of the analysis is to compare the treatment means. Analysis of variance can also be used to analyze the data resulting from an observational study when the study design is similar to an experiment up to the assignment of the units to the treatments. That is, in a designed experiment the treatments are assigned to the experimental units by the researcher, but in an observational study the units come to the researcher already assigned to the treatment groups being studied. However, like an experiment, an observational study can have two or more treatment groups whose means will be compared, there might be blocking factors to control for in the study, and the treatments may have a factorial treatment structure.

Example 12.1
Suppose a retrospective study of survival times of patients diagnosed with melanoma is classified by their cancer stage. In particular, the treatments in this study are Clark Stage I, Clark Stage II, Clark Stage III, and Clark Stage IV. Because the cancer patients come to the researcher with their Clark Stage already assigned, this is an observational study. The patients in the study might be selected using a simple random sample or a stratified random sample from a large pool of melanoma patients and then sorted according to Clark Stage. Analysis of variance could be used to compare the mean survival times using analysis of variance provided the sampling design controlled for as many extraneous factors as possible.

 Analysis of variance is typically used in experiments or observational studies where two or more treatment groups are being compared. In this case, analysis of variance can be used for comparing the means of the treatments. While it would be possible to compare all the means with two-sample *t*-tests, this is neither the most efficient nor the most reliable way to proceed in comparing the treatment means. For example, with 10 treatment groups there would be 45 pairwise two-sample *t*-tests to perform, and therefore, the likelihood of making at least one Type I error would be high. On the other hand, analysis of variance is an efficient approach that can be used to test the simultaneous equality of two or more treatment means and for comparing the treatment means in an efficient way that controls for the probability of making at least one Type I error. In a factorial experiment, analysis of variance can also be used to investigate the interactions and the main effects of the factors making up the treatments.

The general idea behind analysis of variance is to partition the total variation in the observed values of the response variable into sources of variation that are due to treatments, blocking factors, and the experimental error. The sources of variation are summarized in an ANOV table, and by comparing the variation due to the treatments with the variation due to the experimental error, the simultaneous equality of the treatment means can be tested. In Section 12.1, analysis of variance will be discussed for data arising from a completely randomized design experiment or a single-factor observational study; in Section 12.2, the analysis of data arising from a randomized block design will be discussed; and Section 12.3, analysis of variance for data arising from two-factor and three-factor experiments or observational studies will be discussed.

12.1 SINGLE-FACTOR ANALYSIS OF VARIANCE

Single-factor analysis of variance, also referred to as a *one-way analysis of variance*, is the statistical procedure used for analyzing data arising from a completely randomized design experiment or an observational study with treatment groups due to a single factor. In a single-factor analysis of variance, the quantitative response variable Y is believed to depend on the single treatment factor being studied and the primary objective is to compare the treatment means and determine which of the treatment means are different.

The data to be analyzed in a single-factor analysis of variance consists of n observations on the response variable Y that can be sorted into t treatment groups according to the treatments assigned to the experimental units. The number of replicates of the ith treatment is n_i and the total number of experimental units is $n = \sum n_i$. To distinguish the values of the observed response variable from each other, subscripts are often used to identify the treatment a unit received and the replicate of a particular treatment. Thus, in a single-factor analysis of variance, the observed value of the response variable for the jth replicate of the ith treatment is denoted by y_{ij}. The observed values of the response variable for the n experimental units in the experiment are often entered into a spreadsheet in a statistical computing package. The spreadsheet must also include the information on the treatment each experimental unit received. An example of the spreadsheet form of the data resulting in a single-factor study with three treatments is given in Table 12.1.

The linear model fit in a single-factor analysis of variance is $Y = \mu + \tau + \epsilon$ where μ is the overall mean, τ is the treatment effect, and ϵ is the experimental error. The parameters of the model are μ, τ_1, τ_2, ..., and τ_t and the experimental error term ϵ is a random variable. Assumptions required of the single-factor linear model are listed below.

ASSUMPTIONS OF THE SINGLE-FACTOR LINEAR MODEL

AV1 The observations on the response variable are independent random variables.	**AV3** The error terms within each treatment group have the same variance (i.e., constant variance).
AV2 The error terms have mean 0.	**AV4** The error terms are normally distributed.

TABLE 12.1   A Sample of the Spreadsheet Form of the Raw Data for a Single-Factor ANOV

Y	Treatment
y_{11}	1
y_{12}	1
$\vdots$	$\vdots$
y_{1n_1}	1
y_{21}	2
y_{22}	2
$\vdots$	$\vdots$
y_{2n_2}	2
y_{31}	3
y_{32}	3
$\vdots$	$\vdots$
y_{3n_2}	3

Note that the assumptions of the single-factor linear model can also be stated as "the error terms are independently and normally distributed with mean 0 and common variance σ^2."

The first test that is performed in a single-factor analysis of variance is a test of the simultaneous equality of the t treatment means. The null hypothesis for a test of the equality of the treatment means is

$$H_0 : \mu_1 = \mu_2 = \mu_3 = \cdots = \mu_t$$

and the alternative hypothesis is

$$H_A : \text{At least two of the treatment means are different}$$

Note that under the single-factor linear model, the ith treatment mean is $\mu_i = \mu + \tau_i$, and since $\mu_\epsilon = 0$ all of the treatment means will be equal only when all of the treatment effects are equal. Hence, the null hypothesis that all of the treatment means are equal is equivalent to testing all of the treatment effects are equal. Thus, testing

$$H_0 : \mu_1 = \mu_2 = \mu_3 = \cdots = \mu_t$$

is equivalent to testing

$$H_0 : \tau_1 = \tau_2 = \tau_3 = \cdots = \tau_t$$

in a single-factor analysis of variance.

As is the case with any statistical model, the assumptions of the model must be assessed and any violation of the assumptions must be cured before proceeding to use the model for making statistical inferences. Methods for checking the assumptions of the single-factor linear model are discussed in Section 12.1.2.

12.1.1 Partitioning the Total Experimental Variation

A single-factor linear model is fit using the method of least squares and the estimate of the *i*th treatment mean under this model is

$$\hat{\mu}_i = \bar{y}_{i\bullet}$$

Because the response variable has a double subscript, the dot notation is used to identify the factor that the units have been averaged over. For example, $\bar{y}_{i\bullet}$ is the sample mean formed by averaging the replicates of the *i*th treatment (i.e., the units in the *i*th treatment group), and $\bar{y}_{\bullet\bullet}$ is the overall sample mean that is formed by averaging all of the units in the study.

Unlike a linear regression model, the treatment effects (i.e., the τ terms) in a single-factor linear model cannot be uniquely estimated. Fortunately, the difference between two treatment effects, $\tau_i - \tau_j$, that corresponds to the difference of two treatment means can be uniquely estimated. Thus, statistical inferences cannot be made about the individual treatment effects in an analysis of variance; however, statistical inferences about the differences in the treatment effects can be made.

The total variation in the observed values of the response variable is denoted by SSTot and is defined to be the sum of squared deviations from the overall mean. That is,

$$\text{SSTot} = (y_{11} - \bar{y}_{\bullet\bullet})^2 + (y_{12} - \bar{y}_{..})^2 + (y_{13} - \bar{y}_{\bullet\bullet})^2 + \cdots + (y_{tn_t} - \bar{y}_{\bullet\bullet})^2$$

which can also be written using summation notation as

$$\text{SSTot} = \sum\sum(y - \bar{y}_{\bullet\bullet})^2$$

The total variation in the observed values of the response variable is partitioned using the mathematical trick of adding $0 = -\bar{y}_{i\bullet} + \bar{y}_{i\bullet}$ to each deviation involving the *i*th treatment in SSTot. Thus,

$$\text{SSTot} = \sum\sum(y - \bar{y}_{i\bullet} + \bar{y}_{i\bullet} - \bar{y}_{\bullet\bullet})^2 = \sum\sum([y - \bar{y}_{i\bullet}] + [\bar{y}_{i\bullet} - \bar{y}_{\bullet\bullet}])^2$$

and since $(a+b)^2 = a^2 + b^2 + 2ab$, expanding the terms $([y - \bar{y}_{i\bullet}] + [\bar{y}_{i\bullet} - \bar{y}_{\bullet\bullet}])^2$ yields

$$\text{SSTot} = \sum\sum(y - \bar{y}_{i\bullet})^2 + \sum\sum(\bar{y}_{i\bullet} - \bar{y}_{\bullet\bullet})^2 + 2\sum\sum(y - \bar{y}_{i\bullet})(\bar{y}_{i\bullet} - \bar{y}_{\bullet\bullet})$$

But since $2\sum\sum(y - \bar{y}_{i\bullet})(\bar{y}_{i\bullet} - \bar{y}_{\bullet\bullet})$ is always equal to 0, the partitioned form of the total variation is

$$\text{SSTot} = \sum\sum(y - \bar{y}_{i\bullet})^2 + \sum\sum(\bar{y}_{i\bullet} - \bar{y}_{\bullet\bullet})^2$$

Note that the total variation in the observed values of the response variable in a single-factor analysis of variance is partitioned into two separate sums of squares. The first sum of squares component in SSTot is $\sum\sum(y - \bar{y}_{i\bullet})^2$ that measures the variation among the units that were treated alike and is referred to as the *sum of squares due to error*. The sum of squares due to error has $n - t$ degrees of freedom and is denoted by SSE. The value of SSE may also be computed from the sample standard deviations computed from the replicates of each treatment since

$$\text{SSE} = (n_1 - 1)s_1^2 + (n_2 - 1)s_2^2 + (n_3 - 1)s_3^2 + \cdots + (n_t - 1)s_t^2$$

TABLE 12.2   **ANOV Table for a Single-Factor Analysis of Variance**

Source of Variation	DF	SS	MS	F	p
Treatments	$t-1$	SSTR	$\text{MSTR} = \dfrac{\text{SSTR}}{t-1}$	$F_{\text{obs}} = \dfrac{\text{MSTR}}{\text{MSE}}$	p
Error	$n-t$	SSE	$\text{MSE} = \dfrac{\text{SSE}}{n-t}$		
Total	$n-1$	SSTot			

where s_i is the sample standard deviation computed from the replicates of the ith treatment.

The second sum of squares component in SSTot is $\sum\sum(\bar{y}_{i\bullet} - \bar{y}_{\bullet\bullet})^2$ that measures the difference between the treatment means and the overall mean and is called the *sum of squares due to the treatments*. The sum of squares due to the treatments is denoted by SSTR and has $t-1$ degrees of freedom. A simpler form of SSTR is given by

$$\text{SSTR} = \sum n_i(\bar{y}_{i\bullet} - \bar{y}_{\bullet\bullet})^2$$

and when the treatments are equally replicated

$$\text{SSTR} = r\sum(\bar{y}_{i\bullet} - \bar{y}_{\bullet\bullet})^2$$

where r is the number of replicates of each treatment.

Thus, the total variation in the observed values of the response variable in a single-factor analysis of variance is

$$\text{SSTot} = \text{SSE} + \text{SSTR}$$

and the information on the sources of variation, their associated degrees of freedom, sum of squares, and mean squares are typically summarized in an ANOV table of the form given in Table 12.2. ANOV tables are also included in the standard output for an analysis of variance in most of the commonly used statistical computing packages.

The two most important entries in the single-factor ANOV table are MSE that is an unbiased estimator of the standard deviation of the error term in the linear model and the observed F-ratio. The observed F-ratio and its p-value in a single-factor ANOV table are used to test the null hypothesis $H_0 : \mu_1 = \mu_2 = \cdots = \mu_t$; however, the test will only be valid when the assumptions of the model are satisfied. The value of MSE is also used in pairwise comparisons of the treatment means and should only be used when the error term appears to have constant variance σ^2.

12.1.2 The Model Assumptions

Recall the assumptions of the single-factor linear model that the error terms are independent and normally distributed with mean 0 and common standard deviation σ. The results of the F-test of $H_0 : \mu_1 = \mu_2 = \cdots = \mu_t$ and any other comparative test of the treatment means will only be valid when the error assumptions are satisfied. Therefore, the error assumptions must be checked and validated before performing any hypothesis test or computing any confidence interval for comparing the treatment means.

The independence assumption should be dealt with in the planning stages of the experiment or observational study. Randomly allocating the experimental units to the treatment groups usually ensures the observations will be independent as does using a random sample in an observational study. Thus, in a well-designed single-factor study the assumption of the independence of error terms is usually not a problem.

A normal probability plot of the residuals can be used to check the assumption of the normality of the error terms. In a single-factor linear model, the residuals are simply the difference between an observed value and the treatment mean. Thus, the residual for the observed value y_{ij} is

$$e_{ij} = y_{ij} - \bar{y}_{i\bullet}$$

The sum of the squared residuals is SSE (i.e., $\text{SSE} = \sum e^2$) and the residuals contain the relevant information about the distribution of the error term. Thus, a normal plot that passes the fat pencil test will be used as evidence that the errors are approximately normally distributed. Also, when the sample size is sufficiently large, the F-test will be robust to violations of the normality assumption.

The most critical of the analysis of variance assumptions is that the variance of the error term is the same for each of the treatment groups (i.e., constant variance). When the assumption of constant variance is violated, the p-value associated with the observed F-ratio may be inaccurate and the chance of making a type I error may be larger than the specified significance level α. Furthermore, when the treatments do not have a common variance, the value of MSE, which is a pooled estimate of the common treatment variance σ^2, does not estimate any of the individual treatment variances very well. The use of MSE as an estimate of the common treatment group variance when the treatments have grossly different variances also affects the reliability of the pairwise comparisons of the treatment means.

There are two common approaches used to assess the validity of the constant variance assumption. The first approach is to compute the sample variances for each of the treatments groups from the replicates on each treatment. Then, derive the ratio of the largest treatment group variance to the smallest, and when this ratio is less than 4 it will be reasonable to assume that all of the treatment variances are roughly equal. When the ratio is greater than 4, there is sufficient evidence that the treatment variances differ and to reject the constant variance assumption.

Example 12.2

The summary statistics given in Table 12.3 resulted from a balanced completely randomized design experiment with $t = 5$ treatments each replicated $r = 5$ times. On the basis of the summary statistics in Table 12.3, the largest variance is 31.3 and the smallest is 14.0, and therefore, the ratio of the

TABLE 12.3 Summary Statistics for a Balanced Completely Randomized Design Experiment

Treatment	Sample Mean	Sample Variance
1	23.4	16.3
2	28.0	14.0
3	25.2	16.2
4	36.4	31.3
5	33.6	25.3

largest to smallest variance is $\frac{31.3}{14.0} = 2.24$ that is less than 4. Thus, on the basis of the observed sample variances, it appears that the constant variance assumption is satisfied.

The second approach is to formally test the hypothesis $H_0 : \sigma_1 = \sigma_2 = \cdots = \sigma_t$ with Levene's test of the homogeneity of variances. Levene's test is fairly robust to the normality assumption and is available in most of the commonly used statistical computing packages. When the p-value for Levene's test is less than 0.05, there is evidence that the constant variance assumption is not valid, while p-values larger than 0.05 suggest it is reasonable to assume each treatment group has the same variance.

Example 12.3
The p-value for Levene's test of the homogeneity of variances for the raw data used in Example 12.2 is $p = 0.96$, and thus, Levene's test also supports the hypothesis of equal variances. The MINITAB output for Levene's test of the homogeneity of variance is given in Figure 12.1. Note that MINITAB output for Levene's test includes the values of the test statistic and its p-value along with a plot containing confidence intervals for the individual treatment group standard deviations. Since the confidence intervals all overlap, this can be taken as further evidence supporting the constant variance assumption.

In many research studies, it is common for the variation in the response variable to increase as the mean of the treatment group increases, especially when the response variable is a count variable. In this case, there will often be a nonconstant variance problem. When there is sufficient evidence to conclude that the constant variance assumption has been violated, the single-factor model for the response variable Y is not appropriate for making statistical inferences, and the researcher must cure this problem before proceeding with the analysis of variance. A powerful transformation of the response variable Y that often cures a nonconstant variance problem is the natural logarithm transformation $ln(Y)$. Thus, when there is evidence of a nonconstant variance problem, the log-Y model

$$ln(Y) = \mu + \tau + \epsilon$$

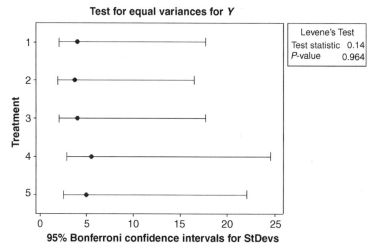

Figure 12.1   MINITAB output for Levene's test of homogeneity of variance for the data in Example 12.2.

should be considered in an attempt to cure the nonconstant variance problem. When the natural log transformation does cure the nonconstant variance problem, the analysis of variance should be on the transformed data; however, when the natural log transformation does not cure the nonconstant variance problem, a trained statistician should be consulted for help in curing this problem.

12.1.3 The *F*-test

Once the model assumptions have been checked and there are no apparent violations of the assumptions, the information in the ANOV table can be used for making inferences about the relationship between the response variable and the treatments. In particular, MSE can be used to estimate the common variance σ^2, and the observed F-ratio and its p-value can be used to test the equality of the treatment means.

The F-ratio is used to test the null hypothesis that all of the treatment means are equal against the alternative hypothesis that at least two of the treatment means are different. Since the ith treatment mean is $\mu_i = \mu + \tau_i$, the F-ratio can also be thought of as a test of the null hypothesis that all treatment effects are equal versus the alternative that at least two treatment effects differ. The test statistic for testing the equality of the treatment means or treatment effects is

$$F = \frac{\text{MSTR}}{\text{MSE}}$$

When the assumptions of the model are satisfied, the sampling distribution of the F-ratio will follow an F distribution with $t - 1$ and $n - t$ degrees of freedom, and the p-value associated with the observed value of the F-ratio is $p = P(F \geq F_{\text{obs}})$.

Large values of the F-ratio support the rejection of $H_0 : \mu_1 = \mu_2 = \cdots = \mu_t$ and occur when MSTR $>>$ MSE. That is, when the mean source of variation due to the difference in the treatments is significantly larger than mean source of variation due to experimental error, the F-ratio will detect a significant difference in at least two of the treatment means. On the other hand, when the mean source of variation due to the difference in the treatments is not significantly larger than mean source of variation due to experimental error, the F-ratio will not detect a significant difference in any of the treatment means. A nonsignificant F-ratio suggests that either the treatment means are all equal or there is too much experimental error to detect any difference in the treatment means. Thus, to ensure that an F-test detects any scientific difference in the treatment means the sample size and number of replicates must be chosen appropriately in designing the study.

Example 12.4
For the data in Example 12.2, a normal probability plot of the residuals is given in Figure 12.2.

Since normal probability plot appears to be linear it passes the fat pencil test and supports the assumption of normality. Also, since no evidence of a nonconstant variance problem was found in Example 12.2, the ANOV table given in Table 12.4 can be used for testing

$$H_0 : \mu_1 = \mu_2 = \mu_3 = \mu_4 = \mu_5$$

The observed F-ratio is 7.41 and has a p-value of $p - 0.001$. Thus, there is sufficient evidence to reject $H_0 : \mu_1 = \mu_2 = \mu_3 = \mu_4 = \mu_5$, and therefore, there at least two of the treatment means are significantly different.

The results of the F-test of the equality of the treatment means dictates the next step in the analysis of variance. In particular, when the F-test for the equality of the treatment means

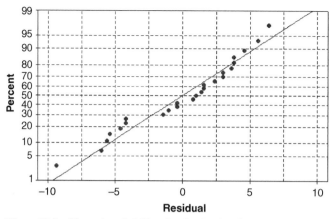

Figure 12.2   Normal probability plot for the data in Example 12.2.

is not significant (i.e., $p > \alpha$), then there are no further tests or mean comparisons that need to be considered. In this case, it is reasonable to conclude that all of the treatment means are equal provided that the experiment or study was designed with a sufficient sample size to detect any scientifically significant difference in the means. On the other hand, when the F-ratio is significant (i.e., $p < \alpha$), the next step in the analysis of variance is to perform pairwise comparisons of the means to determine which of the treatment means are different.

12.1.4 Comparing Treatment Means

When the F-test provides evidence that at least two of the treatment means are significantly different, a researcher will usually want to determine which of the treatment means are different. The comparison of the treatment means following the F-test is referred to as the *separation of the means* and consists of a series of hypothesis tests that compare two means at a time. One approach that could be used for separating the means is to perform two-sample t-tests on each possible pair of means. This approach would consist of $\frac{t(t-1)}{2}$ pairwise mean comparisons for a study having t treatments. The problem with this approach is that the probability of making at least one Type I error in this series of pairwise comparisons will be much larger than is generally preferred. For example, with $t = 8$ treatments there would be 15 pairwise tests, and the probability of making at least one Type I error in these 15 tests is at least 0.265 when each pairwise test is performed at the $\alpha = 0.05$ level.

When multiple comparisons of the treatment means are being made, there are two types of error rates that need to be controlled for. In particular, the *per comparisonwise error rate* that is the probability of making a Type I error in any particular test comparing two treatment means needs to be controlled, as well as the *experimentwise error rate* that is the probability of making at least one Type I error in the series of comparative tests.

TABLE 12.4   The ANOV Table for the Data in Example 12.2

Source	DF	SS	MS	F	P
Treatment	4	611.0	152.8	7.41	0.001
Error	20	412.4	20.6		
Total	24	1023.4			

The experimentwise error rate is denoted by α_E and the per comparisonwise error rate is denoted by α_C. When there are s comparisons being made and each comparative test is performed at the α_C level, the experimentwise error rate is always less or equal to the number of comparisons times the per comparison error rate (i.e., $\alpha_E \leq s \times \alpha_C$). For example, if there are $s = 6$ tests being performed with test using a per comparison error rate of $\alpha_C = 0.01$, then the experimentwise error rate will be less than or equal to $6 \times 0.1 = 0.06$. The experimentwise error rate should be prespecified in the planning stages of the research study and a good rule of thumb is to always chose $\alpha_E \leq 0.10$.

The *Bonferroni multiple comparison procedure* is one of the simplest methods for controlling the experimentwise error rate and is independent of the test statistic being used in the comparisons. The Bonferroni multiple comparison procedure controls the experimentwise error rate by distributing the per comparison error rate α_C equally over the s comparisons being made. That is, in the Bonferroni procedure with a prespecified value of experimentwise error rate of α, the per comparison error rate of $\alpha_C = \frac{\alpha}{s}$ is used so that $\alpha_E \leq s \times \alpha_C = s \times \frac{\alpha}{s} = \alpha$. Note that the Bonferroni multiple comparison procedure is a conservative procedure meaning that the true value of the experimentwise error rate is always less than or equal to the prespecified value of α_E. When s is large, say $s \geq 10$, a less conservative method such as Tukey's multiple comparison method is preferable to the Bonferroni procedure. See *Design and Analysis of Experiments* (Peterson, 1985) for a detailed discussion of Tukey's procedure and several other multiple comparison procedures that can be used for separating the treatment means.

In a single-factor analysis of variance, the mean comparisons are based on the sample treatment means $\bar{y}_{1\bullet}, \bar{y}_{2\bullet}, \bar{y}_{2\bullet}, \ldots, \bar{y}_{t\bullet}$. The sampling distribution of the ith treatment mean, $\bar{y}_{i\bullet}$ has mean μ_i, and hence, is an unbiased estimator of the ith treatment mean. Provided the constant variance assumption is satisfied, the estimated standard error of $\bar{y}_{i\bullet}$ is

$$se(\bar{y}_{i\bullet}) = \sqrt{\frac{MSE}{n_i}}$$

and the estimated standard error of the difference of two sample treatment means, $\bar{y}_{i\bullet} - \bar{y}_{j\bullet}$, is

$$se(\bar{y}_{i\bullet} - \bar{y}_{j\bullet}) = \sqrt{MSE\left(\frac{1}{n_i} + \frac{1}{n_j}\right)}$$

where n_i and n_j are the number of replicates of the ith and jth treatments. Furthermore, when the normality assumption is valid or the sample size is sufficiently large, the sampling distribution of

$$t = \frac{\bar{y}_{i\bullet} - \bar{y}_{j\bullet}}{se(\bar{y}_{i\bullet} - \bar{y}_{j\bullet})}$$

follows a t distribution with the degrees of freedom of MSE.

Thus, when the analysis of variance assumptions are valid, hypothesis tests and confidence intervals for comparing two means can be based on the t distribution. In particular, the Bonferroni multiple comparison procedure for s pairwise comparisons of the treatment means will be based on testing $H_0 : \mu_i = \mu_j$ with the test statistic

$$t = \frac{\bar{y}_{i\bullet} - \bar{y}_{j\bullet}}{se(\bar{y}_{i\bullet} - \bar{y}_{j\bullet})}$$

The two different ways that the Bonferroni multiple comparison procedure is typically used with a statistical computing package are described below.

- **Approach 1:** Using a statistical computing package, compute the p-values of the s pairwise t-tests and reject $H_0 : \mu_i = \mu_j$ when the p-value for this test is less than $\alpha_C = \frac{\alpha_E}{s}$.

- **Approach 2:** Using a statistical computing package, compute a $(1 - \frac{\alpha_E}{s}) \times 100\%$ confidence interval for each of the s pairwise mean comparisons. Reject the null hypothesis $H_0 : \mu_i = \mu_j$ when the confidence interval for $\mu_i - \mu_j$ does not include 0.

Note that since a confidence interval that does not contain 0 corresponds to a t-test with p-value less than α_C, approaches 1 and 2 are equivalent. Furthermore, the Bonferroni multiple comparison procedure is available in most statistical computing packages as an option in their analysis of variance procedures.

Example 12.5

The MINITAB output for the Bonferroni procedure for separating the means for the data in Example 12.2 is given in Figure 12.3.

```
Bonferroni Simultaneous Tests
Treatment = 1  subtracted from:

            Difference      SE of              Adjusted
Treatment   of Means    Difference  T-Value    P-Value
2              4.600       2.872     1.6017     1.0000
3              1.800       2.872     0.6268     1.0000
4             13.000       2.872     4.5266     0.0021
5             10.200       2.872     3.5516     0.0200


Treatment = 2  subtracted from:

            Difference      SE of              Adjusted
Treatment   of Means    Difference  T-Value    P-Value
3             -2.800       2.872    -0.9750     1.0000
4              8.400       2.872     2.9249     0.0838
5              5.600       2.872     1.9499     0.6535


Treatment = 3  subtracted from:

            Difference      SE of              Adjusted
Treatment   of Means    Difference  T-Value    P-Value
4             11.200       2.872     3.900      0.0089
5              8.400       2.872     2.925      0.0838


Treatment = 4  subtracted from:

            Difference      SE of              Adjusted
Treatment   of Means    Difference  T-Value    P-Value
5             -2.800       2.872    -0.9750     1.000
```

Figure 12.3   The MINITAB output for the Bonferroni procedure for separating the means for the data in Example 12.2.

Note that the MINITAB output for the Bonferroni procedure includes the difference of the two means, the standard error of the difference, the t-value for testing the equality of the two means, and an adjusted p-value for the observed t-value. The adjusted p-value reported in the MINITAB output is the minimum value of the experimentwise error rate for which the observed difference in the treatment means will be rejected. Thus, when the adjusted p-value is smaller than the value of α_E being used, the two means are significantly different according to the Bonferroni multiple comparison procedure.

Thus, based on the MINITAB output in Figure 12.3 and using $\alpha_E = 0.05$, the observed data suggests that there are significant differences between μ_1 and μ_4, between μ_1 and μ_5, and between μ_3 and μ_4.

Note that MINITAB's adjusted p-value is not the p-value associated with the t-test. The adjusted p-value is actually an experimentwise p-value that can be used to determine whether or not two treatment means are significantly different. In particular, two means are declared significantly different when the adjusted p-value is less than the prespecified value of the experimentwise error rate α_E. Unfortunately, some statistical computing packages do not include the Bonferroni procedure in their analysis of variance programs; however, the computations in the Bonferroni multiple comparison procedure are simple enough to perform with a calculator as outlined below.

HAND CALCULATIONS FOR THE BONFERRONI PROCEDURE

For the Bonferroni comparison of μ_i and μ_j with $\alpha_C = \frac{\alpha_E}{s}$

1. Compute $D = b_{\text{crit}} \times \sqrt{\text{MSE} \left(\dfrac{1}{n_i} + \dfrac{1}{n_j} \right)}$

   where b_{crit} is the value found in Table A.12 of Bonferroni critical values for s

comparisons and the degrees of freedom associated with MSE.

2. Compute $|\bar{y}_{i\bullet} - \bar{y}_{j\bullet}|$.

3. Reject $H_0 : \mu_i = \mu_j$ when $|\bar{y}_{i\bullet} - \bar{y}_{j\bullet}| > D$.

Note that the value of b_{crit} is the $(1 - \frac{\alpha_C}{2}) \times 100$th percentile of a t distribution with the degrees of freedom of MSE. Also, D is simply the margin of error of the Bonferroni confidence interval for $\mu_i - \mu_j$. When the treatments have balanced replication, a common value of D is used for each of the pairwise mean comparisons. In this case, the value of D is

$$D = b_{\text{crit}} \times \sqrt{\frac{2 \times \text{MSE}}{r}}$$

where r is the number of replicates of each treatment.

Example 12.6
In Example 12.4, the F-ratio has a p-value of $p = 0.001$ suggesting that at least two of the treatment means are different. Using the treatment means given in Example 12.2 and the value of MSE from Example 12.4, separate the treatment means using an experimentwise error rate of $\alpha_E = 0.05$.

Solution From Example 12.4 the value of MSE is 20.6 and has 20 degrees of freedom, and since there are five treatments there are $s = \frac{5(5-1)}{2} = 10$ mean comparisons that need to be performed. The value of b_{crit} for 10 comparisons, 20 degrees of freedom, and $\alpha_E = 0.05$ from Table A.12 is

$b_{crit} = 3.15$, and since all the treatments have $r = 5$ replicates the common value of D is

$$D = 3.15 \times \sqrt{\frac{2 \times 20.6}{5}} = 9.0$$

Thus, any two sample means that differ by a distance of more than 9 are statistically significantly different.

From Example 12.2, the sample treatment means are

$$\bar{y}_1 = 23.4, \ \bar{y}_2 = 28.0, \ \bar{y}_3 = 25.2, \ \bar{y}_4 = 36.4, \ \bar{y}_5 = 33.6$$

Thus, the observed data suggest that there are significant differences between μ_1 and μ_4, between μ_1 and μ_5, and between μ_3 and μ_4.

One method of summarizing the results of the separation of the treatment means is to rank the means from smallest to lowest, list the ranked means in a row, and then underline any means that are not significantly different. For example, the summary of the separation of means in Example 12.6 using this method to summarize the significant differences between the treatment means is shown below.

Treatment	1	3	2	5	4
Sample Mean	23.4	25.2	28.0	33.6	36.4

Finally, confidence intervals for the difference of two treatment means that are significantly different are often included in the summary of an analysis of variance. A $(1 - \alpha) \times 100\%$ confidence interval for the difference of two treatment means, say μ_i and μ_j, is

$$\left(\bar{y}_{i\bullet} - \bar{y}_{j\bullet} \right) \pm t_{crit} \sqrt{MSE \left(\frac{1}{n_i} + \frac{1}{n_j} \right)}$$

where t_{crit} has the degrees of freedom of MSE and is found in Table A.7. Also, a $(1 - \alpha) \times 100\%$ confidence interval for a single treatment mean, say μ_i, can be computed using

$$\bar{y}_{i\bullet} \pm t_{crit} \sqrt{\frac{MSE}{n_i}}$$

Example 12.7
Using the information in Example 12.6, compute a 95% confidence interval for

    a. the difference of μ_4 and μ_1.

    b. for μ_4.

Solution Since $\bar{y}_1. = 23.4$, $\bar{y}_{4\bullet} = 36.4$, and MSE $= 20.6$ with 20 degrees of freedom, a 95% confidence interval for

    a. the difference of μ_4 and μ_1 is

$$(36.4 - 23.4) \pm 2.086 \sqrt{20.6 \left(\frac{1}{5} + \frac{1}{5} \right)}$$

which yields an interval of 7.0–19.0. Thus, it appears that μ_4 is at least seven units larger than μ_1 and possibly as much as 19 units larger.

b. for μ_4 is

$$36.4 \pm 2.086\sqrt{\frac{20.6}{5}}$$

which yields an interval of 32.2–40.6. Thus, it appears that μ_4 is at least 32.2 units and possibly as large as 40.6.

12.2 RANDOMIZED BLOCK ANALYSIS OF VARIANCE

A randomized block design is used to control for an extraneous variable when the experimental units can be sorted into blocks of similar units before the treatments are applied. A randomized block design can also be used in an observational study when the units of the study belong to well-defined strata and the strata factor is an extraneous factor that needs to be controlled for.

The data to be analyzed in a randomized block analysis of variance consists of n observations on the response variable Y that can be sorted into r blocks of t units such that each treatment is replicated exactly once in each block. Thus, the number of units in a randomized block experiment is $n = r \times t$ and the number of replicates on each of the treatments is r. To distinguish the values of the observed response variable from each other, subscripts are often used to identify the treatment a unit received and the block the unit is in. Thus, in a randomized block analysis of variance the observed value of the response variable in the jth block and receiving the ith treatment will be denoted by y_{ij}. The observed data are often entered into a spreadsheet in a statistical package that must also contain the information on the treatment a unit received and the block the experimental unit was in. An example of the spreadsheet form for a randomized block analysis of variance with six treatments and three blocks is given in Table 12.5.

TABLE 12.5   A Sample of the Spreadsheet Form of the Raw Data for a Randomized Block ANOV

Y	Treatment	Block
y_{11}	1	1
y_{12}	1	2
$\vdots$	$\vdots$	$\vdots$
y_{16}	1	6
y_{21}	2	1
y_{22}	2	2
$\vdots$	$\vdots$	$\vdots$
y_{26}	2	6
y_{31}	3	1
y_{32}	3	2
$\vdots$	$\vdots$	$\vdots$
y_{36}	3	6

The linear model for a randomized block analysis of variance is $Y = \mu + \rho + \tau + \epsilon$ where μ is the overall mean, ρ is the block effect, τ is the treatment effect, and ϵ is the experimental error. The parameters of the model are μ and $\tau_1, \tau_2, \ldots, \tau_t$, the block effect is assumed to be a random variable that is normally distributed with mean 0 and standard deviation σ_b, and the experimental error term ϵ is a normal random variable having mean 0 and variance σ^2. Furthermore, the validity of the assumptions placed on the error term must be valid to have reliable hypothesis tests and confidence intervals in an analysis of variance. On the other hand, the validity of the assumptions on the distribution of the block effects does not affect the validity of any hypothesis tests or confidence intervals concerning the treatment means or the treatment effects.

As was the case in a single-factor analysis of variance, the first test that is performed in a randomized block analysis of variance is a test of the simultaneous equality of the t treatment means. The null hypothesis for a test of the equality of the treatment means is

$$H_0 : \mu_1 = \mu_2 = \mu_3 = \cdots = \mu_t$$

and the alternative hypothesis is

$$H_A : \text{At least two of the treatment means are different}$$

Note that under the randomized block model the ith treatment mean is $\mu + \tau_i$ since the mean of the block effects is 0, and therefore, all of the treatment means will be equal only when all of the treatment effects are equal. Hence, the null hypothesis that all of the treatment means are equal is equivalent to testing all of the effects are equal. That is, testing

$$H_0 : \mu_1 = \mu_2 = \mu_3 = \cdots = \mu_t$$

is equivalent to testing

$$H_0 : \tau_1 = \tau_2 = \tau_3 = \cdots = \tau_t$$

in a randomized block analysis of variance as it was in the single-factor analysis of variance.

The assumptions of the randomized block model must be assessed and any violations of the assumptions must be cured before proceeding to use the fitted model for making statistical inferences. Methods for checking the assumptions of the single-factor linear model are discussed in Section 12.2.2.

12.2.1 The ANOV Table for the Randomized Block Design

As was the case in the single-factor linear model, the model for a randomized block design is fit using the method of least squares. The estimate of the ith treatment mean under the randomized block linear model is

$$\widehat{\mu}_i = \bar{y}_{i\bullet}$$

Because the response variable has a double subscript, the dot notation is used to identify the factor that the units have been averaged over. For example, $\bar{y}_{i\bullet}$ is the ith sample treatment mean formed by averaging the values of the experimental units receiving the ith treatment over the b blocks. The other means used in partitioning the total variation in a randomized block analysis of variance are the overall sample mean $\bar{y}_{\bullet\bullet}$ and the block means

$\bar{y}_{\bullet 1}, \bar{y}_{\bullet 2}, \ldots, \bar{y}_{\bullet r}$. Note that in a block mean the dotted subscript is the first subscript because the mean is formed by averaging all of the observations on the treatments within a particular block.

The total variation in the observed values of the response variable is denoted by SSTot and is defined to be the sum of squared deviations from the overall mean. That is, the total variation is

$$\text{SSTot} = \sum \sum (y - \bar{y}_{\bullet \bullet})^2$$

The total variation in a randomized block analysis of variance is partitioned in a fashion similar to that of the partitioning of SSTot in a single-factor analysis of variance. However, in a randomized block analysis of variance, both the block means and the treatment means are used to partition the total sum of squares into three component sum of squares, rather than two. The three-component sum of squares are the sum of squares due to the block differences that will be denoted by SSBL, the sum of squares due to the treatment differences that will again be denoted by SSTR, and the sum of squares due to experimental error that again is denoted by SSE. A summary of the partitioning of the total variation in the observed values of the response variable in a randomized block analysis of variance is listed below.

SS's IN A RANDOMIZED BLOCK ANALYSIS OF VARIANCE

The total variation in the observed values of the response variable in a randomized block analysis of variance is

$$\text{SSTot} = \text{SSBL} + \text{SSTR} + \text{SSE}$$

where the component sum of squares are

$$\text{SSBL} = t \sum (\bar{y}_{\bullet j} - \bar{y}_{\bullet \bullet})^2$$

$$\text{SSTR} = r \sum (\bar{y}_{i \bullet} - \bar{y}_{\bullet \bullet})^2$$

$$\text{SSE} = \text{SSTot} - \text{SSB} - \text{SSTR}$$

The partitioning of SSTot for a randomized block analysis of variance is summarized in an ANOV table of the form given in Table 12.6 that lists the sources of variation, their associated degrees of freedom, sum of squares, mean squares, F-ratio and its p-value for testing the equality of the treatment means.

By controlling for the block factor in a randomized block analysis of variance, the sum of squares due to the block differences is removed from the experimental error. That is, if the block factor was not controlled for the sum of squares, the block differences would be part of the experimental error variation. Thus, controlling for the blocking factor will

TABLE 12.6 ANOV Table for a Single-Factor Analysis of Variance

Source of Variation	DF	SS	MS	F	P
Blocks	$r - 1$	SSBl	$\text{MSBL} = \dfrac{\text{SSBL}}{r - 1}$		
Treatments	$t - 1$	SSTR	$\text{MSTR} = \dfrac{\text{SSTR}}{t - 1}$	$F_{\text{obs}} = \dfrac{\text{MSTR}}{\text{MSE}}$	p
Error	$(r - 1)(t - 1)$	SSE	$\text{MSE} = \dfrac{\text{SSE}}{(r - 1)(t - 1)}$		
Total	$rt - 1$	SSTot			

decrease the experimental error and increase the chance of detecting any differences in the treatment means.

Similar to the information in a single-factor ANOV table, the two most important entries in a randomized block ANOV table are MSE and the observed F-ratio. MSE is an unbiased estimate of the standard deviation of the error term in the linear model, and the observed F-ratio and its p-value in a randomized block ANOV table are used to test the null hypothesis $H_0 : \mu_1 = \mu_2 = \cdots = \mu_t$; hypothesis tests and confidence intervals for comparing the treatment means will be valid only when the assumptions of the model are satisfied.

12.2.2 The Model Assumptions

Recall the assumptions of the randomized block linear model are that the error terms are independent and normally distributed with mean 0 and common standard deviation σ. There is actually another assumption required in a randomized block linear model that the treatment effects and the block effects are additive effects. That is, the additivity assumption states that the treatment effects and the block effects do not interact. When the additivity assumption is violated, the observed value of the F-ratio will be underestimated making more difficult to detect any differences in the treatment means. Since the results of the F-test of $H_0 : \mu_1 = \mu_2 = \cdots = \mu_t$ and any other comparative tests of the treatment means will be valid only when the error assumptions are satisfied, the model assumptions and the additivity assumption must be checked and validated before performing any hypothesis tests or computing any confidence intervals.

The independence assumption and the additivity assumption should be dealt with in the planning stages of the experiment or observational study. Randomly allocating the treatments to the experimental units in a block will usually ensure the error terms will be independent; using a random sample in an observational study usually ensures the independence of the response value, also. The assumption of additivity has more to do with the logistics of the experiment and is usually not a problem in biomedical studies. Thus, in a well-designed experiment, the assumption of the independence of error terms and the additivity do not usually present problems.

To check the assumption of the normality of the error terms, a normal probability plot of the residuals can be used. Thus, a normal plot that passes the fat pencil test will be taken as evidence that the errors are approximately normally distributed. Also, when the sample size is sufficiently large, the F-test will be robust to violations of the normality assumption.

Again, the most critical of the error assumptions is that the variance of the error term is the same for the treatment groups (i.e., constant variance) since a violation of the assumption of constant variance can produce inaccurate p-values and may increase the chance of making a Type I error. Since MSE is a pooled estimate of the common treatment variance σ^2, it will not estimate any of the individual treatment variances well when the treatments do not have a common variance; the use of MSE as an estimate of a treatment group variance when the treatments have grossly different variances would also invalidate the reliability of any pairwise comparison of the treatment means.

Checking the assumption of constant variance in a randomized block analysis of variance is similar to the approach used for checking the constant variance assumption in a single-factor analysis of variance. That is, compute the sample variances for each of the treatment groups from the replicates of each treatment. When the ratio of the largest treatment group variance to the smallest is less than 4, it is reasonable to assume that all of the treatment variances are roughly equal. When the ratio is greater than 4, there is sufficient evidence that the treatment variances differ and the constant variance assumption

TABLE 12.7   Raw Data for Example 12.8

Trial	Treatment			
	I	II	III	IV
1	10.2	13.1	10.5	15.6
2	13.1	13.0	12.1	17.8
3	15.2	19.6	18.1	19.3
4	10.1	13.0	9.5	14.4
5	10.8	13.1	12.3	15.1
6	13.5	15.4	14.1	18.6
Mean	11.88	14.53	12.77	16.80

is not valid. Levene's test can also be used to test the assumption of constant variance. Thus, the constant variance assumption is rejected for Levene's p-values less than 0.05, and Levene's p-values larger than 0.05 suggest it is reasonable to assume each treatment group has the same variance.

Example 12.8

Suppose the data given in Table 12.7 resulted from a randomized block experiment to compare four treatments. Due to physical constraints only four experimental units could be used at any one time, and therefore, the experiment was performed in a series of six trials (i.e., blocks).

A normal probability plot for the randomized block linear model $Y = \mu + \rho + \tau + \epsilon$ is given in Figure 12.4, and on the basis of this normal probability plot it appears that the normality assumption is satisfied.

Figure 12.5 contains the results of Levene's test for constant variance, and since the p-value for Levene's test is $p = 0.946$ there is no evidence of a nonconstant variance problem with the observed data.

Again, when there is sufficient evidence to conclude that the constant variance assumption has been violated, the natural logarithm transformation applied to the response

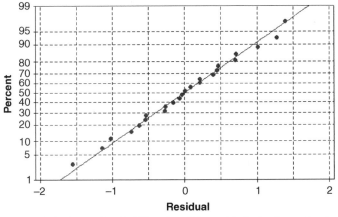

Figure 12.4   Normal probability plot of the residuals for the randomized block model fit to the data in Example 12.8.

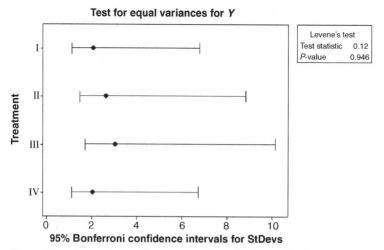

Figure 12.5   Levene's test of constant variance for the randomized block model fit to the data in Example 12.8.

variable (i.e., $\ln(Y)$) will often cure the nonconstant variation problem. Thus, when there is evidence of a nonconstant variance problem, the model

$$\ln(Y) = \mu + \rho + \tau + \epsilon$$

should be fit and assessed in attempting to cure a nonconstant variance problem in a randomized block experiment. If natural log-transformation does cure the nonconstant variance problem, the analysis of variance should on the transformed data; when the natural log-transformation does not cure the nonconstant variance problem, a trained statistician should be consulted for help in curing this problem.

12.2.3 The *F*-test

The *F*-ratio in the ANOV table for a randomized block model is used to test the equality of the treatment means just as it was in the single-factor analysis of variance. Thus, once the model assumptions have been checked and there are no apparent violated assumptions, the information in the *F*-ratio in the ANOV table can be used to test the null hypothesis that all of the treatment means are equal against the alternative hypothesis that at least two of the treatment means are different. Since the *i*th treatment mean is $\mu_i = \mu + \tau_i$, the *F*-ratio can also be thought of as a test of the null hypothesis that all treatment effects are equal versus the alternative that at least two treatment effects differ.

The test statistic for the *F*-test of the equality of the treatment means or treatment effects is

$$F = \frac{\text{MSTR}}{\text{MSE}}$$

which has $t - 1$ and $(r - 1)(t - 1)$ degrees of freedom, and $H_0 : \mu_1 = \mu_2 = \cdots = \mu_t$ is rejected for large values of the *F*-ratio. The *p*-value associated with the observed *F*-ratio is $P(F \geq F_{\text{obs}})$, and the null hypothesis of equal treatment means is rejected when the *p*-value is less than the prespecified value of α.

TABLE 12.8   The ANOV Table for the Data in Example 12.8

Source	DF	SS	MS	F	P
BLK	5	110.752	22.150		
TREATMENT	3	84.755	28.252	33.36	0.000
Error	15	12.703	0.847		
Total	23	208.210			

Example 12.9

The ANOV table for the data in Example 12.8 is given in Table 12.8. The observed F-ratio for testing $H_0 : \mu_{\mathrm{I}} = \mu_{\mathrm{II}} = \mu_{\mathrm{III}} = \mu_{\mathrm{IV}}$ is $F = 33.36$ with p-value $p = 0.000$. Thus, on the basis of the observed data, it appears that at least two of the four treatment means are significantly different.

Most statistical packages will include an F-ratio for testing the equality of the block means; however, because the block factor is an extraneous factor that is being controlled for and not a factor of primary interest, this test is usually ignored. In fact, the reason the randomized block design is used is that block differences are known to exist, and therefore, need not be tested.

Finally, when the F-ratio is significant in a randomized block analysis, the next step in the analysis is to determine which of the treatment means are different with a multiple comparison procedure such as the Bonferroni procedure.

12.2.4 Separating the Treatment Means

The unbiased estimates of the treatment means in a randomized block analysis are

$$\bar{y}_{1\bullet}, \ \bar{y}_{2\bullet}, \ \bar{y}_{3\bullet}, \ \ldots, \ \bar{y}_{t\bullet}$$

and the estimated standard error of the ith treatment mean is

$$\mathrm{se}(\bar{y}_{i\bullet}) = \sqrt{\frac{\mathrm{MSE}}{r}}$$

Note that the estimated standard errors of the treatment means are all the same because a randomized block design is a balanced design. Also, the estimated standard error of the difference between two sample treatment means is

$$\mathrm{se}(\bar{y}_{i\bullet} - \bar{y}_{j\bullet}) = \sqrt{\frac{2\mathrm{MSE}}{r}}$$

The Bonferroni procedure can also be used to separate the means in a randomized block analysis of variance and is used in the same fashion as it was in a single-factor analysis of variance. In particular, for an experimentwise error rate of α_{E} and s pairwise mean comparisons, the test statistic for comparing the ith and jth treatment means is

$$t = \frac{\bar{y}_{i\bullet} - \bar{y}_{j\bullet}}{\sqrt{\frac{2\mathrm{MSE}}{r}}}$$

and $H_0 : \mu_i = \mu_j$ is rejected when the observed p-value for the t-test is less than $\alpha_{\mathrm{C}} = \frac{\alpha_{\mathrm{E}}}{s}$; when a statistical computing package reports the adjusted p-value for testing $H_0 : \mu_i = \mu_j$, H_0 is rejected when the adjusted p-value is less than α_{E}.

Example 12.10

The MINITAB output for the Bonferroni procedure for the data in Example 12.8 is given in Figure 12.6. Based on the output for the Bonferroni procedure, it appears that μ_I is significantly different from μ_{II}, μ_I is significantly different from μ_{IV}, μ_{II} is significantly different from μ_{III}, μ_{II} is significantly different from μ_{IV}, and μ_{III} is significantly different from μ_{IV}. The significant differences between these four treatment means are also summarized using the underline notation.

Treatment	I	III	II	IV
Sample Mean	11.88	12.77	14.53	16.80

Because a randomized block design is a balanced design, performing the Bonferroni multiple comparison procedure by hand is fairly simple. The steps required to perform a Bonferroni separation of means by hand for a randomized block analysis are outlined below.

1. Compute $D = b_{crit} \times \sqrt{\dfrac{2MSE}{r}}$ where b_{crit} is the value found in Table A.12 of Bonferroni critical values for s comparisons and the degrees of freedom of MSE.

2. Compute $|\bar{y}_{i\bullet} - \bar{y}_{j\bullet}|$ for the means being compared.

3. Reject $H_0 : \mu_i = \mu_j$ when $|\bar{y}_{i\bullet} - \bar{y}_{j\bullet}| > D$.

Note that because each treatment is replicated the r times, there is a common value of D used in each of the mean comparisons, and therefore, any two means that differ by more than D are significantly different according to the Bonferroni procedure.

```
All Pairwise Comparisons among Levels of TREATMENT
TREATMENT = I  subtracted from:

           Difference      SE of              Adjusted
TREATMENT  of Means   Difference  T-Value    P-Value
II           2.6500      0.5313     4.988     0.0010
III          0.8833      0.5313     1.663     0.7029
IV           4.9167      0.5313     9.254     0.0000


TREATMENT = II  subtracted from:

           Difference      SE of              Adjusted
TREATMENT  of Means   Difference  T-Value    P-Value
III          -1.767      0.5313    -3.325     0.0277
IV            2.267      0.5313     4.266     0.0041


TREATMENT = III  subtracted from:

           Difference      SE of              Adjusted
TREATMENT  of Means   Difference  T-Value    P-Value
IV            4.033      0.5313     7.591     0.0000
```

Figure 12.6   The MINITAB output for the Bonferroni procedure for the data in Example 12.8.

Example 12.11
Use the data in Example 12.8 with an experimentwise error rate of $\alpha_E = 0.05$ to separate the four treatment means.

Solution The number of pairwise comparisons possible with four treatment means is $s = \frac{4(4-1)}{2} = 6$. Also, the number of blocks in this experiment is $r = 6$, and the value of MSE from the ANOV table in Example 12.9 is MSE $= 0.847$ with 15 degrees of freedom. From Table A.12, the critical value of the Bonferroni t for $s = 6$ comparisons, $\alpha_E = 0.05$, and 15 degrees freedom is $b_{crit} = 3.04$.

Thus, the value of D is

$$D = 3.04 \times \sqrt{\frac{2 \times 0.847}{6}} = 1.62$$

and hence, any two treatment means that differ more than $D = 1.62$ are significantly different.
The treatment means are listed in Table 12.7 and are

$$\bar{y}_{i\bullet} = 11.88, \ \bar{y}_{II.} = 14.53, \ \bar{y}_{III.} = 12.77, \ \text{and} \ \bar{y}_{IV.} = 16.80$$

Thus, except for treatments I and III, all of the means differ by at least 1.62. The separation of these four treatment means is summarized below using the underline notation.

Treatment	I	III	II	IV
Sample Mean	11.88	12.77	14.53	16.80

Confidence intervals for the difference of two treatment means that are often included in the summary of an analysis of variance to convey the scientific difference suggested by the statistical significance. A $(1 - \alpha) \times 100\%$ confidence interval for the difference of two treatment means, say μ_i and μ_j, in a randomized block analysis is

$$\left(\bar{y}_{i\bullet} - \bar{y}_{j\bullet}\right) \pm t_{crit}\sqrt{\frac{2MSE}{r}}$$

where t_{crit} has the degrees of freedom of MSE and is found in Table A.7. Also, a $(1 - \alpha) \times 100\%$ confidence interval for a single treatment mean, say μ_i, can be computed using

$$\bar{y}_{i\bullet} \pm t_{crit}\sqrt{\frac{MSE}{r}}$$

Example 12.12
Using the information in Example 12.8, compute a 95% confidence interval for

a. the difference of μ_{IV} and μ_{II}.

b. for μ_{IV}.

Solutions Since $\bar{y}_{IV.} = 16.80$, $\bar{y}_{II.} = 14.53$, and MSE $= 0.847$ with 15 degrees of freedom a 95% confidence interval for

a. the difference of μ_{IV} and μ_{II} is

$$(16.80 - 14.53) \pm 2.131\sqrt{\frac{2 \times 0.847}{6}}$$

which yields an interval of 1.14–3.40. Thus, it appears that μ_{IV} is at least 1.14 units larger than μ_{II} and possibly as much as 3.40 units larger.

b. for μ_{IV} is

$$16.80 \pm 2.131 \sqrt{\frac{0.847}{6}}$$

which yields an interval of 16.0–17.6. Thus, it appears that μ_{IV} is at least 16.0 units and possibly as large as 17.6.

12.3 MULTIFACTOR ANALYSIS OF VARIANCE

In many biomedical research studies, the treatments are formed from the combinations of the levels of two or more factors in which case the experiment or study is called a *multifactor study*. For example, when the treatment combinations are formed from two factors the study is called a two-factor study, and when the treatment combinations are formed from three factors, the study is called a three-factor study. Multifactor experiments and studies are commonly used to investigate the influence of the individual factors or the response variable and for investigating the interactions between the factors. Also, in many research studies the goal is to determine which combination of the factor levels produces the optimal (i.e., largest or smallest) value of the mean of the response variable.

A multifactor analysis of variance may or may not have a blocking factor and is similar in nature to the analysis of variance procedures used for a single-factor analysis of variance. That is, a multifactor study only differs from a single-factor study and a single-factor randomized block study in the treatment structure used in the study. For example, in a $a \times b$ two-factor study, there are ab treatments and by ignoring the treatment structure the analysis of variance can be performed as a single-factor or randomized block analysis of variance according to the study design. However, because the treatments in a multifactor study have a specific treatment structure, a multifactor analysis of variance is designed to provide information on the sources of variation due to the interactions between the factors and the main effects of the factors.

The assumptions on the error term in a multifactor linear model are the same as the assumptions placed on the error term in a single-factor or randomized block model, and therefore, the assumptions are checked using normal probability plots and Levene's test as before. The Bonferroni procedure can also be used to separate the means in a multifactor analysis of variance. The biggest difference between a single-factor analysis of variance and a multifactor analysis of variance is that there are several F-ratios that must be considered in a multifactor analysis. In particular, the analysis of variance table will contain an F-ratio for each factor used to create the treatment combinations as well as an F-ratio for each of the possible interactions between the factors.

12.3.1 Two-Factor Analysis of Variance

In a $a \times b$ two-factor study, there are ab treatments formed from combinations of the a levels of factor A and the b levels of factor B. For example, in studying the effects of aspirin as a short-term blood thinner when administered at the first sign of a heart attack, the four treatment groups in a retrospective study might be based on combinations of the two factors Sex (Male, Female) and Aspirin (Yes, No). The four treatments in this example are listed in Table 12.9.

TABLE 12.9   The Four Treatments in a Retrospective Study Based on the Factors Sex (Male, Female) and Aspirin (Yes, No)

Treatment	Sex	Aspirin
1	Male	Yes
2	Male	No
3	Female	Yes
4	Female	No

A multifactor study may or may not have a blocking factor, but when there is a blocking factor to be accounted for in the study it is assumed that the blocking factor does not interact with any of the treatment factors. The raw data to be analyzed in a two-factor analysis of variance consists of n observations on the response variable Y distributed over the ab treatment combinations. In a balanced two-factor design, the treatments will be replicated r times, and the number of units in a two-factor experiment is $n = r \times a \times b$. To distinguish the values of the observed response variable from each other, subscripts are used to identify the levels of the factors A and B used to form the treatment combination each experimental unit received and to identify a specific replicate of the treatment. Thus, in a two-factor analysis of variance, the observed value of the response variable for the kth replicate of the treatment combination formed from the ith level of factor A and the jth level of factor B is denoted by y_{ijk}. The observed data is often entered into a spreadsheet in a statistical package identifying the treatment each unit received by its factor A level, its factor B level, and its replicate number. An example of the spreadsheet form for a 2×2 factorial study with three replicates of each treatment is given in Table 12.10.

The linear model for a two-factor analysis of variance without a blocking factor is $Y = \mu + \gamma + \beta + \gamma\beta + \epsilon$ where μ is the overall mean, γ is the factor A main effect, β is the factor B main effect, $\gamma\beta$ is the AB interaction, and ϵ is the experimental error. The model for a two-factor analysis of variance with a blocking factor is $Y = \mu + \rho + \gamma + \beta + \gamma\beta + \epsilon$ where μ is the overall mean, ρ is the random block effect, γ is the factor A main effect, β is the factor B main effect, $\gamma\beta$ is the AB interaction, and ϵ is the experimental error.

Because the only difference between a two-factor linear model and a single-factor model is that the treatment effects (i.e., the τ's) have been replaced by $\gamma + \beta + \gamma\beta$ in the

TABLE 12.10   A Sample of the Spreadsheet Form of the Raw Data for a 2 × 2 Two-Factor ANOV With $r = 3$ Replicates/Blocks

Y	Factor A	Factor B	Replicate/Block
y_{111}	1	1	1
y_{112}	1	1	2
y_{113}	1	1	3
y_{121}	1	2	1
y_{122}	1	2	2
y_{123}	1	2	3
y_{211}	2	1	1
y_{211}	2	1	2
y_{212}	2	1	3
y_{213}	2	2	1
y_{221}	2	2	2
y_{222}	2	2	3

model to represent the treatment structure, it follows that the assumptions of the single-factor and two-factor model are the same. That is, the experimental error term ϵ in both models is a random variable that is assumed to be independently and normally distributed with mean 0 and common variance σ^2. Also, in a randomized block analysis, the block effect is assumed to be a random variable that is normally distributed with mean 0 and standard deviation σ_b that does not interact with treatment effects.

The treatment means in a two-factor study are denoted by μ_{ij} to represent the factor A and factor B levels making up the treatment combination, and therefore,

$$\mu_{ij} = \mu + \gamma_i + \beta_j + \gamma\beta_{ij}$$

where γ_i is the factor A level i main effect, β_j is the factor B level j main effect, and $\gamma\beta_{ij}$ is the interaction effect for the ith level of factor A and the $j$the level of factor B.

Note that when factors A and B interact the effects of the two factors cannot be separated from each other. That is, the difference between two treatment means depends on the level of each factor making up the treatment combinations being compared. On the other hand, when all of the interaction effects are equal to 0, the treatment means are given by $\mu_{ij} = \mu + \gamma_i + \beta_j$. Thus, when the factors A and B do not interact, the treatment means are simply the sum of the main effects of each factor, and in this case, the factors have independent contributions to the values of the response variable . Furthermore, when the factors do not interact, the difference of two treatment means at different levels of factor A but the same level of factor B, say $\mu_{ik} - \mu_{jk}$, is the same for all levels of factor B. Similarly, the difference between two treatment means at different levels of factor B but the same level of factor A, say $\mu_{ki} - \mu_{kj}$, is the same for all levels of factor A.

The first test that will be performed after the model is fit and the assumptions are checked and are satisfied is a test of

$$H_{0_{AB}} : \text{Factors } A \text{ and } B \text{ do not interact}$$

against the alternative hypothesis

$$H_{A_{AB}} : \text{Factors } A \text{ and } B \text{ do interact}$$

Note that in terms of the model parameters, the null hypothesis can be stated as

$$H_{0_{AB}} : \text{All of the } \gamma\beta \text{ terms are equal to 0}$$

Further tests of the main effects of the two factors will depend on the outcome of the F-test of the AB interaction. In particular, when the observed data suggest that factors A and B do not interact, a test of the main effects of each factor can be carried out. When there is a significant interaction between factors A and B, the main effects are meaningless and should not be tested.

As is the case with any statistical model, the assumptions of the model must be assessed and any violation of the assumptions must be cured before proceeding to use the model for making inferences. The normality assumption can again be checked using a normal probability plot of the residuals, and Levene's test for constant variance can be used to check the constant variation assumption. It is important to note that the standard deviations being compared in checking the nonconstant variance assumption are the standard deviations of the $a \times b$ treatment groups.

The total variation in the observed values of the response variable, SSTot, can be partitioned into sources of variation due to factor A, factor B, the interaction between factors A and B, experimental error, and a blocking factor when present. The summary of the partitioning of the total variation is given in an ANOV table containing the degrees of freedom, sum of squares, mean squares, and the F-ratios and their p-values. The ANOV

TABLE 12.11 ANOV Table for a Two-Factor Analysis of Variance

Source of Variation	DF	SS	MS	F	P
A	$a - 1$	SSA	MSA	$F_A = \dfrac{\text{MSA}}{\text{MSE}}$	p_A
B	$b - 1$	SSB	MSB	$F_B = \dfrac{\text{MSB}}{\text{MSE}}$	p_B
AB	$(a - 1)(b - 1)$	SSAB	MSAB	$F_{AB} = \dfrac{\text{MSAB}}{\text{MSE}}$	p_{AB}
Error	$ab(r - 1)$	SSE	MSE		
Total	$abr - 1$	SSTot			

tables for the two-factor analysis of variance without a blocking factor and with a blocking factor are given in Tables 12.11 and 12.12.

As always in an ANOV table, the mean squares for each source of variation are computed by dividing the sum of squares for each source of variation by their degrees of freedom. Also, note that there are three F-ratios given in a two-factor ANOV table. The value of F_{AB} and its p-value are used to test whether or not the factors interact. That is, the null hypothesis tested by F_{AB} is

$$H_{0_{AB}} : \text{Factors } A \text{ and } B \text{ do not interact}$$

which is equivalent to testing

$$H_{0_{AB}} : \text{All of the } \gamma\beta \text{ interaction terms are equal to } 0$$

When the interaction test is not significant (i.e., $p_{AB} \geq \alpha$), the values of F_A and F_B and their p-values are used to test whether the factors A and B are the main effects, and when there is evidence of a significant interaction between the factors (i.e., $p_{AB} < \alpha$), the main effects should not be tested since the factors are not acting independent of each other.

When factors A and B do interact (i.e., $p_{AB} \leq \alpha$), the observed data are suggesting that all of the interaction effects are 0, and therefore, the treatment means are based on only the main effects of the factors. That is, when the interactions are all 0

$$\mu_{ij} = \mu + \gamma_i + \beta_j$$

The null hypothesis tested by F_A is

$$H_{0_A} : \gamma_1 = \gamma_2 = \gamma_3 = \cdots = \gamma_a = 0$$

TABLE 12.12 ANOV Table for a Two-Factor Randomized Block Analysis of Variance

Source of Variation	DF	SS	MS	F	P
Blocks	$r - 1$	SSBL	MSBL		
A	$a - 1$	SSA	MSA	$F_A = \dfrac{\text{MSA}}{\text{MSE}}$	p_A
B	$b - 1$	SSB	MSB	$F_B = \dfrac{\text{MSB}}{\text{MSE}}$	p_B
AB	$(a - 1)(b - 1)$	SSAB	MSAB	$F_{AB} = \dfrac{\text{MSAB}}{\text{MSE}}$	p_{AB}
Error	$(ab - 1)(r - 1)$	SSE	MSE		
Total	$abr - 1$	SSTot			

and rejecting H_{0_A} means that there is significant evidence that factor A is influencing the mean of the response variable. Failing to reject H_{0_A} means that there is no evidence that factor A has any influence on the mean of the response variable. Similarly, the null hypothesis tested by F_B is

$$H_{0_B} : \beta_1 = \beta_2 = \beta_3 = \cdots = \beta_b = 0$$

and rejecting H_{0_A} means that there is significant evidence that factor B is influencing the mean of the response variable; failing to reject H_{0_B} means that there in no evidence that factor B has any influence on the mean of the response variable. The testing procedure for a two-factor analysis of variance is outlined below.

THE TESTING PROCEDURE IN A TWO-FACTOR ANOV

1. Test $H_{0_{AB}}$: Factors A and B do not interact. Reject $H_{0_{AB}}$ when $p_{AB} < \alpha$.

2. When $H_{0_{AB}}$ is rejected, the F-tests for the main effects should be ignored and the $a \times b$ treatment means should be separated.

3. When $p_{AB} \geq \alpha$ there is insufficient evidence to reject H_0 and the main effects can be tested.

   (a) Test H_{0_A} : The factor A main effects are all equal to 0. Reject when $p_A < \alpha$.

   (b) When $p_A < \alpha$ separate the factor A means.

   (c) Test H_{0_B} : The factor B main effects are all equal to 0. Reject when $p_B < \alpha$.

   (d) When $p_B < \alpha$ separate the factor B means.

Example 12.13

In the article "Drug delivery using the endotracheal tube: how much remains inside the tube?" published in *The Internet Journal of Anesthesiology* (Moeller-Bertram et al., 2007), the authors reported the results of a two-factor experiment designed to quantify the critical volume needed to assure 95% drug delivery after injection into an endotracheal tube (ETT).

In the author's experiment delivery room conditions were simulated using endotracheal tubes with internal diameters 2.5, 3.0, and 3.5 mm and five different fluid volumes (0.05, 0.10, 0.25, 0.50, and 1.00 mL) which were tested in a 3×5 factorial experiment. Each of the 15 treatment combinations was replicated 5 times and the ANOV Table given in Table 12.13 was reported.

Assuming that there is no evidence that any of the model assumptions are violated, according to the F-ratios in Table 12.13, there is a significant interaction between endotracheal tube size and volume. Thus, the 15 treatment means should be separated using the Bonferroni procedure.

The Bonferroni procedure can also be used to separate the means in a two-factor analysis of variance, but the type of means that are to be separated will depend on whether or

TABLE 12.13 ANOV Table for the Endotracheal Tube Study

Source of Variation	DF	F	P
Tube	2	21.43	0.000
Volume	4	58.88	0.000
Tube × Volume	8	5.50	0.000
Error	60		

not the AB interaction is significant. In particular, when the AB interaction is significant the treatment means, μ_{ij}, should be separated, and when the AB interaction is not significant the factor A and factor B means are separated. The ith level factor A mean is found by averaging over all of the levels of factor B, and the jth level factor B mean is found by averaging over all of the levels of factor A. In terms of the model parameters, the ith level factor A mean is

$$\mu_{i\bullet} = \mu + \gamma_i$$

and the jth level factor B mean is

$$\mu_{\bullet j} = \mu + \beta_j$$

There are also three types of sample means in a two-factor analysis of variance. The sample treatment means are computed by averaging the observations on each treatment combination over the replicates of each treatment and are denoted by $\bar{y}_{ij\bullet}$. The level i factor A mean is computed by averaging all of the observations having level i of factor A, and the level j factor B mean is computed by averaging all of the observations having level j of factor B. The ith level factor A and jth level factor B means are denoted by $\bar{y}_{i\bullet\bullet}$ and $\bar{y}_{\bullet j\bullet}$, respectively. Note that a treatment mean is found by averaging the r replicates of the treatment, the level i factor A mean is found by averaging the $r \times b$ units having level i of factor A, and the level j factor B mean is found by averaging the $r \times a$ units having level j of factor B.

Thus, when the AB interaction is significant, the sample treatment means, $\bar{y}_{ij\bullet}$, are compared and separated using the Bonferroni multiple comparison procedure, and when the AB interaction is not significant the sample factor A and B means, $\bar{y}_{i\bullet\bullet}$ and $\bar{y}_{\bullet j\bullet}$, are compared and separated using the Bonferroni multiple comparison procedure. The Bonferroni multiple comparison procedure is used just as it was in a single-factor analysis of variance. That is, two means are significantly different when the p-value is less than $\alpha_C = \frac{\alpha_E}{s}$, the adjusted p-value is less than α_E, or the difference between treatment or main effects means is greater than D. The values of D used in a two-factor analysis of variance are listed below.

THE BONFERRONI CRITICAL DISTANCE D

The Bonferroni critical value D in a two-factor study is

1. $D = b_{\text{crit}} \times \sqrt{\frac{2\text{MSE}}{r}}$ for comparing treatment means. The number of possible pairwise comparisons of the treatment means is $s_{AB} = \frac{ab(ab-1)}{2}$.

2. $D = b_{\text{crit}} \times \sqrt{\frac{2\text{MSE}}{rb}}$ for comparing factor A main effect means. The number of

possible pairwise comparisons of the factor A means is $s_A = \frac{a(a-1)}{2}$.

3. $D = b_{\text{crit}} \times \sqrt{\frac{2\text{MSE}}{ra}}$ for comparing factor B main effect means. The number of possible pairwise comparisons of the factor A means is $s_A = \frac{b(b-1)}{2}$.

The Bonferroni separation of means for a two-factor analysis of variance is also often summarized by ordering the means from smallest to largest and then underlining means that are not significantly different.

A $(1 - \alpha) \times 100\%$ confidence interval for the difference of two treatment means, say μ_{ij} and μ_{lm}, can be computed using

$$(\bar{y}_{ij\bullet} - \bar{y}_{lm\bullet}) \pm t_{\text{crit}} \times \sqrt{\frac{2\text{MSE}}{r}}$$

and a $(1 - \alpha) \times 100\%$ confidence interval for a particular treatment mean, say μ_{ij}, can be computed using

$$\bar{y}_{ij\bullet} \pm t_{\text{crit}} \times \sqrt{\frac{\text{MSE}}{r}}$$

When the AB interaction is not significant, confidence intervals for the factor means can be computed, and in this case, a $(1 - \alpha) \times 100\%$ confidence interval for

1. the difference of two factor A means, say $\mu_{i\bullet}$ and $\mu_{l\bullet}$, is

$$(\bar{y}_{i\bullet\bullet} - \bar{y}_{l\bullet\bullet}) \pm t_{\text{crit}} \times \sqrt{\frac{2\text{MSE}}{rb}}$$

2. an individual factor A mean, say $\mu_{i\bullet}$, is

$$\bar{y}_{i\bullet\bullet} \pm t_{\text{crit}} \times \sqrt{\frac{\text{MSE}}{rb}}$$

3. the difference of two factor B means, say $\mu_{\bullet j}$ and $\mu_{\bullet m}$, is

$$(\bar{y}_{\bullet j\bullet} - \bar{y}_{\bullet m\bullet}) \pm t_{\text{crit}} \times \sqrt{\frac{2\text{MSE}}{ra}}$$

4. for an individual factor B mean, say $\mu_{\bullet j}$, is

$$\bar{y}_{\bullet j\bullet} \pm t_{\text{crit}} \times \sqrt{\frac{\text{MSE}}{ra}}$$

Example 12.14

In the article "Drug delivery using the endotracheal tube: how much remains inside the tube?" published in *The Internet Journal of Anesthesiology* (Moeller-Bertram et al., 2007), the authors reported the means given in Table 12.14 for the 3 mm endotracheal tubes and five volumes being studied. Use the Bonferroni procedure to separate these five treatment means with $\alpha_{\text{E}} = 0.05$ and MSE $= 400$.

Solution First, note that there are $s = \frac{5(5-1)}{2} = 10$ pairwise mean comparisons that will need to be performed to separate these five means. The value of D for the Bonferroni multiple comparison

TABLE 12.14 Sample Means for the 3 mm Endotracheal Tube

3 mm Endotracheal Tube	
Volume	Mean
0.05	38
0.10	15
0.25	8
0.50	5
1.00	2

procedure when $\alpha_E = 0.05$, $s = 10$, and MSE $= 400$ is

$$D = 2.91 \times \sqrt{\frac{2 \times 400}{15}} = 21.25$$

Thus, any of these five treatment means that differ by more than $D = 21.25$ are significantly different.

Therefore, the mean for a 3 mm endotracheal tube with volume 0.05 is significantly different from the means for the other four volumes. There are no significant differences between the means of the 3 mm endotracheal tubes for the volumes 0.10, 0.25, 0.50, and 1.00. The separation of these five means is summarized as follows:

Volume (mL)	0.05	0.10	0.25	0.50	1.00
Sample Mean	38	15	8	5	2

In Examples 12.13 and 12.14, there are 15 treatment means, and thus, separating the treatment means in the presence of interaction would involve a large number of pairwise comparisons. In fact, the number of possible pairwise comparisons for 15 treatment means is $s = 105$, and the per comparison wise error rate for an experimentwise error rate of $\alpha_E = 0.05$ would be $\alpha_C = 0.000476$. The value of b_{crit} for the Bonferroni multiple comparison procedure would be almost 4, and therefore, the difference between two treatment means would have to exceed roughly $4 \times$ se to detect a statistically significant difference. Thus, because the Bonferroni procedure is a conservative procedure, it becomes harder and harder to detect significant differences when the number of means being compared is large. Two possible approaches to use when a large number of treatment means are being separated are (1) use a multiple comparison procedure less conservative than the Bonferroni procedure or (2) decide on a predetermined number (i.e., s) of mean comparisons that should reveal important information about the differences in the treatment means yet is much smaller than the total number of possible pairwise mean comparisons.

When the AB interaction is not significant, the number of mean comparisons will be much smaller. That is, at most only the a factor A means and the b factor B means will be compared when the AB interaction is not significant. Example 12.15 illustrates a two-factor analysis of variance and separation of means when the two factors do not have a significant interaction.

Example 12.15
In a study to investigate the effects of the diet and exercise on LDL cholesterol level, a 2×3 factorial experiment was performed on 60 subjects. The factors and factor levels used in this study were

- Diet with the two levels: Mediterranean diet and no change in diet
- Exercise with the three levels: no exercise, 30 min of exercise three times per week, and 30 min of exercise five times per week.

Subjects in the experiment had their LDL cholesterol levels measured on the first day of the experiment and then measured again after one month. The response variable analyzed in this experiment was the change in LDL cholesterol.

Suppose that Levene's test and a normal probability plot of the residuals revealed no evident violation of the model assumption, and the partial ANOV table in Table 12.15 and the means given in Table 12.16 resulted from this two-factor experiment.

Based on the ANOV table there is no evidence of a significant interaction between the factors Diet and Exercise ($F = 1.72$, $p = 0.189$). Thus, the Diet and Exercise main effects can be tested. Because the F-ratio for Diet is not significant ($F = 2.13$, $p = 0.150$), there is no apparent difference between the mean reduction in LDL cholesterol for the Mediterranean diet and no change in a subjects

**TABLE 12.15   ANOV Table for the LDL Study
with Factors Diet and Exercise**

Source of Variation	DF	MS	F	P
Diet	1	48.35	2.13	0.150
Exercise	2	423.80	18.67	0.000
Diet × Exercise	2	39.04	1.72	0.189
Error	54	22.70		
Total	59			

diet. On the other hand, the F-ratio for the Exercise main effects is significant ($F = 18.67$, $p = 0.000$), and therefore, the Exercise main effects means need to be separated.

Note that each exercise regimen was replicated 20 times, and because there are three levels of the factor Exercise, the number of pairwise mean comparisons for separating the Diet means is $s = \frac{3(3-1)}{2} = 3$. The value of D for comparing the mean change in LDL cholesterol for the Exercise factor is

$$D = 2.46 \times \sqrt{\frac{2 \times 22.7}{20}} = 3.71$$

Thus, any two Exercise means that differ by more than $D = 3.71$ are significantly different, and hence, the no exercise mean is significantly different from each of the other two Exercise means. The significant differences between the Exercise means is summarized below.

Exercise	No Exercise	3 × 30 min	5 × 30 min
Sample Mean	1.86	9.39	12.64

Thus, it appears that Diet had no effect on reducing the LDL cholesterol level but Exercise did. In particular, 30 min of exercise either three or five times a week was significantly better at reducing the LDL cholesterol than was no exercise; there was no significant difference between the mean reduction in LDL cholesterol level between the two 30-min exercise regimens.

12.3.2 Three-Factor Analysis of Variance

The analysis of variance for a $a \times b \times c$ three-factor experiment or study is very similar to the two-factor analysis of variance. As in a two-factor analysis of variance, a three-factor analysis of variance may or may not have a blocking factor. The raw data to be analyzed in a three-factor analysis of variance consist of n observations on the response variable Y. The abc treatment combinations are formed from the a levels of factor A, the b levels of factor B, and the c levels of factor C, and since each treatment combinations will be replicated r times, the number of units required to carry out a three-factor experiment or study is $n = r \times a \times b \times c$. Note that the minimum number of treatments that will be compared in a three-factor experiment or study is 8 that results from having only two

TABLE 12.16   Factor Means for the LDL Study

Factor	Means		
Diet	2.63	4.24	
Exercise	1.86	9.39	12.64

TABLE 12.17   A Sample of the Spreadsheet Form of the Raw Data for the First Replicate/Block of a 2 × 2 × 2 Two-Factor ANOV

Y	Factor A	Factor B	Factor C	Replicate/Block
y_{1111}	1	1	1	1
y_{1121}	1	1	2	1
y_{1211}	1	2	1	1
y_{1221}	1	2	2	1
y_{2121}	2	1	1	1
y_{2111}	2	1	2	1
y_{2221}	2	2	1	1
y_{2221}	2	2	2	1

levels of each factor; when each factor is studied at more than two levels, the number of treatments and the number of experimental units required for the study can grow quite large.

To distinguish the values of the observed response variable from each other, subscripts are often used to identify the levels of factors A, B, and C forming the treatment combination a unit received and the replicate of the treatment. Thus, in a three-factor analysis of variance, the observed value of the response variable for the lth replicate of the treatment combination formed from the ith level of factor A, the jth level of factor B, and the kth level of factor C is denoted by y_{ijkl}. Again, the observed data are often entered into a spreadsheet in a statistical package identifying the treatment each unit received. An example of the spreadsheet form for the first replicate of the treatments in a $2 \times 2 \times 2$ three-factor study is given in Table 12.17.

The linear model for a three-factor analysis of variance without a blocking factor is

$$Y = \mu + \gamma + \beta + \delta + \gamma\beta + \gamma\delta + \beta\delta + \gamma\beta\delta + \epsilon$$

where μ is the overall mean, γ is the factor A main effect, β is the factor B main effect, δ is the factor C main effect, $\gamma\beta$ is the AB interaction, $\gamma\delta$ is the AC interaction, $\beta\delta$ is the BC interaction, $\gamma\beta\delta$ is the ABC interaction, and ϵ is the experimental error. The model for a three-factor analysis of variance with a blocking factor is

$$Y = \mu + \rho + \gamma + \beta + \delta + \gamma\beta + \gamma\delta + \beta\delta + \gamma\beta\delta + \epsilon$$

where μ is the overall mean, ρ is the random block effect, γ is the factor A main effect, β is the factor B main effect, δ is the factor C main effect, $\gamma\beta$ is the AB interaction, $\gamma\delta$ is the AC interaction, $\beta\delta$ is the BC interaction, $\gamma\beta\delta$ is the ABC interaction, and ϵ is the experimental error. The AB, AC, and BC interactions are two-way interactions, and the ABC interaction is a three-way interaction, and any of the four interactions between the three factors may be significant in a three-factor analysis of variance.

The assumptions placed on the experimental error term ϵ in both three-factor models is that ϵ is a random variable that is assumed to be independently and normally distributed with mean 0 and common variance σ^2. Also, in a randomized block analysis, the block effect is assumed to be a random variable that is normally distributed with mean 0 and standard deviation σ_b that does not interact with the treatment effects.

The treatment means in a three-factor study are denoted by μ_{ijk}, where i is the level of factor A, j is the level factor B, and k is the level of factor C. In terms of the linear model for a three-factor study, the treatment means are

$$\mu_{ijk} = \gamma_i + \beta_j + \delta_k + \gamma\beta_{ij} + \gamma\delta_{ik} + \beta\delta_{jk} + \gamma\beta\delta_{ijk}$$

In a three-factor analysis of variance where at least two of the factors interact, the effects of the factors cannot be separated from each other. In this case, the difference between two treatment means depends on the particular level of each factor making up the treatment combinations being compared. On the other hand, when all of the interaction effects are equal to 0 the treatment means will be

$$\mu_{ijk} = \mu + \gamma_i + \beta_j + \delta_k$$

Thus, when the factors A, B, and C do not interact, the treatment means are simply the sum of the main effects of each factor, and in this case, each of the factors contributes independently to the mean of the response variable. That is, when none of the factors interacts, the difference of two treatment means at different levels of factor A but the same level of factors B and C, say $\mu_{ijk} - \mu_{mno}$, is the same for all levels of factors B and C. Similar statements can be made for the difference between two treatment means at different levels of factor B or factor C when the other two factors are held constant.

Thus, in a three-factor analysis of variance, the first test that will be performed after the model is fit and the assumptions are checked and are satisfied is a test of

$$H_{0_{ABC}} : \text{Factors } A, B, \text{ and } C \text{ do not interact}$$

against the alternative hypothesis

$$H_{A_{ABC}} : \text{Factors } A, B, \text{ and } C \text{ do interact}$$

Note that in terms of the model parameters the null hypothesis can be stated as

$$H_{0_{ABC}} : \text{All of the } \gamma\beta\delta \text{ terms are equal to 0}$$

Furthermore, in order to have meaningful tests of the factor A, B, and C main effects all of the two-way interaction must also be nonsignificant. The testing procedure for a three-factor analysis of variance will be discussed later in this section.

As is the case with any statistical model, the assumptions of the model must be assessed and any violation of the assumptions must be cured before proceeding to use the model for making inferences. The normality assumption can again be checked using a normal probability plot of the residuals and Levene's test for constant variance can be used to check the constant variation assumption. It is important to note that the standard deviations being compared in checking the nonconstant variance assumption are the standard deviations of the $a \times b \times c$ treatment groups.

The total variation in the observed values of the response variable, SSTot, can be partitioned into sources of variation due to factor A, factor B, factor C, the interactions between factors A, B, C, the experimental error, and the blocking factor when present. The summary of the partitioning of the total variation is given in an ANOV table containing the degrees of freedom, sum of squares, mean squares, F-ratios, and p-values as usual. The ANOV tables for the three-factor analysis of variance without a blocking factor and with a blocking factor are given in Tables 12.18 and 12.19.

Note that there are now seven F-ratios in a three-factor ANOV table. The rules for using the seven F-ratios in a three-factor analysis of variance are outlined below.

TABLE 12.18   ANOV Table for a Three-Factor Analysis of Variance

Source of Variation	DF	SS	MS	F	P
A	$a-1$	SSA	MSA	$F_A = \dfrac{\text{MSA}}{\text{MSE}}$	p_A
B	$b-1$	SSB	MSB	$F_B = \dfrac{\text{MSB}}{\text{MSE}}$	p_B
C	$c-1$	SSB	MSC	$F_C = \dfrac{\text{MSC}}{\text{MSE}}$	p_C
AB	$(a-1)(b-1)$	SSAB	MSAB	$F_{AB} = \dfrac{\text{MSAB}}{\text{MSE}}$	p_{AB}
AC	$(a-1)(c-1)$	SSAC	MSAC	$F_{AC} = \dfrac{\text{MSAC}}{\text{MSE}}$	p_{AC}
BC	$(b-1)(c-1)$	SSBC	MSBC	$F_{BC} = \dfrac{\text{MSBC}}{\text{MSE}}$	p_{BC}
ABC	$(a-1)(b-1)(c-1)$	SSABC	MSABC	$F_{ABC} = \dfrac{\text{MSABC}}{\text{MSE}}$	p_{ABC}
Error	$abc(r-1)$	SSE	MSE		
Total	$abcr-1$	SSTot			

THE TESTING PROCEDURE IN A THREE-FACTOR ANOV

1. Test $H_{0_{ABC}}$: Factors A, B, and C do not interact. Reject $H_{0_{ABC}}$ when $p_{ABC} < \alpha$.

2. When $H_{0_{ABC}}$ is rejected the F-tests for the two-way interactions and main effects should be ignored and the $a \times b \times c$ treatment means should be separated.

3. When $p_{ABC} \geq \alpha$, there is insufficient evidence to reject $H_{0_{ABC}}$; the next step is to test the two-way interactions.

   (a) When any of the two-way interactions are significant, the F-tests for the main effects should be ignored and the $a \times b \times c$ treatment means should be separated.

   (b) When none of the two-way interactions is significant, the factor main effects can be tested.

   i. When a factor main effect is significant, the factor means should be separated.

Because the minimum number of treatments in every three-factor study is 8, the minimum number of pairwise mean comparisons needed to separate the means in the presence of one or more interactions is $s = 28$. Therefore, the Bonferroni multiple comparison procedure should not be used for separating all of the treatment means in a three-factor analysis of variance. However, the Bonferroni procedure can be used to separate the factor means when the three-way and all of the two-way interactions are not significant. Thus, the best approach to use in a three-factor study is to preselect a reasonable number of pairwise mean comparisons (i.e., $s \leq 10$) that will provide relevant information about the treatments and factors and then use the Bonferroni procedure on these planned comparisons.

Because the number of treatment means grows rapidly as the number of levels of each factor is increased in a three-factor study, it is fairly common for researchers to use only two levels of each factor. When each factor in a three-factor study has only two levels, the treatment structure is referred to as a 2^3 *factorial treatment structure*. Another advantage of using a 2^3 factorial treatment structure in a study is that there is no need to use a multiple

TABLE 12.19 ANOV Table for a Three-Factor Randomized Block Analysis of Variance

Source of Variation	DF	SS	MS	F	P
Blocks	$r-1$	SSBL	MSBL		
A	$a-1$	SSA	MSA	$F_A = \dfrac{\text{MSA}}{\text{MSE}}$	p_A
B	$b-1$	SSB	MSB	$F_B = \dfrac{\text{MSB}}{\text{MSE}}$	p_B
C	$c-1$	SSB	MSC	$F_C = \dfrac{\text{MSC}}{\text{MSE}}$	p_C
AB	$(a-1)(b-1)$	SSAB	MSAB	$F_{AB} = \dfrac{\text{MSAB}}{\text{MSE}}$	p_{AB}
AC	$(a-1)(c-1)$	SSAC	MSAC	$F_{AC} = \dfrac{\text{MSAC}}{\text{MSE}}$	p_{AC}
BC	$(b-1)(c-1)$	SSBC	MSBC	$F_{BC} = \dfrac{\text{MSBC}}{\text{MSE}}$	p_{BC}
ABC	$(a-1)(b-1)(c-1)$	SSABC	MSABC	$F_{ABC} = \dfrac{\text{MSABC}}{\text{MSE}}$	p_{ABC}
Error	$(abc-1)(r-1)$	SSE	MSE		
Total	$abcr-1$	SSTot			

comparison procedure to separate the factor means. That is, when the three-way and two-way interactions are not significant in a 2^3 factorial study, because a factor has only two levels, it follows from the significance of the factor main effects that the two factor level means are significantly different.

Example 12.16
Suppose the normal probability plot and Levene's test of nonconstant variance given in Figure 12.7 and ANOV table in Table 12.20 resulted from 2^3 factorial randomized block experiment with $r = 5$ blocks. The normal probability plot and Levene's summary indicate there are no apparent problems with the model assumptions.

The F-ratios in the ANOV table also suggest that none of the interactions is significant. Also, only the factor A and factor C main effects are significant ($p_A = 0.019$ and $p_C = 0.039$). Thus, there are significant differences between the level 1 and level 2 factor means for factors A and C; factor B does not appear to be an important factor ($p = 0.258$). The factor A and C means are given in Table 12.21.

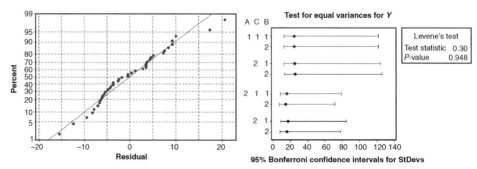

Figure 12.7   The normal probability plot and Levene's summary for Example 12.16.

TABLE 12.20 ANOV Table from the 2^3 Randomized Block Design

Source	DF	SS	MS	F	P
Block	4	11676.4	2919.1	35.73	0.000
A	1	504.1	504.1	6.17	0.019
B	1	108.9	108.9	1.33	0.258
C	1	384.4	384.4	4.71	0.039
A*B	1	115.6	115.6	1.41	0.244
A*C	1	0.1	0.1	0.00	0.972
B*C	1	4.9	4.9	0.06	0.808
A*B*C	1	0.4	0.4	0.00	0.945
Error	28	2287.6	81.7		
Total	39	15082.4			

TABLE 12.21 The Factor A and Factor C Means

Factor	n	Level 1	Level 2
A	20	60.75	53.65
B	20	54.10	60.30

12.4 SELECTING THE NUMBER OF REPLICATES IN ANALYSIS OF VARIANCE

Two methods are presented for determining the number of replicates required to achieve a prespecified level of reliability in an analysis of variance. The first method is based on prespecifying a desired level of power for testing the equality of the treatment means, and the second method is based on a prespecified value of the Bonferroni distance D.

12.4.1 Determining the Number of Replicates from the Power

When the number of replicates is to be determined so that a prespecified power is obtained in the F-test of the equality of the treatment means, the researcher must specify the number of treatments in the study, the desired power, the significance level, the minimum difference in treatment means that is to be detected, and a reasonable guess of the standard deviation associated with the experimental error. In this case, the calculation of the required number of replicates is complicated; however, most of the commonly used statistical computing packages have programs that can be used to compute the number of treatment replicates needed for a given power, significance level, minimum difference, and value of σ.

Example 12.17

The MINITAB output for determining the number of replicates of each treatment in a balanced design for a single-factor analysis of variance with five treatments, $\alpha = 0.05$, desired power of 0.80, (i.e., the probability of a type II is 0.20), and a minimum difference of 10 to be detected with a reasonable guess of $\sigma = 12$ is given in Figure 12.8.

Thus, using $r = 36$ replicates of each treatment will produce an F-test of the equality of the treatment means with power 0.80 for detecting a difference of 10 at the $\alpha = 0.05$ level when $\sigma = 12$. The total number of units needed for this study is $5 \times 36 = 180$.

```
Power and Sample Size

Alpha = 0.05  Assumed standard deviation = 12  Number of Levels = 5

   SS  Sample  Target                      Maximum
Means   Size   Power  Actual Power  Difference
   50     36    0.8       0.808545          10
```
Figure 12.8   The MINITAB output for determining the number of replicates of each treatment in a balanced design for a single-factor analysis of variance.

Most statistical computing packages will also determine the number of replicates needed when the study involves a multifactor factorial treatment structure.

Example 12.18
The MINITAB output for determining the number of replicates of each treatment in a balanced design for a 2^3 factorial analysis of variance $\alpha = 0.05$, desired power of 0.80 (i.e., the probability of a Type II is 0.20), and a minimum difference of 5 to be detected with a reasonable guess of $\sigma = 8$ is given in Figure 12.18.

Thus, using $r = 11$ replicates of each treatment will produce an F-test of the equality of the treatment means with power 0.80 for detecting a difference of 5 at the $\alpha = 0.05$ level when $\sigma = 8$. The total number of units needed for this 2^2 factorial study is $8 \times 11 = 88$.

```
Alpha = 0.05  Assumed standard deviation = 8

Factors:   3   Base Design: 3, 8

Center                  Total  Target
Points  Effect  Reps    Runs   Power   Actual Power
   0       5     11       88    0.8       0.825411
```

12.4.2 Determining the Number of Replicates from D

The second method for determining the number of replicates needed in an analysis of variance is based on the Bonferroni multiple comparison distance D. Recall, the Bonferroni distance D is the minimum distance for which the means will be declared significantly different when using the Bonferroni multiple comparison procedure to separate the treatment means. In a balanced design, the value of D is given by

$$D \approx b_{crit} \times \sqrt{\frac{2 \times \sigma^2}{r}}$$

where σ is the standard deviation of the experimental error, r is the number of replicates of each treatment, and b_{crit} is the Bonferroni critical t-value. Thus, the number of replicates required to produce the desired value of D can be found by solving for the value of r in the equation for D however, because the degrees of freedom of error will be unknown until the number of replicates has been determined, the value of b_{crit} is unknown. When $\alpha_E = 0.05$ and $s \leq 10$, a value of $b_{crit} = 3$ can safely be used to find the approximate number of replicates needed to produce a Bonferroni distance of D. Thus, when a researcher has a prespecified value of D, the number of comparisons s is 10 or less, a reasonable guess of

σ is available, and the experimentwise error rate is $\alpha_E = 0.05$, the approximate number of replicates required to achieve the Bonferroni distance D is

$$r = \frac{18 \times \sigma^2}{D^2}$$

Example 12.19
Suppose that it is important to detect a difference between two treatment means of $D = 10$ in a 3×5 factorial experiment for $s = 6$ preplanned comparisons of the treatment means. With a reasonable guess $\sigma \approx 12$ and $\alpha_E = 0.05$, the number of replicates required for a Bonferroni distance equal to 10 is

$$r = \frac{18 \times 12^2}{10^2} = 25.92$$

Thus, using $r = 26$ replicates of each treatment will produce a Bonferroni distance of $D = 10$ for comparing treatment means with an experimentwise error rate of $\alpha = 0.05$ level when $\sigma \approx 12$. The total number of units needed for this study is $15 \times 26 = 390$.

12.5   SOME FINAL COMMENTS ON ANALYSIS OF VARIANCE

Analysis of variance is a powerful statistical method that can be used to detect differences between the means of two or more populations or treatments. As is the case, any time a statistical model is being fit, it is critical to check and validate the assumptions of the model in an analysis of variance. Statistical inferences based on hypothesis tests or confidence intervals should never be based on a model when one or more of the model's assumptions are violated.

The assumption that most affects the reliability of the tests in an analysis of variance is the assumption of a constant treatment variance. When the constant variance assumption is violated, the statistical inferences based on the F-test of the equality of the treatment means and the Bonferroni separation of means will often be incorrect. Transformations of the response variable such as the natural logarithm can sometimes be used to cure a nonconstant variance problem. The F-test and the Bonferroni procedure for separating the means are fairly robust to the normality assumption, and the normality assumption becomes less important as the degrees of freedom for error increases.

When the model assumptions are valid an F-test can be used to test the equality of the treatment means; however, a significant F-ratio neither does necessarily mean that at least two of the treatment means are scientifically different nor does it determine which of the treatment means are different. Therefore, when the F-ratio for testing the equality of the treatment means is significant, the treatment means should be separated using a multiple comparison procedure. The number of replicates of each treatment should be determined in the planning stages of the study to ensure that a scientifically important difference will be detectable. Confidence intervals for the means being compared can also be used to determine whether or not the statistically significant differences represent scientifically important differences.

In a multifactor analysis of variance, the significance of the factor main effects is important only when none of the interactions in the model is significant. When the interactions are significant, the treatment means should be separated. On the other hand, when there are no significant interactions the factor main effects can be tested, and in this case, the factor means should be separated for the factors having significant main effects.

GLOSSARY

2^k **Factorial Treatment Structure**   A study has a 2^k treatment structure when the treatments are formed from the combinations of the two levels of each of the k factors.

Analysis of Variance Table   The sources of variation are summarized in an analysis of variance (ANOV) table containing a row for each source of variation and its degrees of freedom, sum of squares, mean sum of squares, and where appropriate the observed F-ratio and its p-value.

Analysis of Variance   Analysis of variance is used to partition the total variation in the observed values of the response variable into sources of variation that are caused by the treatments, blocking factors, and the experimental error in a designed study.

Bonferroni Procedure   The Bonferroni multiple comparison procedure is a statistical method that can be used to separate the treatment means when there are significant differences among the treatment means.

Experimentwise Error Rate   The experimentwise error rate is the probability of making at least one Type I error in a series of comparative tests and is denoted by α_E.

Factor Means   In a factorial study, the ith level factor mean is the mean of the response variable averaged over all observations having the ith level of the factor.

Mean Squares   The mean squares, also referred to as the mean sum of squares, for a source of variation are the sum of squares due to the source of variation divided by the degrees of freedom attributed to the source of variation.

$$MS = \frac{SS}{df}$$

MSE   MSE is the mean sum of squares due to the experimental error and is an unbiased estimate of the variance of the error term in an analysis of variance model.

$$MSE = \frac{SSE}{df\ error}$$

Multifactor study   A study with a multifactor treatment structure is called a multifactor study.

Multifactor Treatment Structure   The treatments are said to have a multifactor treatment structure when the treatments are formed from the combinations of the levels of two or more factors.

Per Comparison Wise Error Rate   The per comparison wise error rate is the probability of making a Type I error in any particular test and is denoted by α_C.

Single-Factor Analysis of Variance   A single-factor analysis of variance, also referred to as a one-way analysis of variance, is used for analyzing data arising from a completely randomized design experiment or an observational study with treatment groups due to a single factor.

SSBL   SSBL is the sum of squares due to the blocking factor.

SSE   SSE is the sum of squares due to the experimental error.

SSTot   SSTot is the sum of the squared deviations of the observed values of the response variable from the overall sample mean.

SSTR   SSTR is the sum of squares due to the differences in the treatment means.

EXERCISES

12.1   Why is an experiment preferred over an observational study?

12.2   What is a balanced design?

12.3   In a single-factor analysis of variance what
(a) is the model?
(b) are the assumptions of the model?
(c) does Y_{ij} represent?

12.4   In terms of the parameters of a single-factor analysis of variance model, what is the
(a) ith treatment mean?
(b) difference between the ith and jth treatment means?

12.5   In terms of the parameters of a single-factor analysis of variance model, explain why the difference between two treatment means is equal to the difference of their treatment effects.

12.6   In a single-factor analysis of variance, what are
(a) SSTot?   (b) SSE?
(c) SSTR?

12.7   Describe what each of the sum of squares in Exercise 12.6 measures.

12.8   What parameter does MSE estimate?

12.9   In a single-factor analysis of variance, what is the
(a) estimator of the ith treatment mean?
(b) residual associated with the observation y_{ij}?
(c) unbiased estimator of σ?

12.10   What is the normality assumption in a single-factor model?

12.11   How can the normality assumption of a single-factor model be checked?

12.12   Use the normal probability plot given in Figure 12.9 resulting from a single-factor analysis of variance with four treatments to check the normality assumption. Is it reasonable to assume that the error term is normally distributed? Explain.

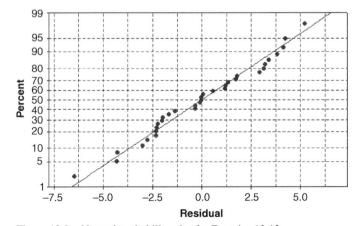

Figure 12.9   Normal probability plot for Exercise 12.12.

TABLE 12.22 Sample Standard Deviations for Exercise 12.16

Treatment	Sample SD
1	24.5
2	33.9
3	19.0
4	28.4

12.13 What is the constant variance assumption in a single-factor model?

12.14 What are the two methods that can be used to check the constant variance assumption in a single-factor model?

12.15 When there is evidence suggesting that there is a nonconstant variance problem in an analysis of variance, which transformation of the response variable is suggested as a potential cure for the nonconstant variance problem?

12.16 Use the sample standard deviations given in Table 12.22 resulting from a single-factor analysis of variance on five treatments to check the constant variance assumption. Is it reasonable to assume that each of the treatment groups has the same variance? Explain.

12.17 Use the sample standard deviations given in Table 12.23 resulting from a single-factor analysis of variance on four treatments to check the constant variance assumption. Is it reasonable to assume that each of the treatment groups has the same variance? Explain.

12.18 Use the summary of Levene's test for nonconstant variance given in Figure 12.10 resulting from a single-factor analysis of variance with four treatments to check the constant variance assumption. Is it reasonable to assume that each of the treatment groups has the same variance? Explain.

12.19 Use the summary of Levene's test for nonconstant variance given in Figure 12.11 resulting from a single-factor analysis of variance with four treatments to check the constant variance assumption. Is it reasonable to assume that each of the treatment groups has the same variance? Explain.

12.20 The partial ANOV table given in Table 12.24 was extracted from the article "Dietary supplement containing mixture of raw curry, garlic, and ginger" published in the *The Internet Journal of Nutrition and Wellness* (Ugwuja et al., 2008). The ANOV

TABLE 12.23 Sample Standard Deviations for Exercise 12.17

Treatment	Sample SD
1	8.5
2	15.1
3	11.8
4	18.4
5	15.6

Test for equal variances for Y

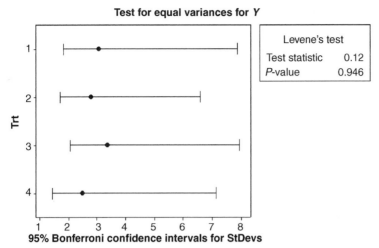

Figure 12.10   Summary of Levene's test of nonconstant variance for Exercise 12.18.

Test for equal variances for Y

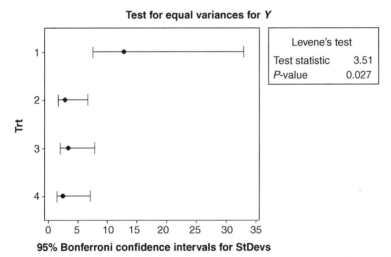

Figure 12.11   Summary of Levene's test of nonconstant variance for Exercise 12.19.

table corresponds to a single-factor experiment with four treatments that were each replicated $r = 5$ times. Use the information in Table 12.24 to answer the following:

(a) Fill in the missing entries in the ANOV table given in Table 12.24.
(b) Estimate the variance of the error term in the model.
(c) Test the hypothesis of equal treatment means at the $\alpha = 0.05$ level.

TABLE 12.24   The ANOV Table for Exercise 12.20

Source of Variation	DF	SS	MS	F	P
Treatments			2.56		0.181
Error					
Total		29.97			

TABLE 12.25   The ANOV Table for Exercise 12.21

Source of Variation	DF	SS	MS	F	P
Treatments				2.26	0.108
Error		295			
Total					

12.21   The partial ANOV table given in Table 12.25 was extracted from the article "Effects of folic acid and combinations of folic acid and vitamin B-12 on plasma homocysteine concentrations in healthy young women" published in the *American Journal of Clinical Nutrition* (Brönstrup et al., 1998). The ANOV table corresponds to a single-factor experiment with three treatments that were replicated 51, 49, and 50 times. Use the information in Table 12.25 to answer the following:

(a) Fill in the missing entries, the ANOV table given in Table 12.25.

(b) Estimate the standard deviation of the error term in the model.

(c) Test the hypothesis of equal treatment means at the $\alpha = 0.01$ level.

12.22   What is the

(a) experimentwise error rate?

(b) per comparisonwise error rate?

12.23   Determine the number of pairwise mean comparisons that would need to be made in separating the treatment means with the Bonferroni procedure when there are

(a) four treatments.   (b) five treatments.

(c) six treatments.   (d) eight treatments.

12.24   Determine the Bonferroni critical t-value for separating the means when there are

(a) three treatments and 25 degrees of freedom for error.

(b) four treatments and 27 degrees of freedom for error.

(c) five treatments and 40 degrees of freedom for error.

(d) $s = 6$ mean comparisons and 60 degrees of freedom for error.

12.25   For a balanced single-factor study, determine the Bonferroni distance D for an experimentwise error rate of $\alpha_E = 0.05$ when

(a) there are three treatments replicated five times and MSE $= 25$.

(b) there are four treatments replicated eight times and MSE $= 50$.

(c) there are 5 treatments replicated 13 times and MSE $= 220$.

12.26   What is an adjusted p-value and how is it used?

12.27   If the adjusted p-value for comparing μ_1 and μ_2 is $p = 0.087$, is there sufficient evidence to reject $H_0 : \mu_1 = \mu_2$ when the Bonferroni multiple comparison procedure is used with $\alpha_E = 0.05$? Explain.

12.28   If the adjusted p-value for comparing μ_1 and μ_2 is $p = 0.037$, is there sufficient evidence to reject $H_0 : \mu_1 = \mu_2$ when the Bonferroni multiple comparison procedure is used with $\alpha_E = 0.05$? Explain.

12.29   Use the MINITAB output for the Bonferroni procedure given in Table 12.26 to determine which of the treatment means in the treatment 1 mean is significantly different from.

TABLE 12.26   MINITAB Output for the Bonferroni Procedure in Exercise 12.29

```
    Treatment 1 subtracted from

                                  Adjusted
    TRT                           P-Value
    2                              0.2030
    3                              0.0004
    4                              0.0070
    5                              0.6709
```

TABLE 12.27   Mean Angle of Hysteresis Value for Four Saliva Substitutes

Treatment	n	Mean Age	SD
Distilled water	40	19.511	2.97
Wet mouth	40	21.161	2.73
AQWET	40	28.399	1.82
SALIVART	40	20.315	2.99
MOUTHKOTE	40	21.346	3.15

MSE = 8.15

12.30   In the article "An *in vitro* comparative study of wettability of four commercially available saliva substitutes and distilled water on heat-polymerized acrylic resin" published in the *Journal of Indian Prosthodontic Society* (Sharma and Chitre, 2008), the authors reported the means given in Table 12.27 and a significant F-ratio ($F = 62.70$, $p = 0.000$) for testing the equality of the treatment means. Use the information in Table 12.27 to separate the treatment means.

12.31   Use the ANOV table given in Table 12.28 for a balanced experiment having three treatments to answer the following:

(a) How many replicates of each treatment were used in this experiment?

(b) Test the hypothesis of the equality of the treatment means at the $\alpha = 0.01$ level.

(c) Estimate the standard deviation of the error term in the model.

(d) Determine the number of pairwise comparisons needed to separate the three treatment means.

(e) Determine the Bonferroni distance D for separating the treatment means when the experimentwise error rate is $\alpha_E = 0.05$.

TABLE 12.28   The ANOV Table for Exercise 12.31

Source of Variation	DF	SS	MS	F	P
Treatments	2	550	275	3.93	0.030
Error	30	2100	70		
Total	32	2550			

TABLE 12.29 Mean Age of Menopause According to Smoking Habits

Number of Cigarettes per day	n	Mean Age	SD
Never smokes	1332	50.05	2.04
Less than 5	214	49.77	2.07
5 to 9	211	47.70	3.10
10 to 19	154	47.79	3.19
More than 20	37	46.98	3.02

(f) If $\bar{y}_{1\bullet} = 12.08$, $\bar{y}_{2\bullet} = 4.31$, and $\bar{y}_{3\bullet} = 13.69$, use the Bonferroni procedure to separate the treatment means with an experimentwise error rate of $\alpha_E = 0.05$.

(g) Summarize the separation of the treatment means using the underline notation.

12.32 In the article "Cigarette smoking and age at natural menopause of women in Poland" published in *The Internet Journal of Biological Anthropology* (Pawlinska-Chmara and Anita Szwed, 2008), the authors reported the results of a retrospective study on smoking and age of menopause for 1948 women. The summary statistics given in Table 12.29 were reported in this article and the ANOV table given in Table 12.30 was reconstructed from the information in Table 12.29. Use Tables 12.29 and 12.30 to answer the following:

(a) On the basis of the information in Table 12.27, is it reasonable to assume the treatment groups have a common variance? Explain.

(b) Test the hypothesis of the equality of the treatment means at the $\alpha = 0.05$ level.

(c) How many pairwise comparisons would be needed to separate the five treatment means?

(d) Determine the Bonferroni distance D for comparing the means for women smoking up to 5 cigarettes a day and women smoking 5–10 cigarettes per day when the experimentwise error rate is $\alpha_E = 0.05$. Are these two means significantly different?

(e) Compute a 95% confidence interval for the difference between the means for women smoking up to 5 cigarettes a day and women smoking 5–10 cigarettes per day.

12.33 In the article "The effect of hydrogel and solution of sodium ascorbate on the bond strength of bleached enamel" published in the *Journal of Conservative Dentistry* (Paul et al., 2007), the authors reported the results of an experiment studying the effects of four different bleaching treatments on the enamel surfaces of maxillary molars. Each of the four treatments was replicated 10 times and Table 12.29

TABLE 12.30 The ANOV Table for Exercise 12.32

Source of Variation	DF	SS	MS	F	P
Treatments	4	1785.95	446.49	83.78	0.000
Error	1943	10355.15	5.33		
Total	1947	12141.10			

TABLE 12.31   Mean Shear Bond Strength After Bleaching

Treatment	n	Mean	SD
No sodium ascorbate	10	21.393	0.862
10% sodium ascorbate solution	10	27.157	0.864
10% sodium ascorbate hydrogel	10	28.684	0.696
20% sodium ascorbate hydrogel	10	28.888	0.576

contains summary statistics reported in the article and the ANOV table given in Table 12.32 was reconstructed from the information in Table 12.31. Use Table 12.31 and 12.32 to answer the following:

(a) On the basis of the information in Table 12.31, is it reasonable to assume the treatment groups have a common variance? Explain.

(b) Test the hypothesis of equal treatment means at the $\alpha = 0.05$ level.

(c) Determine the Bonferroni distance D for separating the treatment means when the experimentwise error rate is $\alpha_E = 0.05$.

(d) Separate the treatment means and summarize the separation of the treatment means using the underline notation.

(e) Compute a 95% confidence interval for the difference between the means of the no-sodium ascorbate treatment and the 20% sodium ascorbate hydrogel treatment.

(f) Compute a 95% confidence interval for the mean of the 20% sodium ascorbate hydrogel treatment.

12.34   In the article "Caudal analgesia in paediatrics: a comparison between bupivacaine and ketamine" published in *The Internet Journal of Anesthesiology* (Siddiqui and Choudhury, 2006), the authors reported the results of a study on the mean time intervals between the recovery from anesthesia and the first dose of analgesia for three treatments. Each of the three treatments was replicated 20 times. Table 12.33 contains the summary statistics that were reported in the article, and the ANOV table given in Table 12.34 was reconstructed from the information in Table 12.33. Use Tables 12.33 and 12.34 to answer the following:

(a) On the basis of the information in Table 12.33, is it reasonable to assume the treatment groups have a common variance? Explain.

(b) Test the hypothesis of the equality of the treatment means at the $\alpha = 0.05$ level.

(c) Determine the Bonferroni distance D for separating the treatment means when the experimentwise error rate is $\alpha_E = 0.05$.

(d) Separate the treatment means and summarize the separation of the treatment means using the underlined notation.

TABLE 12.32   The ANOV Table for Exercise 12.33

Source of Variation	DF	SS	MS	F	P
Treatments	3	369.82	123.27	211.70	0.000
Error	36	20.96	0.58		
Total	39	390.78			

TABLE 12.33   Mean Time Interval Between the Recovery and First Dose of Analgesia

Treatment	n	Mean	SD
Bupivacaine	20	3.26	2.05
Bupivacaine-ketamine	20	12.04	3.31
Ketamine	20	12.70	3.54

TABLE 12.34   The ANOV Table for Exercise 12.34

Source of Variation	DF	SS	MS	F	P
Treatments	2	1110.92	555.46	60.18	0.000
Error	57	526.11	9.23		
Total	59	1637.03			

(e) Compute a 95% confidence interval for the difference between the means of the bupivaciane treatment and the ketamine treatment.

(f) Compute a 95% confidence interval for the mean of the ketamine treatment.

12.35 Why are randomized block designs used?

12.36 In a single-factor randomized block design what
(a) is the model?
(b) are the assumptions of the model?
(c) does Y_{ij} represent?

12.37 In terms of the parameters of a randomized block analysis of variance model, what is the
(a) ith treatment mean?
(b) difference between the ith and jth treatment means?

12.38 How are the assumption of a randomized block model checked?

12.39 Suppose a randomized block experiment is performed with five treatments and eight blocks. If SSBL = 800, SSTR = 1200, and SSTot = 3400, construct an ANOV table for this experiment.

12.40 Use the information in the ANOV table given in Table 12.35 for a randomized block experiment with 6 treatments and 15 blocks to answer the following:
(a) Fill in the missing entries in the ANOV table.
(b) Estimate the variance of the experimental error.

TABLE 12.35   The ANOV Table for Exercise 12.40

Source of Variation	DF	SS	MS	F	P
Blocks		2280			
Treatments				26.4	0.000
Error		560			
Total					

TABLE 12.36   The ANOV Table for Exercise 12.41

Source of Variation	DF	SS	MS	F	P
Blocks			65		
Treatments		810			0.009
Error			60		
Total					

(c) Test the equality of the treatment means.

(d) Compute the value of the Bonferroni distance D for $s = 10$ comparisons and $\alpha_E = 0.05$.

12.41   Use the information in the ANOV table given in Table 12.36 for a randomized block experiment with 4 treatments and 12 blocks to answer the following:

(a) Fill in the missing entries in the ANOV table.

(b) Estimate the variance of the experimental error.

(c) Test the equality of the treatment means.

(d) Compute the value of the Bonferroni distance D used to separate the four means when $\alpha_E = 0.05$.

12.42   Suppose in a randomized block experiment designed to investigate the efficacy of four drugs for reducing the duration of migraine headaches, the observed F-ratio for testing the equality of the treatment means is significant ($p = 0.003$). Use the treatment means given in Table 12.37 to answer the following:

(a) Determine the number of pairwise comparisons that must be carried to separate the treatment means.

(b) Determine the degrees of freedom for the experimental error.

(c) Determine the Bonferroni distance D when the experimentwise error rate is $\alpha_E = 0.05$ and MSE $= 188.2$.

(d) Using the Bonferroni procedure, separate the treatment means and summarize using the underline notation.

(e) Compute a 95% confidence interval for the difference of the treatment A and B means.

12.43   What is a multifactor treatment structure?

12.44   How many treatments are there in a multifactor study when there is a

(a) 3×4 treatment structure?   (b) 4×6 treatment structure?

TABLE 12.37   Mean Duration of Migraine Headache in Minutes

Treatment	n	Mean
A	20	123.1
B	20	232.6
C	20	143.2
D	20	228.7

(c) $2 \times 3 \times 3$ treatment structure?

(d) $3 \times 3 \times 3$ treatment structure?

(e) 2^3 treatment structure?

(f) 2^4 treatment structure?

12.45 How many units are required in each part of Exercise 12.44 when there are

(a) three replicates of each treatment

(b) five blocks of units?

(c) six replicates of each treatment

(d) eight blocks of units?

12.46 In a two-factor analysis of variance what

(a) is the model?

(b) are the assumptions of the model?

(c) does Y_{ijk} represent?

12.47 In a two-factor randomized block analysis of variance what

(a) is the model?

(b) are the assumptions of the model?

(c) does Y_{ijk} represent?

12.48 In a two-factor analysis of variance what does

(a) $\bar{y}_{ij\bullet}$ estimate?

(b) $\bar{y}_{i\bullet\bullet}$ estimate?

(c) $\bar{y}_{\bullet j\bullet}$ estimate?

12.49 In terms of the parameters of a two-factor analysis of variance model, what is the

(a) ijth treatment mean?

(b) difference between the ijth and klth treatment means when the factors interact?

(c) difference between the ijth and klth treatment means when the factors do not interact?

12.50 Explain why the main effects in a two-factor analysis of variance should not be tested when the interaction is significant.

12.51 Use the information in the ANOV table given in Table 12.38 for a two-factor experiment with 2×3 treatment structure and seven replicates of each treatment to answer the following:

(a) Fill in the missing entries in the ANOV table.

(b) Estimate the standard deviation of the experimental error.

(c) Test for the interaction of factors A and B.

(d) Based on the test in part (c), which means should be separated?

TABLE 12.38 The ANOV Table for Exercise 12.51

Source of Variation	DF	SS	MS	F	P
A				5.33	0.027
B				4.00	0.027
AB				7.33	0.002
Error			150		
Total					

TABLE 12.39 The ANOV Table for Exercise 12.52

Source of Variation	DF	SS	MS	F	P
Blocks		1120			
A				12.22	0.000
B				9.01	0.004
AB				1.00	0.399
Error		5548			
Total					

12.52   Use the information in the ANOV table given in Table 12.39 for a randomized block experiment with a 4×2 treatment structure and 10 blocks to answer the following:

(a) Fill in the missing entries in the ANOV table.

(b) Estimate the standard deviation of the experimental error.

(c) Test for the interaction of factors A and B.

(d) Based on the test in part (c), which means should be separated?

12.53   The F-ratios and their p-values for a 5×4 factorial study with five replicates of each treatment are given in Table 12.40. Use the information in Table 12.40 to answer the following:

(a) On the basis of F-ratios and their p-values in Table 12.40, which means should be separated?

(b) How many observations are used in computing each factor A mean?

(c) How many observations are used in computing each factor B mean?

(d) Based on the result of part (a), determine the Bonferroni distance D for separating the means when MSE $= 25$ and $\alpha_E = 0.05$.

12.54   In the article "Effect of irradiation on grip strength" published in the *Journal of Korean Academy of University Trained Physical Therapists* (Sang-hyub, 1999), the author reported the results of a two-factor experiment on grip strength. The two factors in the experiment were dominant hand (Yes, No) and irradiation (ball, no ball), and each of the four treatments was replicated 30 times. The response variable in this study was grip strength. Use the ANOV table given in Table 12.41, which was reported in this article, to answer the following:

(a) Estimate the standard deviation of the experimental error.

(b) On the basis of F-ratios is there sufficient evidence to conclude that the factors interact?

(c) On the basis of their P-values in Table 12.41, is there sufficient evidence to conclude that these two factors affect grip strength? Explain.

TABLE 12.40 The F-Ratios and p-Values for Exercise 12.53

Source of Variation	F	P
A	6.97	0.000
B	2.39	0.075
AB	1.83	0.057

TABLE 12.41   The ANOV Table for the Grip Strength Study

Source of Variation	DF	MS	F	P
Dominant hand	1	285.210	1.140	0.298
Irradiation	1	2501.3	9.998	0.002
Interaction	1	1715.98	6.859	0.010
Error	116	250.18		
Total	119			

TABLE 12.42   The F-Ratios and p-Values for a Dose Uniformity Study

Source of Variation	DF	F	P
Dispersion time	1	3.25	0.070
Zone sampled	4	14.83	0.000
Interaction	4	1.48	0.210

(d) On the basis of their P-values in Table 12.41, which means should be separated?

12.55   In the article "Dose uniformity of samples prepared from dispersible aspirin tablets for paediatric use" published in the *European Journal of Hospital Pharmacy Science* (Broadhurst et al., 2008), the authors reported the results of a two-factor experiment on the dispersion of 75 mg aspirin tablets. The two factors in the experiment were dispersion time (3 or 5 min) and zone sampled (1, 2, 3, 4, or 5), and each of the 10 treatments was replicated 20 times. The response variable in this study was the dose of aspirin sampled with a 2 mL syringe. Use the F-ratios and p-values given in Table 12.42 and the means given in Table 12.43, which were reported in this article, to answer the following:

(a) On the basis of F-ratios and their p-values in Table 12.43, which means should be separated?

(b) On the basis of the result of part (a), determine the Bonferroni distance D for separating the means when MSE $= 5.92$ and $\alpha_E = 0.05$.

(c) Separate the means.

(d) Compute a 95% confidence interval for the difference between the zone 1 and zone 5 means.

12.56   For a 3×4 two-factor analysis of variance with $r = 4$ replicates of each treatment, determine the number of replications of a

(a) factor A mean.   **(b)** factor B mean.

TABLE 12.43   Means for the Dose Uniformity Study

Dispersion Time	Zone Sampled					
	1	2	3	4	5	Row Mean
3 min	9.7	9.2	7.7	6.1	5.4	7.62
5 min	9.4	9.5	7.5	7.9	6.9	8.24
Column Mean	9.55	9.35	7.6	7.00	6.15	7.93

12.57 For a 5×4 two-factor analysis of variance with $r = 3$ replicates of each treatment, if MSE $= 120$, determine the estimated standard error of a

    (a) treatment mean.

    (b) factor A mean.

    (c) factor B mean.

    (d) the difference of two treatment means.

    (e) the difference of two factor A means.

    (f) the difference of two factor B means.

12.58 In a three-factor analysis of variance, what

    (a) is the model?

    (b) are the assumptions of the model?

    (c) does Y_{ijkl} represent?

12.59 In a three-factor randomized block analysis of variance, what

    (a) is the model?

    (b) are the assumptions of the model?

    (c) does Y_{ijkl} represent?

12.60 In a three-factor analysis of variance, what does

    (a) $\bar{y}_{ijk\bullet}$ estimate?

    (b) $\bar{y}_{i\bullet\bullet\bullet}$ estimate?

    (c) $\bar{y}_{\bullet j\bullet\bullet}$ estimate?

12.61 In terms of the parameters of a three-factor analysis of variance model, what is the

    (a) ijkth treatment mean?

    (b) difference between the ijkth and rstth treatment means when none of the factors interact with each other?

12.62 Explain why the main effects in a three-factor analysis of variance should not be tested when there are significant interactions among the factors.

12.63 Use the partial ANOV table given in Table 12.44 for a $2 \times 3 \times 4$ factorial study with four replicates of each treatment to answer the following.

    (a) Fill in the missing entries in the ANOV table.

    (b) Estimate the standard deviation of the experimental error.

TABLE 12.44   ANOV Table for Exercise 12.63

Source of Variation	DF	SS	MS	F	P
A				2.5	0.118
B				4.8	0.011
C				3.6	0.017
AB				2.0	0.143
AC				1.5	0.222
BC				1.8	0.112
ABC				1.2	0.316
Error			8.33		
Total		1008.72			

TABLE 12.45   ANOV Table for Exercise 12.64

Source of Variation	DF	SS	MS	F	P
Blocks		1280			
A				10.1	0.002
B				4.6	0.036
C				1.9	0.174
AB			90		0.163
AC				7.6	0.008
BC				2.8	0.100
ABC			198		0.040
Error			45		
Total		5303			

(c) Based on the F-ratios and their p-values, is it reasonable to test the factor A, B, and C main effects? Explain.

(d) Compute the estimated standard error of a treatment mean.

(e) Compute the estimated standard error of a factor B mean.

12.64 Use the partial ANOV table given in Table 12.45 for a 2^3 randomized block experiment with eight blocks to answer the following:

(a) Fill in the missing entries in the ANOV table.

(b) Estimate the variance of the experimental error.

(c) On the basis of F-ratios and their p-values, is it reasonable to test the factor A, B, and C main effects? Explain.

(d) Compute the estimated standard error of a treatment mean.

(e) Compute the estimated standard error of a factor B mean.

12.65 Use the partial F-ratios and p-values in Table 12.46 for a $2 \times 2 \times 4$ experiment with five replicates of each treatment to answer the following:

(a) Based on the F-ratios and the p-values in Table 12.46, is the three-way interaction significant?

(b) Based on the F-ratios and the p-values in Table 12.46, are any of the two-way interactions significant?

(c) Which means should be separated?

(d) How many replicates are there in a factor A mean?

TABLE 12.46 F-Ratios for Exercise 12.65

Source of Variation	DF	F	P
A	1	5.6	0.021
B	1	2.3	0.134
C	3	4.7	0.005
AB	1	3.2	0.078
AC	3	1.9	0.138
BC	3	2.2	0.097
ABC	3	1.5	0.223

TABLE 12.47   *F*-Ratios for Exercise 12.66

Source of Variation	DF	F	p
A	2	23.8	0.000
B	1	10.9	0.002
C	2	3.1	0.051
AB	2	7.8	0.001
AC	4	4.2	0.004
BC	2	3.8	0.027
ABC	4	2.3	0.068

12.66 Use the partial *F*-ratios and *p*-values in Table 12.47 for a $3 \times 2 \times 3$ randomized block experiment with five blocks to answer the following:

(a) Based on the *F*-ratios and the *p*-values in Table 12.47, is the three-way interaction significant?

(b) Based on the *F*-ratios and the *p*-values in Table 12.47 are any of the two-way interactions significant?

(c) Which means should be separated?

12.67 In the article "Tensile strength of mineralized/demineralized human normal and carious dentin" published in *Journal of Dental Research* (Nishitani et al., 2005), the authors reported the results of a 2^3 three-factor experiment on the ultimate tensile strength (UTS) of human dentin. The factors studied in this experiment were dentin (carious, normal), mineralization (demineralized, mineralized), and direction (parallel, perpendicular), and each of the eight treatments was replicated 10 times. Use the table of *p*-values given in Table 12.48 and the table of means given in Table 12.49 to answer the following:

(a) On the basis of *F*-ratios and *p*-values in Table 12.48, which means should be separated?

(b) How many pairwise comparisons are needed to separate the eight treatment means?

(c) If the Bonferroni critical *t*-value is $b_{crit} = 3.24$, compute the Bonferroni distance *D* for separating the treatment means.

(d) Separate the eight treatment means and summarize using the underline notation.

TABLE 12.48   *P*-Values for the Human Dentin Tensile Strength Experiment

Source of Variation	DF	P
Dentin	1	0.000
Mineralization	1	0.000
Direction	1	0.000
Dentin×mineralization	1	0.000
Dentin×direction	1	0.252
Mineralization×direction	1	0.000
Dentin×mineralization×direction	1	0.000

TABLE 12.49 Treatment Means for the Human Dentin Tensile Strength Experiment

Dentin	Mineralization	Direction	Mean
Carious	Demineralized	Parallel	9.50
Carious	Demineralized	Perpendicular	32.40
Carious	Mineralized	Parallel	51.40
Carious	Mineralized	Perpendicular	60.90
Normal	Demineralized	Parallel	11.50
Normal	Demineralized	Perpendicular	28.60
Normal	Mineralized	Parallel	64.20
Normal	Mineralized	Perpendicular	75.50

MSE $= 33.76$.

12.68 Determine the number of replicates needed to achieve the prespecified Bonferroni distance D when the experimentwise error rate is $\alpha_E = 0.05$ and

(a) $D = 15$ and $\sigma = 10$. (b) $D = 5$ and $\sigma = 2.5$.

(c) $D = 0.5$ and $\sigma = 0.6$. (d) $D = 100$ and $\sigma = 80$.

12.69 Determine the number of replicates needed to achieve the prespecified power when $\alpha = 0.05$ and

(a) there are 5 treatments, $\sigma = 10$, a distance of 5 is to be detected, and the desired power is 0.80.

(b) there are 6 treatments, $\sigma = 45$, a distance of 50 is to be detected, and the desired power is 0.80.

(c) there are 3 treatments, $\sigma = 1.5$, a distance of 2.5 is to be detected, and the desired power is 0.90.

(d) there are 4 treatments, $\sigma = 2.5$, a distance of 5 is to be detected, and the desired power is 0.90.

CHAPTER *13*

SURVIVAL ANALYSIS

$\mathbf{A}$COMMON objective in many medical studies is to investigate the survival time of an individual after being diagnosed with a particular disease or health related condition. *Survival analysis* is the area of statistics that is used to analyze the survival times of the patients in a clinical study. In particular, survival analysis can be used to study with the time to a particular event such as time to death, time to relapse, time to cure, or time to meet a specific goal. In fact, many clinical trials are designed specifically to study whether or not a new drug or procedure prolongs the survival time of an individual. For example, survival analysis may be used to study the time

- to death of an individual after being diagnosed with a disease.
- to death of an individual after receiving an organ transplant.
- to relapse of a drug addict.
- required for an individual to lower their LDL cholesterol by 10%.

The response variable in survival analysis is usually the time to a particular predetermined event that is referred to as the *survival time*. Some of the typical goals in the analysis of survival data are to (1) estimate descriptive parameters such as the mean, median, or percentiles of the survival times, (2) estimate the probability of surviving to a specific time, (3) compare the survival characteristics of two or more populations, or (3) build a model for the survival probability based on a collection of explanatory variables that are believed to influence the survival time of an individual.

In a survival study the subjects are observed until a particular event occurs or the study terminates, and thus, the survival time of a subject is based on the time the subject entered the study to the time the subject left the study. Subjects can leave a study for one of the following three reasons (1) they experience the event of interest, (2) they withdraw from the study, or (3) the study is terminated. Therefore, the observed survival times will consist of either the time to the event of interest or the time at which a subject left the study. For example, in studying the survival times of melanoma patients, patients may be enrolled in the study over a period of 10 years with the subjects survival monitored until they die, withdraw from the study, or the study is terminated.

For simplicity, throughout this chapter a subject experiencing the event of interest will be referred to as a failure. When a subject does not fail in a survival study, the actual survival time for the subject will be unknown. Survival times for the subjects that do not

Applied Biostatistics for the Health Sciences. By Richard J. Rossi
Copyright © 2010 by John Wiley & Sons, Inc.

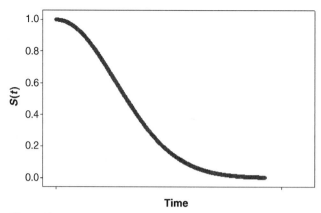

Figure 13.1   The typical shape of a survival function.

fail in a study are said to be *censored*, and the actual survival times of the censored observations will be greater than their observed survival times.

The sample data in a survival analysis generally consists of a random sample of n multivariate observations with variables for the survival time of an observation, information on whether or not an observation was censored before the study terminated, and the information on the explanatory variables being studied. A binary variable is often used to denote whether or not an observation was censored prior to the end of the study. For example, a binary variable C that takes on the value 1 when the observed survival time is censored prior to the termination of the study and 0 otherwise can be recorded for each subject in the study. Also, throughout this chapter it will be assumed that the censoring rules are consistent, the definition of survivorship is constant throughout the study, and the rules for entry into the study do not change over time.

In most survival analysis studies the analysis is based on modeling the probability of survival. When the response variable is the time to a prespecified event (i.e., death, relapse, etc.), represented by the random variable T, the *survival function* or *survivorship function* is the probability that the random variable T exceeds a value t and is denoted by $S(t)$. Thus, the survival function is $S(t) = P(T > t)$ that is always a decreasing function of the time t. An example of the typical shape of a survivor function is given in Figure 13.1.

One of the goals in a survival analysis is usually to model the survival function, and three different approaches for modeling a survival function are presented in this chapter. In particular, in Section 13.1, the Kaplan–Meier method of modeling a survival function is discussed, in Section 13.2, the Cox proportional hazards model for a survivor function is discussed, and in Section 13.3, the use of logistic regression for modeling a binary survival response variable is discussed.

13.1   THE KAPLAN–MEIER ESTIMATE OF THE SURVIVAL FUNCTION

The first method that will be discussed for estimating a survival function is the *Kaplan–Meier product-limit estimator* that is a simple estimator to compute and an estimator that does not assume that the data were drawn from a prespecified probability distribution. Estimators that do not assume that the data were drawn from a prespecified probability distribution are called *nonparametric estimators* or *distribution free estimators*. Thus, the Kaplan–Meier estimator is a nonparametric estimator of the survivor function $S(t)$.

The Kaplan–Meier estimator should be based on a random sample of n individuals that results in k distinct survival times $t_1 < t_2 < \cdots < t_k$; note that some of the survival times will be times of death and some will be times due to censoring. The Kaplan–Meier estimator of the survival function at time t_j is based on the fact that surviving to a time t_j requires that an individual survived all the previous survival times. Thus, let p_j represents the conditional probability that an individual survives beyond the time t_j given that an individual survived beyond time t_{j-1} and S_j represents the probability that an individual survives past time t_j; p_j is called the *survival proportion* and S_j is called the *cumulative survival proportion*. Then, because an individual can only survive to time t_j when they have survived the previous times $t_1, t_2, \ldots, t_{j-1}$, the probability of survival beyond time t_j is

$$S_j = p_1 \times p_2 \times \cdots \times p_j = S_{j-1} \times p_j$$

The Kaplan–Meier estimator is based on estimating conditional probabilities $p_1, p_2, p_3, \ldots, p_k$. The nonparametric estimator of p_j is

$$\widehat{p}_j = \frac{\text{number alive at time } t_j}{\text{number at risk at time } t_j}$$

Then, using the estimated survival proportions $\widehat{p}_1, \widehat{p}_2, \widehat{p}_3, \ldots, \widehat{p}_k$, the Kaplan–Meier estimate of $S(t_j)$ is

$$\widehat{S}(t_j) = \widehat{S}_j = \widehat{p}_1 \times \widehat{p}_2 \cdots \times \widehat{p}_j$$

An alternative form of the Kaplan–Meier estimate of $S(t_j)$ is given by

$$\widehat{S}(t_j) = \widehat{S}_j = \widehat{S}_{j-1} \times \widehat{p}_j$$

Thus, given a random sample of n observations having k distinct survival times $t_1 < t_2 < t_3 \cdots < t_k$, let $d_1, d_2, d_3, \ldots, d_k$ represent the number of deaths at each distinct survival time, $c_1, c_2, c_3, \ldots, c_k$ represent the number censored at each survival time, and $r_1, r_2, r_3, \ldots, r_n$ represent the number of individuals at risk at each of the survival times. Then, in terms of the d, c, and r values, the estimates of p_j and $S(t_j)$ are

$$\widehat{p}_j = \frac{r_j - d_j}{r_j}$$

and

$$\widehat{S}_j = \widehat{S}_{j-1} \times \frac{r_j - d_j}{r_j}$$

The estimated standard error of S_j is

$$\text{se}(\widehat{S}_j) = \widehat{S}_j \times \sqrt{\frac{d_1}{r_1(r_1 - d_1)} + \frac{d_2}{r_2(r_2 - d_2)} + \cdots + \frac{d_j}{r_j(r_j - d_j)}}$$

and for sufficiently large sample sizes the sampling distribution of $\widehat{S}_j$ is approximately normally distributed with mean $S(t_j)$ and standard deviation $\text{se}(\widehat{S}_j)$. Therefore, a $(1 - \alpha) \times 100\%$ large sample confidence interval for $S(t_j)$ is

$$\widehat{S}_j \pm z_{\text{crit}} \times \text{se}(\widehat{S}_j)$$

where z_{crit} is the Z-value for a $(1 - \alpha) \times 100\%$ critical value found in Table A.4.

TABLE 13.1 Hypothetical Data on the Survival Times of $n = 25$ Stage IV Melanoma Patients

Survival Time	Status	Survival Time	Status	Time	Status
3	1	12	1	29	1
5	1	12	1	33	1
7	1	14	1	41	1
7	1	15	1	45	1
9	1	15	1	52	1
11	1	15	0	60	1
11	1	20	1	60	1
12	1	23	1	60	1
				60	1

While the computations required for the Kaplan–Meier estimate of $S(t)$ can easily be computed by hand, it is generally advisable to use a statistical computing package to compute the Kaplan–Meier estimate of the survival function since a statistical computing package will generally provide the Kaplan–Meier estimate of the survival function at the times $t_1, t_2, \ldots, t_k$ and their estimated standard errors. Most statistical computing packages will also provide confidence intervals for the estimate of $S(t_j)$, an estimate of the median survival time, and a plot of the Kaplan–Meier estimate of the survival function over the observed survival times.

Example 13.1

The data given in Table 13.1 represents the hypothetical times of survival for $n = 25$ subjects in a prospective 5-year study of the survival times of individuals diagnosed with Stage IV melanoma. The response variable is time in months from the Stage IV diagnosis to death or censoring, and the censoring variable is

$$\text{Status} = \begin{cases} 1 & \text{Individual died} \\ 0 & \text{Individual was lost to follow-up or survived 5 years} \end{cases}$$

The MINITAB output for the Kaplan–Meier product-limit estimator is given in Table 13.2 and a plot of the estimated survival function is given in Figure 13.2. Note for each of the times of death, the

TABLE 13.2 The MINITAB Output for the Kaplan–Meier Product-Limit Estimator of $S(t)$

```
Kaplan-Meier Estimates

         Number   Number   Survival    Standard    95.0% Normal CI
Time    at Risk   Failed   Probability   Error     Lower      Upper
   3       25       1      0.960000    0.0391918  0.883185   1.00000
   5       24       1      0.920000    0.0542586  0.813655   1.00000
   7       23       2      0.840000    0.0733212  0.696293   0.98371
   9       21       1      0.800000    0.0800000  0.643203   0.95680
  11       20       2      0.720000    0.0897998  0.543996   0.89600
  12       18       3      0.600000    0.0979796  0.407964   0.79204
  14       15       1      0.560000    0.0992774  0.365420   0.75458
  15       14       2      0.480000    0.0999200  0.284160   0.67584
  20       11       1      0.436364    0.0999113  0.240541   0.63219
  23       10       1      0.392727    0.0989917  0.198707   0.58675
  29        9       1      0.349091    0.0971353  0.158709   0.53947
  33        8       1      0.305455    0.0942867  0.120656   0.49025
  41        7       1      0.261818    0.0903523  0.084731   0.43891
  45        6       1      0.218182    0.0851816  0.051229   0.38513
  52        5       1      0.174545    0.0785308  0.020628   0.32846
```

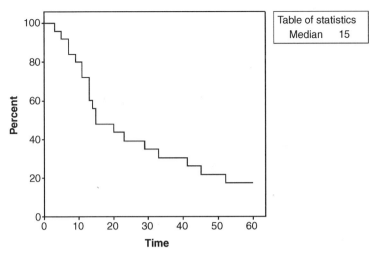

Figure 13.2   Plot of the Kaplan–Meier estimated survival function for Stage IV melanoma patients.

MINITAB output given in Table 13.2 lists the times of death, the number at risk, the number of deaths (i.e., failures), the Kaplan–Meier point estimate of $S(t)$, se($\widehat{S}((t))$), and a 95% confidence interval for $S(t)$. Thus, based on the Kaplan–Meier estimate of the survival function it appears that the median survival time is 15 months and the estimated probability that an individual will live at least 12 months after being diagnosed with Stage IV melanoma is 60%. A 95% confidence interval for the chance that an individual will live at least 12 months after being diagnosed with Stage IV melanoma suggests that the chances of surviving 12 months are at least 41% and possibly as much as 79%.

In many survival studies one of the research goals will be to compare the survival functions for two or more subpopulations. For example, an epidemiologist may be interested in studying the survival times for patients receiving two different treatments or an oncologist may be interested in studying the survival times of male and female patients diagnosed with metastatic liver cancer. A nonparametric test that can be used to test the equality of two or more survival functions is the *log-rank test*.

The test statistic for the log-rank test is based on comparing the observed death rates for each subpopulation against the death rates that would be expected when the survival function is the same for each of the subpopulations. The assumptions required to have a valid log-rank test are the same as the assumptions required for having valid Kaplan–Meier estimates of the survival functions, namely, random samples have been collected from each of the subpopulations. The null hypothesis tested in the log-rank test is

H_0 : The survival function is the same for each subpopulation.

and the alternative hypothesis is

H_0 : At least two of the survival functions for the subpopulations are different.

Thus, when random samples from each subpopulation are collected and the p-value associated with the log-rank test statistic is less than α there is sufficient statistical evidence to reject the null hypothesis, and hence, conclude that at least two of the subpopulations have survival functions that are different. The log-rank test statistic and its p-value will usually be provided by a statistical computing package when the survival functions of two or more subpopulations are being estimated.

TABLE 13.3 Hypothetical Data on the Survival Times of $n = 19$ Stage IV Melanoma Patients Receiving Interferon Treatments

Survival Time	Status	Survival Time	Status	Time	Status
7	1	16	1	41	1
9	1	17	1	47	1
11	1	17	1	51	1
12	1	21	1	58	1
12	0	29	1	60	0
13	1	34	0		
14	1	41	1		

Example 13.2

Suppose in the study of the survival times of Stage IV melanoma patients introduced in Example 13.1 independent random samples on a control group consisting of untreated melanoma patients and a treatment group consisting of patients receiving interferon treatment were collected. The data on the 25 control patients is given in Table 13.1, and the data on the 19 treatment patients is given in Table 13.3. The MINITAB output for the Kaplan–Meier estimates of the survival probabilities for the control and treatment groups are given in Tables 13.4 and 13.5, the results of the log-rank test are given in Table 13.6, and Figure 13.3 contains plots of the estimated survival functions for each population.

While the estimated survival probabilities for the patients receiving interferon are slightly higher than those of the control group for most of the observed survival times (see Figure 13.3), the p-value for the log-rank test is $p = 0.918$ that is not significant. Therefore, there is insufficient statistical evidence to conclude that the survival functions are statistically significantly different for the treatment and control groups.

TABLE 13.4 MINITAB Output for the Kaplan–Meier Estimates of Survival Probabilities for the Control Group in the Study on Stage IV Melanoma

```
Variable: Control
Kaplan-Meier Estimates

        Number    Number    Survival    Standard    95.0% Normal CI
Time    at Risk   Failed    Probability    Error     Lower     Upper
   3       25        1      0.960000    0.0391918   0.883185   1.00000
   5       24        1      0.920000    0.0542586   0.813655   1.00000
   7       23        2      0.840000    0.0733212   0.696293   0.98371
   9       21        1      0.800000    0.0800000   0.643203   0.95680
  11       20        2      0.720000    0.0897998   0.543996   0.89600
  12       18        3      0.600000    0.0979796   0.407964   0.79204
  14       15        1      0.560000    0.0992774   0.365420   0.75458
  15       14        2      0.480000    0.0999200   0.284160   0.67584
  20       11        1      0.436364    0.0999113   0.240541   0.63219
  23       10        1      0.392727    0.0989917   0.198707   0.58675
  29        9        1      0.349091    0.0971353   0.158709   0.53947
  33        8        1      0.305455    0.0942867   0.120656   0.49025
  41        7        1      0.261818    0.0903523   0.084731   0.43891
  45        6        1      0.218182    0.0851816   0.051229   0.38513
  52        5        1      0.174545    0.0785308   0.020628   0.32846
```

TABLE 13.5   MINITAB Output for the Kaplan–Meier Estimates of Survival Probabilities for the Treatment Group in the Study on Stage IV Melanoma

```
Variable: Interferon
Kaplan-Meier Estimates
```

	Number	Number	Survival	Standard	95.0% Normal CI	
Time	at Risk	Failed	Probability	Error	Lower	Upper
7	19	1	0.947368	0.051228	0.846964	1.00000
9	18	1	0.894737	0.070406	0.756744	1.00000
11	17	1	0.842105	0.083655	0.678145	1.00000
12	16	1	0.789474	0.093529	0.606161	0.97279
13	14	1	0.733083	0.102447	0.532290	0.93388
14	13	1	0.676692	0.108987	0.463081	0.89030
16	12	1	0.620301	0.113560	0.397727	0.84287
17	11	2	0.507519	0.117628	0.276972	0.73807
21	9	1	0.451128	0.117299	0.221226	0.68103
34	7	1	0.386681	0.116913	0.157535	0.61583
41	6	2	0.257787	0.107763	0.046576	0.46900
47	4	1	0.193340	0.098221	0.000832	0.38585
51	3	1	0.128894	0.084004	0.000000	0.29354
58	2	1	0.064447	0.061975	0.000000	0.18591

TABLE 13.6   The Results of the Log-Rank Test for Comparing the Survival Functions for the Control and Treatment Groups in the Melanoma Study

```
Comparison of Survival Curves
Test Statistics
```

Method	Chi-Square	DF	P-Value
Log-Rank	0.010555	1	0.918

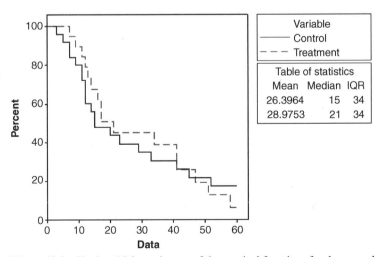

Figure 13.3   Kaplan–Meier estimates of the survival functions for the control and treatment groups in the melanoma study.

As is the case with any hypothesis test, the power of the log-rank test will increase when the sample sizes increase. Thus, it will be easier to detect the differences between two survival functions for larger samples than it is with smaller samples. However, the log-rank test cannot detect the magnitude of the difference between two survival functions, and therefore, it is always important to analyze the Kaplan–Meier estimates and their survival plots to determine whether or not an observed significant difference actually has any scientific importance.

Finally, a disadvantage of using the Kaplan–Meier method to estimate the survival function is that the Kaplan–Meier estimate does not model the survival probabilities as a function of any explanatory variables that may influence the survival times. For example, the survival of melanoma patients is known to depend not only on the stage of melanoma but also on the thickness of the tumor, the age and sex of an individual, and the location of the tumor. Therefore, a survival model that takes into account, relevant explanatory variables should be more informative than the nonparametric Kaplan–Meier survival probabilities.

13.2 THE PROPORTIONAL HAZARDS MODEL

In many survival studies the survival of an individual is known or is expected to depend on a collection of explanatory variables. In this case, a researcher will often wish to model the survival times or the survival probabilities as a function of the explanatory variables to determine how each of the explanatory variables influences the survival times. For example, in a study of the survival of individuals receiving heart transplants, the age, sex, weight, blood pressure, and the compatibility of the heart donor may be expected to influence the survival time of an individual after the transplant. In this case, a model that utilizes the information in the explanatory variables would most likely be more informative than a nonparametric model that does not include any explanatory variables.

One of the most commonly used models for modeling survival times as a function of a collection of explanatory variables is the *Cox proportional hazards model*. One reason that the proportional hazards model is often used is that the proportional hazards model requires no assumptions on the underlying distribution of the survival times. A model involving unknown parameters where the underlying probability distribution is not prespecified is called a *semiparametric* model. On the other hand, a model involving unknown parameters where the underlying probability distribution is prespecified is called a *parametric* model. The Cox proportional hazards model is a semiparametric model for the survival function.

The proportional hazard model is actually a semiparametric model for the *hazard function*, also called the *hazard rate*, associated with a survival function $S(t)$. The hazard function at a time t is the conditional probability that an individual survives a short interval of time after time t given that the individual survived up to time t. That is, the hazard function $h(t)$ is

$$h(t) = P(T > t + \Delta T | T > t)$$

where T is the random variable representing the survival times and Δt is a small time value. The hazard rate can also be thought of as the instantaneous rate of death or failure at a time t. Furthermore, there is a direct relationship between the hazard function $h(t)$ and the survival function $S(t)$, and thus, modeling the hazard function will also provide a model for the survival function.

The Cox proportional hazard model assumes that the hazard function is a function of the survival times and a set of explanatory variables, but no assumptions are made about the underlying distribution of the survival times. The form of the proportional hazards model based on the explanatory variables $X_1, X_2, \ldots, X_p$ is

$$h(t|\vec{x}) = h_0(t) \times e^{\beta_1 x_1 + \beta_2 x_2 + \cdots + \beta_p x_p}$$

where $h_0(t)$ is the *baseline hazard function*, $\vec{x}$ is the set of observed values of the explanatory variables (i.e., $\vec{x} = (x_1, x_2, \ldots, x_p)$), and $\beta_1, \beta_2, \ldots, \beta_p$ are the unknown parameters of the model. The baseline hazard function is the value of $h(t)$ when all of the explanatory variables have the value 0, and the parameters $\beta_1, \beta_2, \ldots, \beta_p$ in a proportional hazards model are called the *proportional hazards regression coefficients*.

The proportional hazards regression model can be simplified by taking the natural logarithm of the hazard function $h(t|\vec{x})$ that yields the following linear model for the natural logarithm of the hazard function

$$\ln[h(t|\vec{x})] = \beta_0(t) + \beta_1 x_1 + \beta_2 x_2 + \cdots + \beta_p x_p$$

where $\beta_0(t) = \ln[h_0(t)]$.

The two assumptions required to have a valid proportional hazards model are listed below.

THE ASSUMPTIONS OF A PROPORTIONAL HAZARDS MODEL

---

1. The natural logarithm of the hazard function is a linear function of the explanatory variables.

2. The ratio of the hazard function for two observed values at time t depends only on the values of the explanatory variables and does not depend on the time t.

The first assumption is often referred to as the *log-linear assumption*, and the second assumption is referred to as the *proportionality assumption*. When the proportional hazards assumptions are valid the explanatory variables have a multiplicative effect on the hazard function, which is the same for each time t. That is, for $\vec{x}_1 = (x_{11}, x_{21}, \ldots, x_{p1})$ and $\vec{x}_2 = (x_{12}, x_{22}, \ldots, x_{p2})$, the ratio of the hazard function at $\vec{x}_1$ and $\vec{x}_2$ at time t under the proportional hazards model is

$$\frac{h(t|\vec{x}_1)}{h(t|\vec{x}_2)} = \frac{h_0(t)e^{\beta_1 x_{11} + \beta_2 x_{21} + \cdots + \beta_p x_{p1}}}{h_0(t)e^{\beta_1 x_{12} + \beta_2 x_{22} + \cdots + \beta_p x_{p2}}}$$

$$= \frac{e^{\beta_1 x_{11} + \beta_2 x_{21} + \cdots + \beta_p x_{p1}}}{e^{\beta_1 x_{12} + \beta_2 x_{22} + \cdots + \beta_p x_{p2}}}$$

$$= e^{\beta_1(x_{11} - x_{12}) + \beta_2(x_{21} - x_{22}) + \cdots + \beta_p(x_{p1} - x_{p2})}$$

$$= e^{\beta_1(x_{11} - x_{12})} \times e^{\beta_2(x_{21} - x_{22})} \times \cdots \times e^{\beta_p(x_{p1} - x_{p2})}$$

Note that in a proportional hazards model the ratio of the hazard function for two different sets of explanatory variables does not depend on the time t. Thus, in a proportional hazards model the ratio of the hazard function for two different sets of explanatory variables will be the same for all of the possible survival times. For example, under a proportional hazards model if the risk of a fatal coronary heart event for males is twice that of females at age 60, then the risk of a fatal coronary heart event for males at age 65, or any other age for that matter, is still twice the risk for females. Also, note that no assumptions are made about the underlying distribution of the survival times or the baseline hazard function $h_0(t)$.

The ith regression coefficient, β_i, in a proportional hazards model represents the change in the natural logarithm of the hazard function when the explanatory variable X_i is increased by one unit and all of the other explanatory variables are held fixed. Furthermore, e^{β_i} is the ratio of the hazard function for two sets of explanatory conditions where only the values of the explanatory variable X_i differ by one unit, and thus, e^{β_i} represents the *risk ratio* associated with a one unit increase in the explanatory variable X_i. Thus, for a binary explanatory variable, the proportional hazard regression coefficient represents the ratio of the risks for the two categories represented by the variable.

Proportional hazards models are fit by determining the regression coefficients that maximize a partial-likelihood function; a partial-likelihood functions is the semiparametric version of the likelihood function used with parametric models. Similar to the maximum likelihood estimates, the estimators that maximize a partial-likelihood function also have well-known large sample properties. In particular, the large sample distribution of an estimated proportional hazards regression coefficient is known to be approximately normal making it possible to perform large sample hypothesis tests and confidence intervals for the unknown regression coefficients in the model. That is, for sufficiently large samples the distribution of

$$Z = \frac{\widehat{\beta}_i - \beta_i}{\text{se}(\widehat{\beta}_i)}$$

can be approximated by a standard normal distribution. Thus, for sufficiently large samples, a Z-test can be used to test the importance of an explanatory variable by testing $H_0 : \beta_i = 0$ with test statistic given by

$$Z = \frac{\widehat{\beta}_i}{\text{se}(\widehat{\beta}_i)}$$

and a $(1 - \alpha) \times 100\%$ confidence interval for the regression coefficient can also be computed using

$$\widehat{\beta}_i \pm z_{\text{crit}} \times \text{se}(\widehat{\beta}_i)$$

where z_{crit} is the Z-value used in a $(1 - \alpha) \times 100\%$ confidence interval and can be found in Table A.4.

The estimated risk ratio associated with a one unit increase in the ith explanatory variable when all of the other explanatory variables are held fixed is $e^{\widehat{\beta}_i}$, and a $(1 - \alpha) \times 100\%$ confidence interval for the risk ratio is computed by exponentiating the lower and upper limits of a confidence interval for β_i. That is, a $(1 - \alpha) \times 100\%$ confidence interval for the risk ratio associated with a one unit increase in the ith explanatory variable when all of the other explanatory variables are held fixed is

$$e^{\widehat{\beta}_i - z_{\text{crit}} \times \text{se}(\widehat{\beta}_i)} \quad \text{to} \quad e^{\widehat{\beta}_i + z_{\text{crit}} \times \text{se}(\widehat{\beta}_i)}$$

A statistical computing package is required for fitting and assessing the fit of a proportional hazards model. The typical output summarizing the fit of a proportional hazards model includes the estimated regression coefficients, the estimated standard errors of the regression coefficients, the observed value of the Z statistic for testing the regression slope is equal to 0, and the p-value associated with the Z statistic. Some statistical computing packages will also provide the estimated risk associated with each explanatory variable along with a 95% confidence interval for the risk ratio. As always, checking assumptions and assessing the fit should be part of any model fitting procedure since making inferences from

TABLE 13.7 The Summary Statistics for a Proportional Hazards Model Fit to the Survival Times of $n = 81$ Patients Having Advanced Nonsmall Cell Lung Cancer

Variable	Coefficient	SE	RR	95% CI	P
Sex(F)	−0.71	0.35	0.49	0.25 to 0.97	0.041
Bone Metastasis(Y)	0.84	0.38	2.31	1.10 to 4.85	0.027
Liver Metastasis(Y)	1.85	0.52	6.36	2.28 to 17.75	0.000
Stable Disease(Y)	1.18	0.43	3.24	1.40 to 7.48	0.006
Progressive Disease(Y)	3.01	0.62	20.35	6.02 to 68.70	0.000
Surgery(Y)	−1.43	0.51	0.24	0.09 to 0.65	0.005

a poorly fitting model often leads to misleading conclusions. Unfortunately, the methods used to check the assumptions and assess the fit of a proportional hazards model are beyond scope of this discussion, and therefore, should be performed by a trained statistician. For a more detailed discussion of the proportional hazards model see *Applied Survival Analysis: Regression Modeling of Time to Event Data* (Hosmer et al., 2008).

Example 13.3

In the article "Prognostic factors for survival in advanced nonsmall cell lung cancer" published in the *Journal of the Medical Association of Thailand* (Laohavinij and Maneechavakajorn, 2004), the reported summary statistics given in Table 13.7 for a proportional hazards model fit to the survival times of $n = 81$ patients having advanced nonsmall cell lung cancer in a retrospecitve study. The explanatory variables in the final model are Sex (female, male), Bone Metastasis (yes, no), Liver Mestastasis (yes, no), Stable Disease (yes, no), Progressive Disease (yes, no), and Surgery (yes, no). Note that all of the variables in the model reported in Table 13.7 are significant since all of the p-values are less than 0.05. The equation of the fitted proportional hazards model is

$$\widehat{\ln}[h(t|\vec{x})] = \widehat{\beta}_0 - 0.71 \times \text{Sex} + 0.84 \times \text{Bone Metastasis}$$

$$+ 1.85 \times \text{Liver Metastasis} + 1.18 \times \text{Stable Disease}$$

$$+ 3.01 \times \text{Progressive Disease} - 1.43 \times \text{Surgery}$$

Note that an estimate of $\beta_0 = \ln[h_0(t)]$ need not be reported because it does not affect the risk ratio associated with any of the explanatory variables since in a proportional hazards model the risk is the same at each time.

Now, the risk ratios listed in Table 13.7 are computed by exponentiating the regression coefficients. For example, the risk ratio for a female compared to a male is $e^{-0.71} = 0.49$ and the 95% confidence interval for the risk ratio is

$$e^{-0.71-1.96\times0.35} = 0.248 \quad \text{to} \quad e^{-0.71+1.96\times0.35} = 0.976$$

Since the risk ratio is more meaningful than the regression coefficients are in medical research, many biomedical articles report the risk ratio associated with an explanatory variable rather the regression coefficient. In this case, the estimated standard errors of the risk ratios or confidence intervals for the risk ratios should also be reported so that the reliability of the reported estimates can be assessed.

Example 13.4

In the article "The role of microsatellites as a prognostic factor in primary malignant melanoma" published in the *Archives of Dermatology*, (Shaikh et al., 2005), the authors reported the estimated risk ratios given in Table 13.8 for a proportional hazards model for the survival times of $n = 504$ melanoma patients in a retrospective study. The explanatory variables in the proportional hazards model were Tumor Thickness, Age, Ulceration (yes, no), Location , Sex (male, female), Microsatellites (yes, no), and Clark Level.

TABLE 13.8 The Estimated Risk Ratios and their *p*-Values for a Proportional Hazards Model for the Survival Times of *n* = 504 Melanoma Patients in a Retrospective Study

Variable	Risk Ratio	P
Tumor thickness	1.73	< 0.001
Age	1.24	< 0.001
Ulcertion	1.66	0.010
Location	1.59	0.050
Sex	1.30	0.160
Microsatellites	1.48	0.130
Clark level	1.14	0.340

Note that the explanatory variables Sex, Microsatellites, and Clark Level are not significant at the $\alpha = 0.05$ level while Tumor Thickness, Age, Ulceration, and Location are significant. Thus, there is no apparent increase in the risk of death for males when compared to females nor for the presence of microsatellites, or for a higher Clark Level. On the other hand, for every millimeter increase in the tumor thickness, the risk of death is roughly 1.7 times higher when all of the other explanatory variables are held constant; note that for a two millimeter increase in tumor thickness, the risk of death would be $1.73^2 = 2.99$ times higher when all of the other explanatory variables are held constant.

Note that in Example 13.4, the authors only reported the risk ratio and the *p*-value for each explanatory variable. Since a *p*-value does not measure the size of the effect due to an explanatory variable it is always advisable to report a confidence interval for the risk ratio along with *p*-value and the estimated risk ratio.

Finally, there are statistical methods that can be used for two comparing proportional hazards models of variable selection that are analogous to those used in linear and logistic regression. For example, the Bayes Information Criterion (BIC) can be used for screening the importance of the variables in a variable selection procedure with a proportional hazards model.

13.3 LOGISTIC REGRESSION AND SURVIVAL ANALYSIS

In many epidemiological studies the goal is to study the survival rates for a fixed survival time such as the 1, 5, or 10-year survival rate. For example, in studies of the survival of heart transplant patients the 1-year survival rate is often studied and for most types of cancer the 5-year survival rate is studied. The Kaplan–Meier estimator and the Cox proportional hazards model can be used for estimating the survival probabilities at a predetermined survival time when the actual times to the event of interest are observed, however, in some studies the actual times to the event of interest are not available. When the only information available to the researcher is whether or not an individual has experienced the event of interest in the period up to a predetermined survival time logistic regression can be used for modeling the survival rate at the predetermined survival time of interest. For example, retrospective studies often contain much less information on the survival times than do well-designed prospective studies, and therefore, logistic regression is often used to model the survival rates at for fixed survival times such as 5 and 10-year survival rate in a retrospective study.

When logistic regression is used to model the survival rate at a predetermined time, say t^*, the response variable will be a binary variable taking on the value 1 when an individual has survived to time t^* and 0 when the individual has not survived to time t^*. Note that the observations that were censored because an individual is lost to follow-up before the time t^* cannot be used in fitting a logistic regression model. The logistic regression model is a *parametric model* since it is assumed that the underlying distribution of the response variable follows a binomial distribution with the binomial probability p depending on the explanatory variables in the model.

Recall, a logistic regression model is a model of the logit of $p(\vec{X}) = P(Y = 1|\vec{X})$ and is given by

$$\text{logit}\left[p(\vec{X})\right] = \beta_0 + \beta_1 X_1 + \beta_2 X_2 + \cdots + \beta_p X_p$$

where $\vec{X} = (X_1, X_2, \ldots, X_p)$ and $\beta_0, \beta_1, \beta_2, \ldots, \beta_p$ are the logistic regression coefficients. Logistic regression models can be used to investigate the influence of the explanatory variables on the probability of survival at time t^* and for estimating the odds ratios associated with the explanatory variables. However, unlike the proportional hazards model, a logistic regression model for the survival probability at time t^* cannot be used to determine how the explanatory variables may affect the probability of survival at any survival times other than t^*.

Example 13.5

In the article "Predictive 5-year survivorship model of cystic fibrosis" published in the *American Journal of Epidemiology* (Liou et al., 2001), the authors reported the results given in Table 13.9 for the logistic regression model fit for a study on the 5-year survival of cystic fibrosis patients. The authors also reported that the p-value for the Hosmer–Lemeshow goodness of fit test was $p = 0.54$, and thus, there is no evidence of a significant lack of fit for the fitted logistic regression model.

Note that all of the explanatory variables in the model are significant with the exception of pancreatic sufficiency ($p = 0.147$) and *Staphylococcus aureus* ($p = 0.080$). Also, the interaction between the variables *Burkholderia cepacia* and the number of acute exacerbations is significant ($p = 0.001$).

Since the explanatory variables Age, Gender, Diabetes mellitus, *Burkholderia cepacia*, and No. of acute exacerbations have negative coefficients, the survival probability decreases with the age and the number of acute exacerbations, and the survival probability is smaller for females than males, individuals having diabetes mellitus, and individuals having *Burkholderia cepacia*. Using the estimated logistic regression coefficients given in Table 13.9, the probability of the 5-year survival can be estimated with

$$\widehat{p}(\vec{x}) = \frac{e^{\widehat{\text{logit}(\vec{x})}}}{1 + e^{\widehat{\text{logit}(\vec{x})}}}$$

TABLE 13.9   Logistic Regression Model the 5-year Survival for Cystic Fibrosis Patients

Variable	Coefficient	SE	Odds Ratio	P
Intercept	1.93	0.27	6.88	0.000
Age (per year)	−0.028	0.0060	0.97	0.000
Gender (male = 0, female = 1)	−0.23	0.10	0.79	0.022
FEV1% (per %)	0.038	0.0028	1.04	0.000
Weight-for-age z score	0.40	0.053	1.50	0.000
Pancreatic sufficiency (0 or 1)	0.45	0.31	1.58	0.147
Diabetes mellitus (0 or 1)	−0.49	0.15	0.61	0.001
Staphylococcus aureus (0 or 1)	0.21	0.12	1.24	0.080
Burkholderia cepacia (0 or 1)	−1.82	0.30	0.16	0.000
No. of acute exacerbations (0 to 5)	−0.46	0.031	0.63	0.000
No. of acute exacerbations *B. cepacia*	0.40	0.12	1.49	0.001

For example, estimated logit for a 50-year-old male, with an FEV1% of 60%, a weight-for-age z score of 2, with pancreatic sufficiency and diabetes mellitus, but no *Staphylococcus aureus* or *Burkholderia cepacia*, and 0 acute exacerbations is

$$\widehat{\text{logit}} = 1.93 - 0.028 \times 50 + 0.038 \times 60 + 0.40 \times 2 + 0.45 - 0.49 = 3.57$$

and therefore, the corresponding estimate of the 5-year survival probability is

$$\widehat{p} = \frac{e^{3.57}}{1 + e^{3.57}} = 0.97$$

An important difference between a proportional hazards model and a logistic regression model for the survival function is that the proportional hazards model uses the actual survival times and the logistic regression model does not. More importantly, when the actual survival times are measured in the sampling process the survival probabilities can be estimated at a wide range of survival times. On the other hand, when the observed response variable is a binary variable noting whether or not a subject survived to the time $t^\star$, the only survival probability that can be modeled is the survival probability at time $t^\star$. Thus, a proportional hazards model will provide more information on the survival probabilities than will a logistic regression model, and therefore, whenever possible the sampling plan should be designed so that the actual survival times are observed.

13.4   SOME FINAL COMMENTS ON SURVIVAL ANALYSIS

Three different approaches have been discussed for modeling the survivor functions in this chapter. In particular, a nonparametric approach using the Kaplan–Meier model, a semiparametric approach using the Cox proportional hazards model, and a parametric approach using logistic regression have been discussed as means of estimating the survival probabilities and for investigating the influence of the explanatory variables. In general,

- the Kaplan–Meier product-limit estimator is used in exploratory studies to find estimates of the unadjusted survival probabilities and for comparing the survival functions of two or more subpopulations.

- the proportional hazards model is used for exploring the influence of the explanatory variables on the survival function.

- logistic regression is used to model the survival probability for a fixed survival time and can be used to investigate the influence of the explanatory variables on the survival probability at a fixed time.

It is important to note that the proportional hazards model is based on the actual survival times and the explanatory variables, a proportional hazards model will provide more information about the survival probabilities than will either the Kaplan–Meier model or a logistic regression model.

No matter which approach is used for estimating the survival function or the survival probabilities, it is critical that the rules for entry into the study and the censoring of the subjects be consistent throughout the study. As always, the assumptions and the fit of a model should be assessed before making inferences with the fitted model. Also, each of the modeling approaches used to model the survival times uses large sample hypothesis tests and confidence intervals, and thus, the sampling plan in a survival study must be designed to ensure that the sample is sufficiently large to that it will provide reliable statistical inferences.

GLOSSARY

Censoring Survival times for the subjects that do not fail in a survival study are said to be censored observations.

Hazard Function The hazard function, also called the hazard rate, associated with a survival function $S(t)$ is the conditional probability that an individual survives a short interval of time after time t given that the individual survived to time t. That is, the hazard function $h(t)$ is

$$h(t) = P(T > t + \Delta T | T > t)$$

where T is the random variable representing the survival times and Δt is a small time value.

Kaplan–Meier Estimator The Kaplan–Meier product-limit estimator is a nonparametric estimator of the survivor function.

Log-linear Assumption The log-linear assumption in a proportional hazards model is that the natural logarithm of the hazard function is a linear function of the explanatory variables.

Log-rank Test The log-rank test is a nonparametric test used to test the equality of two or more survival functions.

Nonparametric Estimators Estimators that do not assume that the data were drawn from a prespecified probability distribution are called nonparametric estimators or distribution free estimators.

Parametric Model A parametric model is a model involving unknown parameters where the underlying probability distribution is prespecified.

Proportional Hazard Regression Coefficients The coefficients $\beta_1, \beta, \ldots, \beta_p$ in a proportional hazards model are called the proportional hazards regression coefficients.

Proportional Hazards Model The Cox proportional hazards model is a semiparametric model for the hazard function of a survival function. The form of the model is

$$h(t|\vec{x}) = h_0(t) \times e^{\beta_1 x_1 + \beta_2 x_2 + \ldots + \beta_p x_p}$$

where $h_0(t)$ is the baseline hazard that is the value of $h(t)$ when all of the explanatory variables have the value 0, $\vec{x}$ is the set of observed values of the explanatory variables (i.e., $\vec{x} = x_1, x_2, \ldots, x_p$), and $\beta_1, \beta_2, \ldots, \beta_p$ are the unknown parameters of the model.

Proportionality Assumption The proportionality assumption in a proportional hazards model is that the ratio of the hazard function for two observed values at time t depends only on the values of the explanatory variables and does not depend on the time t.

Risk Ratio The risk ratio for the ith explanatory variable in a proportional hazards model is the ratio of the hazard function for two sets of explanatory conditions where the explanatory variable X_i differs by only one unit.

Semiparametric Model A semiparametric model is a model involving unknown parameters where the underlying probability distribution is not prespecified.

Survival Analysis Survival analysis is the area of statistics that is used to analyze the survival times of the patients in a clinical study.

Survival Function The survival function, also called the survivorship function, is the probability of surviving past the time t (i.e., $S(t) = P(T > t)$).

Survival Time The time to a particular predetermined event is referred to as the survival time.

EXERCISES

13.1   What is the survival function $S(t)$?

13.2   What happens to the survival function as the value of t increases?

13.3   If $S(10) = 0.42$, is $S(20)$ larger or smaller than 0.42? Explain.

13.4   What is a censored survival time?

13.5   What are two reasons that cause the censoring of a survival time?

13.6   Under what conditions is an estimator a nonparametric estimator?

13.7   Which estimator of the survival function is a nonparametric estimator?

13.8   What is the formula for estimating the survival function with the Kaplan–Meier estimator?

13.9   Suppose the fourth survival time is $t_4 = 12$ months and there are 42 patients alive out of 47 who were at risk at time t_4. If $\widehat{S}(t_3) = 0.82$, compute the Kaplan–Meier estimate of the survival probability at 12 months.

13.10   Suppose the fourth survival time is $t_4 = 12$ months and there are 12 patients alive out of 13 who were at risk at time t_4. If $\widehat{p}_1 = 0.97$, $\widehat{p}_2 = 0.91$, and $\widehat{p}_3 = 0.85$, compute the Kaplan–Meier estimate of the survival probability at 12 months.

13.11   Use the information in Table 13.10 to answer the following:
(a) How many patients were censored at time t_2 and at time t_3?
(b) Estimate p_1, p_2, p_3, p_4, p_5, and p_6.
(c) Estimate $S(t_1)$, $S(t_2)$, $S(t_3)$, $S(t_4)$, $S(t_5)$, and $S(t_6)$.
(d) Plot the estimated survival function.

13.12   Use the information in Table 13.11 to answer the following:
(a) Estimate $S(t_1)$, $S(t_2)$, $S(t_3)$, $S(t_4)$, and $S(t_5)$.
(b) Plot the estimated survival function.
(c) If $\mathrm{se}(\widehat{S}(23)) = 0.049$, compute an approximate 95% confidence interval for the value of $S(23)$.
(d) Is the median survival time greater than 30 months? Explain.

13.13   Use the information in Table 13.12 to answer the following:
(a) Estimate $S(t_1)$, $S(t_2)$, $S(t_3)$, $S(t_4)$, $S(t_5)$, $S(t_6)$, $S(t_7)$, and $S(t_8)$.
(b) Plot the estimated survival function.

TABLE 13.10   Summary Statistics for Exercise 13.11

Time	Patients at Risk	Patients Alive
$t_1 = 5$	29	25
$t_2 = 7$	23	22
$t_3 = 11$	22	18
$t_4 = 13$	17	15
$t_5 = 17$	15	13
$t_6 = 21$	12	10

TABLE 13.11   Summary Statistics for Exercise 13.12

Time	$\widehat{p}_i$
$t_1 = 5$	0.98
$t_2 = 11$	0.95
$t_3 = 14$	0.94
$t_4 = 23$	0.83
$t_5 = 30$	0.75

TABLE 13.12   Summary Statistics for Exercise 13.13

Time	$\widehat{p}_i$
$t_1 = 6$	0.98
$t_2 = 9$	0.92
$t_3 = 14$	0.94
$t_4 = 18$	0.86
$t_5 = 22$	0.72
$t_6 = 25$	0.74
$t_7 = 29$	0.68
$t_8 = 30$	0.62

    (c) If $\text{se}(\widehat{S}(30)) = 0.072$, compute an approximate 95% confidence interval for the value of $S(30)$.

    (d) Is the median survival time greater than 30 months? Explain.

13.14   Use the Kaplan–Meier estimate in Figure 13.4 to answer the following:

    (a) Estimate the median survival time.

    (b) Estimate $S(50)$.

    (c) If $\text{se}(\widehat{S}(50)) = 0.058$, compute an approximate 95% confidence interval for the value of $S(50)$.

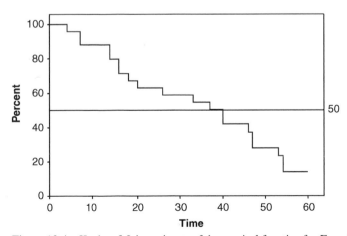

Figure 13.4   Kaplan–Meier estimate of the survival function for Exercise 13.14.

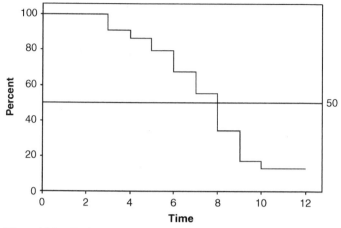

Figure 13.5   Kaplan–Meier estimate of the survival function for Exercise 13.15.

13.15   Use the Kaplan–Meier estimate given in Figure 13.5 to answer the following:
(a) Estimate the median survival time.
(b) Estimate $S(5)$.
(c) If $se(\widehat{S}(5)) = 0.082$, compute an approximate 95% confidence interval for the value of $S(5)$.

13.16   Which hypothesis test is used to test the equality of two or more survival functions?

13.17   What does it mean when the p-value associated with the log-rank test for comparing two survival functions is

(a) less than α?   (b) larger than α?

13.18   Use the Kaplan–Meier estimates given in Figure 13.6 and the summary of the log-rank test given in Table 13.19 to answer the following:
(a) Is there sufficient evidence in the observed sample data to conclude the survival functions are different for the treatment and control groups? Explain.

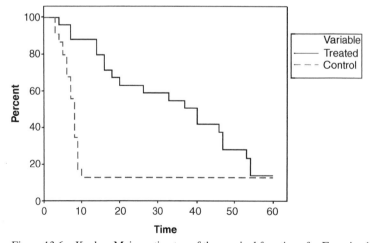

Figure 13.6   Kaplan–Meier estimates of the survival functions for Exercise 13.18.

TABLE 13.13   Summary of the Log-Rank Test for Exercise 13.18

```
Test Statistic
Method     Chi-Square   DF   P-Value
Log-Rank     27.9271     1    0.000
```

TABLE 13.14   Summary of the Log-Rank Test for Exercise 13.19

```
Test Statistics
Method     Chi-Square   DF   P-Value
Log-Rank     3.30388     2    0.192
```

(**b**) Estimate the probability of surviving 10 months, $S(10)$, for the treatment group.

(**c**) Estimate the probability of surviving 10 months, $S(10)$, for the control group.

13.19 The Kaplan–Meier estimates of the survival functions for three treatments used in treating ovarian cancer are given in Figure 13.7, and the results of the log-rank test are given in Table 13.14. Use the information given in Figure 13.7 and Table 13.14 to answer the following:

(**a**) Is there sufficient evidence to reject the equality of the survival functions for the three treatments? Explain.

(**b**) Which treatment appears to have the highest survival probability for $t = 36$ months and for $t = 48$ months?

(**c**) Which treatment appears to have the smallest median survival time?

13.20 Under what conditions is a model a semiparametric model?

13.21 What is the hazard function?

13.22 What is the proportional hazards model for

(**a**) a single explanatory variable?   (**b**) p explanatory variables?

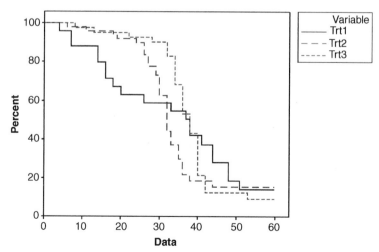

Figure 13.7   Kaplan–Meier estimates of the survival functions for three treatments in Exercise 13.18.

13.23   What is the risk ratio?

13.24   What is the risk ratio in a proportional hazards model?

13.25   When a proportional hazards coefficient is negative, does this indicate that risk ratio increases or decreases when the value of the explanatory variable is increased?

13.26   In the proportional hazards model

$$\ln [h(t)] = \ln [h_0(t)] + \beta_1 X_1 + \beta_2 X_2 + \cdots + \beta_p X_p$$

what does

(**a**) β_i represent?   (**b**) e^{β_i} represent?

13.27   When fitting a proportional hazards model, what is the large sample distribution of $\dfrac{\widehat{\beta_i}}{se(\widehat{\beta_i})}$ when $\beta_i = 0$?

13.28   For the proportional hazards model $\ln [h(t)] = \ln [h_0(t)] + \beta_1 X_1 + \beta_2 X_2$ suppose that $\widehat{\beta_1} = 1.68$ and $se(\widehat{\beta_1}) = 0.56$.
(**a**) Test $H_0 : \beta_1 = 0$ at the $\alpha = 0.05$ level. Be sure to compute the p-value for this test.
(**b**) Compute a 95% confidence interval for β_1.
(**c**) Estimate the risk ratio associated with a one unit increase in X_1.
(**d**) Compute a 95% confidence interval for the risk ratio associated with a one unit increase in X_1.

13.29   For the proportional hazards model $\ln [h(t)] = \ln [h_0(t)] + \beta_1 X_1 + \beta_2 X_2$ suppose that $\widehat{\beta_1} = 0.87$, $se(\widehat{\beta_1}) = 0.61$, $\widehat{\beta_2} = -2.07$, and $se(\widehat{\beta_2}) = 0.69$.
(**a**) Test $H_0 : \beta_1 = 0$ at the $\alpha = 0.05$ level. Be sure to compute the p-value for this test.
(**b**) Test $H_0 : \beta_2 = 0$ at the $\alpha = 0.05$ level. Be sure to compute the p-value for this test.
(**c**) Based on the hypothesis tests in parts (a) and (b) is there sufficient evidence suggesting that both X_1 and X_2 are needed in the model? Explain.

13.30   In the article "Enhanced survival in patients with multiple primary melanoma" published in the *Archives of Dermatology* (Doubrovsky and Menzies, 2003), the authors reported the results of a study on the survival probabilities of patients with three or more multiple primary melanomas. The authors fit a proportional hazards model to $n = 4952$ survival times of patients with a single primary melanoma. The explanatory variables in the model are tumor thickness (Thickness), tumor location with axial coded as 1 and extremal coded as 0 (Location), ulcerated tumor with absence coded as 1 and presence coded as 0, the sex of the patient with males coded as 1 and females as 0 (Sex), age at diagnosis (Age), and the interaction between the variables Sex and Thickness. Use the summary of the fitted proportional hazards coefficients given in Table 13.15 to answer the following:
(**a**) Are there any explanatory variables in the fitted model that are not significant? Explain.
(**b**) Compute the estimate of the risk ratio for the explanatory variable Sex.
(**c**) Based on part (b) does the risk appear to be higher or lower for a male? Explain.
(**d**) Compute a 95% confidence interval for the risk ratio associated with a 1 year increase in the explanatory variable Age.

TABLE 13.15   Summary of the Proportional Hazards Regression Model for $n = 4952$ Patients with a Single Primary Melanoma

Variable	Coefficient	SE	P-value
Thickness	0.640	0.079	< 0.001
Location	−0.381	0.098	< 0.001
Ulceration	0.754	0.102	< 0.001
Sex	−0.410	0.155	0.008
Age	0.010	0.003	0.001
Sex*Thickness	0.273	0.119	0.020

13.31   In the article "Biological determinants of cancer progression in men with prostate cancer" published in the *Journal of the American Medical Association* (Stamey et al., 1999), the authors reported the results of a study on whether prostate cancer progression is associated with % Gleason grade 4/5. The authors fit a proportional hazards model to the times to progression of prostate cancer for $n = 379$ patients. The explanatory variables in the model are tumor volume (Log10 volume), percent Gleason grade 4/5 (Log10 gleason grade 4/5), positive findings in the lymph nodes coded as 1 for yes and 0 for no (Positive findings in lymph nodes), and the amount of vascular invasion (Log10 vascular invasion). Use the summary of the fitted proportional hazards coefficients given in Table 13.16 to answer the following:

(a) Compute the estimate of the risk ratio associated with a 1% increase in the explanatory variable Log10 Gleason grade 4/5 cancer.

(b) Compute a 95% confidence interval for the risk ratio associated with a 1% increase in the explanatory variable Log10 Gleason grade 4/5 cancer.

(c) Does a positive finding in the lymph nodes increase or decrease the estimated value of the risk ratio? Explain.

(d) Compute a 95% confidence interval for the risk ratio associated with a one unit increase in the explanatory variable Log10 volume.

(e) Compute a 95% confidence interval for the risk ratio associated with a one unit increase in the explanatory variable Log10 vascular invasion.

13.32   Use the results of the Bayes Information Criterion variable selection procedure for screening three explanatory variables in a proportional hazards model given in Table 13.17 to answer the following:

(a) Which two models are the best fitting models according to the Bayes Information Criterion?

TABLE 13.16   Summary of the Proportional Hazards Model Fit to $n = 379$ Men with Peripheral Zone Cancers

Variable	Coefficient	SE	Z	P
Log10 volume, cm3	1.687	0.254	6.63	<0.001
Log10 Gleason grade 4/5 cancer, %	1.494	0.220	6.79	<0.001
Positive findings in lymph nodes	1.004	0.245	4.11	<0.001
Log10 vascular invasion	0.793	0.192	4.13	<0.001

TABLE 13.17   Summary of the BIC Variable Selection
for the Explanatory Variables X_1, X_2, and X_3 in a
Proportional Hazards Model

Variables in Model	BIC
X_3	128.671
X_1	132.089
X_2	158.114
X_3, X_1	117.490
X_3, X_2	119.176
X_1, X_2	129.026
X_3, X_1, X_2	118.193

(b) If there are no prespecified scientific reasons for including any of the explanatory variables in the model, which model should be selected as the final model?

(c) If there are scientific reasons for including the explanatory variable X_2 in the model, which model should be selected as the final model?

13.33 Under what conditions is a model a parametric model?

13.34 Under what conditions would it be appropriate to use a logistic regression model to model the survival probability at a fixed time $t^\star$?

13.35 What is the response variable in a logistic regression model of the 5-year survival probability?

13.36 How are the observations that are censored before time $t^\star$ used in a logistic regression model for estimating $S(t^\star)$?

13.37 In terms of the logit function what is the survival probability at time $t^\star$?

13.38 What are the differences between a logistic regression model of a survival probability and the proportional hazards model of the hazard function?

13.39 In the logistic regression model

$$\text{logit}(p(\vec{X})) = \beta_0 + \beta_1 X_1 + \beta_2 X_2 + \cdots + \beta_p X_p$$

what does

(a) β_i represent?   **(b)** e^{β_i} represent?

13.40 When fitting a logistic regression model, what is the large sample distribution of $\dfrac{\widehat{\beta_i}}{\text{se}(\widehat{\beta_i})}$ when $\beta_i = 0$?

13.41 For the logistic regression model $\text{logit}(p(\vec{X})) = \beta_0 + \beta_1 X_1 + \beta_2 X_2$ suppose that $\widehat{\beta_1} = 2.39$ and $\text{se}(\widehat{\beta_1}) = 0.83$.

(a) Test $H_0 : \beta_1 = 0$ at the $\alpha = 0.05$ level. Be sure to compute the p-value for this test.

(b) Compute a 95% confidence interval for β_1.

(c) Estimate the odds ratio associated with a one unit increase in X_1.

(d) Compute a 95% confidence interval for the odds ratio associated with a one unit increase in X_1.

TABLE 13.18   Summary of the Logistic Regression Model for the 10-year Survival Probability for Melanoma Patients

Variable	Coefficient	95% CI for the Odds Ratio
Intercept	−1.1984	
Lesion thickness < 0.76	3.7433	16.7–106.5
Lesion thickness 0.76–1.69	2.0366	4.4–13.4
Lesion thickness 1.70–3.60	0.7463	1.2–3.6
Primary lesion on extremity	1.0717	1.9–4.5
Age ≤ 60	0.6844	1.3–3.1
Female	0.1950	0.8–1.8

13.42   In the article "Predicting 10-year survival of patients with primary cutaneous melanoma: corroboration of a prognostic model" published in *Cancer* (Sahin, 1997), the authors reported a logistic regression model for the 10-year survival probability of melanoma patients. The variables in the model are age coded as 1 when a patients age is ≤ 60 and 0 otherwise, sex coded as 1 for female and 0 for male, lesion thickness entered as three dummy variables for the intervals < 0.76, 0.76–1.69, and 1.70–3.60, and a dummy variable for the location of the lesion coded as 1 for a lesion on an extremity and 0 otherwise. The model was fit using the data from $n = 780$ melanoma patients. Use the summary of the fitted logistic regression model given in Table 13.18 to answer the following:

(a) Determine the odds ratios associated with each of the explanatory variables.

(b) How many times more likely is it for female to survive 10-years than for a male, assuming all of the other explanatory variables are the same?

(c) Estimate the 10-year survival probability for a 65-year-old female with a primary extremity lesion of tumor depth 1 mm.

(d) Estimate the 10-year survival probability for a 65-year-old male with a primary extremity lesion of tumor depth 1 mm.

(e) Estimate the 10-year survival probability for a 55-year-old-female with a primary extremity lesion of tumor depth 4 mm.

(f) Estimate the 10-year survival probability for a 55-year-old male with a primary extremity lesion of tumor depth 4 mm.

13.43   In the article "Validation of a melanoma prognostic model" published in the *Archives of Dermatology* (Margolis et al., 1998), the authors reported a logistic regression model for the 5-year probability of death for melanoma patients. The variables in the model are age coded as 1 if greater than 60 and 0 otherwise, sex coded as 1 for male and 0 for female, tumor thickness entered as three dummy variables for the intervals 0.76–1.69, 1.70–3.60, and > 3.60, and a dummy variable for the location of the lesion coded as 1 for a truncal lesion and 0 otherwise. The model was fit using the data from $n = 1261$ melanoma patients. Use the summary of the odds ratios for the fitted logistic regression model given in Table 13.19 to answer the following:

(a) Determine the coefficients of the fitted logistic regression model.

(b) Estimate the 5-year probability of death for a 50-year-old male with a truncal lesion of tumor depth 2 mm.

TABLE 13.19   Odds Ratios for Death from Melanoma Within 5-Years of Diagnosis

Prognostic Factor	Odds Ratio	95% CI
Intercept	5.25	
Truncal lesion	3.02	1.90–4.79
Age > 60	1.93	1.30–2.88
Sex	1.26	0.84–1.87
Tumor thickness 0.76–1.69	5.57	2.50–12.44
Tumor thickness 1.70–3.60	25.20	11.83–53.70
Tumor thickness > 3.60	56.76	25.40–126.83

(c) Estimate the 5-year probability of survival for a 50-year-old male with a truncal lesion of tumor depth 2 mm.

(d) Estimate the 5-year probability of death for a 50-year-old female with a truncal lesion of tumor depth 2 mm.

(e) Estimate the 5-year probability of survival for a 50-year-old female with a truncal lesion of tumor depth 2 mm.

(f) How many times more likely is an individual with a tumor thickness of > 3.6 mm to die from the melanoma within 5-years than is a patient with a tumor thickness ≤ 3.6 mm, assuming all of the other prognostic factors are the same?

REFERENCES

Asayama, K., Hayashibe, H., Dobashi, K., Uchida, N., Nakane, T., Kodera, K., and Shirahata, A. (2002). Increase serum cholesterol ester transfer protein in obese children. *Obesity Research*, **10**, 439–446.

Aspirin Myocardial Infarction Study Research Group. (1980). A randomised controlled trial of aspirin in persons recovered from myocardial infarction. *Journal of the American Medical Association*, **243**, 661–669.

Bernard, P., Chosidow, O., and Vaillant, L. (2002). Oral pristinamycin versus standard penicillin regimen to treat erysipelas in adults: randomized, non-inferiority, open trial. *British Medical Journal*, **325**, 864–866.

Borrel, L. N., Crespo, C. J., and Garcia-Palmieri, M. R. (2007). Skin color and mortality risk among men: The Puerto Rico Heart Program. *Annals of Epidemiology*, **17**, 335–341.

Boruk, M., Chernobilsky, B., Rosenfeld, R. M., and Har-El, G. (2005). Age as a prognostic factor for complications of major head and neck surgery. *Archives of Otolaryngology—Head & Neck Surgery*, **131**, 605–609.

Box, G. E. P., and Draper N. R. (1987). *Empirical Model-Building and Response Surfaces*, John Wiley & Sons, Inc., New York, p. 424.

Broadhurst, E. C., Ford, J. L., Nunn, A. J., Rowe, P. H., and Roberts, M. (2008). Dose uniformity of samples prepared from dispersible aspirin tablets for paediatric use. *European Journal of Hospital Pharmacy Science*, **14**, 27–31.

Brönstrup, A., Hages, M., Prinz-Langenohl, R., and Pietrzik, K. (1998). Effects of folic acid and combinations of folic acid and vitamin B-12 on plasma homocysteine in healthy, young women. *American Journal of Clinical Nutrition*, **68**, 1104–1110.

Carroll, R. J., Ruppert, D., Stefanski, L. A., and Crainiceanu, C. M. (2006). *Measurement Error in Nonlinear Models*, Chapman & Hall, Boca Raton.

Chatterjee, S., Hadi, A. S., and Price, B. (2006). *Regression Analysis by Example*, John Wiley & Sons, Inc., Hoboken.

Cheung, N., Tikellis, G., Saw, S. M., Islam, F. M. A., Mitchell, P., Wang, J. J., and Wong, T. Y. (2007). Relationship of axial length and retinal vascular caliber in children. *American Journal of Ophthalmology*, **144**, 658–662.

Craven, R. B., Quan, T. J., Bailey, R. E., Dattwyler, R., Ryan, R. W., Sigal, L. H., Steere, A. C., Sullivan, B., Johnson, B. J. B., Dennis, D. T., and Gubler, D. J. (1996). Improved serodiagnostic testing for lyme disease: results of a multicenter serologic evaluation. *Emerging Infectious Diseases*, **2**, 136–140.

Das, A. K., Olfson, M., Gameroff, M. J., Pilowsky, D. J., Blanco, C., Feder, A., Gross, R., Neria, Y., Lantigua, R., Shea, S., and Weissman, M. M. (2005). Screening for bipolar disorder in a primary care practice. *Journal of the American Medical Association*, **293**, 956–963.

Davis, C. and Fox, J. (2008). Sensitivity to reward and body mass index (BMI): evidence for a non-linear relationship. *Appetite*, **50**, 43–49.

De Catarina, R., Lanza, M., Manca, G., Strata, G. B., Maffei, S., and Salvatore, L. (1994). Bleeding time and bleeding: an analysis of the relationship of the bleeding time test with parameters of surgical bleeding. *Blood*, **84**, 3363–3370.

Dell, J. L., Whitman, S., Shah, A. M., Silva, A., and Ansell, M. (2005). Smoking in 6 diverse Chicago communities—a population study. *American Journal of Public Health*, **95**, 1036–1042.

de Lorgeril, M., Renaud, S., Mamelle, N., Salen, P., Martin, J. L., Monjaud, I., Guidollet, J., Touboul, P., and Delaye, J. (1994). Mediterranean alpha-linolenic acid-rich diet in secondary prevention of coronary heart disease. *Lancet*, **343**, 1454–1459.

Doubrovsky, A. and Menzies, S. W. (2003). Enhanced survival in patients with multiple primary melanoma. *Archives of Dermatology*, **139**, 1013–1018.

Efron, B. and Tibshirani, R. J. (1993). *An Introduction to the Bootstrap*. Chapman & Hall, New York.

Eide, M. J. and Weinstock, M. A. (2005). Association of UV index, latitude, and melanoma incidence in nonwhite populations—US surveillance, epidemiology, and end results (SEER) program, 1992 to 2001. *Archives of Dermatology*, **141**, 477–481.

El Sahly, H. M., Teeter, L. D., Pan, X., Musser, J. M., and Graviss, E.A. (2007). Mortality associated with central nervous system tuberculosis. *Journal of Infection*, **55**, 502–509.

Exposure to secondhand smoke among students aged 13–15 years—worldwide, 2000–2007. (2007). *Morbidity and Mortality Weekly Report*, **56**, 497–500.

Fagan, J. F. and Detterman, D.K. (1992). The Fagan test of infant intelligence: a technical summary. *Journal of Applied Developmental Psychology*, **13**, 173–193.

Firestone, J. A., Smith-Weller, T., Franklin, G., Swanson, P., Longstreth, W. T., and Checkoway, H. (2005). Pesticides and risk of Parkinson disease: a population-based case–control study. *Archives of Neurology*, **62**, 91–95.

Fisher, R. A. (1925) *Statistical Methods for Research Workers*, First Edition, Oliver and Boyd Ltd., Edinburgh.

Fisher, R. A. (1947) *The Design of Experiments*, Fourth Edition, Hafner Publishing Co., Inc, New York.

Fort, J. G. (2007). Improving the health of African American men: experiences for the targeting cancer in Blacks (TCiB) project. *The Journal of Men's Health & Gender*, **4**, 428–439.

Frequency of vaccine-related and therapeutic injections—Romania, 1998. (1998). *Morbidity and Mortality Weekly Report*, **48**, 271–274.

Furey, M. L. and Drevets, W. C. (2006). Antidepressant efficacy of the antimuscarinic drug scopolamine: A randomized, placebo-controlled clinical trial. *Archives of General Psychology*, **63**, 1121–1129.

Ghandehari, K. and Izadimoud, Z. (2007). Evaluation of cerebral microembolic signals in patients with mechanical aortic valves. *The Internet Journal of Neuromonitoring*, **4**(2).

Hajjar, I. and Kotchen, T. A. (2003). Trends in prevalence, awareness, treatment, and control of hypertension in the United States, 1988–2000. *Journal of the American Medical Association*, **290**, 199–206.

Hartz, A. J., Daly, J. M., Kohatsu, N. D., Stromquist, A. M., Jogerst, G. J., and Kukoyi, O. A. (2007). Risk factors for insomnia in a rural population. *Annals of Epidemiology*, **17**, 940–947.

Harvey, R. L., Roth, E. J., Yarnold, P. R., Durham, J. R., and Green, D. (1996). Deep Vein Thrombosis in Stroke: The use of plasma D-dimer level as a screening test in the rehabilitation setting. *Stroke*, **27**, 1516–1520.

He, J., Whelton, P. K., Vu, B., and Klag, M. J. (1998). Aspirin and risk of hemorrhagic stroke. *Journal of the American Medical Association*, **280**, 1930–1935.

Healthy weight, overweight, and obesity among U.S. adults. (2003). NHANES Report 03-0260.

Henin, A., Savage, C. R., Rauch, S. L., Deckersbach, T., Wilhelm, S., Baer, L., Otto, M. W., and Jenike, M. A. (2001). Is age at symptom onset associated with severity of memory impairment in adults with obsessive-compulsive disorder? *American Journal of Psychiatry*, **158**, 137–139.

Hennessey, K. A., Schulte, J. M., Cook, L., Collins, M., Onorato, I. M., and Valway, S. E. (1998). Tuberculin skin test screening practices among US colleges and universities. *Journal of the American Medical Association*, **280**, 2008–2012.

Hernandez, L., Chaubey, R., Cork, R. C., Brandt, S., Alexander, L., and Saleemi, S. (2003). Treatment of Piriformis syndrome with Botox, *The Internet Journal of Anesthesiology*, **6**.

Hommel, A., Bjorkelund, K. B., Thorngren, K., and Ulander, K. (2007). A study of a pathway to reduce pressure ulcers for patients with a hip fracture. *Journal of Orthopaedic Nursing*, **11**, 151–159.

Hosmer, D. W. and Lemeshow, S. (2000). *Applied Logistic Regression*, 2nd Edition, John Wiley & Sons, New York.

Hosmer, D., Lemeshow, S., and May, S. (2008.) *Applied Survival Analysis: Regression Modeling of Time to Event Data*, Second Edition, John Wiley & Sons, Inc., New York.

Hron, G. Kollars, M., Binder, B. R., Eichinger, S., and Kyrle, P. A. (2006). Identification of patients at low risk for recurrent venous thromboembolism by measuring thrombin generation. *Journal of the American Medical Association*, **296**, 397–402.

Jacobson, C. C., Nguyen, J. C., and Kimball, A. B. (2004). Gender and parenting significantly affect work hours of recent dermatology program graduates. *Archives of Dermatology*, **140**, 191–196.

Johnson, R. W. (1996). Fitting percentage of body fat to simple body measurements. *Journal of Statistics Education*, **4**.

Jones-Smith, J. C., Fernald, L. C. H., and Neufeld, L. M. (2007). Birth size and accelerated growth during infancy are associated with increased odds of childhood overweight in Mexican children. *Journal of the American Dietetic Association*, **107**, 2061–2069.

Kelley, M. C., Jones, R. C., Gupta, R. K., Yee, R., Stern, S., Wanek, L., and Morton, D. L. (1998). Tumor-associated antigen TA-90 immune complex assay predicts subclinical metastasis and survival for patients with early stage melanoma. *Cancer*, **83**, 1355–1361.

Kleiner-Fisman, G., and Fisman, D. N. (2007). Risk factors for the development of pedal edema in patients using pramipexole. *Archives of Neurology*, **64**, 820–824.

Koizumi, H., Ferraraa, D. C., Bruła, C., and Spaide, R. F. (2007). Central retinal vein occlusion case–control study. *American Journal of Ophthalmology*, **144**, 858–863.

Krumholz, H. M., Chen, Y., and Radford, M. J. (2001). Aspirin and the treatment of heart failure in the elderly. *Archives of Internal Medicine*, **161**, 577–582.

Kuczmarski, R. J., Carroll, M. D., Flegal, K. M., and Troiano, R. P. (1997). Varying body mass index cutoff points to describe overweight prevalence among U.S. adults: NHANES III (1988 to 1994). *Journal of Obesity*, **5**, 542–8.

Laessle, R. G., Lehrke, S., and Dückers, S. (2007). Laboratory eating behavior in obesity. *Appetite*, **49**, 399–404.

Laohavinij, S. and Maneechavakajorn, J. (2004). Prognostic factors for survival in advanced non-small cell lung cancer. *Journal of the Medical Association of Thailand*, **87**, 1056–64.

Lasater, L. M., Davidson, A. J., Steiner, J. F., and Mehler, P. S. (2001). Glycemic control in English-vs Spanish-speaking hispanic patients with Type 2 diabetes mellitus. *Archives of Internal Medicine*, **161**, 77–82.

Leitzmann, M. F., Willett, W. C., Rimm, E. B., Stampfer, M. J., Spiegelman, D., Colditz, G. A., and Giovannucci, E. (1999). A prospective study of coffee consumption and the risk of symptomatic gallstone disease in men. *Journal of the American Medical Association*, **281**, 2106–2112.

Lie, D. (2003). Standard of care for pap screening. *Medscape Today*, **5**.

Lin, S., Lin, Y., Chen, D., Chu, P., Hsu, C., and Halperin, M. L. (2004). Laboratory tests to determine the cause of hypokalemia and paralysis. *Archives of Internal Medicine*, **164**, 1561–1566.

Liou, T. G., Adler, F. R., FitzSimmons, S. C., Cahill, B. C., Hibbs, J. R., and Marshall, B. C. (2001). Predictive 5-year survivorship model of cystic fibrosis. *American Journal of Epidemiology*, **153**, 345–352.

Lonn, E. (2005). Effects of long-term vitamin E supplementation on cardiovascular events and cancer: a randomized controlled trial. *Journal of the American Medical Association*, **293**, 1338–1347.

Macknin, M. L., Piedmonte, M., Calendine, C., Janosky, J., and Wald, E. (1998). Zinc gluconate lozenges for treating the common cold in children: a randomized controlled trial. *Journal of the American Medical Association*, **279**, 1962–1967.

Margolis, D. J., Halpern, A. C., Rebbeck, T., Schuchter, L., Barnhill, R. L., Fine, J., and Berwick, M. (1998). Validation of a melanoma prognostic model. *Archives of Dermatology*, **134**, 1597–1601.

McMurray, J. J. V., Teerlink, J. R., Cotter, G., Bourge, R. C., Cleland, J. G. F., Jondeau, G., Krum, H., Metra, M., OŠConnor, C. M., Parker, J. D., Torre-Amione, G., van Veldhuisen, D. J., Lewsey, J., Frey, A., Rainisio, M., and Kobrin, I. (2007). Effects of tezosentan on symptoms and outcomes in patients with acute heart failure: the VERITAS randomized controlled trials. *Journal of the American Medical Association*, **298**, 2009–2019.

Medscape Family Medicine/Primary Care (2003), **5**.

Miller, C. D., Phillips, L. S., Ziemer, D. C., Gallina, D. L., Cook, C. B., and El-Kebbi, I. M. (2001). Hypoglycemia in patients with Type 2 diabetes mellitus. *Archives of Internal Medicine*, **161**, 1653–1659.

Misciagna, G., Guerra, V., Di Leo, A., Correale, M., and Trevisan, M. (2000). Insulin and gall stones: a population case control study in southern Italy. *Gut*, **47**, 144–147.

Moeller-Bertram, T., Greenberg, M., Schulteis, G., Hayes, J., and Finer, N. (2007). Drug delivery using the endotracheal tube: how much remains inside the tube? *The Internet Journal of Anesthesiology*, **12**(1).

Monnier, L., Mas, E., Ginet, C., Michel, F., Villon, L., Cristol, J., and Colette, C., (2006). Activation of oxidative stress by acute glucose fluctuations compared with sustained chronic hyperglycemia in patients with Type 2 diabetes. *Journal of the American Medical Association*, **295**, 1681–1687.

Muramoto, M. L., Leischow, S. J., Sherrill, D., Matthews, E., and Strayer, L. J. (2007). Randomized, double-blind, placebo-controlled trial of 2 dosages of sustained-release bupropion for adolescent smoking cessation. *Archives of Pediatrics & Adolescent Medicine*, **161**, 1068–1074.

Muss, H. B., Woolf, S., Berry, D., Cirrincione, C., Weiss, R. B., Budman, D., Wood, W. C., Henderson, I. C., Hudis, C., Winer, E., Cohen, H., Wheeler, J., and Norton, L. (2005). Adjuvant chemotherapy in older and younger women with lymph node—positive breast cancer. *Journal of the American Medical Association*, **293**, 1073–1081.

Nassar, M. F., Gomaa, S. M., and El Batrawy, S. R. (2007). Low ghrelin level affects bone biomarkers in childhood obesity. *Nutrition Research*, **27**, 605–611.

Nishitani, Y., Yoshiyama1, M., Tay, F. R., Wadgaonkar, B., Waller, J., Agee, K., and Pashley, D. H. (2005). Tensile strength of mineralized/demineralized human normal and carious dentin. *Journal of Dental Research*, **84**, 1075–1078.

Ockene, J. K., Adams, A., Hurley, T. G., Wheeler, E. V., and Hebert, J. R. (1999). Brief physician- and nurse practitioner-delivered counseling for high-risk drinkers: does it work? *Archives of Internal Medicine*, **159**, 2198–2205.

Ownby, D. R., Johnson, C. C., and Peterson, E. L. (2000). Passive cigarette smoke exposure of infants. *Archives of Pediatric and Adolescent Medicine*, **154**, 1237–1241.

Paul, P., Rosaline, H., and Balagopal, S. (2007). The effect of hydrogel and solution of sodium ascorbate on the bond strength of bleached enamel. *Journal of Conservative Dentistry*, **10**, 43–47.

Pawlinska-Chmara, R. and Szwed, A. (2008). Cigarette smoking and age at natural menopause of women in Poland. *The Internet Journal of Biological Anthropology*, **2**(1).

Penrose, K. W., Nelson, A. G., and Fisher, A. G. (1985). Generalized body composition prediction equation for men using simple measurement techniques. *Medicine and Science in Sports and Exercise*, **17**, 189.

Percentage distribution of blood pressure categories among adults aged ≥ 18 years, by race/ethnicity—National Health and Nutrition Survey, United States, 1999–2004. (2007). *Morbidity and Mortality Weekly Report*, **56**, 611.

Petersen, R. (1985). *Design and Analysis of Experiments*, Marcel Dekker, Inc.

Pillar, G., Shahar, E., Peled, N., Ravid, S., Lavie, P., and Etzioni, A. (2000). Melatonin improves sleep–wake patterns in psychomotor retarded children. *Pediatric Neurology*, **23**, 225–228.

Power, D. M., Bhadra, A., Bhatti, A., Forshaw, M. J. (2006). Xylocaine spray reduces patient discomfort during nasogastric tube insertion. *The Internet Journal of Surgery*, **8**(2).

Prescott, E., Hippe, M., Schnohr, P., Hein, H. O., and Vestbo, J.(1998). Smoking and risk of myocardial infarction in women and men: longitudinal population study. *British Medical Journal*, **316**, 1043–1047.

Presnell, K., Stice, E., and Tristan, J. (2008). Experimental investigation of the effects of naturalistic dieting on bulimic symptoms: moderating effects of depressive symptoms. *Appetite*, **50**, 91–101.

Prevalence of overweight among persons aged 2–19 years, by sex—National Health and Nutrition Examination Survey (NHANES), United States, 1999–2000 through 2003–2004. (2006). *Morbidity and Mortality Weekly Report*, **55**, 1229.

Price, R. K., North, C. S., Wessely, S., and Fraser, V. J. (1992), Estimating the prevalence of chronic fatigue syndrome and associated symptoms in the community. *Public Health Reports*, **107**, 514–522.

Rahimi, A. R., Spertus, J. A., Reid, K. J., Bernheim, S. M., and Krumholz, H. M. (2007), Financial barriers to health care and outcomes after acute myocardial infarction. *Journal of the American Medical Association*, **297**, 1063–1072.

Ramsey, F. and Schafer, D. (2002). *Statistical Sleuth: A Course in Methods of Data Analysis*, Second Edition, Duxbury Press.

Rohlfing, C. L., Wiedmeyer, H., Little, R. R., England, J. D., Tennill, A., and Goldstein, D. E. (2002). Defining the relationship between plasma glucose and HbA1c: analysis of glucose profiles and HbA1c in the diabetes control and complications trial. *Diabetes Care*, **25**, 275–278.

Sahin, S., Rao, B., Kopf, A. F., Lee, E., Rigel, D. S., Nossa, R., Rahman, I. J., Wortzel, H., Marghoob, A. A., and Bart, R. S. (1997). Predicting ten-year survival of patients with primary cutaneous melanoma: corroboration of a prognostic model. *Cancer*, **80**, 1426–31.

Sang-hyub, L. (1999). Effect of irradiation on grip strength. *Journal of Korean Academy of University Trained Physical Therapists*, **6**, 8–14.

Sasso, F. C., Carbonara, O., Nasti, R., Campana, B., Marfella, R., Torella, M., Nappi, G., Torella, R,, and Cozzolino, D. (2004). Glucose metabolism and coronary heart disease in patients with normal glucose tolerance. *Journal of the American Medical Association*, **291**, 1857–1863.

Schmults, C. D., Phelps, R., and Goldberg, D. J. (2004). Nonablative facial remodeling erythema reduction and histologic evidence of new collagen formation using a 300-microsecond 1064-nm Nd:YAG laser. *Archives of Dermatology*, **140**, 1373–1376.

Schober, S. E., Sinks, T. H., Jones, R. L., Bolger, P. M., McDowell, M., Osterloh, J., Garrett, E. S., Canady, R. A., Dillon, C. F., Sun, Y., Joseph, C. B., and Mahaffey, K. R. (2003). Blood mercury levels in US children and women of childbearing age, 1999–2000. *Journal of the American Medical Association*, **289**, 1667–1674.

Shaikh, L., Sagebiel, R. W., Ferreira, C. M. M., Nosrati, M., Miller, J. R., and Kashani-Sabet, M. (2005). The role of microsatellites as a prognostic factor in primary malignant melanoma. *Archives of Dermatology*, **141**, 739–742.

Sharma, N. and Chitre, V. (2008). An in-vitro comparative study of wettability of four commercially available saliva substitutes and distilled water on heat-polymerized acrylic resin. *Journal of Indian Prosthodontic Society*, **8**, 30–35.

Siddiqui, Q. and Chowdhury, E. (2006). Caudal analgesia in paediatrics: a comparison between bupivacaine and ketamine. *The Internet Journal of Anesthesiology*, **11**(1).

Siri, W. E. (1956). Gross composition of the body. *Advances in Biological and Medical Physics* (Vol. IV), eds. J. H. Lawrence and C. A. Tobias. Academic Press, New York, pp. 239–280.

Stamey, T. A., McNeal, J. E., Yemoto, C. M., Sigal, B. M., and Johnstone, I. M. (1999). Biological determinants of cancer progression in men with prostate cancer. *Journal of the American Medical Association*, **281**, 1395–1400.

Stan, S., Levy, E., Delvin, E. E., Hanley, J. A., Lamarche, B., OŠLoughlin, J., Paradis, G., and Lambert, M. (2005). Distribution of LDL particle size in a population-based sample of children and adolescents and relationship with other cardiovascular risk factors. *Clinical Chemistry*, **51**, 1192–1200.

Stearns, V., Beebe, K. L., Iyengar, M., and Dube, E. (2003). Paroxetine controlled release in the treatment of menopausal hot flashes: a randomized controlled trial. *Journal of the American Medical Association*, **289**, 2827–2834.

Strandberg, T. E., Strandberg, A. Y., Pitkälä, K. H., Salomaa, V. V., Tilvis, R. S., and Miettinen, T. A. (2006). Cardiovascular risk in midlife and psychological well-being among older men. *Archives of Internal Medicine*, **166**, 2266–2271.

Sulheim, S., Holme, I., Ekeland, A., and Bahr, R. (2005). Helmet use and risk of head injuries in alpine skiers and snowboarders. *Journal of the American Medical Association*, **295**, 919–924.

Thomson, W. M., Poulton, R., Broadbent, J. M., Moffitt, T. E., Caspi, A., Beck, J. D., Welch, D., and Hancox, R. J. (2008). Cannabis smoking and periodontal disease among young adults. *Journal of the American Medical Association*, **299**, 525–531.

Tolga, K., Burcu, C., Taskin, T., and Ziya, O. M., (2007). Effects of tonsillectomy on acoustic parameters. *The Internet Journal of Otorhinolaryngology*, **6**(2).

Tsai, S. P., Ahmed, F. S., Wendt, J. K., Bhojani, F., and Donnelly, R. P. (2008). The impact of obesity on illness absence and productivity in an industrial population of petrochemical workers. *Annals of Epidemiology*, **18**, 8–14.

Ugwuja, E. I., Ugwu, N. C., and Nwibo, A. N. (2008). Dietary supplement containing mixture of raw curry, garlic, and ginger. *The Internet Journal of Nutrition and Wellness*, **5**(2).

Villanueva, E. V. (2001). The validity of self-reported weight in US adults: a population based cross-sectional study. *BMC, Public Health*, **1**.

Villareal, D. T., Banks, M., Sinacore, D. R., Siener, C., and Klein, S. (2006). Effect of weight loss and exercise on frailty in obese older adults. *Archives of Internal Medicine.*, **166**, 860–866.

Villarino, M. E., Burman, W., Wnag, Y., Ludergan, L., Catanzaro, A., Bock, N., Jones, C., and Nolan,

C. (1999). Comparable specificity of 2 commercial tuberculin reagents in persons at low risk for tuberculosis infection. *Journal of the American Medical Association*, **281**, 169–171.

Vogeser, M., Briegel, J., and Zachoval, R. (2002). Dialyzable free cortisol after stimulation with synacthen. *Clinical Biochemistry*, **35**, 539–543.

Ward, A., Pollock, M. L., Jackson, A. S., Ayres, J. J., and Pape, G., (1978). A comparison of body fat determined by underwater weighing and volume displacement. *American Journal of Physiology*, **234**, E94–E96.

Weil, M., Bressler, J., Parsons, P., Bolla, K., Glass, T., and Schwartz, B. (2005). Blood mercury levels and neurobehavioral function. *Journal of the American Medical Association*, **293**, 1875–1882.

Weitzel, J. N., Lagos, V. I., Cullinane, C. A., Gambol, P. J., Culver, J. O., Blazer, K. R., Palomares, M. R., Lowstuter, K. J., and MacDonald, D. J. (2007). Limited family structure and BRCA gene mutation status in single cases of breast cancer. *Journal of the American Medical Association*, **297**, 2587–2595.

Wiszniewska, M., Devuyst, G., Bogousslavsky, J., Ghika, J., and van Melle, G. (2000). What is the significance of leukoaraiosis in patients with acute ischemic stroke? *Archives of Neurology*, **57**, 967–973.

Zingmond, D. S., McGory, M. L., and Ko, C. Y. (2005). Hospitalization before and after gastric bypass surgery. *Journal of the American Medical Association*, **294**, 1918–1924.

APPENDIX A

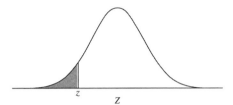

Figure A.1   Standard normal cumulative probabilities for $-3.49 \le z \le 0$.

TABLE A.1   Cumulative Probabilities for the Standard Normal for $-3.49 \le z \le 0$

z	0.00	0.01	0.02	0.03	0.04	0.05	0.06	0.07	0.08	0.09
−3.4	0.0003	0.0003	0.0003	0.0003	0.0003	0.0003	0.0003	0.0003	0.0003	0.0002
−3.3	0.0005	0.0005	0.0005	0.0004	0.0004	0.0004	0.0004	0.0004	0.0004	0.0003
−3.2	0.0007	0.0007	0.0006	0.0006	0.0006	0.0006	0.0006	0.0005	0.0005	0.0005
−3.1	0.0010	0.0009	0.0009	0.0009	0.0008	0.0008	0.0008	0.0008	0.0007	0.0007
−3.0	0.0013	0.0013	0.0013	0.0012	0.0012	0.0011	0.0011	0.0011	0.0010	0.0010
−2.9	0.0019	0.0018	0.0017	0.0017	0.0016	0.0016	0.0015	0.0015	0.0014	0.0014
−2.8	0.0026	0.0025	0.0024	0.0023	0.0023	0.0022	0.0021	0.0021	0.0020	0.0019
−2.7	0.0035	0.0034	0.0033	0.0032	0.0031	0.0030	0.0029	0.0028	0.0027	0.0026
−2.6	0.0047	0.0045	0.0044	0.0043	0.0041	0.0040	0.0039	0.0038	0.0037	0.0036
−2.5	0.0062	0.0060	0.0059	0.0057	0.0055	0.0054	0.0052	0.0051	0.0049	0.0048
−2.4	0.0082	0.0080	0.0078	0.0075	0.0073	0.0071	0.0069	0.0068	0.0066	0.0064
−2.3	0.0107	0.0104	0.0102	0.0099	0.0096	0.0094	0.0091	0.0089	0.0087	0.0084
−2.2	0.0139	0.0136	0.0132	0.0129	0.0125	0.0122	0.0119	0.0116	0.0113	0.0110
−2.1	0.0179	0.0174	0.0170	0.0166	0.0162	0.0158	0.0154	0.0150	0.0146	0.0143
−2.0	0.0228	0.0222	0.0217	0.0212	0.0207	0.0202	0.0197	0.0192	0.0188	0.0183
−1.9	0.0287	0.0281	0.0274	0.0268	0.0262	0.0256	0.0250	0.0244	0.0239	0.0233
−1.8	0.0359	0.0352	0.0344	0.0336	0.0329	0.0322	0.0314	0.0307	0.0301	0.0294
−1.7	0.0446	0.0436	0.0427	0.0418	0.0409	0.0401	0.0392	0.0384	0.0375	0.0367
−1.6	0.0548	0.0537	0.0526	0.0516	0.0505	0.0495	0.0485	0.0475	0.0465	0.0455
−1.5	0.0668	0.0655	0.0643	0.0630	0.0618	0.0606	0.0594	0.0582	0.0571	0.0559
−1.4	0.0808	0.0793	0.0778	0.0764	0.0749	0.0735	0.0722	0.0708	0.0694	0.0681
−1.3	0.0968	0.0951	0.0934	0.0918	0.0901	0.0885	0.0869	0.0853	0.0838	0.0823
−1.2	0.1151	0.1131	0.1112	0.1093	0.1075	0.1056	0.1038	0.1020	0.1003	0.0985
−1.1	0.1357	0.1335	0.1314	0.1292	0.1271	0.1251	0.1230	0.1210	0.1190	0.1170
−1.0	0.1587	0.1562	0.1539	0.1515	0.1492	0.1469	0.1446	0.1423	0.1401	0.1379
−0.9	0.1841	0.1814	0.1788	0.1762	0.1736	0.1711	0.1685	0.1660	0.1635	0.1611
−0.8	0.2119	0.2090	0.2061	0.2033	0.2005	0.1977	0.1949	0.1922	0.1894	0.1867
−0.7	0.2420	0.2389	0.2358	0.2327	0.2296	0.2266	0.2236	0.2206	0.2177	0.2148
−0.6	0.2743	0.2709	0.2676	0.2643	0.2611	0.2578	0.2546	0.2514	0.2483	0.2451
−0.5	0.3085	0.3050	0.3015	0.2981	0.2946	0.2912	0.2877	0.2843	0.2810	0.2776
−0.4	0.3446	0.3409	0.3372	0.3336	0.3300	0.3264	0.3228	0.3192	0.3156	0.3121
−0.3	0.3821	0.3783	0.3745	0.3707	0.3669	0.3632	0.3594	0.3557	0.3520	0.3483
−0.2	0.4207	0.4168	0.4129	0.4090	0.4052	0.4013	0.3974	0.3936	0.3897	0.3859
−0.1	0.4602	0.4562	0.4522	0.4483	0.4443	0.4404	0.4364	0.4325	0.4286	0.4247
−0.0	0.5000	0.4960	0.4920	0.4880	0.4840	0.4801	0.4761	0.4721	0.4681	0.4641

For $z \le -3.5$, $P(X \le z) = 0$.

Applied Biostatistics for the Health Sciences. By Richard J. Rossi
Copyright © 2010 by John Wiley & Sons, Inc.

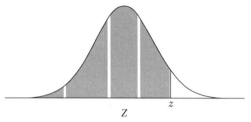

Figure A.2   Standard normal cumulative probabilities for $0 \leq z \leq 3.49$.

TABLE A.2   Cumulative Probabilities for the Standard Normal for $0 \leq z \leq 3.49$

z	0.00	0.01	0.02	0.03	0.04	0.05	0.06	0.07	0.08	0.09
0.0	0.5000	0.5040	0.5080	0.5120	0.5160	0.5199	0.5239	0.5279	0.5319	0.5359
0.1	0.5398	0.5438	0.5478	0.5517	0.5557	0.5596	0.5636	0.5675	0.5714	0.5753
0.2	0.5793	0.5832	0.5871	0.5910	0.5948	0.5987	0.6026	0.6064	0.6103	0.6141
0.3	0.6179	0.6217	0.6255	0.6293	0.6331	0.6368	0.6406	0.6443	0.6480	0.6517
0.4	0.6554	0.6591	0.6628	0.6664	0.6700	0.6736	0.6772	0.6808	0.6844	0.6879
0.5	0.6915	0.6950	0.6985	0.7019	0.7054	0.7088	0.7123	0.7157	0.7190	0.7224
0.6	0.7257	0.7291	0.7324	0.7357	0.7389	0.7422	0.7454	0.7486	0.7517	0.7549
0.7	0.7580	0.7611	0.7642	0.7673	0.7704	0.7734	0.7764	0.7794	0.7823	0.7852
0.8	0.7881	0.7910	0.7939	0.7967	0.7995	0.8023	0.8051	0.8078	0.8106	0.8133
0.9	0.8159	0.8186	0.8212	0.8238	0.8264	0.8289	0.8314	0.8340	0.8365	0.8389
1.0	0.8413	0.8438	0.8461	0.8485	0.8508	0.8531	0.8554	0.8577	0.8599	0.8621
1.1	0.8643	0.8665	0.8686	0.8708	0.8729	0.8749	0.8770	0.8790	0.8810	0.8830
1.2	0.8849	0.8869	0.8888	0.8907	0.8925	0.8944	0.8962	0.8980	0.8997	0.9015
1.3	0.9032	0.9049	0.9066	0.9082	0.9099	0.9115	0.9131	0.9147	0.9162	0.9177
1.4	0.9192	0.9207	0.9222	0.9236	0.9251	0.9265	0.9278	0.9292	0.9306	0.9319
1.5	0.9332	0.9345	0.9357	0.9370	0.9382	0.9394	0.9406	0.9418	0.9429	0.9441
1.6	0.9452	0.9463	0.9474	0.9484	0.9495	0.9505	0.9515	0.9525	0.9535	0.9545
1.7	0.9554	0.9564	0.9573	0.9582	0.9591	0.9599	0.9608	0.9616	0.9625	0.9633
1.8	0.9641	0.9649	0.9656	0.9664	0.9671	0.9678	0.9686	0.9693	0.9699	0.9706
1.9	0.9713	0.9719	0.9726	0.9732	0.9738	0.9744	0.9750	0.9756	0.9761	0.9767
2.0	0.9772	0.9778	0.9783	0.9788	0.9793	0.9798	0.9803	0.9808	0.9812	0.9817
2.1	0.9821	0.9826	0.9830	0.9834	0.9838	0.9842	0.9846	0.9850	0.9854	0.9857
2.2	0.9861	0.9864	0.9868	0.9871	0.9875	0.9878	0.9881	0.9884	0.9887	0.9890
2.3	0.9893	0.9896	0.9898	0.9901	0.9904	0.9906	0.9909	0.9911	0.9913	0.9916
2.4	0.9918	0.9920	0.9922	0.9925	0.9927	0.9929	0.9931	0.9932	0.9934	0.9936
2.5	0.9938	0.9940	0.9941	0.9943	0.9945	0.9946	0.9948	0.9949	0.9951	0.9952
2.6	0.9953	0.9955	0.9956	0.9957	0.9959	0.9960	0.9961	0.9962	0.9963	0.9964
2.7	0.9965	0.9966	0.9967	0.9968	0.9969	0.9970	0.9971	0.9972	0.9973	0.9974
2.8	0.9974	0.9975	0.9976	0.9977	0.9977	0.9978	0.9979	0.9979	0.9980	0.9981
2.9	0.9981	0.9982	0.9982	0.9983	0.9984	0.9984	0.9985	0.9985	0.9986	0.9986
3.0	0.9987	0.9987	0.9987	0.9988	0.9988	0.9989	0.9989	0.9989	0.9990	0.9990
3.1	0.9990	0.9991	0.9991	0.9991	0.9992	0.9992	0.9992	0.9992	0.9993	0.9993
3.2	0.9993	0.9993	0.9994	0.9994	0.9994	0.9994	0.9994	0.9995	0.9995	0.9995
3.3	0.9995	0.9995	0.9995	0.9996	0.9996	0.9996	0.9996	0.9996	0.9996	0.9997
3.4	0.9997	0.9997	0.9997	0.9997	0.9997	0.9997	0.9997	0.9997	0.9997	0.9998

For $z \geq 3.5$, $P(Z \leq z) = 1$.

TABLE A.3 Percentiles of the Standard Normal Distribution

Percent	0	1	2	3	4	5	6	7	8	9
Percentile	NA	−2.33	−2.05	−1.88	−1.75	−1.645	−1.56	−1.48	−1.41	−1.34
Percent	10	11	12	13	14	15	16	17	18	19
Percentile	−1.28	−1.23	−1.18	−1.13	−1.08	−1.04	−0.99	−0.95	−0.92	−0.88
Percent	20	21	22	23	24	25	26	27	28	29
Percentile	−0.84	−0.81	−0.77	−0.74	−0.71	−0.67	−0.64	−0.61	−0.58	−0.55
Percent	30	31	32	33	34	35	36	37	38	39
Percentile	−0.52	−0.50	−0.47	−0.44	−0.41	−0.39	−0.36	−0.33	−0.31	−0.28
Percent	40	41	42	43	44	45	46	47	48	49
Percentile	−0.25	−0.23	−0.20	−0.38	−0.35	−0.33	−0.30	−0.08	−0.05	−0.03
Percent	50	51	52	53	54	55	56	57	58	59
Percentile	0.00	0.03	0.05	0.08	0.10	0.13	0.15	0.18	0.20	0.23
Percent	60	61	62	63	64	65	66	67	68	69
Percentile	0.25	0.28	0.31	0.33	0.36	0.39	0.41	0.44	0.47	0.50
Percent	70	71	72	73	74	75	76	77	78	79
Percentile	0.52	0.55	0.58	0.61	0.64	0.67	0.71	0.74	0.77	0.81
Percent	80	81	82	83	84	85	86	87	88	89
Percentile	0.84	0.88	0.92	0.95	0.99	1.04	1.08	1.17	1.23	1.23
Percent	90	91	92	93	94	95	96	97	98	99
Percentile	1.28	1.34	1.41	1.48	1.56	1.645	1.75	1.88	2.05	2.33

TABLE A.4 The z_{crit} Values for the Large Sample Z Confidence Intervals

Confidence Level	90%	95%	98%	99%
Two-sided z_{crit}	1.645	1.96	2.326	2.576
One-sided z_{crit}	1.282	1.645	2.054	2.326

TABLE A.5 The $z_{crit,\alpha}$ Values for the Upper-, Lower-, and Two-Tailed Z-Tests

α	Upper-tail $z_{crit,\alpha}$	Lower-tail $z_{crit,\alpha}$	Two-tail $z_{crit,\alpha}$
0.15	1.036	−1.036	1.440
0.10	1.282	−1.282	1.645
0.05	1.645	−1.645	1.96
0.01	2.326	−2.326	2.576

TABLE A.6 The Values of z_β Used in Determining the Sample Size n in the One- and Two-Tailed Z-Tests for a Prespecified Values of α and β

β	z_β
0.15	1.036
0.10	1.282
0.05	1.645
0.01	2.326

TABLE A.7 The Critical Values of the *t* Distribution Used in Confidence Intervals and Hypothesis Tests

Two-sided confidence level	80%	90%	95%	98%	99%	99.8%	99.9%
One-sided confidence level	90%	95%	97.5%	99%	99.5%	99.9%	99.95%
One-tailed α	0.10	0.05	0.025	0.01	0.005	0.001	0.0005
Two-tailed α	0.20	0.10	0.05	0.02	0.01	0.002	0.001
Percentile	90	95	97.5	99	99.5	99.9	99.95
df (ν)							
1	3.078	6.314	12.706	31.82	63.66	318.31	636.62
2	1.886	2.920	4.303	6.965	9.925	22.362	31.598
3	1.638	2.353	3.182	4.541	5.841	10.213	12.924
4	1.533	2.132	2.776	3.747	4.604	7.173	8.610
5	1.476	2.015	2.571	3.365	4.032	5.893	6.869
6	1.440	1.943	2.447	3.143	3.707	5.208	5.959
7	1.415	1.895	2.365	2.998	3.499	4.785	5.408
8	1.397	1.860	2.306	2.896	3.355	4.501	5.041
9	1.383	1.833	2.262	2.821	3.250	4.297	4.781
10	1.372	1.812	2.228	2.764	3.169	4.144	4.587
11	1.363	1.796	2.201	2.718	3.106	4.025	4.437
12	1.356	1.782	2.179	2.681	3.055	3.930	4.318
13	1.350	1.771	2.160	2.650	3.012	3.852	4.221
14	1.345	1.761	2.145	2.624	2.977	3.787	4.140
15	1.341	1.753	2.131	2.602	2.947	3.733	4.073
16	1.337	1.746	2.120	2.583	2.921	3.686	4.015
17	1.333	1.740	2.110	2.567	2.898	3.646	3.965
18	1.330	1.734	2.101	2.552	2.878	3.610	3.922
19	1.328	1.729	2.093	2.539	2.861	3.579	3.883
20	1.325	1.725	2.086	2.528	2.845	3.552	3.850
21	1.323	1.721	2.080	2.518	2.831	3.527	3.819
22	1.321	1.717	2.074	2.508	2.819	3.505	3.792
23	1.319	1.714	2.069	2.500	2.807	3.485	3.767
24	1.318	1.711	2.064	2.492	2.797	3.467	3.745
25	1.316	1.708	2.060	2.485	2.787	3.450	3.725
26	1.315	1.706	2.056	2.479	2.779	3.435	3.707
27	1.314	1.703	2.052	2.473	2.771	3.421	3.690
28	1.313	1.701	2.048	2.467	2.763	3.408	3.674
29	1.311	1.699	2.045	2.462	2.756	3.396	3.659
30	1.310	1.697	2.042	2.457	2.750	3.385	3.646
40	1.303	1.684	2.021	2.423	2.704	3.307	3.551
60	1.296	1.671	2.000	2.390	2.660	3.232	3.460
120	1.289	1.658	1.980	2.358	2.617	3.160	3.373
∞	1.282	1.645	1.960	2.326	2.576	3.090	3.291

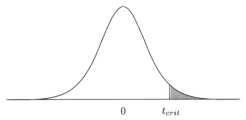

Figure A.3   Upper tail probabilities for the *t* distribution.

TABLE A.8   Upper Tail Probabilities for the *t* Distribution $P(t_{\nu} > t)$

df (ν)	*t*								
	1.7	1.8	1.9	2.0	2.1	2.2	2.3	2.4	2.5
1	0.169	0.161	0.154	0.148	0.141	0.136	0.131	0.126	0.121
2	0.116	0.107	0.099	0.092	0.085	0.079	0.074	0.069	0.065
3	0.094	0.085	0.077	0.070	0.063	0.058	0.052	0.048	0.044
4	0.082	0.073	0.065	0.058	0.052	0.046	0.041	0.037	0.033
5	0.075	0.066	0.058	0.051	0.045	0.040	0.035	0.031	0.027
6	0.070	0.061	0.053	0.046	0.040	0.035	0.031	0.027	0.023
7	0.066	0.057	0.050	0.043	0.037	0.032	0.027	0.024	0.020
8	0.064	0.055	0.047	0.040	0.034	0.029	0.025	0.022	0.018
9	0.062	0.053	0.045	0.038	0.033	0.028	0.023	0.020	0.017
10	0.060	0.051	0.043	0.037	0.031	0.026	0.022	0.019	0.016
11	0.059	0.050	0.042	0.035	0.030	0.025	0.021	0.018	0.015
12	0.057	0.049	0.041	0.034	0.029	0.024	0.020	0.017	0.014
13	0.056	0.048	0.040	0.033	0.028	0.023	0.019	0.016	0.013
14	0.056	0.047	0.039	0.033	0.027	0.023	0.019	0.015	0.013
15	0.055	0.046	0.038	0.032	0.027	0.022	0.018	0.015	0.012
16	0.054	0.045	0.038	0.031	0.026	0.021	0.018	0.014	0.012
17	0.054	0.045	0.037	0.031	0.025	0.021	0.017	0.014	0.011
18	0.053	0.044	0.037	0.030	0.025	0.021	0.017	0.014	0.011
19	0.053	0.044	0.036	0.030	0.025	0.020	0.016	0.013	0.011
20	0.052	0.043	0.036	0.030	0.024	0.020	0.016	0.013	0.011
21	0.052	0.043	0.036	0.029	0.024	0.020	0.016	0.013	0.010
22	0.052	0.043	0.035	0.029	0.024	0.019	0.016	0.013	0.010
23	0.051	0.042	0.035	0.029	0.023	0.019	0.015	0.012	0.010
24	0.051	0.042	0.035	0.028	0.023	0.019	0.015	0.012	0.010
25	0.051	0.042	0.035	0.028	0.023	0.019	0.015	0.012	0.010
26	0.051	0.042	0.034	0.028	0.023	0.018	0.015	0.012	0.010
27	0.050	0.042	0.034	0.028	0.023	0.018	0.015	0.012	0.009
28	0.050	0.041	0.034	0.028	0.022	0.018	0.015	0.012	0.009
29	0.050	0.041	0.034	0.027	0.022	0.018	0.014	0.012	0.009
30	0.050	0.041	0.034	0.027	0.022	0.018	0.014	0.011	0.009
40	0.048	0.040	0.032	0.026	0.021	0.017	0.013	0.011	0.008
60	0.047	0.038	0.031	0.025	0.020	0.016	0.012	0.010	0.008
120	0.046	0.037	0.030	0.024	0.019	0.015	0.012	0.009	0.007
∞	0.045	0.036	0.029	0.023	0.018	0.014	0.011	0.008	0.006

TABLE A.9 Upper Tail Probabilities for the t Distribution $P(t_{\nu} > t)$

df (ν)	t								
	2.6	2.7	2.8	2.9	3.0	3.1	3.2	3.3	3.4
1	0.117	0.113	0.109	0.106	0.102	0.099	0.096	0.094	0.091
2	0.061	0.057	0.054	0.051	0.048	0.045	0.043	0.040	0.038
3	0.040	0.037	0.034	0.031	0.029	0.027	0.025	0.023	0.021
4	0.030	0.027	0.024	0.022	0.020	0.018	0.016	0.015	0.014
5	0.024	0.021	0.019	0.017	0.015	0.013	0.012	0.011	0.010
6	0.020	0.018	0.016	0.014	0.012	0.011	0.009	0.008	0.007
7	0.018	0.015	0.013	0.011	0.010	0.009	0.008	0.007	0.006
8	0.016	0.014	0.012	0.010	0.009	0.007	0.006	0.005	0.005
9	0.014	0.012	0.010	0.009	0.007	0.006	0.005	0.005	0.004
10	0.013	0.011	0.009	0.008	0.007	0.006	0.005	0.004	0.003
11	0.012	0.010	0.009	0.007	0.006	0.005	0.004	0.004	0.003
12	0.012	0.010	0.008	0.007	0.006	0.005	0.004	0.003	0.003
13	0.011	0.009	0.008	0.006	0.005	0.004	0.003	0.003	0.002
14	0.010	0.009	0.007	0.006	0.005	0.004	0.003	0.003	0.002
15	0.010	0.008	0.007	0.005	0.004	0.004	0.003	0.002	0.002
16	0.010	0.008	0.006	0.005	0.004	0.003	0.003	0.002	0.002
17	0.009	0.008	0.006	0.005	0.004	0.003	0.003	0.002	0.002
18	0.009	0.007	0.006	0.005	0.004	0.003	0.002	0.002	0.002
19	0.009	0.007	0.006	0.005	0.004	0.003	0.002	0.002	0.002
20	0.009	0.007	0.006	0.004	0.004	0.003	0.002	0.002	0.001
21	0.008	0.007	0.005	0.004	0.003	0.003	0.002	0.002	0.001
22	0.008	0.007	0.005	0.004	0.003	0.003	0.002	0.002	0.001
23	0.008	0.006	0.005	0.004	0.003	0.003	0.002	0.002	0.001
24	0.008	0.006	0.005	0.004	0.003	0.002	0.002	0.002	0.001
25	0.008	0.006	0.005	0.004	0.003	0.002	0.002	0.001	0.001
26	0.008	0.006	0.005	0.004	0.003	0.002	0.002	0.001	0.001
27	0.007	0.006	0.005	0.004	0.003	0.002	0.002	0.001	0.001
28	0.007	0.006	0.005	0.004	0.003	0.002	0.002	0.001	0.001
29	0.007	0.006	0.004	0.004	0.003	0.002	0.002	0.001	0.001
30	0.007	0.006	0.004	0.003	0.003	0.002	0.002	0.001	0.001
40	0.006	0.005	0.004	0.003	0.002	0.002	0.001	0.001	0.001
60	0.006	0.004	0.003	0.003	0.002	0.001	0.001	0.001	0.001
120	0.005	0.004	0.003	0.002	0.002	0.001	0.001	0.001	0.000
∞	0.005	0.003	0.003	0.002	0.001	0.001	0.001	0.000	0.000

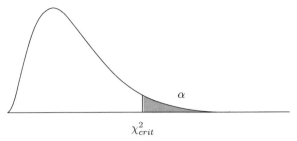

Figure A.4   The critical value of the chi-square distribution.

TABLE A.10   The Critical Values of the Chi-Square Distribution

df	0.10	0.05	0.01	0.005	0.001
1	2.71	3.84	6.63	7.88	10.83
2	4.61	5.99	9.21	10.60	13.82
3	6.25	7.81	11.34	12.84	16.27
4	7.78	9.49	13.28	14.86	18.47
5	9.24	11.07	15.09	16.75	20.52
6	10.64	12.59	16.81	18.55	22.46
7	12.02	14.07	18.48	20.28	24.32
8	13.36	15.51	20.09	21.95	26.12
9	14.68	16.92	21.67	23.59	27.88
10	15.99	18.31	23.21	25.19	29.59
11	17.28	19.68	24.72	26.76	31.26
12	18.55	21.03	26.22	28.30	32.91
13	19.81	22.36	27.69	29.82	34.53
14	21.06	23.68	29.14	31.32	36.12
15	22.31	25.00	30.58	32.80	37.70
16	23.54	26.30	32.00	34.27	39.25
17	24.77	27.59	33.41	35.72	40.79
18	25.99	28.87	34.81	37.16	42.31
19	27.20	30.14	36.19	38.58	43.82
20	28.41	31.41	37.57	40.00	45.31
25	34.38	37.65	44.31	46.93	52.62
30	40.26	43.77	50.89	53.67	59.70
40	51.81	55.76	63.69	66.77	73.40
50	63.17	67.50	76.15	79.49	86.66
60	74.40	79.08	88.38	91.95	99.61
70	85.53	90.53	100.43	104.21	112.32
80	96.58	101.88	112.33	116.32	124.84
90	107.57	113.15	124.12	128.30	137.21
100	118.50	124.34	135.81	140.17	149.45

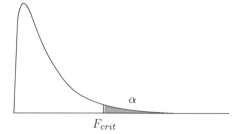

Figure A.5 The critical value of the F distribution.

TABLE A.11 The Critical Values of the F Distribution for $\alpha = 0.05$ and 0.01

Denominator df	α	Numerator df								
		2	3	4	5	6	7	8	9	10
10	0.05	4.10	3.71	3.48	3.33	3.22	3.14	3.07	3.02	2.98
	0.01	7.56	6.55	5.99	5.64	5.39	5.20	5.06	4.94	4.85
11	0.05	3.98	3.59	3.36	3.20	3.09	3.01	2.95	2.90	2.85
	0.01	7.21	6.22	5.67	5.32	5.07	4.89	4.74	4.63	4.54
12	0.05	3.89	3.49	3.26	3.11	3.00	2.91	2.85	2.80	2.75
	0.01	6.93	5.95	5.41	5.06	4.82	4.64	4.50	4.39	4.30
13	0.05	3.81	3.41	3.18	3.03	2.92	2.83	2.77	2.71	2.67
	0.01	6.70	5.74	5.21	4.86	4.62	4.44	4.30	4.19	4.10
14	0.05	3.74	3.34	3.11	2.96	2.85	2.76	2.70	2.65	2.60
	0.01	6.51	5.56	5.04	4.69	4.46	4.28	4.14	4.03	3.94
15	0.05	3.68	3.29	3.06	2.90	2.79	2.71	2.64	2.59	2.54
	0.01	6.36	5.42	4.89	4.56	4.32	4.14	4.00	3.89	3.80
16	0.05	3.63	3.24	3.01	2.85	2.74	2.66	2.59	2.54	2.49
	0.01	6.23	5.29	4.77	4.44	4.20	4.03	3.89	3.78	3.69
17	0.05	3.59	3.20	2.96	2.81	2.70	2.61	2.55	2.49	2.45
	0.01	6.11	5.18	4.67	4.34	4.10	3.93	3.79	3.68	3.59
18	0.05	3.55	3.16	2.93	2.77	2.66	2.58	2.51	2.46	2.41
	0.01	6.01	5.09	4.58	4.25	4.01	3.84	3.71	3.60	3.51
19	0.05	3.52	3.13	2.90	2.74	2.63	2.54	2.48	2.42	2.38
	0.01	5.93	5.01	4.50	4.17	3.94	3.77	3.63	3.52	3.43
20	0.05	3.49	3.10	2.87	2.71	2.60	2.51	2.45	2.39	2.35
	0.01	5.85	4.94	4.43	4.10	3.87	3.70	3.56	3.46	3.37
25	0.05	3.39	2.99	2.76	2.60	2.49	2.40	2.34	2.28	2.24
	0.01	5.57	4.68	4.18	3.85	3.63	3.46	3.32	3.22	3.13
30	0.05	3.32	2.92	2.69	2.53	2.42	2.33	2.27	2.21	2.16
	0.01	5.39	4.51	4.02	3.70	3.47	3.30	3.17	3.07	2.98
35	0.05	3.27	2.87	2.64	2.49	2.37	2.29	2.22	2.16	2.11
	0.01	5.27	4.40	3.91	3.59	3.37	3.20	3.07	2.96	2.88
40	0.05	3.23	2.84	2.61	2.45	2.34	2.25	2.18	2.12	2.08
	0.01	5.18	4.31	3.83	3.51	3.29	3.12	2.99	2.89	2.80
60	0.05	3.15	2.76	2.53	2.37	2.25	2.17	2.10	2.04	1.99
	0.01	4.98	4.13	3.65	3.34	3.12	2.95	2.82	2.72	2.63
90	0.05	3.10	2.71	2.47	2.32	2.20	2.11	2.04	1.99	1.94
	0.01	4.85	4.01	3.53	3.23	3.01	2.84	2.72	2.61	2.52
120	0.05	3.07	2.68	2.45	2.29	2.18	2.09	2.02	1.96	1.91
	0.01	4.79	3.95	3.48	3.17	2.96	2.79	2.66	2.56	2.47
200	0.05	3.49	3.10	2.87	2.71	2.60	2.51	2.45	2.39	2.35
	0.01	5.85	4.94	4.43	4.10	3.87	3.70	3.56	3.46	3.37
∞	0.05	3.00	2.60	2.37	2.21	2.10	2.01	1.94	1.88	1.83
	0.01	4.61	3.78	3.32	3.02	2.80	2.64	2.51	2.41	2.32

Problem Solutions

SOLUTIONS FOR CHAPTER 1

1.1   Biostatistics is the area of statistics that deals with the methodology for collecting and analyzing biomedical or healthcare data.

1.3   NIH, CDC, FDA

1.4   (a) The population of interest; (b) A subset of units of the target population; (c) A sample consisting of the entire target population.

1.6   (a) A numerical measure of a population characteristic; (b) A value computed from only the sample and known values.

1.7   A statistic is computed from a sample while a parameter is computed from a census.

1.8   (a) Use a census; (b) From a sample.

1.9   A statistic.

1.10 A parameter.

1.14 (a) Hospitals in the United States; (b) A statistic.

1.15 (a) Doctors belonging to the AMA; (b) A parameter; (c) A statistic.

1.16 (a) Blood stored in 500 ml bags; (b) A statistic.

1.17 (a) People aged 50 or older with mild to moderate Alzheimer's disease; (b) People; (c) Placebo, Omega-3 fatty acids; (d) 300; (e) Yes; (f) Yes.

1.18 (a) People with colds; (b) Lenght of a cold; (c) 1000 mg vitamin C, placebo; (d) 0 Yes.

1.19 (a) Prostate cancer patients; (b) Individual with prostate cancer; (c) Percentages surviving 5 years for each treatment; (d) Age, sex, race; (e) Surgery, hormone therapy, radiation therapy.

1.21 A prospective study follows subjects to see what happens in the future while a retrospective study looks at what has already happened to the subjects.

1.29 (a) A study where the researcher assigns the units to the treatments or comparison groups; (b) A study where the units come to the researcher already assigned to the treatments or comparison groups.

1.30 The researcher assigns the units to the treatments or comparison groups.

1.31 Experiments can be designed to control for external and confounding factors.

Applied Biostatistics for the Health Sciences. By Richard J. Rossi
Copyright © 2010 by John Wiley & Sons, Inc.

1.33 (a) Not ethical; (b) Ethical; (c) Not ethical; (d) Ethical.

1.38 Phases I, II, and III.

1.39 To further investigate the long-term safety and efficacy of the drug.

1.40 Safety reasons, the drug is clearly beneficial, the drug is clearly not beneficial.

1.41 No.

SOLUTIONS FOR CHAPTER 2

2.1 A quantitative variable takes on numerical values while a qualitative variable takes on nonnumeric values.

2.2 A continuous variable takes on any value in one or more intervals while a discrete variable takes on any value in a finite or countable set.

2.3 The values of a ordinal variable have a natural ordering that is meaningful while the order of the values of a nominal variable do not have any meaning.

2.4 (a) Quantitative; (b) Quantitative; (c) Qualitative; (d) Qualitative; (e) Qualitative.

2.5 (a) Qualitative, nominal; (b) Qualitative, ordinal; (c) Quantitative, discrete; (d) Quantitative, continuous; (e) Quantitative, discrete; (f) Quantitative, continuous; (g) Qualitative, nominal; (h) Quantitative, continuous; (i) Quantitative, discrete; (j) Quantitative, discrete.

2.6 (a) Nominal; (b) Ordinal; (c) Nominal; (d) Ordinal; (e) Nominal; (f) Ordinal; (g) Ordinal.

2.9 (a) D; (b) C; (c) B; (d) E; (e) B; (f) A.

2.10 58.

2.11 (a) Long tailed right; (b) 1; (c) B; (d) 0.

2.12 Modes.

2.13 Subpopulations.

2.14 The proportion of individuals having the disease.

2.17 When the distribution is symmetric.

2.18 (a) Yes; (b) No.

2.19 (a) 35.2%; (b) 26%; (c) 25.6%; (d) 31.2%, 42.8%, 26%; (e) 41–55.

2.21 (a) Mean, median, mode; (b) Vriance, standard deviation, interquartile range.

2.23 (a) 140 to 240; (b) 0.132 or 13.2%.

2.24 (a) 95%; (b) 0.5%; (c) 16%.

2.26 (a) The distribution is highly variable; (b) the distribution has a long tail to the right.

2.27 (a) 0.043 or 4.3%; (b) 0.105 or 10.5%; (c) 0.034 or 3.4%; (d) 0.110 or 11.0%; (e) Males; (f) Females.

2.29 The strength of the linear relationship between two quantitative variables.

2.30 The correlation coefficient is unitless.

2.31 $P(A|B) = P(A)$ or $P(B|A) = P(B)$.

2.32 When A and B are disjoint.

2.33 When A and B are independent.

2.34 (a) 0.064; (b) 0.069; (c) 0.31; (d) 0.353; (e) 0.5.

2.35 (a) 0.6; (b) 0.9; (c) 0.1; (d) 0; (e) 0.

2.36 (a) 0.6; (b) 0.2; (c) 0.8; (d) 0.4; (e) 0.5.

2.37 (a) 0.59; (b) 0.635; (c) 0.825.

2.38 (a) 0.96; (b) 0.926; (c) 0.075.

2.39 (a) 0.033; (b) 0.088; (c) 0.912.

2.40 (a) 0.291; (b) 0.003.

2.41 (a) 0.00015; (b) 0.62742; (c) 0.31019.

2.42 (a) 0.25; (b) 0.75; (c) 0.25.

2.44 (a) $X = 2$; (b) 0.0035; (c) 0.0197; (d) 0.4709.

2.45 (a) $\mu = 20$ and $\sigma = 2$; (b) $\mu = 24$ and $\sigma = 3.1$; (c) $\mu = 5$ and $\sigma = 2.12$.

2.46 (a) $p > 0.5$; (b) $p < 0.05$; (c) $p = 0.5$; (d) $p = 0.5$.

2.47 (a) 0.0000; (b) 0.0046; (c) 0.0060; (d) 10.

2.48 (a) 0.1216; (b) 0.6769.

2.49 (a) 0.0256; (b) 0.4096.

2.51 (a) 0.1869;   (b) 0.9950; (c) 0.80; (d) 0.849.

2.52 (a) 0.7939; (b) 0.9767; (c) 0.0207; (d) 0.4940; (e) 0.9929; (f) 0.0007; (g) 0.8522; (h) 0.0662; (i) 0.0203; (j) 0.9411.

2.53 (a) -1.645; (b) -0.67; (c) 0.67; (d) 2.05; (e) 1.34.

2.54 (a) 0.0038; (b) 0.0918; (c) 0.3231; (d) 124.675.

2.55 (a) 0.0228; (b) 0.0082; (c) 0.8904; (d) 3820.

2.56 (a) 0.0808; (b) 0.0548; (c) 0.9911; (d) 122.8.

2.57 (a) 0.2743; (b) 0.7257; (c) 0.6469; (d) 28.175.

2.58 A z score is unitless.

2.59 1.5.

2.61 (a) -1.645; (b) -1.645 and 1.04; (c) 1.04 and 1.645; (d) 1.645.

2.62 (a) 3.65; (b) 1.68; (c) 10 year old.

2.63 (a) 0.55; (b) 1.00; (c) Female.

SOLUTIONS FOR CHAPTER 3

3.1   The distribution of the sampled units is similar to the distribution of population units.

3.3   A sample is only a subset of the population units.

3.4   A parameter is computed from the entire population of units while a statistic is computed from only a sample of the population units.

3.6   The list of population units available for sampling.

3.7   The sampling frame contains only the population units that are available for sampling.

3.12   No.

3.13   (a) No;   (b) No.

3.15   A well-defined subpopulation.

3.17   (a) Stratified random sample;   (b) Stratified random sample;   (c) Simple random sample;   (d) Simple random sample.

3.18   (a) Systematic random sample;   (b) Stratified random sample;   (c) Simple random sample;   (d) Stratified random sample;   (e) Cluster random sample.

3.19   (a) Systematic random sample;   (b) Cluster random sample;   (c) Cluster random sample;   (d) Stratified random sample.

3.20   In a simple random sample population units are selected while in a cluster random sample clusters of the population units are sampled.

3.22   There is no periodic, systematic, or cyclical pattern in the sampling frame.

3.25   (a) $n = 400$;   (b) $n = 200$;   (c) $n = 50$.

3.26   (a) 250;   (b) 100;   (c) 50;   (d) 25.

3.32   From a pilot study or previous research.

3.33   (a) 250;   (b) 1.25;   (c) 10.

3.36   (a) 1213;   (b) 286;   (c) 7144;   3093.

3.37   (a) $6565;   (b) $1930;   (c) $36,200;   (d) $20,015.

3.38   (a) 1600;   (b) 2500;   (c) 2500;   (d) 3600.

3.39   (a) $26,500;   (b) $40,000;   (c) $40,000;   (d) $56,500.

3.40   (a) 371;   (b) 385;   (c) 1064;   (d) 589.

3.41   (a) 400;   (b) 625;   (c) 1112;   (d) 1600.

3.42   (a) $ 20,500;   (b) $26,125;   (c) $38,300;   (d) $25,225.

3.43   (a) 20;   (b) 400;   (c) $10,500.

3.44   (a) 817;   (b) $44,085.

3.45   Proportional and optimal allocation.

3.47   (a) $w_1 = 0.4$, $w_2 = 0.15$, $w_3 = 0.25$, $w_4 = 0.2$;   (b) $n_1 = 1000$, $n_2 = 38$, $n_3 = 62$, $n_4 = 50$;   (c) \$4086.

3.48   (a) $w_1 = 0.33$, $w_2 = 0..50$, $w_3 = 0.17$;   (b) $n = 555$;   (c) $n_1 = 185$, $n_2 = 278$, $n_3 = 92$;   (c) \$13303.

3.49   (a) $w_1 = 0.24$, $w_2 = 0.59$, $w_3 = 0.17$; (b) $n = 295$; (c) $n_1 = 71$, $n_2 = 174$, $n_3 = 50$.

3.50   (a) $w_1 = 0.18$, $w_2 = 0.82$;   (b) $n = 285$;   (c) $n_1 = 51$, $n_2 = 234$;   (d) \$7850.

3.51   (a) $w_1 = 0.29$, $w_2 = 0.71$;   (b) $n = 279$;   (c) $n_1 = 81$, $n_2 = 198$.

3.52   (a) $w_1 = 0.07$, $w_2 = 0.93$;   (b) $n = 312$;   (c) $n_1 = 22$, $n_2 = 290$;   (d) \$9340.

3.53   (a) $w_1 = 0.15$, $w_2 = 0.85$;   (b) $n = 633$;   (c) $n_1 = 95$, $n_2 = 538$;   (d) \$13,280.

3.54   (a) $n = 233$;   (b) $k = 10$;   (c) \$14,025.

3.55   (a) $n = 376$;   (b) $k = 15$;   (c) \$2558.

3.56   (a) $n = 1575$;   (b) $k = 63$;   (c) \$43,375.

SOLUTIONS FOR CHAPTER 4

4.1   To obtain a sample that is representative of the target population.

4.2   No.

4.3   A parameter is computed from a census of the population while a statistic is computed from a sample.

4.4   No.

4.5   (a) Bar chart, pie chart;   (b) Boxplot, histogram, normal probability plot

4.6   Simple bar chart, side-by-side bar chart, stacked bar chart.

4.7   Proportion, relative frequency, or percentage.

4.8   Side-by-side bar chart,

4.9   (a) Roughly 28%;   (b) Roughly 72%.

4.10   (a) 56.8%;   (b) 25.2%;   (c) 18.0%.

4.11   (a) 10%;   (b) 6%;   (c) 54%.

4.13   The minimum, 25th percentile, median, 75th percentile, and the maxixum of the sample.

4.14   The first, second, and third.

4.15   Any observation that falls more than $1.5 \times \widehat{\text{IQR}}$ below the sample 25th percentile or above the 75th sample percentile.

4.19   (a) Long tail right;   (b) 140;   (c) 40.

4.20   No.

4.21   No.

4.23   Histogram.

4.24   (a) $\mu > \tilde{\mu}$;   (b) $\mu < \tilde{\mu}$.

4.25   (a) 18%;   (b) 0.72% or 0.0072.

4.27   (a) Yes;   (b) Yes.

4.28   (a) Bimodal;   (b) 69 and 21;   (c) No.

4.29   (a) The histogram of the case subjects appears mound shaped, the histogram of the controls appears long tail right;   (b) No;   (c) Case subjects.

4.32   The normal probability plot in (a) supports normality, the normal probability plot in (b) does not.

4.33   (a) Yes;   (b) Yes;   (c) 1.052;   (d) 1.08.

4.34   (a) Yes;   (b) Yes;   (c) 130;   (d) 187.

4.38   (a) 0.01;   (b) 0.62;   (c) 13;   (d) 12.95;   (e) 12.

4.39   (a) 0.90;   (b) 0.93.

4.40   (a) 0.87;   (b) 0.07;   (c) 0.93;   (d) 0.87 and 0.93;   (e) 0.11.

4.41   (a) 0.989;   (b) 0.982.

4.42   1.44.

4.43   1.35.

4.44   Long tail right.

4.46   (a) $\tilde{x}$, $\widehat{IQR}$;   (b) $\bar{x}$, s, s^2.

4.49   (a) No;   (b) Yes;   (c) No;   (d) No;   (e) Yes.

4.50   (a) $\bar{x} = 20.48$, $s^2 = 20.75$, $s = 4.56$, $\widehat{CV} = 0.22$;
(b) $\bar{x} = 120.5$, $s^2 = 225$, $s = 15$, $\widehat{CV} = 0.12$;
(c) $\bar{x} = 0.36$, $s^2 = 0.13$, $s = 0.36$, $\widehat{CV} = 1.00$;
(d) $\bar{x} = 21.9$, $s^2 = 483.79$, $s = 22.00$, $\widehat{CV} = 1.00$.

4.51   No.

4.52   (a) 3.04;   (b) 0.41;   (c) 0.13;   (d) 48.5;   (e) 1.96;   (f) 0.04.

4.53   (a) 6.69, 0.902, 0.13;   (b) 19.09, 0.77, 0.04.

4.54   The coefficient of variation is independent of the units of measurement.

4.58   220 and 30.

4.59   213.375 and 29.412.

4.63 ρ is a parameter and r is a statistic.

4.66   The correlation coefficient is unitless.

4.68   (a) $r > 0$;   (b) $r < 0$;   (c) Nothing;   (d) $r \approx 0$.

4.69   (a) All of the points lie on a line sloping upward;   (b) There is no apparent linear relationship between Y and X;   (c) The points are tightly clustered around a line sloping upward;   (d) The points are tightly clustered around a line sloping downward.

4.70   (a) Yes;   (b) $\widehat{y} = 42.12 - 1.72X$.

SOLUTIONS FOR CHAPTER 5

5.1   The probability distribution of the statistic for all possible samples of size n that can be drawn from a particular target population.

5.4   The mean of the sampling distribution is the parameter that the estimator estimates on the average and the standard deviation of the sampling distribution measures the precision of the estimator.

5.5 $\text{Bias}(T) = 0$ or T does not systematically over or under estimate θ on the average.

5.6 $\bar{x}, s^2, \widehat{p}$.

5.7 $\text{Bias}(T, \theta) = \mu_T - \theta$.

5.8   (a) T tends to over estimate θ;   (b) T tends to under estimate θ;   (c) T is unbiased.

5.9   The standard error of a statistic is the standard deviation of the sampling distribution of the statistic.

5.11   Mean squared error.

5.12 $\text{MSE}(T, \theta) = \text{SE}(T)^2 + \text{Bias}(T, \theta)^2$.

5.13   MSE includes the bias.

5.14 $\text{SE}(T) = \sqrt{\text{MSE}(T, \theta)}$ when T is unbiased.

5.15   (a) Yes;   (b) Yes;   (c) T_1.

5.16   (a) -0.02θ;   (b) 0;   (c) $25.0004\theta^2$;   (d) $30.25\theta^2$;   (e) T_1.

5.18 $B = 2 \times \text{SE}$.

5.20   (a) 68%;   (b) 95%;   (c) 95%.

5.22 $f\text{pc} = \sqrt{\frac{N-n}{N-1}}$, use when $\frac{n}{N} \geq 0.05$.

5.23 p and $\sqrt{\frac{N-n}{N-1}} \times \sqrt{\frac{p(1-p)}{n}}$.

5.24   Yes.

5.27   (a) 0.033, 0.066;   (b) 0.033, 0.066;   (c) 0.010, 0.020;   (d) 0.006, 0.012;   (e) 0.009, 0.018.

5.28   (b) 0.034;   (e) 0.009.

5.29 $p = 0.4$.

5.30   (a) 0.047;   (b) 0.018;   (c) 0.015;   (d) 0.018;   (e) 0.010.

5.31   0.056.

5.32 (a) 0.30; (b) 0.008; (c) 0.284 to 0.316; (d) No.

5.33 (a) 0.22; (b) 0.018; (c) 0.184 to 0.256; (d) No.

5.34 (a) 0.81; (b) 0.078; (c) 0.67; (d) 0.093; (e) No.

5.35 (a) 286; (b) 1213; (c) 702; (d) 625; 1112.

5.36 (a) $3930; (b) $8564; (c) $6010; (d) $5625; (e) $8069.

5.39 (a) 0.2358; (b) 0.3328; (c) 0.7698.

5.40 (a) 0.8664; (b) 0.9876.

5.41 μ and $\sqrt{\frac{N-n}{N-1}} \times \frac{\sigma}{\sqrt{n}}$.

5.42 Yes.

5.45 (a) 0.480, 0.96; (b) 2.08, 4.16; (c) 1.18, 2.36; (d) 11.90, 23.80; (e) 0.05, 0.10.

5.46 (a) 0.50; (b) 2.23; (c) 1.26; (d) 12.91; (e) 0.05.

5.47 (a) 100; (b) 65.

5.48 (a) 2.37; (b) 2.64; (c) 0.027; (d) 5.28; (e) 0.24.

5.49 (a) 0.32; (b) 0,64; (c) 0.29; (d) 0.58.

5.50 (a) 0.73; (b) 1.46; (c) 0.71; (d) 1.42.

5.51 (a) 385; (b) 763; (c) 2927; (d) 196; (e) 1296.

5.52 (a) $ 13,770; (b) $22,086; (c) $69,694; (d) $9612; (e) $33,812.

5.55 (a) 0.8164; (b) 0.9412.

5.56 0.6826.

5.57 (a) 0.6826; (b) 0.9010; (c) 0.9544; (d) 0.9974.

5.59 t distribution with $n - 1$ degrees of freedom.

5.60 Approaches a Z distribution.

5.61 $p_X - p_Y$ and $\sqrt{\frac{p_X(1-p_X)}{n_X} + \frac{p_Y(1-p_Y)}{n_Y}}$.

5.64 (a) 0.073; (b) 0.090; (c) 0.066.

5.65 (a) 0.146; (b) 0.180; (c) 0.132.

5.66 (a) 0.369; (b) 0.137; (c) 0.232; (d) 0.066; (e) 0.132.

5.67 (a) 50, 50; (b) 45, 55; (c) 50, 50.

5.68 (a) $2150; (b) $2165; (c) $2150.

5.69 (a) $n = 2071, n_X = 986, n_Y = 1085$; (b) $n = 1735, n_X = 902, n_Y = 833$; (c) $n = 2500, n_X = 1250, n_Y = 1250$.

5.70 (a) $26,450; (b) $22,550; (c) $32,050.

5.71 (a) $n = 202, n_X = 106, n_Y = 96$; (b) $n = 78, n_X = 36, n_Y = 42$; (c) $n = 250, n_X = n_Y = 125$.

5.72   (a) $n = 1887, n_X = 941, n_Y = 946$;   (b) $n = 924, n_X = 527, n_Y = 397$;   (c) $n = 5833, n_X = 2546, n_Y = 3287$.

5.73 $\mu_X - \mu_Y$ and $\sqrt{\frac{\sigma_X^2}{n_X} + \frac{\sigma_Y^2}{n_Y}}$.

5.76   (a) 0.95;   (b) 3.32;   (c) 77.79.

5.77   (a) 1.90;   (b) 6.64;   (c) 155.58.

5.78   (a) −0.61;   (b) 0.20;   (c) 0.40.

5.79   (a) $n_X = 143, n_Y = 107$;   (b) $n_X = 114, n_Y = 136$.

5.80   (a) \$6072;   (b) \$5956.

5.81   (a) $n = 441, n_X = 126, n_Y = 315$;   (b) $n = 502, n_X = 179, n_Y = 323$.

5.82   (a) \$5310;   (b) \$5674.

5.83   (a) $n = 324, n_X = 175, n_Y = 149$;   (b) $n = 153, n_X = 147, n_Y = 106$.

5.84   (a) $n = 470, n_X = 233, n_Y = 237$;   (b) $n = 180, n_X = 78, n_Y = 102$.

SOLUTIONS FOR CHAPTER 6

6.1   An estimator than produces an interval of estimates.

6.2 $T \pm B$.

6.3   An interval estimator that captures the true value of the parameter of interest with a prespecified probability.

6.4 $(1 - \alpha) \times 100\%$.

6.5   The confidence level.

6.7   (a) 0.95;   (b) 0 or 1.

6.9   95%.

6.10   50.

6.11   118 to 129.

6.14 $\widehat{p} \pm z_{\text{crit}} \times se(\widehat{p})$.

6.15   (a) 1.645;   (b) 2.576.

6.17   (a) 0.46 to 0.66;   (b) 0.12 to 0.30;   (c) 0.81 to 0.95;   (d) 0.95 to 0.97.

6.18   (a) 406;   (b) 801;   (c) 1037;   (d) 1537.

6.19   (a) \$2830;   (b) \$4805;   (c) \$5985;   (d) \$8485.

6.21   (a) 1.282;   (b) 1.645.

6.22   (a) $p \geq 0.55$;   (b) $p \geq 0.80$;   (c) $p \leq 0.13$;   (d) $p \leq 0.25$.

6.23   (a) 384;   (b) 415;   (c) 1503;   (d) 1083.

6.24   (a) \$4980;   (b) \$5212.5;   (c) \$13,372.5;   (d) \$10,222.5.

6.25 0.11 to 0.31.

6.26 0.23 to 0.29.

6.28 (a) $t_{crit} \times se(\bar{x})$; (b) $z_{crit} \times se(\bar{x})$.

6.31 (a) 1.645; (b) 1.96; (c) 2.576.

6.32 (a) 26.1 to 28.5; (b) 119.5 to 124.3; (c) 4.24 to 4.36.

6.33 (a) 33.2 to 34.4; (b) 477.4 to 518.8; (c) 102.9 to 105.7.

6.34 (a) 31.1 to 36.5; (b) 999.3 to 1103.1; (c) 0.32 to 0.36.

6.35 (a) $\mu \geq 105.0$; (b) $\mu \geq 48.1$.

6.36 (a) $\mu \leq 78.6$; (b) $\mu \leq 91.3$.

6.37 (a) 1.699; (b) 2.093; (c) 2.064; (d) 2.947.

6.38 (a) 1.671; (b) 2.000; (c) 1.96.

6.39 A normal probability plot.

6.40 (a) Yes; (b) No.

6.41 (a) 68.3 to 87.3; (b) 19.9 to 23.9; (c) 192.1 to 216.5.

6.42 (a) 112 to 142; (b) 48.2 to 54.6; (c) 2.1 to 2.5.

6.43 (a) $\mu \geq 20.6$; (b) $\mu \geq 219.9$; (c) $\mu \leq 1334.0$; (d) $\mu \leq 27.1$.

6.44 (a) $\mu \geq 46.0$; (b) $\mu \geq 784.5$; (c) $\mu \geq 13.2$.

6.45 (a) $\mu \leq 3.01$; (b) $\mu \leq 98.7$ (c) $\mu \leq 1.34$.

6.48 3.91 to 4.77.

6.50 (a) 171; (b) 97; (c) 385; (d) 43.

6.51 (a) 121; (b) 68; (c) 423; (d) 31.

6.52 (a) 121; (b) 68.

6.53 (a) 106; (b) 68.

6.57 18 to 67.

6.60 (a) No; (b) Yes; (c) Yes.

6.63 (a) -0.23 to 0.09; (b) -0.05 to 0.19; (c) -0.15 to 0.09; (d) -0.16 to -0.02.

6.64 (a) No; (b) No; (c) No; (d) Yes.

6.65 (a) $p_X - p_Y \geq -0.21$; (b) $p_X - p_Y \geq 0.04$; (c) $p_X - p_Y \leq 0.04$; (d) $p_X - p_Y \leq -0.02$.

6.66 (a) 829; (b) 588; (c) 846.

6.67 (a) 961; (b) 1105; (c) 1201.

6.68 (a) 762; (b) 673; (c) 846.

6.69 (a) 724; (b) 724; (c) 846.

6.70 (a) 0.07 to 0.11; (b) Yes; (c) -0.44 to 0.004; (d) No.

6.71 (a) 0.14 to 0.36.

6.74 0 and ∞.

6.77 (a) 4.88; (b) 1.41; (c) 2.92 to 5.75.

6.78 (a) 2.24; (b) 0.099; (c) 1.84 to 2.72.

SOLUTIONS FOR CHAPTER 7

7.1 The null and alternative hypotheses. The research hypothesis is the alternative hypothesis.

7.3 (a) By rejecting a true null hypothesis; (b) By failing to reject a false null hypothesis.

7.5 (a) 0.05; (b) Reject H_0; (c) Yes, a Type I error.

7.6 (a) No error; (b) Type I error; (c) Type II error; (d) No error.

7.11 When β is known and is small.

7.12 $1 - \beta(\theta)$.

7.14 $1 - \beta(\theta)$.

7.16 (a) Reliable, unreliable; (b) Unreliable, reliable; (c) Reliable, reliable; (d) Reliable, unreliable; (e) Unreliable, reliable; (f) Reliable, reliable.

7.17 (a) Nothing; (b) β decreases; (c) The power increases.

7.27 (a) Fail to reject H_0; (b) Reject H_0; (c) Reject H_0; (d) Fail to reject H_0; (e) Fail to reject H_0; (f) Fail to reject H_0.

7.29 $H_0 : p \leq p_0$ versus $H_A : p > p_0$; $H_0 : p \geq p_0$ versus $H_A : p < p_0$; $H_0 : p = p_0$ versus $H_A : p \neq p_0$.

7.31 $np_0 \geq 5$ and $n(1 - p_0) \geq 5$.

7.32 (a) Yes; (b) No; (c) Yes; (d) No; (e) Yes; (f) No.

7.33 $\dfrac{\widehat{p} - p_0}{\sqrt{\dfrac{p_0(1-p_0)}{n}}}$.

7.35 (a) $z < -z_{\text{crit}}$; (b) $z > z_{\text{crit}}$; (c) $|z| > z_{\text{crit}}$.

7.36 (a) -1.645; (b) -2.326.

7.37 (a) 1.645; (b) 2.326.

7.38 (a) 1.96; (b) 2.576.

7.39 (a) $z_{\text{obs}} > 1.645$; (b) $z_{\text{obs}} < -2.326$; (c) $z_{\text{obs}} < -2.326$; (d) $|z_{\text{obs}}| > 1.96$; (e) $|z_{\text{obs}}| > 1.96$; (f) $z > 1.282$.

7.40 (a) 0.2302; (b) 0.0014; (c) 0.1292; (d) 0.0048; (e) 0.0174; (f) 0.0026.

7.41 (a) Reject H_0 for parts b, d, e, and f; (b) Reject H_0 in parts b, d, and f.

7.42   (a) $|z_{obs}| > 1.96$, $z_{obs} = -0.58$, $p = 0.5620$, Fail to reject H_0.
        (b) $z_{obs} < -1.645$, $z_{obs} = -1.73$, $p = 0.0418$, Reject H_0.
        (c) $z_{obs} > 1.645$, $z_{obs} = 1.00$, $p = 0.1587$, Fail to reject H_0.
        (d) $|z_{obs}| > 2.576$, $z_{obs} = 6.00$, $p = 0.000$, Reject H_0.
        (e) $z_{obs} > 1.645$, $z_{obs} = 1.29$, $p = 0.0985$, Fail to reject H_0.

7.44   (a) 335; (b) 845; (c) 498; (d) 2954; (e) 298; (f) 992.

7.50   (a) $z_{obs} > 1.45$; (b) $z_{obs} > 2.326$; (c) $z_{obs} < -1.645$; (d) $z_{obs} < -2.326$; (e) $|z_{obs}| > 1.96$; (f) $|z_{obs}| > 2.576$.

7.51   (a) 0.0118; (b) 0.0015; (c) 0.0838.

7.52   (a) Fail to reject H_0; (b) Reject H_0; (c) Fail to reject H_0.

7.53   (a) 0.52; (b) 0.14; (c) 0.22.

7.54   (a) $|z_{obs}| > 1.96$, $z_{obs} = -0.85$, $p = 0.3954$, Fail to reject.
        (b) $z_{obs} > 2.326$, $z_{obs} = 2.23$, $p = 0.0129$, Fail to reject.
        (c) $z_{obs} < -1.645$, $z_{obs} = -3.40$, $p = 0.0003$, Reject.
        (d) $|z_{obs}| > 2.576$, $z_{obs} = -1.32$, $p = 0.1868$, Fail to reject.
        (e) $z_{obs} > 1.645$, $z_{obs} = 2.53$, $p = 0.0057$, Reject.

7.56   (a) 1796; (b) 542; (c) 429; (d) 542; (e) 1714; (f) 10710.

7.57   (a) 0.396; (b) 0.376; (c) Fail to reject; (d) 0.7872; (e) -0.12 to 0.16.

7.58   (a) Reject; (b) 0; (c) 0.22 to 0.36.

7.59   (a) Fail to reject; (b) 0.0108; (c) -0.19 to -0.03.

7.60   (a) Reject; (b) 0.0138; (c) -0.23 to -0.03.

7.61   (a) Fail to reject; (b) 0.234.

7.65 H_0: The two variables are independent; H_A: The two variables are not independent.

7.68 $X^2 > \chi^2_{crit}$ with 1 degree of freedom.

7.69   1.

7.70   (a) $X^2 > 6.63$; (b) $X^2 > 3.84$.

7.71   (a) Yes; (b) Reject; (c) 0.16 to 0.24.

7.72   (a) Yes; (b) Reject.

7.73   (a) Yes; (b) Reject.

7.77 $X^2 > \chi^2_{crit}$ with $(r-1)(c-1)$ degrees of freedom.

7.78   2.

7.79   8.

7.80   12.

7.81   (a) $X^2 > 16.81$; (b) $X^2 > 12.59$.

7.82   (a) $X^2 > 13.28$; (b) $X^2 > 9.49$.

7.83   (a) $X^2 > 21.67$; (b) $X^2 > 16.92$.

7.84 (a) Yes; (b) Fail to reject.

7.85 (a) Yes; (b) Reject.

7.86 (a) Yes; (b) Reject.

7.87 $\dfrac{T - \theta}{\text{se}(T)}$.

7.88 (a) $H_0 : \mu \geq \mu_0$, $H_A : \mu < \mu_0$; (b) $H_0 : \mu = \mu_0$, $H_A : \mu \neq \mu_0$; (c) $H_0 : \mu \leq \mu_0$, $H_A : \mu > \mu_0$.

7.89 (a) $t_{\text{obs}} < -1.725$; (b) $t_{\text{obs}} > 2.485$; (c) $|t_{\text{obs}}| > 2.179$.

7.90 (a) 0.010; (b) 0.009; (c) 0.002; (d) 0.002; (e) < 0.001.

7.91 $\dfrac{\bar{x} - \mu_0}{\frac{s}{\sqrt{n}}}$.

7.93 (a) $t_{\text{obs}} < -1.701$; (b) $t_{\text{obs}} > 2.518$; (c) $|t_{\text{pbs}}| > 2.000$; (d) $|t_{\text{obs}}| > 1.96$.

7.94 No.

7.96 (a) $|t_{\text{obs}}| > 2.074$, $t_{\text{obs}} = -7.19$, Reject, $p < 0.001$.
(b) $t_{\text{obs}} > 1.697$, $t_{\text{obs}} = 3.44$, Reject, $p < 0.001$.
(c) $t_{\text{obs}} < -2.492$, $t_{\text{obs}} = -3.36$, Reject, $p < 0.001$.
(d) $|t_{\text{obs}}| > 2.000$, $t_{\text{obs}} = 2.01$, Reject, $p < 0.050$.

7.97 (a) 66; (b) 253; (c) 24; (d) 44.

7.99 Matched pairs and within-subject sampling.

7.100 $\dfrac{\bar{d}}{\frac{s_d}{\sqrt{n}}}$.

7.102 (a) $t_{\text{obs}} < -1/701$; (b) $t_{\text{obs}} > 2.518$; (c) $|t_{\text{obs}}| > 2.000$; (d) $|t_{\text{obs}}| > 1.96$.

7.103 Yes.

7.104 (a) $|t_{\text{obs}}| > 2.064$, $t_{\text{obs}} = 1.98$, Fail to reject, $p = 0.056$.
(b) $|t_{\text{obs}}| > 2.750$, $t_{\text{obs}} = 2.07$, Fail to reject, $p = 0.044$.
(c) $t_{\text{obs}} > 2.086$, $t_{\text{obs}} = 2.67$, Reject, $p = 0.007$.
(d) $t_{\text{obs}} < -2.064$, $t_{\text{obs}} = -3.70$, Reject, $p < 0.001$.

7.106 (a) 52; (b) 116; (c) 52; (d) 68.

7.110 $\dfrac{\bar{x} - \bar{y}}{\text{se}(\bar{x} - \bar{y})}$.

7.112 $\sqrt{\dfrac{s_x^2}{n_X} + \dfrac{s_y^2}{n_Y}}$.

7.115 $0.5 \leq \frac{s_x}{s_y} \leq 2$.

7.116 (a) $s_P = \sqrt{\dfrac{(n_X - 1)s_x^2 + (n_Y - 1)s_Y^2}{n_X + n_Y - 2}}$; (b) $\text{se}(\bar{x} - \bar{y}) = \sqrt{S_p^2 \left(\frac{1}{n_X} + \frac{1}{n_Y} \right)}$;
(c) $n_X + n_Y - 2$.

7.117 (a) Yes; (b) Yes; (c) No; (d) No.

7.118   (a) 45/09; (b) 2.65; (c) 9.07; (d) 0.12.

7.120   (a) $|t_{\text{obs}}| > 2.485$; (b) $|t_{\text{obs}}| > 1.96$; (c) $t_{\text{obs}} < -2.423$; (d) $t_{\text{obs}} > 1.671$.

7.121   (a) Yes; (b) 136.47; (c) Reject; (d) $p < 0.001$; (e) 329 to 871.

7.122   (a) Yes; (b) 1.55; (c) Reject; (d) $p < 0.001$; (e) 5.09 to 11.51.

7.123   (a) Yes; (b) 1.10; (c) Reject; (d) $p < 0.001$; (e) -8.23 to -3.77.

7.124   (a) Yes; (b) 0.08; (c) Reject; (d) $p = 0.000$; (e) -0.46 to -0.14.

7.125   (a) Yes; (b) 66.11; (c) Fail to reject;   (d) $p > 0.096$; (e) -224.6 to 41.6.

7.127   (a) $n_X = n_Y = 68$; (b) $n_X = n_Y = 20$; (c) $n_X = n_Y = 49$; (d) $n_X = n_Y = 54$;
 (e) $n_X = n_Y = 208$; (f) $n_X = n_Y = 27$.

SOLUTIONS FOR CHAPTER 8

8.1   Simple linear regression model.

8.2   Linear sloping upward, linear sloping downward, curvilinear, or no pattern.

8.3   The linear relationship between two quantitative variables.

8.4 ρ is a parameter while r is a statistic.

8.6   (a) b, d; (b) a, c; (c) b; (d) a.

8.8   (a) Weak positive; (b) Very strong positive; (c) No obvious linear relationship;
 (d) Strong positive; (e) Moderate negative;   (f) No obvious linear relationship.

8.10   There may be a nonlinear relationship.

8.11   (a) Decrease; (b) Increase.

8.14 $y = \beta_0 + \beta_1 x$.

8.15 $y = \beta_0 + \beta_1 x + \epsilon$.

8.16 β_0, β_1.

8.21   Constant variance.

8.24   (a) $\widehat{\beta}_0 = \bar{y} - \widehat{\beta}_1 \bar{x}$; (b) $\widehat{\beta}_1 = r \times \frac{s_x}{s_y}$; (c) $\widehat{y} = \widehat{\beta}_0 + \widehat{\beta}_1 x$.

8.25 β_0 is a parameter and $\widehat{\beta}_0$ is a statistic.

8.26 β_1 is a parameter and $\widehat{\beta}_1$ is a statistic.

8.27   (a) $\widehat{\beta}_0 = 53.56, \widehat{\beta}_1 = 2.01$; (b) $\widehat{\beta}_0 = 162.00, \widehat{\beta}_1 = -1.57$.

8.29   (a) Moderate; (b) $\widehat{\beta}_1 = 44.595$; (c) $\widehat{\beta}_0 = -112.92$; (d) 44.595.

8.30 $e = y - \widehat{y}$.

8.31 A residual divided by its standard deviation.

8.33 According to the three standard deviation Empirical Rule only 1% of the standardized residuals should fall below -3 or above 3.

8.34 A plot of the standardized residuals versus either the fitted values or the X values.

8.36 (a) No obvious pattern; (b) Funneling pattern; (c) Curvilinear pattern; (d) A standardizes residual will be greater than 3 or less than -3.

8.37 The model does not fit this observation very well.

8.40 Natural logarithm.

8.41 Examine a normal probability plot of the standardized residuals and apply the fat pencil test.

8.43 (a) No; (b) Yes.

8.46 $s_e = \sqrt{\text{MSE}}$.

8.47 $s_e = \sqrt{\dfrac{\sum e^2}{n-2}}$.

8.48 $n - 2$.

8.49 (a) $\sum (y - \bar{y})^2$; (b) $\text{sum}(\widehat{y} - \bar{y})^2$; (c) $\text{sum}(y - \widehat{y})^2$; (d) $\dfrac{\text{SSReg}}{\text{SSTot}}$.

8.51 (a) 0.75; (b) 0.625.

8.52 (a) 0.6084; (b) 0.2025.

8.53 (a) -0.923; (b) 0.773.

8.56 $H_0 : Y = \beta_0 + \epsilon$, $H_A : Y = \beta_0 + \beta_1 X + \epsilon$.

8.59 (a) $\beta_1 \neq 0$; (b) $\beta_1 = 0$.

8.60 $\text{SSReg} = 310$, $\text{MSReg} = 310$, $\text{df}_{\text{err}} = 117$, $\text{MSE} = 20.94$, $F_{\text{obs}} = 14.8$.

8.61 (a) 1.64; (b) Yes; (c) 0.09; (d) 9%; (e) $r = -0.30$.

8.64 (a) $\dfrac{\widehat{\beta_0}}{\text{se}(\widehat{\beta_0})}$; (b) $\dfrac{\widehat{\beta_1}}{\text{se}(\widehat{\beta_1})}$; (c) $\dfrac{\widehat{\beta_0} - 10}{\text{se}(\widehat{\beta_0})}$; (d) $\dfrac{\widehat{\beta_1} - 2}{\text{se}(\widehat{\beta_1})}$.

8.65 (a) $t_{\text{obs}} > t_{\text{crit}}$; (b) $|t_{\text{obs}}| > t_{\text{crit}}$; (c) $t_{\text{obs}} < -t_{\text{crit}}$.

8.66 (a) $\widehat{\beta_0} \pm t_{\text{crit}} \times \text{se}(\widehat{\beta_0})$; (b) $\widehat{\beta_1} \pm t_{\text{crit}} \times \text{se}(\widehat{\beta_1})$.

8.67 (a) -17.30 to -7.4; (b) 1276.9 to 1898.7.

8.68 (a) -5.35 to -2.38; (b) 26.9 to 119.3.

8.69 (a) Yes; (b) Yes.

8.70 (a) Reject; (b) Fail to reject; (c) Reject; (d) Reject.

8.72 (a) Reject; (b) $p < 0.001$; (c) 97.2 to 156.8.

8.73 (a) $\widehat{\beta}_0 = -110$, $\widehat{\beta}_1 = 4.86$, se$(\widehat{\beta}_0) = 10.46$, se$(\widehat{\beta}_1) = 0.1754$;
(b) $\widehat{y} = -110 + 4.86$Thigh; (c) 14.5870; (d) 75.5%; (e) Reject; (f) 4.52 to 5.2;
(g) $r = 0.869$.

8.74 (a) $\widehat{\beta}_0 = -53.813$, $\widehat{\beta}_1 = 0.73033$, se$(\widehat{\beta}_0) = 5.775$, se$(\widehat{\beta}_1) = 0.05766$;
(b) $\widehat{y} = -53.8 + 0.73$Hip; (c) 6.54; (d) 0.391%; (e) 39.1%; (f) Reject;
(g) 4.52 to 5.2.

8.78 Estimating $\mu_{Y|X=x_0}$ and predicting the value of Y when $X = x_0$.

8.79 (a) $\widehat{\mu}_{Y|X=x_0} = \widehat{\beta}_0 + \widehat{\beta}_1 x_0$; (b) $\widehat{Y}_{X=x_0} = \widehat{\beta}_0 + \widehat{\beta}_1 x_0$.

8.81 $\text{pe}(\widehat{y}_{x_0}) = \sqrt{s_e^2 + \text{se}(\widehat{\mu}_{Y|X=x_0})}$.

8.83 Gets wider.

8.84 Gets wider.

8.85 $\text{pe}(\widehat{y}_{x_0}) \geq \text{se}(\widehat{\mu}_{Y|X=x_0})$.

8.86 (a) 91.65 to 93.71; (b) 5.22; (c) 82.45 to 102.91.

8.87 (a) 84.499 to 86.737; (b) 92.629 to 94.353.

8.88 (a) 6.95; (b) 71.996 to 99.24; (c) 6.94; (d) 79.889 to 107.093.

SOLUTIONS FOR CHAPTER 9

9.1 A data set with two or more variables measured on each unit sampled.

9.2 Pairwise scatterplots.

9.3 $Y = \beta_0 + \beta_1 X_1 + \beta_2 X_2 + \cdots + \beta_p X_p + \epsilon$.

9.4 $Y = \beta_0 + \beta_1 X + \beta_2 X^2 + \epsilon$.

9.5 (a) $\beta_0, \beta_1, \beta_2, \ldots, \beta_p$; (b) $\beta_0, \beta_1, \beta_2, \ldots, \beta_p$; (c) $\beta_1, \beta_2, \ldots, \beta_p$.

9.6 (a) β_1; (b) β_2; (c) $\beta_1 + \beta_2$.

9.7 (a) Linear; (b) Nonlinear; (c) Linear; (d) Nonlinear; (e) Nonlinear.

9.9 Multiple regression has a collinearity assumption.

9.11 (a) $\beta_0 + 3\beta_1 + 10\beta_2 + 2\beta_3$; (b) $\beta_0 + 5\beta_2 + 10\beta_3$.

9.13 No.

9.15 Yes.

9.16 Examine VIF values and pairwise correlations.

9.17 VIF ≥ 10 indicates a possible collinearity problem.

9.18 X_2 and X_3.

9.19 Yes.

9.20 (a) $y - \widehat{y}$; (b) A residual divided by its standard deviation.

9.22 $|e_s| > 3$.

9.23 The model does not fit this observation very well.

9.27 (a) Nonconstant variance; (b) Natural logarithm of Y.

9.28 (a) Curvilinear relationship; (b) X^2.

9.29 (a) Curvilinear pattern; (b) 6.66; (c) 0.64.

9.30 Examine a normal probability plot and apply the fat pencil test.

9.31 Confidence intervals and hypothesis tests.

9.32 Yes.

9.33 Cook's distance.

9.34 1.

9.40 $s_e = \sqrt{\dfrac{\sum e^2}{n - p - 1}}.$

9.41 $n - p - 1$.

9.42 $R^2 = \dfrac{\text{SSReg}}{\text{SSTot}}.$

9.44 $R^2_{\text{adj}} = 1 - \dfrac{\text{MSE}}{\text{MSTot}}.$

9.45 R^2_{adj} penalizes a model for including uninformative variables.

9.47 (a) 0.79; (b) 0.66; (c) 0.78; (d) 0.57.

9.48 (a) SSRe = 1632, $\text{df}_{\text{reg}} = 4$, MSReg = 408, $\text{df}_{\text{err}} = 120$, MSE = 50.42, $F_{\text{obs}} = 8.09$; (b) 7.10; (c) $R^2 = 0.21$ and $R^2_{\text{adj}} = 0.19$.

9.50 $H_0 : \beta_1 = \beta_2 = \cdots = \beta_p = 0$ and H_A: At least one of the regression slopes is not 0.

9.53 (a) Reject; (b) Reject.

9.54 An unimportant variable is being included in the model.

9.55 (a) t distribution with $n - p - 1$ degrees of freedom; (b) Standard normal distribution.

9.56 (a) $\widehat{\beta}_i \pm t_{\text{crit}} \times \text{se}(\widehat{\beta}_i)$; (b) $t = \dfrac{\widehat{\beta}_i}{\text{se}(\widehat{\beta}_i)}$; (c) $F = \dfrac{\text{MSReg}}{\text{MSE}}.$

9.57 (a) Reject; (b) 0.0144; (c) Reject; (d) 0.0057 to 0.0231.

9.58 (a) No; (b) Reject; (c) 0.00005135; (d) Reject; (e) 0.000033 to 0.000069; (f) S.

9.60 Estimating the mean value of Y when $X = x_0$ and predicting the value of Y when $X = x_0$.

9.61 $\text{pe}(Y_{X=\vec{x}}) = \sqrt{s_e^2 + \text{se}(\widehat{\mu}_{Y|X=\vec{x}})}.$

9.62 (a) 8.6; (b) 6.0 to 11.2; (c) 8.6; (d) 5.7 to 11.5.

9.63 (a) 7.11; (b) 5.74 to 8.48; (c) 7.11; (d) 4.51 to 9.77.

9.65 Extra sums of squares F-test.

9.66 Fail to reject.

9.67 Fail to reject.

9.70 A binary variable taking on the values 0 and 1.

9.71 (a) 3; (b) 4; (c) 2.

9.73 (a) $Y = \beta_0 + \beta_1 X_1 + \beta_2 X_2 + \beta_3 X_3 + \beta_4 Z + \epsilon$.
(b) $Y = \beta_0 + \beta_1 X_1 + \beta_2 X_2 + \beta_3 X_3 + \beta_4 Z + \beta_5 X_1 Z + \beta_6 X_2 Z + \beta_7 X_3 Z + \epsilon$.

9.74 (a) $Y = \beta_0 + \beta_1 Z_1 + \beta_2 Z_2 + \beta_3 X + \beta_4 Z_1 X + \beta_5 Z_2 X + \epsilon$; (b) $\beta_3 + \beta_4 + \beta_5$;
(c) β_3; (d) $\beta_3 + \beta_4$.

9.75 (a) $\widehat{y} = 10.2 + 4.5x$; (b) $\widehat{y} = 8.1 + 5.6x$; (c) 2.3.

9.77 (a) No; (b) No; (c) Not with the given information; (d) CCI score and TUGA.

9.78 (a) No; (b) No; (c) No; (d) Extra sums of squares F-test.

9.79 (a) Fail to reject; (b) 3.34.

9.80 R^2_{adj} and BIC.

9.85 $\text{BIC} = n \ln \left[\frac{\text{SSE}}{n} \right] + (k + 1) \ln(n)$ and $\text{BIC} = n \ln \left[\frac{n-k-1}{n} \times s^2_e \right] + (k + 1) \ln(n)$.

9.86 (a) The model with all 10 variables; (b) The model with X_2, X_4, X_5, X_6, X_9, and X_{10}.

SOLUTIONS FOR CHAPTER 10

10.1 A binary variable can only take on the values 0 and 1.

10.2 Linear regression is used to model a quantitative response variable while logistic regression is used to model a dichotomous qualitative variable.

10.3 $Z = \begin{cases} 1 & \text{when BMI} \geq 30 \\ 0 & \text{when BMI} < 30 \end{cases}$

10.4 $\dfrac{P(Y = 1)}{P(Y = 0)}$

10.5 (a) The event $Y = 1$ is five times as likely as the event $Y = 0$; (b) $\frac{5}{6}$.

10.6 (a) 1; (b) 4; (c) 0.111; (d) 9; (e) 4; (f) 0.515.

10.7 $\dfrac{\text{odds}(Y = 1 | X = x_1)}{\text{odds}(Y = 1 | X = x_2)}$.

10.9 3.

10.10 9.

10.11 (a) 0.2; (b) 0.068; (c) 2.94.

10.12 (a) 0.43; (b) 0.08; (c) 2.25.

10.13 5.89.

10.15 $\text{logit}(p) = \ln \left(\frac{p}{1-P} \right)$.

10.16 (a) -1.10; (b) 2.20.

10.17 (a) $\text{logit}(p) = \beta_0 + \beta_1 X$.
(b) $\text{logit}(p) = \beta_0 + \beta_1 X_1 + \beta_2 X_2 + \beta_3 X_3$.
(c) $\text{logit}(p) = \beta_0 + \beta_1 Z + \beta_2 X + \beta_3 X Z$.
(d) $\text{logit}(p) = \beta_0 + \beta_1 Z_1 + \beta_2 Z_2 + \beta_3 X + \beta_4 X Z_1 + \beta_5 X Z_2$.

10.18 (a) $\beta_0 + \beta_1 X_1 + \beta_2 X_2 + \cdots + \beta_p X_p$; (b) $\dfrac{e^{\beta_0 + \beta_1 X_1 + \beta_2 X_2 + \cdots + \beta_p X_p}}{1 + e^{\beta_0 + \beta_1 X_1 + \beta_2 X_2 + \cdots + \beta_p X_p}}$.

10.19 (a) 0.45; (b) 0.029; (c) Decreases; (d) 15.52.

10.23 By examining the VIF values and pairwise correlations.

10.24 $\text{Var}(Y|\vec{X}) = \sigma^2 \times p(\vec{X})(1 - p(\vec{X}))$ and $\sigma^2 > 1$.

10.25 Maximum likelihood estimation.

10.28 1.138.

10.29 (a) 0.059; (b) 0.846; (c) 1.06; (d) 1.34.

10.30 (a) $\text{logit}(p) = -0.768 - 0.075X$; (b) No evidence of lack of fit; (c) 0.93; (d) 0.242.

10.31 (a) $\text{logit}(p) = -1.761 - 0.086X_1 + 0.032X_2$; (b) No evidence of lack of fit; (c) 1.03; (d) 0.010.

10.35 $\Delta\chi^2$ and $\Delta\beta$.

10.38 (a) $\widehat{\beta}_1 \pm z_{\text{crit}} \times \text{se}(\widehat{\beta}_1)$; (b) $e^{\widehat{\beta}_1 - z_{\text{crit}} \times \text{se}(\widehat{\beta}_1)}$ to $e^{\widehat{\beta}_1 + z_{\text{crit}} \times \text{se}(\widehat{\beta}_1)}$.

10.39 (a) 1.19 to 2.69; (b) 0.07 to 0.36.

10.40 (a) $z_{\text{obs}} = 2.76$, Reject, $p = 0.0058$; (b) $z_{\text{obs}} = -4.46$, Reject, $p = 0.0000$.

10.41 (a) No evidence of lack of fit; (b) Significant; (c) HRA; (d) 1.01 to 1.05.

10.42 (a) No evidence of lack of fit; (b) Significant; (c) No; (d) 0.975 to 0.998.

10.43 (a) No; (b) No; (c) Male sex, Race-white, Race-hispanic, Race-other, Diabetes duration.

10.45 deviance $= -2 \times$ loglikelihood.

10.47 3.

10.48 Reject.

10.49 Fail to reject.

10.54 $\text{BIC} = \text{deviance} + (k + 1)\ln(n)$.

10.55 The three variable model.

SOLUTIONS FOR CHAPTER 11

11.1 A study where the researcher assigns the units to the treatments or comparison groups.

11.2   A study where the units come to the researcher already assigned to the treatments or comparison groups.

11.3   Whether or not the researcher assigns the units to the treatments or comparison groups.

11.5   The effects of one variable cannot be distinguished from the effects of the other variable.

11.6   (a) Observational study; (b) Observational study; (c) Experiment; (d) Experiment.

11.7   Extraneous variables can be controlled for.

11.9   No.

11.10   Observational study.

11.11   (a) Experiment; (b) 10% increase in fiber intake and 15% increase in fiber intake; (c) People; (d) Change in cholesterol level.

11.12   (a) Experiment; (b) Echinacea, vitamin C, placebo; (c) People; (d) Length of common cold; (e) Yes.

11.13   (a) Experiment; (b) Weight training, quatic exercise, walking; (c) Knee surgery patients; (d) Change in condition score; (e) No.

11.17   To make the groups as alike as possible before the treatments are applied.

11.18   Inherent variability in the experimental units and variability induced by carrying out the experiment.

11.19   A pre-existing characteristic of the experimental units that is not assigned by the researcher which needs to be controlled for.

11.20   To control for the differences in the units due to the blocking factor.

11.21   (a) Homogeneous or heterogeneous units; (b) Units align in well-defined blocks.

11.23   (a)

SOV	df
Treatments	3
Error	21
Total	24

(b)

SOV	df
Treatments	2
Error	22
Total	24

(c)

SOV	df
Treatments	2
Error	24
Total	26

(d)

SOV	df
Treatments	3
Error	28
Total	31

11.24

(a)

SOV	df
Treatments	3
Error	32
Total	35

(b)

SOV	df
Treatments	4
Error	45
Total	49

(c)

SOV	df
Treatments	2
Error	27
Total	29

(d)

SOV	df
Treatments	9
Error	30
Total	39

11.25 (a) 6; (b)

SOV	df
Treatments	3
Error	20
Total	23

11.26 (a) 7; (b)

SOV	df
Treatments	5
Error	36
Total	41

11.27 (a) 30; (b) 5; (c) 6.

11.28 (a) 72; (b) 6; (c) 12.

11.30

(a)

SOV	df
Blocks	5
Treatments	3
Error	15
Total	23

(b)

SOV	df
Blocks	4
Treatments	2
Error	8
Total	14

(c)

SOV	df
Blocks	6
Treatments	2
Error	12
Total	20

(d)

SOV	df
Blocks	3
Treatments	4
Error	12
Total	19

11.31 (a)

SOV	df
Blocks	3
Treatments	5
Error	15
Total	23

(b)

SOV	df
Blocks	3
Treatments	5
Error	15
Total	23

(c)

SOV	df
Blocks	7
Treatments	6
Error	42
Total	55

(d)

SOV	df
Blocks	9
Treatments	9
Error	81
Total	99

11.32 (a) 8; (b)

SOV	df
Blocks	7
Treatments	4
Error	28
Total	39

11.33 (a) 6; (b)

SOV	df
Blocks	5
Treatments	7
Error	35
Total	47

11.35 Controls for a blocking factor.

11.37 Randomized block design.

11.38 (a)

SOV	df
Blocks	9
Treatments	1
Error	9
Total	19

(b)

SOV	df
Blocks	24
Treatments	1
Error	24
Total	49

11.39 (a) Subject; (b) 20; (c) No alcohol and alcohol.

11.41 (a) Low and low, low and high, medium and low, medium and high, high and low, high and high.
(b) 10% and water, 10% and alcohol, 10% and glycerine, 15% and water, 15% and alcohol, 15% and glycerine, 20% and water, 20% and alcohol, 20% and glycerine,

11.43 (a) 8; (b) 12; (c) 16; (d) 20; (e) 16; (f) 32.

11.44   (a) 4; (b) 2; (c) 16

11.45   (a)

SOV	df
A	3
B	2
AB	6
Error	60
Total	71

(b)

SOV	df
A	2
B	2
AB	4
Error	36
Total	44

(c)

SOV	df
A	1
B	4
AB	4
Error	90
Total	99

11.46   (a) 5;   (b)

SOV	df
A	3
B	1
AB	3
Error	32
Total	39

11.47   (a) 5;   (b)

SOV	df
A	4
B	1
AB	4
Error	40
Total	49

11.48   (a)

SOV	df
Blocks	3
A	1
B	2
AB	2
Error	15
Total	23

(b)

SOV	df
Blocks	4
A	3
B	3
AB	9
Error	60
Total	79

(c)

SOV	df
Blocks	11
A	2
B	5
AB	10
Error	187
Total	215

11.49   (a) 8;   (b)

SOV	df
Blocks	7
A	1
B	2
AB	2
Error	35
Total	47

11.50 (a) 6; (b)

SOV	df
Blocks	5
A	2
B	2
AB	4
Error	40
Total	53

11.53 (a)

SOV	df
A	3
B	2
C	1
AB	6
AC	3
BC	2
ABC	6
Error	96
Total	119

(b)

SOV	df
A	2
B	2
C	1
AB	4
AC	2
BC	2
ABC	4
Error	90
Total	107

(c)

SOV	df
A	1
B	1
C	4
AB	1
AC	4
BC	4
ABC	4
Error	140
Total	159

11.54 (a) 3; (b)

SOV	df
A	3
B	1
C	2
AB	3
AC	6
BC	2
ABC	6
Error	48
Total	71

11.55 (a) 5; (b)

SOV	df
A	1
B	1
C	1
AB	1
AC	1
BC	1
ABC	1
Error	32
Total	39

11.56 (a)

SOV	df
Blocks	4
A	1
B	2
C	2
AB	2
AC	2
BC	4
ABC	4
Error	68
Total	89

(b)

SOV	df
Blocks	7
A	1
B	3
C	3
AB	3
AC	3
BC	9
ABC	9
Error	217
Total	255

(c)

SOV	df
Blocks	9
A	2
B	1
C	1
AB	2
AC	2
BC	1
ABC	2
Error	99
Total	119

11.57 (a) 4; (b)

SOV	df
Blocks	3
A	1
B	2
C	1
AB	2
AC	1
BC	2
ABC	2
Error	33
Total	47

11.58 (a) 6; (b)

SOV	df
Blocks	5
A	1
B	1
C	1
AB	1
AC	1
BC	1
ABC	1
Error	35
Total	47

11.62 (a) $(\alpha_i - \alpha_j) + (\beta_k - \beta_l) + (\alpha\beta_{ik} - \alpha\beta_{jl})$; (b) $(\alpha_i - \alpha_j) + (\beta_k - \beta_l)$

11.65 (a) $\text{logit}(p) = \mu + \tau$
(b) $\text{logit}(p) = \mu + \rho + \tau$
(c) $\text{logit}(p) = \mu + \alpha + \beta + \alpha\beta$
(d) $\text{logit}(p) = \mu + \rho + \alpha + \beta + \alpha\beta$
(e) $\text{logit}(p) = \mu + \alpha + \beta + \gamma + \alpha\beta + \alpha\gamma + \beta\gamma + \alpha\beta\gamma$
(e) $\text{logit}(p) = \mu + \rho + \alpha + \beta + \gamma + \alpha\beta + \alpha\gamma + \beta\gamma + \alpha\beta\gamma$

SOLUTIONS FOR CHAPTER 12

12.1 An experiment can be designed to control for external variables.

12.2 Equal replication of the treatments.

12.3 (a) $Y = \mu + \tau + \epsilon$; (b) The ϵs are independently normally distributed with mean 0 and common standard deviation σ; (c) The observation on the response variable for the jth replicate of the ith treatment.

12.4 (a) $\mu + \tau_i$; (b) $\tau_i - \tau_j$.

12.6 (a) $\sum\sum(y_{ij} - \bar{y}_{\bullet\bullet})^2$; (b) $\sum(n_i - 1)s_i^2$ or SSTot − SSTR; (c) $\sum n_i(\bar{y}_{i\bullet} - \bar{y}_{\bullet\bullet})^2$.

12.8 σ^2.

12.9 (a) $\bar{y}_{i\bullet}$; (b) $y_{ij} - \bar{y}_{i\bullet}$; (c) $\sqrt{\text{MSE}}$

12.11 By examining a normal probability plot of the residuals.

12.12 Yes.

12.13 Each treatment group has the same variance.

12.14 The ratio of the largest sample standard deviation to the smallest sample standard deviation and Levene's test.

12.15 Natural logarithm.

12.16 Yes.

12.17 No.

12.18 Yes.

12.19 No.

12.20 (a) $df_{\text{TRT}} = 3$, $df_{\text{err}} = 16$, SSTR $= 7.68$, SSE $= 22.29$, MSE $= 1.39$, $F_{\text{obs}} = 1.84$; (b) 1.18; (c) Fail to reject.

12.21 $df_{\text{TRT}} = 2$, $df_{\text{err}} = 147$, SSTR $= 4.52$, SSE $= 299.52$, MSE $= 2.01$, $F_{\text{obs}} = 1.12$; (b) 1.42; (c) Fail to reject.

12.23 (a) 6; (b) 10; (c) 15; (d) 28.

12.24 (a) 2.57; (b) 2.85; (c) 2.97; (d) 2.73.

12.25 (a) 8.79; (b) 10.04; (c) 16.94.

12.26 The smallest experimentwise error rate for which the two treatment means are declared significantly different.

12.27 No.

12.28 Yes.

12.29 Treatments 3 and 4.

12.30 $D = 1.79$, 1 and 3, 2 and 3, 3 and 4, 4 and 5.

12.31 (a) 11; (b) Reject; (c) 8.37; (d) 3; (e) 9.06; (f) 2 and 3 are significantly different.

12.32 (a) Yes; (b) Reject; (c) 10; (d) $D = 0.63$; (e) 1.63 to 2.51.

12.33 (a) Yes; (b) Reject; (c) 0.95; (d) 1 is significantly different from 2, 3, and 4, 2 is significantly different from 3 and 4; (e) -8.183 to -6.807; f) 28.356 to 28.420.

12.34 (a) Yes; (b) Reject; (c) 2.36; (d) 1 is significantly different from 2 and 3; (e) -11.36 to -7.52; (f) 11.34 to 14.06.

12.35 To control for a blocking factor.

12.36 (a) $Y = \mu + \rho + \tau + \epsilon$; (b) The ϵ's are independently normally distributed with mean 0 and common standard deviation σ, the blocks do not interact with the treatments; (c) The response variable for the unit receiving the ith treatment in the jth block.

12.37 (a) $\mu + \tau_i$; (b) $\tau_i - \tau_j$.

12.39

SOV	df	SS	MS	F
Blocks	7	800	114.29	
Treatments	4	1200	300	6
Error	28	1400	50	
Total	39	3400		

12.40 (a) $df_{blk} = 14$, $df_{TRT} = 5$, $df_{err} = 70$, $df_{tot} = 89$, SSTR $= 132$, SSTot $= 2972$, MSBLK $= 162.86$, MSTR $= 26.4$, MSE $= 8$, $F_{obs} = 3.3$; (b) 8; (c) Reject; (d) 3.01.

12.41 (a) $df_{blk} = 11$, $df_{TRT} = 3$, $df_{err} = 33$, $df_{tot} = 47$, SSBL $= 715$, SSE $= 1980$, SSTot $= 3505$, MSTR $= 270$, $F_{obs} = 4.5$; (b) 60; (c) Reject; (d) 6.92.

12.42 (a) 6; (b) 76; (c) $D = 11.41$; (d) A is significantly different from B and D; (e) -118.18 to -100.82.

12.44 (a) 12; (b) 24; (c) 18; (d) 27; (e) 8; 16.

12.45 (a) 36; (b) 120; (c) 108; (d) 216.

12.46 (a) $Y = \mu + \alpha + \beta + \alpha\beta + \epsilon$; (b) The ϵs are independently normally distributed with mean 0 and common standard deviation σ; (c) The value of the response variable for the kth replicate of the treatment formed from the ith level of factor A and the jth level of factor B.

12.49 (a) $\alpha_i + \beta_j + \alpha\beta_{ij}$; (b) $(\alpha_i - \alpha_k) + (\beta_j - \beta_l) + (\alpha\beta_{ij} - \alpha\beta_{kl})$; (c) $(\alpha_i - \alpha_k) + (\beta_j - \beta_l)$.

12.51 (a) $df_A = 1$, $df_B = 2$, $df_{AB} = 2$, $df_{err} = 36$, $df_{tot} = 41$, SSA $= 799.5$, SSB $= 1200$, SSAB $= 2199$, SSE $= 5400$, SSTot $= 9598.5$, MSA $= 799.5$, MSB $= 600$, MSAB $= 1099.5$; (b) 12.25; (c) Significant; (d) The treatment means.

12.52 (a) $df_{blk} = 9$, $df_A = 3$, $df_B = 1$, $df_{AB} = 3$, $df_{err} = 63$, $df_{tot} = 79$, SSA $= 3228.27$, SSB $= 793.42$, SSAB $= 264.18$, SSTot $= 10953.9$, MSBL $= 124.44$, MSA $= 1076.09$, MSB $= 793.42$, MSAB $= 88.06$; (b) 9.38; (c) Not significant; (d) The A and B main effects means.

12.53 (a) Only the A main effect means; (b) 20; (c) 25; 4.60.

12.54 (a) 15.82; (b) Yes; (c) Yes; (d) The treatment means.

12.55 (a) Zone means; (b) 1.53; (c) 1 and 2 are is significantly different from 3, 4, and 5, 3 and 4 are significantly different from 5; (d) 2.33 to 4.47.

12.56 (a) 16; (b) 12.

12.57 (a) 6.32; (b) 3.16; (c) 2.83; (d) 8.94; (e) 4.47; (f) 4.00.

12.61 (a) $\mu + \alpha_i + \beta_j + \gamma_k + \alpha_i\beta_j + \alpha\gamma_k + \beta_j\gamma_k + \alpha_i\beta_j\gamma_k$; (b) $(\alpha_i - \alpha_r) + (\beta_j - \beta_s) + (\gamma_k - \gamma_t)$.

12.63 (a) $\mathrm{df}_A = 1$, $\mathrm{df}_B = 2$, $\mathrm{df}_C = 3$, $\mathrm{df}_{AB} = 2$, $\mathrm{df}_{AC} = 3$, $\mathrm{df}_{BC} = 6$, $\mathrm{df}_{ABC} = 6$, $\mathrm{df}_{err} = 72$, $\mathrm{df}_{tot} = 95$, $\mathrm{SSA} = 20.825$, $\mathrm{SSB} = 79.968$, $\mathrm{SSC} = 89.964$, $\mathrm{SSAB} = 333.32$, $\mathrm{SSAC} = 37.485$, $\mathrm{SSBC} = 89.964$, $\mathrm{SSABC} = 9.976$, $\mathrm{SSE} = 599.76$, $\mathrm{MSA} = 20.825$, $\mathrm{MSB} = 39.984$, $\mathrm{MSC} = 29.998$, $\mathrm{MSAB} = 16.60$, $\mathrm{MSAC} = 12.495$, $\mathrm{MSBC} = 14.994$, $\mathrm{MSABC} = 9.996$; (b) 2.89; (c) Yes; (d) 1.44; (e) 0.51.

12.65 (a) No; (b) No; (c) The factor A and the factor C main effect means; (d) 40.

12.66 (a) No; (b) Yes; (c) The treatment means.

12.67 (a) The treatment means; (b) 28; (c) 8.42.

12.68 (a) 8; (b) 5; (c) 26; (d) 12.

SOLUTIONS FOR CHAPTER 13

13.1 $S(t) = P(\text{Survival time is greater than } t) = P(T > t)$.

13.2 $S(t)$ decreases.

13.3 Smaller.

13.7 Kaplan–Meier estimator.

13.8 $\widehat{S}(t_j) = \widehat{S}(t_{j-1}) \times \widehat{p}_j$ or $\widehat{S}(t_j) = \widehat{p}_1 \times \widehat{p}_2 \times \cdots \times \widehat{p}_j$.

13.9 0.73.

13.10 0.69.

13.11 (a) 2, 0; (b) $\widehat{p}_1 = 0.86$, $\widehat{p}_2 = 0.96$, $\widehat{p}_3 = 0.82$, $\widehat{p}_4 = 0.88$, $\widehat{p}_5 = 0.87$, $\widehat{p}_6 = 0.83$; (c) $\widehat{S}_1 = 0.86$, $\widehat{S}_2 = 0.83$, $\widehat{S}_3 = 0.68$, $\widehat{S}_4 = 0.60$, $\widehat{S}_5 = 0.52$, $\widehat{S}_6 = 0.43$.

13.12 (a) $\widehat{S}_1 = 0.98$, $\widehat{S}_2 = 0.93$, $\widehat{S}_3 = 0.88$, $\widehat{S}_4 = 0.73$, $\widehat{S}_5 = 0.54$; (c) 0.44 to 0.64; (d) Yes.

13.13 (a) $\widehat{S}_1 = 0.98$, $\widehat{S}_2 = 0.90$ $\widehat{S}_3 = 0.85$, $\widehat{S}_4 = 0.73$, $\widehat{S}_5 = 0.52$, $\widehat{S}_6 = 0.39$, $\widehat{S}_7 = 0.26$, $\widehat{S}_8 = 0.16$; (c) 0.02 to 0.30; (d) No.

13.15 (a) 8; (b) 0.85; (c) 0.69 to 1.00.

13.16 Log-rank test.

13.17 (a) There is a significant difference in at least two of the survival functions; (b) There is no significant difference between the survival functions.

13.18 (a) Yes; (b) 0.88; (c) 10.

13.19   (a) No; (b) Treatment 3, treatment 1; (c) Treatment 2.

13.22   (a) $\ln[\,h(t|X)\,] = \beta_0 + \beta_1 X$.
(b) $\ln[\,h(t|\vec{X})\,] = \beta_0 + \beta_1 X_1 + \beta_2 X_2 + \cdots + \beta_p X_p$.

13.25   Decreases.

13.26   (a) The change in $\ln[\,h(t|\vec{X})\,]$ for a 1 unit increase in X_i when all of the other variables are held fixed; (b) The risk ratio for a 1 unit increase in X_i when all of the other variables are held fixed.

13.27   Standard normal.

13.28   (a) Reject; (b) 0.58 to 2.78; (c) 5.37; (d) 1.79 to 16.12.

13.29   (a) Fail to reject; (b) Reject; (c) No.

13.30   (a) No; (b) 0.66; (c) Lower; (d) 1.004 to 1.016

13.31   (a) 4.45; (b) 1.06 to 6.86; (c) Increases; (d) 3.28 to 8.89; (e) 1.52 to 3.22.

13.32   (a) X_3, X_1 and X_3, X_1, X_2; (b) X_3, X_1; (c) X_3, X_1.

13.39   (a) The change in $logit(p)$ for a 1 unit increase in X_i when all of the other variables are held fixed; (b) The odds ratio for a 1 unit increase in X_i when all of the other variables are held fixed.

13.40   Standard normal.

13.41   (a) Reject; (b) 0.76 to 4.02; (c) 10.91; (d) 2.14 to 55.70.

13.42   (a) 42.10, 7.69, 2.12, 2.92, 1.97, 1.22; (b) 1.22; (c) 0.90; (d) 0.68; (e) 0.64.

13.43   (a) $\widehat{\beta}_0 = 1.658, \widehat{\beta}_1 = 1.105, \widehat{\beta}_2 = 0.658, \widehat{\beta}_3 = 0.231, \widehat{\beta}_4 = 1.717, \widehat{\beta}_5 = 3.227,$ $\widehat{\beta}_6 = 4.039$; (b) 0.886; (c) 0.114; (d) 0.875; (d) 0.125; (e) 56.76.

INDEX

Applied Biostatistics for the Health Sciences. By Richard J. Rossi
Copyright © 2010 by John Wiley & Sons, Inc.